HIV AND AIDS IN AFRICA

HIV and AIDS
in Africa

Beyond Epidemiology

Edited by

Ezekiel Kalipeni, Susan Craddock,
Joseph R. Oppong, and Jayati Ghosh

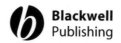

© 2004 by Blackwell Publishing Ltd

BLACKWELL PUBLISHING
350 Main Street, Malden, MA 02148-5020, USA
9600 Garsington Road, Oxford OX4 2DQ, UK
550 Swanston Street, Carlton, Victoria 3053, Australia

First published 2004 by Blackwell Publishing Ltd

5   2006

Library of Congress Cataloging-in-Publication Data

HIV and AIDS in Africa: beyond epidemiology / edited by Ezekiel Kalipeni … [et al.].
    p. cm.
Includes bibliographical references and index.
    ISBN 0-631-22356-8 (alk. paper) — ISBN 0-631-22357-6 (alk. paper)
1. AIDS (Disease) —Africa.   I. Kalipeni, Ezekiel, 1954–

RA643.86.A35H554 2004
616.97′92′0096—dc21

                                                        2003000322

ISBN-13: 978-0-631-22356-6 (alk. paper) — ISBN-13: 978-0-631-22357-3 (alk. paper)

A catalogue record for this title is available from the British Library.

Set in 9 / 11 pt Palatino
by Kolam Information Services Pvt. Ltd, India
Printed and bound in Singapore
by COS Printers Pte Ltd

The publisher's policy is to use permanent paper from mills that operate a sustainable forestry policy, and which has been manufactured from pulp processed using acid-free and elementary chlorine-free practices. Furthermore, the publisher ensures that the text paper and cover board used have met acceptable environmental accreditation standards.

For further information on
Blackwell Publishing, visit our website:
www.blackwellpublishing.com

Contents

---

1 Part introductions by Susan Craddock

About the Authors

Samuel Agyei-Mensah is a Senior Lecturer in Geography in the Department of Geography and Resource Development at the University of Ghana, Legon. He did his graduate studies at the Norwegian University of Science and Technology where he obtained M.Phil. and Ph.D. degrees in 1992 and 1997 respectively. Dr. Agyei-Mensah's area of specialization is population and the geography of health. Current research interests include: fertility in sub-Saharan Africa, the demography of fatherhood in Ghana, and the geo-epidemiology of disease in Ghana. He has published research articles dealing with fertility and health in journals such as the *Norwegian Journal of Geography*, *Bulletin of the Ghana Geographical Association*, *Scandinavian Journal of Development Alternatives*, and *Geografiska Annaler*. Greenwood Publishing recently published his book *Fertility Decline in Developing Countries, 1960–1997: An Annotated Bibliography*.

Anne V. Akeroyd is a lecturer in the Centre for Southern African Studies, the Centre for Women's Studies and the Department of Sociology, University of York, England. She took a Ph.D. in social anthropology at University College London. Recent papers include "Gender, Food Production and Property Rights: Constraints on Women Farmers in Southern Africa" in *Women, Development and Survival in the Third World* (1991); "Personal Information and Qualitative Research Data: Some Practical and Ethical Problems Arising from Data Protection Legislation" in *Using computers for Qualitative Research* (1991); and "Sociocultural Aspects of AIDS in Africa: Occupation and Gender Issues" in *AIDS in Africa and the Caribbean* (1997).

Carolyn Baylies is a Senior Lecturer in Sociology and former Director of the Centre for Development Studies at the University of Leeds. She received a Ph.D.

in Sociology and a Master's degree in Rural Sociology from the University of Wisconsin and has taught at universities in Zambia, California, and Leeds. Her interests lie in the areas of health, gender, and socio-political change, with a regional focus on southern Africa. She has carried out research on gender aspects of AIDS as well as processes of democratization in Zambia. Recent publications include *AIDS, Sexuality and Gender in Africa* (2000, with J. Bujra); Special issue on AIDS (2000, *Review of African Political Economy*, edited with J. Bujra); "The Impact of HIV on Family Size Preference in Zambia" (2000, *Reproductive Health Matters*); "HIV/AIDS in Africa, Global and Local Inequalities and Responsibilities" (2000, *Review of African Political Economy*); and "Safe Motherhood in the Time of AIDS" (2001, *Gender and Development*).

Lynn R. Brown is a rural development specialist at the World Bank. She graduated from the University of Warwick, England, undertook postgraduate work at the same university and at Cornell University, USA, and holds a Master's degree in quantitative development economics. She is a specialist in gender, food policy, and AIDS and food security as they relate to international development. She has carried out extensive research on these issues, resulting in a number of publications, including a book edited with Joanna Kerr, *The Gender Dimensions of Economic Reforms in Ghana, Mali and Zambia* (1998). Selected other publications include *The Role of Labor in Household Food Security: Implications of AIDS in Africa* (1994), *Gender, Property Rights and Natural Resources* (1997), *The Importance of Gender Issues for Environmentally and Socially Sustainable Rural Development* (1998), and *Women and Food Security: Roles, Constraints, and Missed Opportunities* (2001).

Catherine Campbell is a Reader in Social Psychology at the London School of Economics and an Adjunct Professor at the University of Natal, Durban. She has published widely on the psycho-social and community-level determinants of HIV/AIDS transmission and prevention. Her latest work is *Letting Them Die: Why HIV/AIDS Prevention Programmes Often Fail* (Bloomington: Indiana University Press; Oxford: James Currey, 2003).

Susan Craddock is an Associate Professor in the Institute for Global Studies and Women's Studies at the University of Minnesota. She holds Ph.D. and M.A. degrees from the University of California at Berkeley. Her research interests include social geography of health, health policy, women's health in historical and geographical perspective, the US, eastern Africa, and India. Her book titled *City of Plagues: Disease, Poverty, and Deviance in San Francisco* was recently published by University of Minnesota Press. She has published articles dealing with the AIDS epidemic in Malawi and elsewhere in eastern Africa.

David Eaton is an Assistant Professor of Anthropology at Middlebury College in Vermont. He received his M.P.H. in International Population and Family Health from UCLA in 1991 and his Ph.D. in Medical Anthropology from UC Berkeley in 2001. His research has focused on men's lives and the politics of AIDS in the Republic of Congo, Cameroon, Zaire (now D. R. Congo), and Rwanda. His essay "A Brazzaville Friendship" appeared in the journal *Ethnography* in 2000.

Alex C. Ezeh directs the African Population and Health Research Center (APHRC). He has been actively involved in policy-oriented analysis and evaluation of health, social, and demographic issues in Africa for more than ten years. At APHRC, Dr. Ezeh implements the Center's research agenda and establishes linkages with research institutions, donor agencies, policymakers, program managers, and collaborators within and outside the region. Dr. Ezeh manages a number of projects at APHRC, including the Nairobi Reproductive Health and Poverty Project and the Onset of Fertility Transition Project. Prior to joining APHRC, Dr. Ezeh worked with Macro International Inc. for six years where he provided technical expertise to governmental and nongovernmental institutions in several African countries in the design and conduct of demographic and health surveys (DHS). Dr. Ezeh received his Ph.D. in Demography from the University of Pennsylvania in 1993. Recent publications include "Polygyny Level, Gender Relations, and Reproductive Behavior in Ghana," *Journal of Comparative Family Studies*, Vol. XXXI, No. 4 (2000), pp. 427–441 (with Victor Agadjanian); "Unmet Need for Couples: An Analytical Framework and Evaluation with DHS data," *Population Research and Policy Review*, Vol. 18 (1999), pp. 579–605 (with Akin Bankole); and "Some Insights into the Relationship between Spousal Discussion and Prediction of Both Partner Approval and Disapproval among Married Kenyan Men: A Behavioural Paradox?," *Population Studies* (forthcoming) (Alex C. Ezeh and Tom O. Owour).

Francis Nii-Amoo Dodoo is Professor in the Afro-American Studies Program and an affiliated Professor of the Department of Sociology at the University of Maryland, College Park. He was formerly Director of the African Population and Health Research Center and has been actively involved in African population and health research for about 14 years. He holds a Ph.D. (1988) in Demography from the University of Pennsylvania and has Master's degrees in Economics and Demography. Much of his work has been in the area of gender, power, and reproductive/health decision making, and on urban poverty and health issues. He has sat on a number of advisory boards and committees of prestigious organizations. His other research interests have involved the analysis of US Census data to explicate patterns of stratification and inequality, particularly of black immigrants, in American society. Recent publications include "Some Evidence against the Assumption that Approval of Family Planning is Associated with Frequency of Spouses' Discussion of the Subject," *Population Studies*, 55 (2), July 2001 (with Alex C. Ezeh and Tom O. Owour); "AIDS-Related Knowledge and Behavior among Married Kenyan Men: A Behavioral Paradox?," *Journal of Health and Human Services Administration* (Forthcoming 2001) (with Akosua A. Ampofo); and "Gender, Power, and Reproduction: Rural-Urban Differences in the Relationship between Fertility Goals and Contraceptive Use in Kenya," *Rural Sociology*, Vol. 67 (forthcoming 2002) (with Maria Tempenis).

Jayati Ghosh is Associate Professor of International Business and Interdisciplinary studies at the Dominican University of California. She holds a Ph.D. degree in Geography from the University of Waterloo in Canada. She received her M.A. from Wilfrid Laurier University, Canada, and M.Sc. from the University of Calcutta, India. Her research interests are in the areas of economic development, health, women's health in Africa and Asia from an economic and social perspective. She has written a number of articles dealing with the AIDS epidemic and economic development in India. Some of her research has appeared in *Geography, Wisconsin Geographer*, and *Geographical Review*. Currently she is working on a comparative project of HIV/AIDS on the Indian population in India and the Indian diaspora in eastern and southern Africa.

Emma Guest is a freelance writer on AIDS-related issues. She has lived in South Africa and traveled extensively in Africa, and she now lives in London.

Percy C. Hintzen is Professor and Chair of African American Studies at the University of California, Berkeley. He teaches political and economic development of the Global South and immigrant identity in the Global North. Among his publications are *The Costs of Regime Survival* (Cambridge University Press), *West Indian in the West* (New York University Press), and *Invisible Others: Active Presences in U.S. "Black Community,"* edited with Jean Rahier (Routledge, forthcoming).

A physiotherapist by profession, **Noerine Kaleeba** helped found The AIDS Support Network Organization (TASO) in Kampala, Uganda, in 1987 and served as its director until 1995. She is now Patron of the organization. TASO quickly became a model for community-based AIDS organizations across Africa, offering information, counseling, medical and nursing care, and material assistance to people living with HIV/AIDS and their families. Mrs. Kaleeba is currently the community mobilization specialist at the Joint United Nations Program on HIV/AIDS (UNAIDS) in Geneva, Switzerland. She was awarded an honorary doctorate of Humane Letters (honoris causa) by Nkumba University of Social Sciences, Kampala, in 2000 in recognition of her pioneering work in the response to HIV/AIDS. Noerine also serves in a voluntary capacity as vice Chair of ActionAid UK Board of Trustees.

Ezekiel Kalipeni is Associate Professor of Geography and African Studies at the University of Illinois at Urbana-Champaign. He holds both a Ph.D. degree and a Master's degree in Geography from the University of North Carolina at Chapel Hill. He is a population/medical/environmental geographer interested in demographic, health, environmental, and resource issues in sub-Saharan Africa. He has in the past taught at the University of Malawi (1986–8), University of North Carolina at Chapel Hill (1988–91), and Colgate University (1991–4). He has carried out extensive research on the population dynamics of Malawi and Africa in general, concentrating on fertility, mortality, migration, and health care issues. Some of the books he has published include *Population Growth and Environmental Degradation in Southern Africa* (1994); *Issues and Perspectives on Health Care in Contemporary Sub-Saharan Africa* (1997, edited with Philip Thiuri); *AIDS, Health Care Systems and Culture in Sub-Saharan Africa: Rethinking and Re-Appraisal* (special issue of *African Rural and Urban Studies* (1998, edited with Joseph Oppong)); and *Sacred Spaces and Public Quarrels: African Cultural and Economic Landscapes* (edited with Paul T. Zeleza, 1999).

Mike Kesby is a Lecturer in Geography at the University of St Andrews, Scotland. He holds a B.A. from the University of Manchester and a Ph.D. from the University of Keele. He is a gender/health geographer interested in the social embeddedness of HIV in sub-Saharan Africa and the use of participatory approaches to address this. His work on gender and on HIV has hitherto concentrated on Zimbabwe, but is presently extending to neighboring countries and to African migrants in the UK. Papers he has published focus on the spatial dimensions of gender relations in Zimbabwe and the use of participatory methods in HIV research.

Robert A. Lowe, M.D., M.P.H., is Associate Professor of Emergency Medicine, Associate Professor of Public Health and Preventive Medicine, and Associate Professor of Informatics and Medical Outcomes at Oregon Health and Science University. He is a Senior Scholar at the Leonard Davis Institute of Health Economics, University of Pennsylvania. An emergency physician and health services researcher, he received his undergraduate degree in Sociology from the University of California, Santa Cruz, his M.D. from University of California, Davis, and his Master's in Public Health from University of California, Berkeley.

Peter Lurie, M.D., M.P.H. is Deputy Director of Public Citizen's Health Research Group, a Ralph Nader-founded advocacy group in Washington, DC. He has held faculty positions at the University of California, San Francisco (UCSF), and the University of Michigan. After obtaining his medical degree from the Albert Einstein College of Medicine, he completed residencies in Family Practice at UCSF and in Preventive Medicine at the University of California, Berkeley, where he also obtained an M.P.H. He was the principal investigator of a three-volume, 700-page study of needle exchange programs for the Centers for Disease Control and Prevention. He has written on the subject of needle exchange programs in the *Lancet* and on ethical aspects of mother-to-infant HIV transmission studies and HIV vaccine trials in developing countries in the *New England Journal of Medicine* and the *Journal of the American Medical Association*. He has also examined the impact of economic development policies on the spread of HIV and conducted a number of HIV epidemiology studies in Africa, Asia, and Brazil. At Public Citizen, he has been involved in efforts to ban or re-label multiple drugs (e.g., Propulsid, Lotronex, Arava) and has sought to increase access to anti-HIV drugs in the developing world. He has filed petitions to ban certain unsafe needles, to ban candles with lead wicks, to reduce worker exposure to beryllium, and to lower medical resident work hours. He was a member of the Food and Drug Administration's Transmissible Spongiform Encephalopathy Advisory Committee and is conducting several studies related to pharmaceutical company influence in clinical care and medical education.

Maryinez Lyons Works for HIV/AIDS Focal Point in Nairobi, Kenya. She received her Ph.D. in history at the University of California at Los Angeles in 1987. She has written numerous articles, the most recent of which is entitled "Foreign Bodies: the History of Labour Migration as a Threat to Public Health in Uganda" in *African Boundaries, Barriers, Conduits and Opportunities* (1996) edited by Paul Nugen; and "The Point of View: Perspectives on AIDS in Uganda" in *AIDS in Africa and the Carribean* (1997). She has also published several books: *The Colonial Disease: Sleeping Sickness in the Early Colonial Belgian Congo, 1890–1940* (1992), and *Histories of Sexually Transmitted Diseases and HIV/AIDS in Sub-Saharan Africa* (with Philip Setel and Milton James Lewis, 1999).

John Lloyd Lwanda is a Fellow of the Royal College of Physicians of Edinburgh and a Member of the Faculty of Family Planning (UK). Dr. Lwanda is a practicing medical practitioner (Glasgow), clinical tutor (Department of General Practice, University of Glasgow), writer, and researcher. His research interests include music, politics, and traditional and popular culture. He is currently working on a social science doctoral thesis on "Culture, Politics and HIV/AIDS" at the Center of African Studies, University of Edinburgh. He has worked in the Department of Genitourinary Medicine (1982–97), Glasgow Royal Infirmary and Medicine, and College of Medicine, University of Malawi (1994–5). Lwanda's books include *Promises, Power Politics and Poverty: Democratic Transition in Malawi (1961–1999)* (Glasgow, Dudu Nsomba Publications, 1996) and *Kamuzu Banda of Malawi – A Study in Promise, Power and Paralysis; Malawi Under Dr Banda, 1961 to 1993* (Glasgow, Dudu Nsomba Publications, 1993). He has contributed a number of articles on popular and traditional music, including the Malawi chapter in *The Rough Guide to World Music* (Penguin Rough Guides, 1999). His research interests in music have led to the compilation, editing, and publication of a series of six cassettes, five CDs, and seven videos of Malawi popular, folk, and traditional music.

Njeri Mbugua grew up in Kenya, where she received her Bachelors degree (1987) in Social Work and her Master's degree (1992) in Sociology from The University of Nairobi. She received her Ph.D. (1999) in Sociology from Indiana University. Between 1988 and 1992, Dr. Mbugua worked in several nongovernmental agencies as a researcher and consultant. Her scholarly interests focus on the interaction of women and health with cultural, social, economic, and political factors. This is reflected in her dissertations: M.A. (*The Impact of Marriage and Motherhood on University Female Students*) and Ph.D. (*Strategies for HIV/AIDS Prevention Among High School Female Students*). Some of her recent publications include: "The Global Healthcare Challenge" in *Sociology For a New Century* published by Pine Forge Press (2001); *Empowerment of Third World Women Against AIDS With Special Reference to East and Central Africa* published by Indiana University African Studies Program (1997); and "Fighting AIDS by Tracing its Origin," *Social Focus*, 2 (1), 1996, pp. 6–7.

Joseph R. Oppong is an Associate Professor of Geography at the University of North Texas. He holds a Ph.D. degree in medical geography from the University of Alberta, Canada. He has published extensively on health care issues and the AIDS epidemic in Africa. His most recent book is *AIDS, Health Care Systems and Culture in Sub-Saharan Africa: Rethinking and Re-Appraisal* (special issue of *African Rural and Urban Studies* (1998, edited with Ezekiel Kalipeni)). Some of his recent work has appeared in journals such as *Socio-Economic Planning Sciences*, *Social Science & Medicine*, *Applied Geographic Studies*, *African Geographical Review*, and *The Professional Geographer*. He chaired the Africa Specialty Group of the Association of American Geographers and is currently Chair of the Medical Geography Specialty Group of the Association of American Geographers.

Oliver Phillips grew up in Zimbabwe and South Africa and is now a senior lecturer at the School of Law, University of Westminster, London, England. From September 2000 to August 2001, he was Rockefeller Fellow at the Program for the Study of Sexuality, Gender, Health, and Human Rights at Columbia University,

New York, USA. He has written widely on sexuality, human rights, and the law in southern Africa and has worked with a number of sexual rights advocacy organizations in southern Africa. In 1997 he received the Socio-Legal Studies Association/Dartmouth Prize for best Socio-Legal Article. He has a Bachelor's degree from the University of Cape Town, and a Ph.D. from the Institute of Criminology at the University of Cambridge, and has worked at the Universities of Keele, London, and Zimbabwe.

Gabriel Rugalema works for the International Institute for Education Planning, Paris, France. He obtained his Ph.D. from the Institute of Social Studies, The Hague, Netherlands. He has conducted field work on AIDS and rural livelihoods in Bukoba District, NW Tanzania and in Kenya. His work also explores the language and concepts used by respondents in describing and explaining AIDS.

Brooke G. Schoepf (Ph.D. Columbia University, 1969) is a medical and economic anthropologist with an interest in human rights and development. She is a Lecturer in the Department of Social Medicine at Harvard Medical School, and a Fellow at the Institute for Health and Social Justice. Following early fieldwork, Schoepf taught at the University of Connecticut Medical School. In 1974 she joined the Rockefeller Foundation's Education for Development team at the University of Zaire, and taught at Tuskegee Institute in Alabama from 1978 to 1982. Following a sabbatical in Zimbabwe and further research, Schoepf led Project CONNAISSIDA's AIDS prevention research in Kinshasa, Zaire (now DRC) from 1985 to 1990. She has led research and training teams in ten African countries, and consulted on AIDS prevention in various UN organizations. In 1990 she was a recipient of the Evelyn Green Davis fellowship at Radcliffe's Bunting Institute. Her recent publications include the Africa chapter in *Dying for Growth: Global Inequality and the Health of the Poor* (co-authored with C. Schoepf and J. V. Millen for Common Courage Press, 2000), and a review essay on international AIDS research in Annual Review of Anthropology (2001). Her book *Gender, Sex and Power: A Social History of AIDS* is forthcoming from Blackwell (2004).

Zena Stein is Professor of Public Health (Epidemiology) at Columbia University, Associate Dean for Research in the Columbia University School of Public Health, Director of the Epidemiology of Brain Disorders Department of New York State Psychiatric Institute, and Co-Director of the HIV Center for Behavioral and Clinical Sciences at Columbia University. She received her medical degree in 1950, from the University of Witwatersrand in Johannesburg, South Africa. Since 1987, she has been co-director of the NIMH-funded HIV Center for Clinical and Behavioral Studies at the New York State Psychiatric Institute and Columbia-Presbyterian Medical Center. She has written extensively on epidemiological issues, with over 197 papers and four books to her credit. Over the past few years she has spearheaded and led the conceptualization and implementation of Methods Women Can Use in the battle against HIV infection.

Ida Susser received her Ph.D. in anthropology from Columbia University. She is currently Professor of Anthropology at Hunter College and in the Doctoral Program of Anthropology at the Graduate Center for the City University of

New York. She is the Director of the International Anthropology of AIDS Group in the HIV Center for Behavioral and Clinical Sciences, Columbia University. She has conducted research with respect to health and HIV prevention in New York City, Puerto Rico, and South Africa, and in addition to her book, *Norman Street: Poverty and Politics in an Urban Neighborhood*, has published numerous articles concerning issues of poverty, gender, and political mobilization. She is also co-editor of a recent book titled *AIDS in Africa and the Caribbean* (with George C. Bond, John Kreniske, and Joan Vincent, 1997).

Eliya Msiyaphazi Zulu is a Senior Research Scientist at the African Population and Health Research Center, which he joined in 1997 after completing his doctoral studies at the University of Pennsylvania. Before his doctoral studies, Zulu worked at the Demographic Unit, University of Malawi, as a Lecturer in Demography. Zulu's research centers on reproductive change in sub-Saharan Africa, with particular emphasis on the interplay between modern and traditional reproductive regimes. He is currently involved in a longitudinal research project, in collaboration with the University of Pennsylvania, to understand the role of ideation in fertility and sexual behavior in Malawi and Kenya. He is also a Principal co-investigator in the study of the Onset of Fertility Decline in Kenya and the Nairobi Reproductive Health and Poverty Project which involves continuous demographic surveillance of slum residents in Nairobi City. Zulu has extensive field experience in carrying out both qualitative and quantitative studies. Some of his recent publications include: "Mothers, Fathers and Children: Regional Patterns in Child–Parental Living Arrangements in Sub-Saharan Africa," *African Population Studies*, No. 11, pp. 1–28 (October 1996) (with MacDaniel Antonio); "Gender and Husband–Wife Survey Responses in Malawi," *Studies in Family Planning* (forthcoming) (with Kate Miller and Susan Cotts Watkins); and "Ethnic Variations in Rationale and Observance of Postpartum Sexual Abstinence in Malawi," *Demography* (forthcoming).

Acknowledgments

The meeting in Champaign-Urbana in 1999 that originally brought together many of the contributors to this book would not have been possible without grants from the National Science Foundation and several organizations at the University of Illinois at Urbana-Champaign which included the International Programs and Studies, the Critical Research Initiative, the Center for African Studies, the Department of Veterinary Pathobiology, and the Department of Geography. We also wish to acknowledge the support received from the Departments of Geography at the University of North Texas, the University of Arizona at Tucson, and the University of Wisconsin at Whitewater. We want to thank those individuals who attended the meeting and gave their time and expert thoughts on the subject which subsequently formed the focus of this book.

  The editors would like to thank all of the contributors for their time and expertise, and for their patience in seeing this project through to fruition. We also want to thank Shirley Lindenbaum, Joan Vincent, Ida Susser, and Ibulaimu Kakoma for their insightful comments on early stages of the manuscript, and for their willingness to give of their time and energy to the project. Their own commitments to understanding and confronting AIDS in Africa have been inspirational to our efforts in producing this book. Our several anonymous reviewers provided invaluable comments on the questions a book on AIDS in Africa should address and why, and to these individuals we give our hearty thanks and a hope that the final product comes somewhere close to their expectations. We would also like to gratefully acknowledge the help received from many individuals which inevitably led to the successful completion of this book. In particular, we would like to mention the assistance received from Barbara Bonnell and Gerry Gallagher of the Department of Geography at the University of Illinois who were very instrumental in organizing and running the meeting that took place in July 1999 at the University of Illinois.

But most of all we thank Jane Huber, the Acquisitions Editor for Anthropology and Archaeology at Blackwell Publishing, for believing in the project and in us, for her acuity in knowing what was needed to make this the best book possible, and for her willingness to work with us well beyond the call of editorial duty. Without her, this book would not have happened. The dedicated and experienced staff at Blackwell Publishing facilitated the timely production of this book. We are particularly grateful to Annie Lenth of Blackwell Publishing for ensuring that an exceptionally high standard of professionalism was involved in the production of the book.

Acknowledgments

The editor and publisher wish to thank the following for permission to use copyright material:

1 Lurie, Peter, Hintzen, Percy and Lowe, Robert A., 1995 Socioeconomic Obstacles to HIV Prevention and Treatment in Developing Countries: the Roles of the International Monetary Fund and the World Bank. AIDS 9 (36):539–46. Reprinted with the permission of Lippincott, Williams & Wilkins, a Wolters Kluwer Company.

2 Susser, Ida and Stein, Zena, 2000 Culture, Sexuality, and Women's Agency in the Prevention of HIV/AIDS in Southern Africa. American Journal of Public Health 2000, 90 (6), July:1042–1048. Copyright © 2000 by American Public Health Association. Reprinted with the permission of the American Public Health Association.

3 Kaleeba, Noerine with Sunanda Ray, 2002 We Miss You All. SAfAIDS, 2nd edn, pp. 1–122 (excerpted). Copyright © 2002 by Noerine Kaleeba and Sunanda Ray. Reprinted with the permission of Noerine Kaleeba and Sunanda Ray.

4 Guest, Emma, 2001 Children of AIDS: Africa's Orphan Crisis. London: Pluto Press, Chapter 9: A Mother to her Brothers, pp. 131–143. Reprinted with the permission of Pluto Press.

5 Campbell, Catherine, 1997 Migrancy, Masculine Identities and AIDS: The Psychosocial Context of HIV Transmission on the South African Gold Mines. Social Science and Medicine 45(2): 273–83. Reprinted with the permission of Pergamon Press.

Every effort has been made to trace copyright holders and to obtain their permission for the use of copyright material. The authors and publishers will gladly receive any information enabling them to rectify any error or omission in subsequent editions.

Introduction

Beyond Epidemiology:
Locating AIDS in Africa

Susan Craddock

AIDS in Africa. The phrase itself has come to signal an almost apocalyptic level of devastation. Broadcast from television, photojournals, and newspapers, images of the epidemic as it has progressed through sub-Saharan Africa are by now mind-numbingly familiar: painfully wasted bodies; haunted eyes; isolation; fear; imminent death. The words accompanying these images are also becoming predictable in their descriptions of "plague," "horror," "calamity," "conflagration," and deaths that are "biblical" in number and proportion.[1] The basis of these representations lies in the fact that with less than 8 percent of the world's population, sub-Saharan Africa encompasses an estimated two-thirds of global AIDS cases (UN Population Institute 2001; UNAIDS 2001a). As the maps in Figure 0.1 show, sub-Saharan Africa accounts for an estimated 28 million individuals living with HIV/AIDS out of a total of 40 million as of 2001; it has experienced over 17 million deaths since the beginning of the epidemic, and 2.3 million in 2001 alone. Five hundred thousand of these deaths have been children (UNAIDS 2001a).

With only a few exceptions such as Uganda and Senegal, the epidemic in sub-Saharan Africa continues to get worse instead of better. Over the past 15 years, more countries in southern and central Africa have joined eastern Africa in recording infection rates among adult populations of 20 percent or more (Figure 0.1). In Swaziland, Botswana, and parts of South Africa, the most recent statistics for pregnant women attending antenatal clinics reveal seropositivity rates of over 30 percent. In urban areas of Botswana, that figure was 43.9 percent (UNAIDS 2001a). In Burkina Faso, Cameroon, Côte d'Ivoire, Nigeria, Ethiopia, and Togo, national adult prevalence rates exceeded 5 percent in 2000, far lower than in southern Africa but much higher than the same region a decade ago (UNAIDS 2001a; Donnelly 2002).

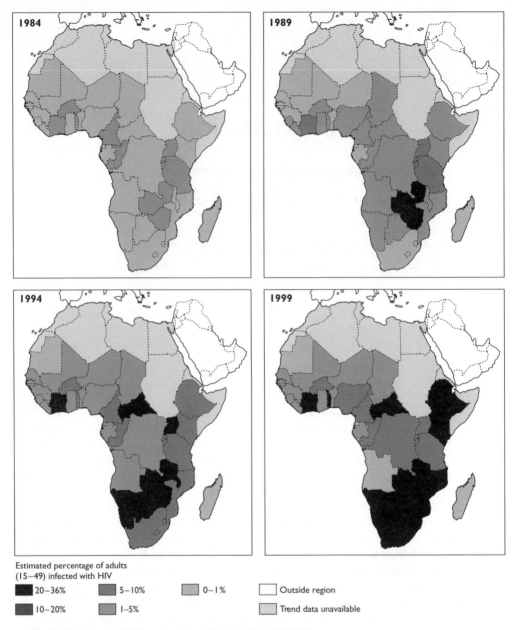

Figure 0.1 *Spread of HIV over time in sub-Saharan Africa, 1984–99*

Nigeria and Ethiopia together constitute nearly a third of sub-Saharan Africa's population, adding further alarm to their ascending rates of HIV (Donnelly 2002). For the most affected countries especially, high mortality from AIDS is reflected in steep drops in life expectancies (Figure 0.2). From the 1950s until about 1990, life expectancies for many African countries rose more or less steadily. Botswana achieved a peak of almost 63 in 1990. For South Africa, life expectancies peaked at just over 60 in 1990 and by 2000 were projected to reach 66 without AIDS. Since

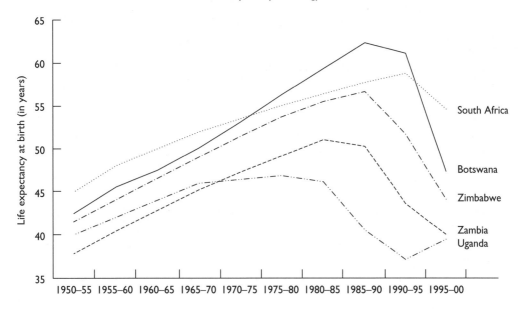

Figure 0.2 *Projected changes in life expectancy in selected African countries with high HIV prevalence, 1995–2000*
Source: UNAIDS 2000

1990, these rates have plummeted to 37 and 47, respectively. Malawi, Mozambique, and Swaziland also have life expectancies of less than 40 today (UNAIDS 2001a:7).

The magnitude and trajectory of the AIDS epidemic in sub-Saharan Africa in part underlie the reason for this book. But it is not just the fact of AIDS' existence that led the four of us to bring together a diversely experienced group of AIDS researchers in the social sciences to contribute to this volume. It was also our mutual frustration at dominant interpretations of how AIDS came to be in Africa, how it has progressed, and why it does not diminish. Media representations in the U.S. have been one significant source making AIDS in Africa an "epidemic of significations" (Treichler 1999). Though these sources on the one hand bring visibility to an epidemic remaining too long in relative obscurity in the West, they have often done so by couching the epidemic in terms that too often resonate with neocolonialist under standings of African culture. In a prominent *Time Magazine* cover story on AIDS in Africa in February of 2001, AIDS is said to be a spark in the "dry timber" of African societies, with reporters venturing into "the heart of the heart" of the epidemic in southern Africa where "ignorance, promiscuity, and denial help generate HIV transmission" (McGeary, 2001:36). In a 1998 *New York Times* series on AIDS in Africa dramatically titled "Dead Zones," stories tell of incomprehensible denial, shame, and stigma in the face of AIDS (Daley 1998; Specter 1998). Though such denials and stigma undoubtedly exist and require scrutiny, the elision of ongoing struggles with stigma and denial in the experience of AIDS in the U.S. suggests a singular pathology in the way Africans deal with epidemic. Though these and other news accounts highlight the numbing magnitude of human suffering involved in African AIDS, they also tend toward unreflexive depictions of cultural practices as causal factors. AIDS in these accounts exists because of entrenched fear and ignorance. Such representations, damaging enough by themselves, in turn imbricate with and help

reproduce vestigial colonial images of Africans as ignorant, hypersexual, and culturally backward (Packard and Epstein 1991; Schoepf 1991a; Watney 1989).

Within academic paradigms, funding priorities have determined that biomedical models remain dominant in generating understandings of AIDS in Africa (see
Schoepf and Baylies this volume). Early in the epidemic, biomedical researchers
focused largely on particular "risk" groups such as military men, truck drivers,
and prostitutes visible for their mobility or for sexual practices involving multiple
partners. In attempts to discern the driving mechanisms of the epidemic, the
precise sexual practices of members of these occupations were explored, including numbers of partners per day or month, geographic origins of clients, usual
patterns of travel, STD rates, and level of condom use.[2] There is no question that
these studies have provided relevant information on HIV infection rates and
practices of individuals within these prescribed occupations. They found, for
example, that even by the 1980s some urban-based commercial sex workers
were experiencing incomprehensibly high rates of infection. They have added
to our base knowledge about the links between STDs and HIV risk. Yet the
tendency in these studies to focus on sexual practices devoid of socioeconomic
contexts, and the emphasis on rational action models of behavior change, have
led to implications that Africans only need to be more aware of AIDS in order to
change their behavior. Underlying many studies is the assumption that Western-
centric norms of marital-based sexual conduct either do or should pertain in
differing regions of sub-Saharan Africa. The emphasis on risk groups also gives
the impression that anyone outside of these occupations need not worry about
their HIV status, elides ambiguous and culturally-bound definitions of "prostitute" (Akeroyd 1997 this volume), and leaves unexamined the vulnerability of
individuals outside of these "risk groups."

The dividing line here is not simply between biomedical researchers on the one
hand and social scientists on the other. As Schoepf makes clear (this volume),
there are plenty of physicians and epidemiologists who recognize the social
embeddedness of vulnerability and who contest the dominant biomedical paradigms with nuanced studies of sexuality and social practice. Until current
funding patterns change, however, these studies will remain in the shadow of
larger "scientifically based" epidemiological studies. Unfortunately, most national AIDS prevention programs are designed according to these biomedical
models of individual risk and rational behavior change, and their lack of success
in intervening into the epidemic is evident.

This book, then, intervenes into these predominant understandings of AIDS in
Africa. It addresses, inter alia, a concern over how Africa as well as AIDS has
come to be "known," what knowledge is privileged, and how it gets deployed.
We are concerned, for example, that dominant interpretations of AIDS are aiding
in the reproduction of problematic colonial and postcolonial African representations, practices, and social politics. This is not only troubling from a moral or
geopolitical standpoint. Problematic gender and racialized representations of
sexual practices, social behaviors, and government actions generated within
and outside of Africa are proving detrimental to the lives of millions currently
affected by HIV/AIDS. Women are "reservoirs of infection," Africans are promiscuous, AIDS victims are depraved, African governments are incompetent (see

Oppong and Kalipeni this volume). The aggregate effects of such interpretations are insidious for the stigmatization, misguided interventions, and indifference they help to produce as well as the lives that continue to be lost. The representations cited above from the U.S. have undoubtedly influenced national ambivalence about African AIDS, raising into question not only whether it should be our concern but whether there is any point in expensive interventions. An example within an African context is problematic postcolonial discourses associating AIDS with Western immorality and locating subsequent interventions in "traditional" patriarchal heterosexual praxis (Forster 1994; Lwanda, Schoepf, Philips this volume).

Intersecting with these representations are conflicts that sometimes emerge over how much preeminence biomedical models of AIDS should have in the highly varied and complex contexts in which the disease gets played out. This is especially true when biomedical solutions have thus far proven miserably inadequate in turning the tide of infections and helping those already infected. Perhaps the most visible example of what is at stake in conflicting interpretations of AIDS is still playing out in South Africa. South African President Thabo Mbeki's controversial stance on AIDS as a disease of poverty rather than an epidemic driven by HIV has caused profound consternation among international researchers as well as frustration among physicians and AIDS activists within South Africa (cf. Treatment Action Campaign at www.tac.za.org). While these concerns are more than understandable given Mbeki's refusal to provide antiretrovirals to affected populations, the incontrovertible dominance of biomedical models placing HIV front and center have silenced Mbeki's more insightful statements on poverty's role in creating AIDS in the South African context. AIDS is no exception, then, to Charles Rosenberg's contention that disease is itself a social actor (1992:xvi). AIDS continues to serve as a tool for diverse interests in and outside of Africa.

Our departure from these paradigms comes in striving to uncover the various ways AIDS is embedded within social, economic, cultural, political, and ideological contexts. The contributors to this volume largely disagree with the representation of AIDS as multiple instances of individual risk resulting from lack of information or poor decisions. We understand it rather as deeply rooted in historical antecedents, geopolitical relations, global financial configurations, government policies, local institutions, and cultural politics. From our own and others' collective research, it is clear that AIDS has been exacerbated by deepening poverty experienced by the majority of African countries over the past 20 years; that it has spread in the aftermath of war, civil unrest, and refugee movements; that migration patterns necessitated by underemployment in chronically underfinanced economies ensure both an increase in rates of transmission and a spread from urban to rural areas; and that governments shackled by poor terms of trade and crippling debts have neither the finances nor the personnel to address the problem adequately. Our purpose, then, is to offer in the chapters provided a more nuanced exploration of the multivalent forces shaping HIV/ AIDS in Africa. In doing so, we have included multidisciplinary approaches focusing on many of the critical foci of current AIDS research in the social sciences. The organization of the book suggests our understanding of the most trenchant conceptual and theoretical points of analysis concerning transmission, treatment, interpretation, and repercussions of AIDS. Our five sections of history, regional perspectives, social terms, methods and ethics, and impacts convey in effect that AIDS is not just a biological phenomenon affecting humans but a phenomenon whose relationship to economics, social ideologies, geography, corporate practices, and government policies is both constantly shifting and profound. Yet within these categories we have also attended to the importance of multiple voices in elucidating diverse perspectives of AIDS, a strategy that replicates the complexity of the epidemic and recognizes the partiality and situatedness of knowledge produced about it (Haraway 1988). Our conscious interventions into the biomedical status quo mean allowing a range of perspectives that do not necessarily agree with each other.

Though the contributors vary in their conceptual approaches to understanding AIDS, they employ for the most part variations of a cultural political economy of vulnerability framework that reflects their understanding of AIDS as resulting from material, symbolic, and discursive forces effectively constraining the opportunities and choices available to individuals and potentially creating conditions of vulnerability for large sectors of regional populations. Within this general framework, however, the contributors take different points of entry, focusing primary attention on individuals and the varying means by which they interpret, shape, and negotiate structural parameters defining their lives (Rugalema, Mbugua); elucidating the uneven deployment of structural constraints with the consequence that some groups are at higher risk than others (Zulu, Akeroyd, Schoepf, Campbell, Lurie et al.); exploring various interventions into HIV, including designs for more effective prevention programs (Kesby) and potential intervention technologies (Susser and Stein); sketching ethical implications of funding parameters (Baylies) or intellectual property laws (Craddock); and outlining the social experiences of AIDS (Guest) and its various impacts and community responses (Brown, Kalipeni and Ghosh, Kaleeba). Though no single book can be exhaustive on a subject with so many ongoing permutations, we have tried hard to cover those topics we felt were the most compelling and which together constituted a relatively well-rounded exploration.

Evident explicitly and implicitly throughout the book is also the elucidation of interconnecting global, national, regional, and local factors in creating patterns of vulnerability to and experience of AIDS. Most contributors to this book recognize the epidemic as in part an outcome of globalization defined by balances of power privileging industrial nations, and the economic and political policies instrumental in maintaining that balance of power. This means in part that the effects of colonialism need greater scrutiny in epidemic investigations for the long-term impacts to vulnerability of shifts in local social practices, gender politics, community cohesion, economic livelihoods, and types of and access to medical care. Many of the migration patterns extant today in parts of southern, eastern, and western Africa, for example, began as a result of colonial policies undermining rural livelihoods and channeling labor into regional industries with high labor demands (Packard 1989; Turshen 1984). Depressed economies and struggling agricultural sectors resulting in part from African countries' location in global economies today (addressed further below) underlie continued migratory circuits that heighten vulnerability to HIV primarily through family dissolution and concomitant shifts in sexual economies towards casual, extramarital, or remunerated relationships (Campbell, Schoepf, Oppong and Agyei-Mensah this volume). Chronic overcrowding and deepening immiseration in urban areas signal as well the failure of agricultural sectors, diminished civic spending, and governments' lack of resources for addressing issues of sanitation, health care, and employment. The results once again are conditions of extreme vulnerability to HIV among the poorest and most precarious urban populations (Zulu this volume).

Structural adjustment programs implemented in the 1980s by the World Bank and International Monetary Fund are a key equation in the various supranational antecedents of AIDS in Africa. Designed to jump-start devastated economies after the 1970s oil debacle, structural adjustment requires governments to deflate their currencies, curtail public spending, improve infrastructure, privatize industries, and gear national economies towards international markets. The result frequently has been increased impoverishment among the already-poor through lower wages coupled with higher prices for food and housing, fewer employment options, and diminished access to education and medical care (Brown, Schoepf, Lurie et al. this volume; Lele 1990). All of these consequences together generate varying degrees of heightened vulnerability to HIV in affected communities where individuals face fewer choices for generating enough money to feed themselves and their families. By most accounts, structural adjustment programs (SAPs) have immiserated women and girls disproportionately since girls are usually the first to be taken out of schools forced to initiate fees for attendance, and women have fewer employment options, face lower wages, and have more tenuous access to land and agricultural resources (Lele 1990; Schoepf et al. 2000). With heightened vulnerability and exposure to HIV comes even greater poverty. When an adult succumbs to AIDS, their already strapped household not only does without the added income, but has to find the resources for medical fees. According to UNAIDS, one-quarter of households in Botswana can expect to lose an income earner to AIDS within the next ten years, while the incomes of the poorest households across Africa are expected to fall 13 percent (UNAIDS 2001a:5). Debt forgiveness, not more structural adjustment, has become a rallying cry of organizations who recognize not only the detrimental impact of SAPs on communities, but understand as well that as long as governments are consigning prohibitive portions of their national budgets to debt repayments, they cannot possibly have the resources to intervene adequately into HIV/AIDS (cf. Jubilee 2000 campaign, www.jubilee2000uk.org).

The World Trade Organization has emerged recently as another significant player in producing global inequalities with repercussions for AIDS. By defining terms of trade within an economic jargon of fairness and "free markets," the WTO has in effect catered primarily to multinationals by forcing poor countries to open up their markets to imports, an action that frequently results in the decline of local manufacturing and a consequent reliance upon foreign products. The 1994 Trade-Related Investment Measures (TRIMS) of the WTO, for example, were designed to alleviate obligations of multinational corporations to invest in local resources in poor countries while exploiting cheap local labor for product manufacturing and assembly (Stiglitz 2002). Meanwhile, many industrial countries, including the U.S., continue to pass tariff and subsidy legislation making it difficult for nonindustrial countries to compete. Particularly in the context of already overwhelming debt burdens among poor countries, the need to increase imports while exports face insurmountable obstacles creates further economic devastation rather than the greater equity to which the WTO and national governments pay lip-service. One recent controversy surrounding WTO policies emerges from regulation of drug prices within its Trade-Related Intellectual Property Rights (TRIPS) agreement of 1999. Under the auspices of protecting corporate innovation and competition, TRIPS has effectively guaranteed pharmaceuticals the right to charge what they want for on-patent AIDS and other drugs, with the predictable result that the vast majority of AIDS patients in Africa and other poor regions have no way of affording antiretrovirals (Craddock this volume). Critiques of the WTO's role in producing and maintaining global inequalities and privileging corporate interest over human rights, public health, and the environment are mounting (cf. Soros 2002; Kim et al. 2000; Faux 2002; Dommen 2002). Far more studies are needed that attend to the impact of WTO and national trade policies on HIV transmission and AIDS treatment.

What is becoming clear is that global forces recognized as playing significant roles in producing global inequalities also play a significant role in generating AIDS in regions such as Africa (Schoepf this volume). The ways in which these broader forces play out, though, are complex and multivalent. Their diverse regional manifestations shape what might be called a series of AIDS microepidemics that are localized in their precise patterns, causal factors, and meanings. In other words, the broader brushstrokes of structural adjustment and WTO policies at global and national levels of analysis take on different coordinates as they intersect with local economies, government policies, social practices, and structures of meaning. Even where impoverishment appears to be a consistent outcome across regions, poverty itself needs to be disaggregated as to its precise definition and variable relationship with HIV risk, as Akeroyd argues in this volume. Not all poor individuals are equally vulnerable, even though across regions some groups tend to be more vulnerable. Women, for example, currently constitute 55 percent of HIV/AIDS cases in sub-Saharan Africa (UNAIDS 2001a). Young women and girls especially suffer disproportionately, sometimes experiencing rates of infection four to five times higher than boys in the same age group (Stock 1995). The reasons behind this have in part to do with the ways in which poverty, resource allocation, and community norms play out differently along gender and generational lines (see Akeroyd, Schoepf, Mbugua, and Kesby this volume). It is clear, at any rate, that the pervasive and multidirectional relations among global, national, and regional factors suggest that we can understand neither why HIV is transmitted in particular areas nor how to respond to it without comprehending the relevance of multiple scales of analysis.

This is not to suggest, however, that investigations need to include all levels of analysis equally. In-depth, bottom-up studies focusing on specific communities are necessary for illuminating the ways AIDS is experienced, interpreted, and made meaningful. While acknowledging the role of more distal contributions to regional patterns of vulnerability, recent studies are illuminating the critical importance of ethnographic approaches to fully understanding the place-specific cultural multivalence of AIDS (Farmer 1992a). In this book, ethnographic tactics were used to trace accommodations of HIV/AIDS within regional east African belief systems (Rugalema), to describe the impact of household dynamics on teenage sexual exploration (Mbugua), to highlight case studies in gendered vulnerability (Schoepf), to discern Zambian women's own priorities in intervention (Kesby), and to sketch the capacity of music stars to erode the walls of silence surrounding AIDS (Eaton). Critical, too, are those nuanced studies of sexualities and their importance to understanding the nature and durability of sexual practices (Campbell this volume; Setel 1996), as well as to the construction of national identities and supranational norms of behavior and belonging (Philips this volume). The relative absence of such ethnographic explorations until recently has meant sustained consternation from researchers and public health officials over why individuals do not or can not change behaviors despite increased knowledge, or has left invisible those groups not residing within self-consciously "traditional" definitions of a heteronormative mainstream. Instead, better prevention and treatment programs can only be determined by understanding the meanings individuals and governments have constructed about AIDS, sexual identities, sexual practices, risk, and treatment. Whereas anthropologists and historians of medicine have recognized for decades the deep social and political rootedness of sexual practice and disease interpretations, such understandings have been slow to intrude upon biomedical research on AIDS. Nevertheless, ethnographies exploring systems of meaning, their means of reproduction, and their flexibility in accommodating possibilities for change in social practices are increasingly recognized as critically important complements to a political economy of AIDS vulnerability.

The impacts of and community responses to AIDS constitute another important arena of inquiry, though as Brown's chapter suggests, defining impact is more difficult than it might seem in the context of national and regional economies. As Brown suggests, the way in which economic output, labor loss, agricultural production, and well-being are measured determines conclusions on just how devastated African economies are now or might be in the future because of AIDS. More certain is the growing problem of AIDS orphans experienced especially by countries hard hit by the epidemic. As Kalipeni and Ghosh outline in their chapter, the number of AIDS orphans continues to grow at a staggering pace, leaving communities and governments struggling to accommodate so many children in need of food, clothing, housing, school, medical care, and psychological support. Often the burden lands on extended families and communities already stretched beyond endurance by epidemic loss. Governments also do not usually have the economic resources to adequately address the issue, with the result that orphans frequently suffer mentally, physically, and emotionally. Yet, as Guest's chapter suggests, communities and orphans themselves are amazingly resilient in finding ways to build lives, muster resources, and provide caring environments for those so closely affected by the devastation of AIDS. Kaleeba's chapter, too, is a moving testament not only to the pain of losing a loved one, but to the determination involved in creating grassroots movements that disrupt cultural stigmas and make life easier for those affected by AIDS.

Community and nongovernmental organizations have clearly made significant differences in regional experiences and treatments of HIV/AIDS. Yet the unspoken message of this book is that the epidemic cannot be stopped by communities themselves. The primary emphasis throughout this book is that we need to understand the precise combination of global politics, financial policies, national priorities, and community politics maintaining ascendant rates of HIV / AIDS in order to understand what it will take to intervene effectively into transmission and treatment. Given the global complexity of causes, the burden of solutions cannot be left to affected communities alone. This point and others lead the majority of contributors to this volume to conceptualize AIDS in Africa and elsewhere as a human rights issue (Mann et al. 1999; Farmer 1999a). Contrary to the World Health Organization's 1978 Alma Ata declaration of health as a universal human right, Africans are being systematically denied their health by increasing impoverishment and chronic inequities that create conditions of vulnerability. As many of the following chapters illustrate, persistent inequities mean not only that more individuals will be vulnerable to HIV, but that they will be equally unable to determine their HIV status or, in the transition to AIDS, will have few if any options available to them for effective treatment. AIDS prevention, then, is not a matter simply of infusing large amounts of international aid into educational outreach and condom subsidization. Until global, national, and community antecedents of chronic inequity are recognized and meaningfully addressed, AIDS will persist across much of sub-Saharan Africa.

The extent of devastation in Africa on the one hand has at least awakened governments of industrial nations to the idea that AIDS is unlikely to disappear in Africa without outside assistance. The nature and degree of that assistance, however, are in question. As frequently happens with high-level policy decisions concerning poor countries, there remains a significant if unspoken opinion that Africa and its interminable plights are beyond the purview of foreign aid and irrelevant to foreign policy interests. Such thinking, of course, strategically elides historical and contemporary Western participation in creating problems such as AIDS in Africa and elsewhere. Kofi Annan's call for international humanitarian intervention into AIDS in Africa and other hard-hit countries, and the subsequent establishment within UNAIDS auspices of a Global Fund to fight AIDS, TB, and malaria, were commendable. Yet it is not surprising that only $800 million has been collected out of an annual targeted budget of $10 billion.[3] Whether the Global Fund can actually make a difference is itself debatable given the bureaucratic morass typical of high-level aid. In the face of such telling international indifference, however, this does not seem to be the most important question. Rather, the stinginess of global contributions raises the much more disturbing question of why 17 million deaths and 28 million individuals living with AIDS in Africa have generated such international apathy.

NOTES

1. These were taken from *Time Magazine*'s cover story, February 12, 2001, as well as from various issues of the *New York Times*.
2. The biomedical literature on AIDS in Africa is too vast to cite. Representative examples would be Ndinya-Achola et al. 1997, Slutsker et al. 1994.
3. As this book goes to press, President Bush has pledged $15 billion for the fight against AIDS in Africa. Yet the nature and distribution of these funds remain questionable.

Part I

History

Introduction to Part I

Historical investigations into impacts of colonialisms on African economies and social practices are pivotal to understanding regional patterns of HIV transmission today. Though research on health and medical systems in colonial Africa is relatively prolific,[1] studies examining the relevance to AIDS of Africa's colonial history are fewer (cf. Vaughan 1991). The two chapters within this section provide very different accounts of why history is important to understanding the emergence and development of AIDS. Both exemplify the growing acknowledgment that socio-economic conditions conducive to HIV transmission were largely created during colonial administrations that, though highly differentiated in form and function according to region, were nevertheless virtually universal in disrupting economic livelihoods, social practices, and community cohesion. With the appropriation of arable land by white settlers, colonial control of agricultural production, and distribution of resources toward urban centers came the rural impoverishment and migration patterns currently playing a role in HIV transmission. Lwanda's chapter examines colonial influences on HIV/AIDS in Malawi, but focuses attention primarily upon the impact of colonial medical systems and social practices on indigenous medical beliefs and cultural traditions. Lwanda's observations suggest that colonialism drove indigenous practices into rural pockets where they continue to function, while urban areas are more Western-influenced in their medical and cultural practices. Rather than a hybridity of Western and indigenous practices, then, he suggests that a duality still pertains in much of Malawi in the areas of medical care, initiation rites, and sexual conduct. In particular, those practices in rural areas that place individuals at greater risk need scrutiny, even if it means increased flexibility in the interpretations of "tradition." His study is highly nuanced in its appreciation of the tensions inherent between colonial aftermath and postcolonial nationalisms as these are reflected in leaders' grappling with AIDS and its implications for a post-independence unity.

Equally important to colonial antecedents is how Africans and the international community responded in the early days of AIDS. Much early response focused on finding the origins of the virus within Africa, an endeavor that proved controversial around what an answer about origins of HIV would tell us about the disease and its distribution. For some, knowing the origins would tell us more about the virus and its evolution over time; for others, origins would do little in the way of scientific elucidation but much more in the way of creating discourses of blame. In this case, such discourses were especially damaging because they imbricated with existing neocolonial perceptions of Africa as the cradle of disease, famine, and other disasters of apocalyptic magnitude (Chirimuuta and Chirimuuta 1989; Helen Epstein 1999). According to Chirimuuta and Chirimuuta (1989), origins investigations targeting Africa resulted in strained geopolitical relations, diminutions in international aid to African countries, and damage to regional tourist industries. Though still inconclusive, the most recent evidence from genetic "fingerprinting" still suggests central Africa as the original birthplace of HIV, where it began as Simian Immunodeficiency Virus in chimpanzees and eventually spread to humans. Questions remain about how and when this leap from simian to human retrovirus occurred (cf. Hooper 1999; Epstein 1999).

Another trenchant question, as Schoepf points out, is why it took so long for the international community to respond to the growing epidemic, and why biomedical knowledge was privileged among the interpretations eventually circulating. Recognizing the interactions of discursive representations and material practices, Schoepf decries biomedical research that focused on prostitutes as "reservoirs of infection" for the misguided policies it has informed and the damaging misunderstandings it has generated of the epidemic. Simultaneous with growing biomedical interest in and predominance over behavioral models of HIV transmission in Africa in the 1980s was the initiation of structural adjustment programs by the World Bank and the International Monetary Fund. Designed to boost economies by diverting resources into export industries and curtailing domestic spending, these programs were implemented across sub-Saharan Africa with the result, argues Schoepf, of not only exacerbating poverty in almost every instance, but consequently of catapulting thousands of individuals into heightened vulnerability (see also Lurie et al. this volume). Only by understanding these separate but related spheres of influence in the early years of AIDS in Africa can we comprehend the pattern of epidemic today.

NOTE

1. Examples include Turshen 1999b, 1984; Feierman and Janzen 1992; Ernst and Harris 1999; Vaughan 1991.

Chapter 1

AIDS, History, and Struggles over Meaning

Brooke Grundfest Schoepf

Introduction

Disease epidemics are social processes. The spread of infection is propelled by history, political economy, and culture. Beset by grinding poverty, AIDS, drought, rampant malnutrition, genocide, and war, the world's poorest continent has suffered a quarter century of profound, multiplex crisis. Structural violence is a term used to encompass the concatenation of adverse social, economic, and political conditions in which the world's poor live out their lives. The destructive impact of ongoing economic crisis on the health of poor communities takes forms less dramatic than violent conflict, yet which may be just as devastating. Structural and social violence has contributed decisively to the dissemination of the Human Immunodeficiency Virus (HIV) on the African continent. As economic crisis spread across the continent in the late 1970s, the HIV virus silently spread as well. Seemingly unrelated, the two phenomena are in fact intimately entwined. The effects of poverty accelerated the spread of the virus in the 1980s. By the 1990s the ravages of AIDS in turn plunged afflicted regions deeper into economic crisis.

Internationally, as in the United States, AIDS is "an epidemic of signification." Many responses have been moralizing and stigmatizing. Initially recognized among elites in many countries, HIV rapidly spread along "the fault-lines of society" to the poor and disinherited. Response to AIDS is political everywhere, in Africa no less than in the West. Knowledge is socially situated, built on previous knowledges with the power to define how we know, and to determine what facts shall be considered "real." Public health action takes place on a terrain of contested meanings and unequal power, where different forms of knowledge struggle for control. In the case of AIDS in Africa, the defining power lay in the international biomedical arena, but these definitions met with enduring disease representations and practices, especially with respect to contagion and "disordered" sexuality in afflicted societies. The contradictions between situational need and societal response have been particularly sharp. This can be explained, at least in part, by discourses surrounding the appearance and spread of the new virus. AIDS brings forth representations that support and reproduce already constituted gender, color, class, and national hierarchies. Societal responses to AIDS, including disease control policies, are propelled by cultural politics forged in the history of relations between Africa and the West.

My understanding of the cultural politics of AIDS comes from participation in the struggle to discover and reshape meanings of AIDS in Africa and the West. In 1985 I joined with colleagues to form the transdisciplinary CONNAISSIDA Project in what was then Zaire (now Democratic Republic of Congo, or DRC).[1] Formed from the French words *connaisance* (knowledge) and *Sida* (AIDS), CONNAISSIDA means "knowledge of AIDS." We investigated popular representations of and responses to AIDS, and compared these with what was known in the biomedical research community. Grounded in medical and economic anthropology, the project incorporated understandings from several other fields, including social psychology, public health, and development studies.

From February 1985 through June 1990, CONNAISSIDA conducted more than 1,800 open-ended interviews, mainly in Kinshasa and Lubumbashi, but also in the smaller cities of Matadi and Kikwit. Interviews with many individuals and groups were repeated over time, and supplemented by participant-observation in several popular neighborhoods and elite networks, and collection of life-history narratives.[2] For the most part, researchers lived as accepted members of the communities where they worked. Topics ranged widely, as people variously situated socially were asked what they knew about AIDS, what problems they saw in ensuring their own protection and that of persons close to them, and, given their understanding of their culture, how obstacles might be overcome. Results were used to design community-based education using participatory empowerment methods based on group dynamics (Schoepf, Walu, Rukarangira et al. 1991; Schoepf 1993).[3] The action-research generated local attempts at social change, some of which were successful, and led to new understandings of the dynamics of social structure, agency, and negotiated couple relations.[4, 5]

This research is related to current theoretical and methodological advances in anthropology. It is especially attuned to listening to knowledge "from below" and to viewing culture through the lens of gender relations. Linking macro-level political economy to micro-level ethnography, case studies illuminate women's risk. They show how racism, poverty, inequality, and gendered discourses about AIDS hamper prevention (Schoepf, Rukarangira et al. 1988a, b; Schoepf 1988, 1992a). Many findings have been replicated by research undertaken elsewhere in sub-Saharan Africa.

An Historical Note

The cultural politics of AIDS are now well understood; their effects were to increase the velocity of the pandemic, rather than to slow it. At the outset, epidemiologists in government agencies designated entire populations as "risk groups," obscuring differences among people assigned to the categories. A focus on risk groups implies that everyone not included within the boundaries of stigma is not at risk. Common in public health discourse, such constructions are part of a "hegemonic process" that helps dominant groups to maintain, reinforce, reconstruct, and obscure the workings of the established social order.

In the 1980s Western epidemiologists and health planners in the development agencies greatly underestimated the potential magnitude of HIV/AIDS in Africa. The risk group paradigm fostered belief in AIDS as an urban disease, in both biomedical and popular circles. High risk was believed to be limited to bounded groups of "core transmitters." These included sex workers and their clients, the military, and long-distance truckers, all of whom were recognized as having multiple sex partners. A corollary was that rural areas, with "traditional" sexual morality and practices, would be spared. Since Africa's populations were mainly rural, they reasoned, the impact of AIDS would be limited. Critical social scientists argued against this view, which we call the "merrie Africa" paradigm. Charles Hunt, a sociologist, Randall Packard and Leroy Vail, historians, pointed to linkages between AIDS and a century of extensive male labor migration in central and southern Africa that brought about the transformation of family relations.

Conditions were somewhat different in Kinshasa and other cities of Zaire, where sex ratios were virtually equal. Our previous research had indicated the importance of gender in the context of deepening poverty. We noted the pertinence of cosmology related to constructions of sexuality, reproduction, and health discovered in previous research. Given the powerful socio-economic and cultural forces driving the epidemic, we argued that information and education (IEC) campaigns could increase knowledge, but would not suffice to reduce the spread of HIV. We feared that without broad social mobilization a heterosexual epidemic of long-delayed manifestation would attain catastrophic proportions. We identified groups in civil society that we proposed to involve in determining the changes necessary to stop HIV infection that could promote changes in social relations among their members. We submitted project proposals to the Zaire government, official agencies, and foundations in 1986 and 1987.

Dismissing concerns about a potentially catastrophic pandemic, officials in control of American AIDS funds proposed to control AIDS by targeting prevention efforts to those identified as "core transmitters." The rationale was that as these were the people who would transmit HIV to more than one other person, such targeting would be cost-effective. In contrast, they reasoned, infected women in long-term relationships would only risk transmission to one other person: their next infant.[6] The epidemiological model was largely driven by unwillingness to commit funds to a wider effort. One recent report states blandly that the wives of men with AIDS are likely to become infected.

Prevention was essentially viewed as a technocratic problem of behavior change based on access to information and condoms. STD treatment was later added on a pilot basis. Only rarely were free diagnosis and antibiotics made widely available, most often to sex workers. Where they were, incidence of new infection was significantly reduced in the populations served. A few research projects have included counseling of "discordant couples" in which only one partner was HIV positive. Their labor-intensive efforts were most successful in promoting consistent condom use when the infected partner was female. None of these employed the participatory action-research methodology or other devices that CONNAIS-SIDA found so useful. Most prevention efforts to date have been limited in scope, and merely paid lip-service to the economic and cultural constraints that prevent many Africans from protecting themselves and their children from AIDS.

Ignoring declining health services, gender inequality, and mounting poverty, planners funded "KAP" surveys of AIDS knowledge, attitudes, and sexual practices around the world. They acted as though increased information would be sufficient to change complexly determined actions and as though individuals could exercise control over the social and cultural constraints to prevention. They focused on individuals in special "risk groups" and their "high risk behaviors," rather than on processes of economic empowerment and sociocultural change. The result of this blindness, as noted above, is what is now recognized: the effects of AIDS in Africa are already in some countries, and will be in still others, nothing short of catastrophic.

The question addressed here is: why did it take so long for the potential of the AIDS pandemic to be recognized in the international community? Or to put it another way: by what processes was the scientific imagination stifled? My questions are related to a question posed recently by Professor Donna Haraway, who asked: "What does it take for facts to be recognized as 'real'?"[7] The answer, of course, is that the facts must be put about by those who are socially authorized to do so. In the domain of epidemic disease, these persons are epidemiologists and specialists in public health, not social scientists, and above all, not ethnographers who use qualitative methods to examine culture: social relations, meanings, and their contexts.

But this short answer is misleading. From the early 1990s, critical anthropologists and other social scientists were joined by physicians, epidemiologists, and health planners in describing social forces propelling the HIV epidemic in Africa. These physicians, however, were not those conducting biomedical research in big labs with multimillion-dollar government and foundation grants. That, too, is part of Haraway's answer. Only members of the research "establishment" are socially authorized to produce knowledge. The critical physicians were public health specialists of a particular kind, dedicated to social medicine and community health. They sought to read social patterns from seroprevalence numbers, rather than simply seeing individual "risk factors." They also sought to dispel the racist assumptions and the moralizing that accompanied constructions of "African sexuality."

Full responsibility for moralizing discourses and resulting social demobilization cannot be laid solely at the feet of biomedical policymakers, for the discourses and policy are embedded in the public culture of late 20th-century Western societies and exported to Africa. The currently dominant biomedical model incorporates capitalist economic assumptions about health resulting from individually chosen lifestyles. It leaves little scope for understanding how behaviors are related to social conditions, or how communities shape the lives of their members. The officially situated epidemiologists' focus on individual sexual behavior, their claim to exclusive, value-neutral objectivity, and reliance on surveys as the sole method of "science" are very much their responsibility, however. The late Dr. Jonathan Mann, architect of the World Health Organization's Special (later Global) Program on AIDS, was self-critical when he wrote:

> The focus on individual risk reduction was simply too narrow, for it was unable to deal concretely with the lived social realities... applying classical epidemiological methods to HIV/AIDS ensures – pre-determines – that "risk" will be defined in terms of individual determinants and individual behavior... (Mann 1996:3)

The epistemological failure was political rather than disciplinary, however. Critical traditions in epidemiology and social medicine long have "situated the primary origins of epidemic diseases in economic misery," beginning in the mid-19th century with Rudolph Virchow (Dubos 1965:394):

> the history of epidemic diseases must form part of the cultural history of mankind. Epidemics correspond to large signs of warning which tell the true statesman that a disturbance has oc-

curred in the development of his people which even a policy of unconcern can no longer overlook (Virchow 1848, cited by Dubos 1965:393).

Virchow developed a concept of health as what economists today would call a "public good," a public rather than an individual responsibility. He maintained that governments have a responsibility to preserve the public's health, and conversely, that medicine must intervene in social and political affairs to prevent epidemics. It took another century for health to be considered a human right, enshrined in UN convention, although honored more by rhetorical flourishes than by actual resource allocation. By the 1980s, this concept was no longer part of mainstream discourse. Privatization became the watchword in the West, as in structural adjustment programs (SAPs) mandated in the south. Struggles over meaning were international and interdisciplinary, as African and Western researchers contested the narrow paradigm and its implications. They were ignored.

CONNAISSIDA's research, with its examples of empowering community-based prevention based on cultural understandings, failed to gain credence in official circles. Perhaps the international community had decided that Africans (or African men) were too culture-bound and too driven by sex to change. Obviously, Western dictates could not make the changes happen. But African intellectuals with deep roots in popular culture could use forms of "consciousness-raising" to work out with others ways to reduce risks. For some effects of the dominant paradigm, see my critical assessment in *Annual Review of Anthropology* (Schoepf 2001).

Mann (who was provided with pre-publication copies of CONNAISSIDA's results in February 1988) noted two reasons for limiting the focus to individual risk behaviors. One was medical dominance: "...a desire by public health workers to 'own' the problem...by keeping the discourse at a medical and public health level...." Another was to avoid "...the inevitable accusation that public health is 'meddling' in societal issues which 'go far beyond' its scope and competence and inevitably puts [researchers]...potentially 'at odds' with governmental and other sources of power in the society" (Mann 1996:6).

In other words, marginalization of the critical social sciences, including social medicine and public health, was a consciously chosen strategy, deliberately maintained. Ethnographic research on the political and economic inequalities that drive the pandemic was kept from the *tables de partage* where AIDS funds were apportioned.[8] Reid (1992) charged that the physicians who crafted international AIDS policy lacked "epistemic responsibility" in their neglect of gender inequality. Mann concurred that sexism in the GPA caused them to overlook risk to women.[9] Upon leaving World Health Organization (WHO) to found an independently funded institute, Mann became a leading proponent of health and human rights.

Discourses of Stigma and Racism

In the U.S. and Western Europe, the focus on "risk groups" reverberated in discourse about risk and responsibility. Once placed in a risk category, individuals are separated from other sources of identity, henceforward stigmatized and degraded by definition. Creation of alterity, or "otherness," allows those in power to dehumanize, to scapegoat, to blame, and thus to avoid responsibility for sufferers. Accused witches, lepers, and other people who are assigned the status of "dangerous others" in various times and places are believed to be morally contagious and often sexually polluting. The results are broadly similar: such people may be consigned to limbo and to social or corporeal death. The struggles of people with HIV and AIDS to resist this "othering" process were charted from the beginning of ethnographic research on AIDS.

Homosexual men, Haitians, and Africans were placed on the "other" side of the social fault-line and stigmatized as "promiscuous" – a notion so imprecise and value-laden that it cannot be used scientifically. Stigma rapidly led to discrimination, in what Farmer (1992b) calls a "geography of blame." Haitians were denied housing, dismissed from jobs, and required to undergo tests to enter the United States. In Europe, Africans were targeted. In Russia, several African students were killed by mobs; others interrupted their studies and fled home (Osman Kabia, personal communica-

tion, May 2000). In Britain, African sex workers were hounded from their homes and denied service in local shops (Sabatier 1996).

With respect to Africa, some early writers, novices to African Studies, produced rapid assessments and cobbled-together surveys. The worst literature searches tore bits of erotica from context. Sweeping statements were made about a special "African sexuality," based on "traditional" (i.e., unchanging) marriage patterns that were different from those of Europe and Asia. Culture was designated as the culprit of HIV spread. But while culture was the concept most bandied about, social scientists specialized in the study of culture were left out of the loop. African and Africanist anthropologists were ignored by biomedical researchers and by major funding agencies. This, too, was a political stance. Blaming cultural differences for situations clearly linked to economic and political inequality supports the status quo. Social scientists of my generation will recall the 1960s struggle against the "culture of poverty" notion that became a substitute for understanding the socio-economic and psychological effects of racism and poverty on families in the inner cities of the U.S. and elsewhere in North America. As a result, the victims were blamed for causing their woes.

When anthropologists *were* taken on board in AIDS research, they were not full partners in the setting of the research agenda. Most were asked to conduct KAP surveys. Frankenberg (1995) describes the travails of anthropologists struggling with the categories imposed by epidemiologists in interdisciplinary teams. Anthropologists were "... token members on research projects [directed] by scientists who regarded 'culture' as an obstacle" (Obbo 1999:69). Some, like myself, worked on small grants without salaries in order to maintain their independence.

Critics disputed the premises and methods of authors who misapplied genetics and ethology (studies of animal behavior) to human populations. They challenged racist representations surrounding heterosexual transmission of HIV. They showed how elements of *raciologie* used to justify slavery and colonial domination were adapted in AIDS discourse. They contested notions of culture as fixed and immutable, posing insurmountable barriers to protection from HIV. These critics included anthropologists, historians, biologists, and physicians.

Emphasis on the supposed uniqueness of heterosexual transmission in Africa, published in scientific journals and sensationalized in the mass media, supported the contention of some critics that AIDS was being blown out of proportion by Western governments. Many criticized the statements about promiscuity, redolent of colonial discourse. Some researchers argued that the sexual transmission paradigm had closed off the search for organic co-factors that made weakened bodies unable to fend off HIV infection. Others viewed concern with AIDS and sex in Africa as a diversionary ploy by conservative Western politicians strongly influenced by the moralizing of the Christian right, who sought to justify drastically reduced assistance to Africa in the 1980s. The moralizing resonated within African churches, where clergymen proclaimed AIDS to be "the wages of sin" and assured women that they would be in no danger if they remained faithful to their husbands. Many African leaders and intellectuals also adopted moralist discourses, and refused to countenance the wide distribution of condom publicity and supplies. Not unexpectedly, stigma aroused defensive reactions among African officials, intellectuals, and journalists, not only making it difficult to conduct culturally sensitive, in-depth, qualitative research on contemporary sexuality. In the early years, one could be called to task for supplying condoms to adults who requested them on the grounds that "condoms promote immorality" (field notes, Kinshasa, November 1987; Kampala, February 1992).

In Africa, the dominance of bio-power was limited by competing representations in several arenas. The example of Zaire is instructive. AIDS was first diagnosed among Zairians in Europe in 1983, and international biomedical research of Projet SIDA began in Kinshasa in 1984. Still, AIDS remained a politically tabooed subject. Public discussion was muted and little information appeared in national news media. Prodded by international donors, however, the government campaign began in 1987. As health officials, mass media, and voluntary organizations cautiously began to provide information, people started talking more about AIDS. Ideas

regarding transmission and prevention, disease origins and etiology varied widely and changed over time. Urban elites, who had access to television, international publications, and friends in the health professions, were most informed. On the other hand, most people's knowledge was sketchy, and misinformation common. For example, the media told of insect transmission and, despite later disclaimers, people continued to cite it. On the other hand, few were aware of the risk of mother – infant transmission.

Popular constructions of AIDS changed over time. At first, people denied that AIDS was "real." Since some rich and powerful men widely reputed for their sexual exploits apparently were unaffected, people said that AIDS could not be too serious in Kinshasa. Several jokes spread on *radio trottoir*, the "sidewalk radio" that carries popular culture in Africa's cities, reinforced this denial. Beginning with university students in Kinshasa in 1985, then spreading elsewhere, the acronym for AIDS was given a humorous meaning. AIDS (SIDA, in French) was dubbed a *Syndrome Imaginaire pour Décourager les Amoureux*, "an imaginary syndrome to discourage lovers." People were aware that many Westerners stigmatized Africans for "having [what Westerners, poor benighted things, considered] too much sex, and too many children." Belittled by this clever phrase, the potential danger of the epidemic could be denied, and its implications avoided. This dismissive political construction was elaborated and spread along the *radio trottoir* in numerous other countries across Africa.

Skepticism also was related to unfamiliarity with people with AIDS (PWAs). Women and youth, especially, suspected that churches and government officials sought to control their sexuality. When AIDS was recognized as real, it was declared to have come from "elsewhere." Not only in Africa, but elsewhere in the Third World, American military men, businessmen, and sex tourists were made into plausible sources; deliberate biological warfare seemed a possibility to many during the cold war; a laboratory accident or a result of vaccine testing, all had their supporters. There were also fantasmic scenarios, some drawn from the wells of history. For example, Euro-American suggestions of monkey's blood, used in love magic or voodoo rites, were matched in Africa by attribution of AIDS' origin to European men who paid African women to have sex with dogs (or chimpanzees, or horses). The latter built on an old construction of STD origins found across the continent and recirculated in relation to AIDS.

While sophisticates could joke about Europeans' notions, the emphasis in public health advice and in Western mass media on promiscuity and on sex with prostitutes reinforced the perception that Westerners continued to stigmatize Africans' sexuality as "excessive," "diseased," and "dirty." Depiction of prostitutes as "a reservoir of infection" fueled local constructions of AIDS as "a disease of women," or of the "lower orders," from whom the "morally pure" required protection.[10] Advice to "avoid prostitutes" was heard, but just who is a prostitute? Some working-class men believed themselves to be free of risk even while they engaged in risky behavior. For example, two garage mechanics in their twenties said that AIDS is not a danger for them, because: "We are too poor to travel to all those foreign places. Anyway, our girlfriends are young and healthy schoolgirls."

Advice to "stay faithful to one partner" was impractical for many and misleading for those whose partners were already infected. Advice about safer sex was extremely limited and seldom cited by the public. As predicted, messages of the mass campaign created considerable awareness of AIDS, but relatively few people changed their sexual behavior sufficiently to reduce their own risk of infection or to protect partners. Mass media campaigns did not adequately inform the public about the slow action of the virus. People found it difficult to grasp that a healthy-looking person could harbor a fatal HIV infection, could infect others, and would be likely to die in a few years. Failure to comprehend the lengthy and variable incubation period contributed to confusion and blame-casting. CONNAISSIDA designed exercises to promote these understandings. The most successful was the metaphor of a tree that harbors unseen termites. The tree goes on living for many years, until slowly it begins to lose its leaves. Once that happens it is too late to smoke them out, and

the tree dies. Trees are potent symbols of life. Represented by graphics, the death of a tree can provoke expression of concern and discussion about how to avoid HIV.[11]

In mid-1987 the most common reaction to AIDS in Kinshasa was denial. At the same time that most HIV prevention interventions targeted low-status and stigmatized groups, wealthy and powerful high-status men were rarely mentioned in official discourse. Yet, as holders of "the triptych of masculinity, seniority and renown" (Eboko 1999:47), such men possessed the means to attract (and discard) multiple sexual partners. They could have triggered an early sea-change in situations that put women and children at risk. Instead, many denied their risk and their responsibility. The Zairian cabinet minister, who in August 1986 told me that "I just don't want to think about AIDS," expressed a commonly held view. Another cabinet minister took home an informational leaflet handed out in a cabinet meeting in June 1987.[12] He placed it on his wife's night table, but avoided discussion. His wife wondered if he was indirectly accusing her of infidelity (field notes, Kinshasa, July 1987; see Schoepf 1992a).

In April 1987 I devised a game called "scoreboard" to help men break through their denial of risk as a way to opening small group discussion about risk and responsibility. Players chart their total number of partners for the previous month, the last year, and the past five years. The result is often a gasp of astonishment. Without showing their slips to the group, they then discuss HIV risks and ways to lower them. Initially, I had titled the exercise "Russian roulette," but as the participants were unfamiliar with that game, I changed it to "scoreboard." At the end of the exercise, I explained the original title. Participants immediately understood that without condoms, they were playing sexual Russian roulette. Most men in the groups with whom this exercise was used expressed resolve to change. Some, however, said that they could not. One man who said that he would stop hitting on students, later confessed somewhat shamefacedly that he only did so after his blood was tested for a transfusion donation and found negative.

Brooke Grundfest Schoepf

Denial was not simply a Congolese predilection. Each country appears to have gone through a stage of refusal early in the epidemic. For example, a Zanzibari cabinet minister interviewed during a planning mission focused on AIDS risk to sailors and fishermen. When I asked him if government officials are likely to sleep alone when they travel, his face turned gray. He managed a small smile and turned to other matters (field notes, Zanzibar, October 1991). At the time, seroprevalence in the islands was quite low.

Many people across the continent construe AIDS as "a disease of women." The attitudes expressed by one highly educated Zairian university official interviewed over a three-year period evolved from skepticism to blame. In 1985 the informant considered AIDS to be an invention of Western propagandists seeking to discredit Africans. He believed that this "imaginary syndrome" was intended not only to discourage African lovers, but also to discourage European and Japanese tourists and investors whose money is needed to redress the economic crisis. Why else, he reasoned, would scientists engage in irresponsible speculation about an African origin for AIDS? In 1987 this informant said that since he became aware of the danger, he had limited his sexual relations to three current wives. If he should find himself infected he "knew" that it would be due to their infidelity. He did not believe that he might have been infected by previous partners. "Women are the major transmitters of AIDS, because they are more promiscuous than men, who if they desire a woman, marry her." By 1988 his fear of AIDS had increased. He said that seropositive women should be quarantined. The prospect of interning thousands of women for many years did not give him pause. Nor did he recognize that infected men would continue to spread the virus. It was difficult to record his views without starting an argument. I went into the kitchen to help his third wife, whom he was visiting that afternoon, prepare his meal.

The identification of AIDS as an STD made it plausible to blame "promiscuous" women for its spread, as many African cultures attribute such conditions to a wife's adultery or failure to observe various cleansing rituals. The wife of a former cabinet minister related:

Several of my neighbors are said to have died of AIDS. There is Doctor [X]'s first wife and her last child, as well as his second wife. He is still well and though he might be a healthy carrier, people suspect the women of infidelity. A professor down the street also died of AIDS. Since his wife is a long-distance trader, people are sure that she gave him the disease. (Interview with Mme. Miriam Lobho, August 1996)

As the epidemic went on, deaths from this "long and painful sickness" mounted in Kinshasa. By 1987, the popular imagination began to reflect the epidemic's economic roots. Another phrase built from the acronym expressed the evolving understanding of AIDS' (SIDA's) social epidemiology: "*Salaire Insuffisant Depuis des Années.*"[13] In anglophone Africa the same causal relationship was expressed as "the Acquired Income Deficiency Syndrome." That is, although still constructed as a "disease of women," AIDS came to be widely understood as a disease brought on by poverty, unemployment, and the strategies that poor women commonly adopted for survival. In Zaire, as in Uganda, Tanzania, and Senegal, resistance from many religious leaders and community elders continued strong into the early 1990s. Alarmed governments nevertheless instituted imaginative forms of education and made free STD treatment and condoms widely available. These, and growing awareness of deaths from "a long and painful illness," understood as AIDS, rendered protection acceptable and possible among young people. Crisis notwithstanding, infection prevalence apparently has remained stable in Kinshasa from 1988, while in Uganda people aged 15–29 registered declines from 1996. More recently, the epidemic seems to have stabilized in Zambia and Zimbabwe. Elsewhere in DRC and other countries the virus continues to spread, not only in cities, but in rural towns and in countries apparently HIV-free in the 1980s.

High Politics

The racism and moralizing texts were "words that kill," for prevention was retarded by reluctance to address the issues. The defensive response of many governments was to try to keep the lid on news of AIDS. Scientists in Kinshasa were periodically told not to talk to the press. The official response reverberated in international policy circles. Many in the U.S. feared that the biomedical projects would be shut down. USAID and other bilateral lenders channeled most funds for AIDS research and prevention through the World Health Organization. The latter, as a UN agency, at the time worked only with governments. Funds remained centralized in health ministries. Governments insisted on the assurance that programs be closely controlled, centralized, and vertical. African Health Ministries, perennially short of funds and especially starved by structural adjustment programs (SAPs), welcomed AIDS programs as a major source of international funds bringing perquisites such as foreign travel, vehicles, cash, and patronage jobs. Among the weaker ministries in terms of policy implementation, this frequently meant that AIDS prevention largely remained confined to the capital. It also over-determined the focus on politically powerless risk groups. International biomedical research offered Western and African professionals opportunities for advancement in careers and for multiple roles in the national political economy. Some of the silences within Africa that made it difficult to conduct social research on AIDS were linked to economic interests of policymakers, who feared their business would be harmed. Like many authoritarian states, Zaire prevented community-based mobilization of imaginative educational responses rooted in popular culture.

AIDS and Accusation

Stigma not only retarded prevention campaigns. By fostering social isolation, it added to the suffering endured by sick people and their families. In several countries, "free women," living without male protection, were made scapegoats, rounded up and deported to rural areas where they were unable to make a living; others were imprisoned and raped. Women whose HIV/AIDS was known or suspected were evicted from their homes and deprived of livelihoods and children. Some were accused as witches. While witchcraft may be an "imagined violence," accusations often have social and material effects.

Accusations of blame are related to older representations of disease as "sent sickness." AIDS became part of the many "reinventions" of tradition, including sorcery accusations, that increased with socio-economic changes, including labor migration, markets, and sharp competition for jobs, housing, and other resources in the cities. Some link AIDS to witchcraft and to illnesses believed to be sexually transmitted and caused by "polluted" women. Although some African healers were cautious in the face of a new, fatal disease, many claimed to cure AIDS. Across the continent, too, there were healers who told their older male clients to have sex with a virgin to rid themselves of AIDS, transposing old ideas about "sickness in the blood," contagion, and cure.

New healers have emerged as desperately sick people search both for cures that biomedicine cannot offer, and for explanations of why they have fallen sick. The numbers of "traditional" practitioners expanded markedly.[14] While many have knowledge of herbal remedies, the claims of others to treat a wide variety of unrelated symptoms, and diseases such as cancers, tuberculosis, and AIDS, suggest charlatanism. Evangelical Christian "healing churches" have attracted numerous converts in this crisis period. Their pastor-prophets claim to heal by means of prayer and the laying on of hands. Some healers combine various forms of herbal medicine with spirit mediumship and divination. The newest trend is a bricolage of these elements with prophetism, and New Age discourse, replete with dietary fads, healing crystals, and notions of balance (field notes, Kinshasa 1985–9). While such constructions are perhaps harmless in themselves, and may bring some comfort to those for whom biomedicine has little to offer, they come at a price. Many families have expended scarce resources in the search for cures, and following the death of the sufferer, poor survivors are often left penniless. Home care of the sick and dying places additional burdens on women in their role as caretakers.

Given the material and psychological burdens of so much fatal disease, reliance upon poor extended families and communities to shoulder the burdens of caring for AIDS orphans (or for those who have lost parents in Africa's civil wars and genocide) is unrealistic. Due to the stigma surrounding the deaths of their parents, AIDS orphans may be shunned and left to roam the streets. Even when they are accepted by relatives, poverty makes many of these children vulnerable to HIV infection in their turn.

Another old belief has been entwined with new practices applied to the AIDS tragedy. Despite the efforts of many extended families and communities, many are unable to cope. Some orphans who are fostered in poor families have been accused of killing their parents through sorcery. They are believed to be "witch children," who kill, not out of evil intent, but as a result of bewitchment by a sorcerer, an enemy of the parent. One young man accused by his aunt was set upon by neighbors, who attempted to burn him alive by "necklacing" with a gasoline-filled tire. This method, used on suspected police informers in South Africa, became part of the ethnic cleansing of Tutsi in Kinshasa in 1998. Accusations of children became a socially acceptable way to rid a family of troublesome orphans whom they are expected to foster, but who constitute an intolerable burden. More than 2,000 such children were living on the streets of Kinshasa in 1999 (MSF 2000).

Community care, cast as a "traditional practice," is one more panacea, a salve to the consciences of those who leave Africa to cope with AIDS without adequate support from the international community. A recent World Bank report estimates that quality orphan care and education requires expenditure of about $450 per child when provided in a group home. This puts a price to the reproductive labor that women do without pay. It is more than many entire families in Congo see in a year, and more than the government's per capita expenditure for health and education combined.

Social Medicine, Structural Violence and AIDS

Despite some prevention successes in a few countries, the AIDS crisis gathers momentum. Few governments seriously address the problems involved in a comprehensive manner; the international community provides limited assistance. HIV/AIDS strikes with special severity in poor African communities struggling under the burdens of continent-wide economic crisis. From the 1980s the institutions of international finance (IFIs) began to impose a series of "structural adjustment programs," which they claimed would restore health to stagnant African economies. The IFIs imposed SAPs on 38 governments in sub-Saharan Africa in the 1980s and 1990s as a condition for new loans. In Africa the goals were to further debt reimbursement and create profitable conditions for new foreign investment in the resources the Western world needs from Africa, namely oil and minerals. Their policies contributed to deepening a global economic and political crisis, and during this time, HIV, AIDS, and tuberculosis gained a stranglehold on the countries of east and southern Africa. In many countries AIDS further slowed the already unfavorable per capita income growth (see Schoepf, Schoepf, and Millen 2000).

My second chapter in this book shows how the forces of SAPs, poverty, and gender inequality come together in the life of a poor woman in Kinshasa, Zaire, now the Democratic Republic of Congo (DRC). This section summarizes the macro-level political and economic processes that cause suffering and death for so many people, emphasizing the international context in which these patterns emerged. In 1980 leaders of conservative alliances won elections that put them in control of governments in western Europe, Britain, Japan and the U.S. Neoclassical economic theory became dogma in the "conservative revolution." Their claim to authoritative wisdom rested upon the power embodied in the conservative alliance, and their social positioning in the institutions of international finance (IFIs). Their neutral-sounding technical calculus was similar to the dominant public health discourse of the period. It re-presented policies discredited in the late 1960s and 70s by extensive scholarly research on development. Their discourse masked the convergence of economic prescriptions with circles of power and interest. Firmly under the sway of large corporate interests, they made concerted assaults on the welfare state, "downsizing" government bureaucracies in the name of efficiency. They set about restructuring production systems in aid of increasing the share of the product accruing to capital and management, reducing labor's share and leaving many unemployed and the poor without a social safety net. De-industrialization and civil service shrinkage threw many out of work. At the same time that they imposed "fiscal discipline" on African governments, the IFIs in effect operated "bailouts" for private banks that had made bad loans and governments that insured the loans. Bilateral development lending was drastically reduced. The IFIs became African governments' most important source of foreign funds, and the "enforcer" of debt reimbursement. Much of Africa stagnated, while such growth as occurred failed to "trickle down" to ordinary people.

SAPs not only failed to remedy the deep causes of Africa's crises. They visited the brunt of austerity measures on the most vulnerable and powerless people. Successive currency devaluations and cheap food imports undermined the viability of rural peasant economies, prompting massive labor migration. Free trade led to de-industrialization that, coupled with downsized governments, worsened urban unemployment, degraded the condition of poor women, and left health systems to founder. Privatization of all public services became a dogma of SAPs. Support for primary health care was jettisoned. In severely affected countries, three decades of achievement in health – including longer life expectancies and reduced mortality among infants and young children – were annulled in the 1990s due to the mutually reinforcing effects of poverty and AIDS.

Health was no longer viewed as an entitlement, as a motor of development, or as a public good. Instead, discourse about health as a human right was relegated to the margins. The goal of "Health for all by the Year 2000" proclaimed in 1978 became an empty slogan. Two decades of "reforms" left more Africans poorer and less healthy than in the early years following independence. The gap between rich and poor widened not only within Africa, but between Africa and the West, and created a postmodern world that Professor Ida Susser calls a "new world *dis*order." As a result of these dislocations, of the social violence and civil wars to which they have given rise in many areas, vast numbers of people are at increased risk for HIV infection. Such economic and social factors, rather than hormones raging out of control or a special "African sexuality," explain why HIV spreads so rapidly on the continent.

Somewhat belatedly, the World Bank acknowledged AIDS as a key development issue, not simply a health problem; that is, AIDS is exerting a dramatic impact in sub-Saharan Africa by increasing poverty and reducing life expectancy and productivity (World Bank 1999). Yet a project paper by one Bank health analyst, who drew on a pre-publication copy of my *Canadian Journal* article, framed HIV/AIDS in these terms in 1988. The project proposed for Zaire was shelved (interview, Kinshasa, May 1988). The foremost proponent of SAPs is now the single largest lender for AIDS prevention efforts in Africa.

Zaire/Democratic Republic of Congo

The crisis in Zaire was among the earliest and most profound (see Nzongola-Ntaladja 2002). Renamed the Democratic Republic of Congo following Mobutu's ousting in 1997, the country continues to suffer the legacy of the Mobutu years. The everyday popular practices of survival strategies do not suffice to maintain health. Structural violence once more has turned into corporeal violence, as it has at different political junctures in the Congo's past. Resumption of the name of the first republic is thus far an empty promise, for DRC has yet to undergo a democratic transition. In the 1990s, while the Western powers criticized Mobutu for his corrupt administration, they refused to support the pro-democracy forces, and allowed political terrorism to prevail. In 1997, in the aftermath of genocide in Rwanda, as Zaire played host to armed perpetrators and their political leaders, Mobutu was overthrown. DRC remains riven by civil war and autocratic repression.

Government health services are weak or non-existent over much of the territory. Privatization had serious consequences for the quality of care provided to the approximately 30 percent (mainly in cities) who could obtain it. According to a joint WHO/UNICEF report:

Right now in Congo, the vast majority of the health and education services is a business in which struggling workers have to play off their family's survival against that of patients and pupils...Rational treatment and prescribing are abandoned where giving fewer drugs or more appropriate drugs can be detrimental to [the health worker's] income. (cited WHO 2001)

Actually, the situation described in this report has been ongoing since the mid-1980s; it was exacerbated with SAPs and the neglect of public health. The general features of social decay are compounded in eastern DRC, where the grinding poverty of the Mobutu era, and conflict over land, has been made even more desperate by six years of civil wars. Armed men terrorize a broad swath of eastern Congo, the site of "Africa's First World War." The pursuit of genocide terrorists by Rwanda has turned into general anarchy. Leaders of armed men from eight other countries, some quite distant, seek to get rich from the DRC's mineral wealth (see *Review of African Political Economy*, Nos. 93–94, 2002). Gender violence, including rape and mutilation by armed gangs, and increasingly by neighbors, as well, is sure to increase the numbers of the infected, as it has wherever rape is used as a weapon of war (Brittain 2002). Withdrawal of Rwanda's army leaves the field to local gangs that continue the chaos. The poisoned legacy of the Mobutu era constitutes an enormous challenge.

This bleak economic and political picture does not mean that nothing can be done. Infection prevalence has declined in several countries, and in specific populations, over the past five years. There are also some indications of reduced incidence of new infections. These successes have occurred despite extremely harsh conditions. Where peace prevails, it may be possible to use primary health care (PHC) organization as a focal point for democratic change, as was intended in the early 1980s by social medicine proponents who framed the 1978 Alma Ata Declaration. Social mobilization is crucial both for health maintenance and for behavior change. Gender and power issues will have to be addressed, and ways found to circumvent cultural constraints.

Conclusion

Just as the international health institutions avoided and delayed recognition of the social causes of AIDS, so the international financial institutions avoided and delayed recognition of the effects of policy reforms on poverty. While AIDS, corruption, and civil war appear to be internal African problems, the power wielded by the IFIs, Western governments, and transnational corporations over African governments, economies, and peoples remains decisive. Economic recovery depends upon transformation of the enduring legacy of distorted production and power structures that keep Africa a supplier of cheap raw materials. Recovery from AIDS depends upon reconstituting public health systems to treat classic sexually transmitted infections and distribute condoms, to find and treat tuberculosis, to deliver and monitor antiretroviral drugs. Making health services available is crucial, but not sufficient. Prevention also depends on changing moral and material constructions of gender relations that impede recognition of risk and responsibility. At some levels gender relations are subject to negotiation, but women's efforts to improve their condition take place in circumstances not of their own making. Poverty, violence, and pervasive gender inequality continue to make it especially difficult for women and girls to avoid unsafe sex. Change can be preceded and supported by imaginative mass media communications, but community-based problem solving in high-prevalence areas is crucial to reduce stigma and enable effective prevention and treatment.

In DRC and in many other countries, health systems, education, and social services must be rebuilt from the ground up. The challenge is to institute successful prevention methods on a national scale in quantities matched to need, without deadening people's creativity in the bureaucratic process and without becoming mired in corruption. A recent study commissioned by WHO estimates that it will take $25 billion annually to support health systems that can rid the world's poor of major diseases, including HIV/AIDS, tuberculosis, and malaria, and to render motherhood safe (Sachs 2001). Those resources must come from outside. While it may sound like a huge sum, it pales in comparison with the resources currently devoted to war. Despite pledges of support for the fight against AIDS, Africa's debt and international donors' reluctance continue to impede effective response. AIDS control cannot be done on the cheap.

AUTHOR'S NOTE

Many citations to the comparative literature have been omitted. They can be found in earlier cited publications. Initial funding for this research was provided by my family. In 1987 the Rockefeller Foundation's Health Sciences Division awarded a three-year grant that allowed us to expand the work. Additional funds came from small grants from OXFAM/UK, the Wenner Gren Foundation, and IAME-NEH in 1988, and the Bunting Institute of Radcliffe College in 1989.

NOTES

1. Founding members of CONNAISSIDA were Professor Pascal Ntsomo Payanzo, sociologist; Dr. Alphonse wa Nkera Rurarangira, public health specialist; and Mme. (now Dr.) Veronique Engundu Walu, medical and economic anthropologist. The project was back-stopped in the U.S. by Claude Schoepf, an agricultural economist.
2. These include ethnographic studies using participant-observation of household economics and family life by Walu and myself. In 1987 Dr. Walu recorded 18 month-long women's budgets in a World Bank sponsored project (Schoepf and Walu 1991; Schoepf, Walu, Russell and Schoepf 1991). Dr. Rukarangira conducted participant-observation in the informal economy and cross-border trade in southeastern Katanga between 1983 and 1987, under my direction. The final month of his research was funded by the World Bank (Rukarangira and Schoepf 1991). I also collected life histories of women in Lubumbashi and Kinshasa between 1975 and 1990 with the aid of Dr. Walu and the late Mmes. Beatrice Hateyana Makyla, Bernadette Nsengimana, and Noella M'Nkulira Ngirabakunzi.
3. Professor Payanzo contributed his extensive knowledge of Kinshasa, its civil society and national politics. He was President of Kinshasa Region's parliamentary caucus in the National Legislative Council from 1984 to 1987. In 1989–90 he was consultant to the USAID-funded Social Marketing Project, and in 1991 became Minister for Higher Education and Scientific Research. At that time it would have been possible to restart CONNAISSIDA, but I was chary of the violence in Kinshasa, and unwilling to continue dealing with the Mobutu regime. At the time, Drs. Rukarangira and Walu were abroad, the former as a consultant to WHO, the latter pursuing graduate studies. At present, Professor Payanzo teaches sociology at the University of Kinshasa, and once more serves as a consultant to PSI. He is seeking funds to reestablish Projet CONNAISSIDA.
4. For descriptions of CONNAISSIDA's action research, see Schoepf, Walu, Rukarangira et al. 1991; Schoepf 1993, 1995.
5. The Zaire Department of Health officially closed the CONNAISSIDA Project in April 1987, despite its evident success. Thus we were unable to benefit from international funds. Research continued with the tacit approval of the Ministry for Higher Education and Scientific Research.

The Coordinator of the National AIDS Control Program later offered to have CONNAISSIDA hold workshops for government leaders and businessmen instead of poor and working-class people. He was killed shortly thereafter, allegedly murdered because, as a protégé of the late Dr. Jonnathan Mann, founding Director of the WHO Global Program on AIDS, he had tried to keep a firm hand on the purse-strings.
6. Dr. Joseph Foumbi, UNICEF's AIDS coordinator for Africa, personal communication, December 1991.
7. Public lecture at the Radcliffe Institute, Harvard University, Cambridge, MA, April 24, 2002.
8. CONNAISSIDA's exclusion was systematic. Despite encouraging letters from Dr. Mann and his collaborators from 1996, I was told privately by a Tanzanian sociologist, who had spent time in Geneva at the WHO/GPA, that there was no way CONNAISSIDA would get funds, for our perspective was considered "too radical" (Professor Eustace Muhondwa, pers. comm. February 1988). In 1988, Dr. Rukarangira and I presented a paper on the action-research at a conference on AIDS education in Mexico. The editor of a WHO-supported newsletter asked to publish it as an example of a successful intervention. Two years later, we received word that Dr. Mann had rejected the paper on the grounds that since not every woman had been able to convince her husband, or all her clients, to use condoms, it was not a "success story."

The organizer of a conference sponsored by two leading foundations and held in my home town initially failed to invite me. When I pointed out how odd that would look, a collaborator prevailed upon the organizer to admit me to the first (public) session. This professor neglected to mention in his Department's yearly activities' roster the talk on women and AIDS that I had presented in his department.

9. Response to a question posed by the author following his Harvard lecture on "AIDS and Human Rights," Department of Social Medicine, April 1996.

10. The stigmatizing depiction of sex workers is not limited to central Africa. It is found among many people in Europe, Africa, Latin America, Asia, the Caribbean, and the United States.

11. Adapted from a poster published by the Ethiopian national campaign.

12. Financed by OXFAM/UK, the leaflet, written in French, was first distributed to government officials. Later that year, OXFAM passed on a request to Dr. Rukarangira to write a series of brochures for the Catholic Diocese of Kinshasa. These were the first public information made generally available in Kinshasa, where seroprevalence had already reached 6 percent of adults in 1985.

13. Meaning "insufficient salaries for many years."

14. B. G. Schoepf, interviews, Abidjan, May 1997; Professor Seri Dedy, personal communication, June 1997. See Schoepf 1986, 1991b.

Chapter 2

Politics, Culture, and Medicine: An Unholy Trinity? Historical Continuities and Ruptures in the HIV/AIDS Story in Malawi

John Lloyd Lwanda

Balala! balala! (Scatter! Scatter!)
Mabvuto mbuyomo! (Trouble follows behind!)
Tiyeni tithawe! (Let us all run away!)[1]

Introduction

The relationship between culture, social medicine, and politics in Malawi and Africa has been noted (Baker 1975; Feierman and Janzen 1992; Lwanda 1993; Mitchell 1952; K. Phiri 1998; Schoffeleers 1997; Vaughan 1991). Some (Chavunduka 1973; Hours 1986; Ciekawy and Geschieri 1998) view traditional medicine in terms of power – socially healing, cohesive, accumulative, or destructive. Traditional medicine and allied cultural practices emerge as important pillars supporting various socially cohesive constructs. I argue that these constructs, inherited from precolonial traditions, continue to inform indigenous attitudes to Western medicine, particularly in the case of HIV/AIDS. This chapter, using some markers, reflects on traditional medicine's historical ability to treat and "prevent," in the broad sense, illness, and takes a more robust and holistic view of traditional beliefs and medicine. Traditional medicine had, and has, purely medical [and surgical] function[s] independent of the social dimensions (Johnston 1897:439–452; Msonthi 1982:81–85; Roles 1966:570–594; Werner 1906:80–81). The markers include: malaria (*malungo*), a "classical disease" (Karlen 1995); rheumatism (*Nyamakazi*), a symptom of musculoskeletal disease;[2] fortification against disease, failure, or enemies (*kukwima*), a preventive power act; witchcraft (*ufiti*); and HIV/AIDS (*Edzi*), a disease new to both traditions.

A Brief Precolonial Cultural and Political History of Malawi

A southern African Bantu cultural context is supported by historical, linguistic, and archaeological work (cf. Guthrie 1967–71). The Maravi (Malawi) – Mang'anja, Chewa, Nyanja, Lomwe, Yao, etc. – share oral historical traditions, linguistic and settlement patterns, and some cultural practices (Mitchell 1956; K. Phiri 1983; Schoffeleers and Roscoe 1985) show similarities. In this context, I include the Yao in the Maravi group. Cultural similarities with the Ngoni (Thompson 1995) are also noted.

Given their successively hunter-gatherer, nomadic, pastoral, and agricultural lifestyles, we can argue that the precolonial political, social, and medical culture of the Maravi was significantly affected by the question of land (Pachai 1975). The possession of adequate un-contested land tended to contribute to ad-equate food, better health, and stability. The "ownership" of land (*mwini wa dziko*), as now, was vested in the religious and/or secu-lar head of the community, a communal rather than individualistic ownership. Religious and cosmological ideas pertained to the rituals of harvesting, planting, births, puberty, deaths, prayers for rain, etc., reflecting their depend-ence on nature. Inevitably, religious authority, held by mediums and practitioners, became intimately connected to the political author-ity it legitimized (Amanze 1982:37–50; Gaga 1982:61–63; Schoffeleers 1979:1–46). This intim-acy shaped the evolution of complex socially formative and normative constructs, myths, beliefs, rituals, and taboos integrating reli-gious, economic, political, and cultural elem-ents.

The Maravi believed in the High God (*Chauta*) worshipped through territorial cults, spirit (ancestral) worship, and witchcraft (McCracken 1977:13–14; Thompson 1995), and disease causality theories mirrored this reli-gious trichotomy. They had a comprehensive medical service and were aware of diseases not caused by witchcraft (Feierman and Janzen 1992:214–215; Morris 1985:34–35). Early colo-nial writers also noted, sometimes favorably, "the ability to effect" preventive "fortifica-tion" (*kukwima*). Thus precolonial Malawi had the ability to recognize and treat malaria (*mal-ungo*), as the "fever," and rheumatism (*nyama-kazi*) (M. King and E. King 1992:6).

Perhaps for reasons of ethnocentrism, sor-cery and witchcraft discourses dominated co-lonial literature (cf. Parrinder 1956:142–150) as negative forces that led to "antisocial, nefari-ous acts." The "positive" and "socially con-structive" aspect of "sorcery" (i.e., controlling mechanisms, via taboos) in pre-industrial soci-eties was largely ignored. Yet comparisons to modern governmental constructs, taboos, se-crecy, and control should be made. A case for

a pre-Foucault (1977) communal "panopticism and disciplinary power" to aspects of sorcery and witchcraft can be made by replacing "abil-ity to observe" with "ability to deter." Pre-colonial witchcraft practices can be viewed as originating from socially positive taboos and medical practices that became corrupted. Bongmba (1998:165–191) offers a useful her-meneutic of Wimbum *Tfu* (a "witchcraft" prac-tice that can be negative or positive), using power, economic and religious discourse (cf. Ciekawy and Geschieri 1998). Given the "cor-ruptibility" of all three, we favor the concept of a negative practice arising from an original positive one.

Public health control was achieved by appeals to territorial spirits, witchcraft, and sorcery, enforcing public taboos and medical measures like variolation for smallpox (Waite 1992:215). To this can be added the formative rituals, music, and dances.

Taboos were important in sexual health. The concept of *Tsempho* or *mdulo* diseases, caused by transgressing various sexual taboos via promiscuity, infidelity, or sexual relations at prohibited or "hot" times, is common in Mar-avi societies (Drake 1976). The prevention was clearly fidelity. Contagious illnesses, like lep-rosy, associated with "heat" were likely to "infect" and heat others. The leprosy skin manifestations (neuropathic ulcers, swollen tissues) signified "heat." This "heat" resonates with the AIDS manifestations of shingles, skin ulcers, and tumors.

The Maravi concept of disease prevention was, therefore, a mixture of morality, social and political engineering, and religion – con-sistent with Hughes' (1963:157) definition of public health as all illness that affects the public as well as all activity that the public under-takes to influence its health status. Given that "public health is the meeting ground between politics and medicine" (Waite 1992:213), it is the power and authority of this construct in dealing with epidemics and social order that interests us. Thus smallpox outbreaks in precolonial Kenya could be caused by social reactions to famine: "raiding, trading, migration, disrup-tion of preventive variolation and the disrup-tion of the traditional ceremonies to drive away epidemics" (Dawson 1992:93–97). A simi-lar reaction was seen among the Maravi. The traditional song quoted at the beginning of this chapter has echoes of this.

To prevent *balala! balala!* (Scatter! Scatter!), authorities had to prevent or control epidemics. Significantly, in 1992 the (U.S.) National Institute of Medicine identified six similar major causes of disease emergence as: "*Breakdown of public health measures*, economic development and *land use*, international *travel and trade*, technology and industry, *human demographics* and *behaviour*" (Karlen 1995:217–218), and microbial adaptation and change.

We note, therefore, that precolonial Malawi societies had measures for combating epidemics like smallpox, rituals for leprosy, and measures to combat famine (migration). They also had medical practices to cope with "every ill likely to befall mankind"; and used fortification (*kukwima*) as a preventive measure and "witchcraft practices" (*ufiti*) both positively, as taboos, and negatively in corrupted forms. Of greater relevance here is the fact that they had taboos, like *mdulo* and *tsempho*, for preventing sexually transmitted diseases. We have also noted the intimate connection between public health, political governance, and religious activity.

A Survey of the Sociocultural Colonial History of Malawi

The colonial phase is dominated by the impact of Christianity and European culture on, and the resistance of, the indigenous cultures. For example, compared to Christianity, Islam achieved "easier" syncresis with Yao traditions (Alpers 1972:169–175; Bone 1982:126–138; Msiska 1995:49–86). Islamic and Yao funeral rites syncretized to produce *sadaka*, as did Islamic and Yao *lupanda* and *chiputu* rites of passage to produce the *unyago* (initiation) customs of *jando* (boys) and *nsondo* (girls).

In the context of the HIV/AIDS debate, these cherished localized *unyago* rites are of relevance. When Yao chiefs succumbed to colonialism, their communities split into smaller units (Mitchell 1956:2) or localities from where they resisted "Christian cultural colonialism" until after 1945, by refusing "Christian education," for example. Small village units were crucial in resisting cultural change among the Maravi too.

Missionaries and settlers followed Livingstone's arrival in 1859, and a British Protectorate was declared in 1891 (A. Ross 1996:13–16). African opposition was overcome by persuasion or force (Pachai 1973:57). The settlers appropriated the best land for agricultural estates, using African labor, some of it under *thangata* (indentured labor) conditions (Kandawire 1979).

Compounding the loss of land was the loss of African independent status and, in the case of the estates, village/area units. Here the cultural restrictions were resisted; daytime village culture, suppressed by hard work and governance, reasserted itself at night. These constraints placed on traditional medical and cultural practices, given their social construction role, were, in effect, attacks on the very basis of Maravi culture. The removal of the legitimacy of land – hence economic power – from the chiefs threatened the precolonial "preventive medicine" structures and upset local order. The "guardians of the land" maintained their legitimacy by becoming protectors of culture, reflected in the intense conflict with colonialists. These early, rural-led, anti-colonial resistances were for land and cultural rights (Linden and Linden 1974; McCracken 1977).

Conflict between Western medicine and the indigenous culture was also colored by racism predicated by European "Darwinian assumptions" (Vaughan 1991:33). European "individualism" and culture equated with "civilization," ignoring African concepts of *umuntu* (Musopole 1996:27).[3] Traditional medicine and cultural practices became significant parts of the resistance to colonialism and, later, to the postcolonial hegemony. This resistance in village localities, we argue, persists and promotes the survival of traditional medicine. Given the colonial hegemony over land, borders, travel, etc., which reduced the ability of the traditional authorities to respond coherently over large areas to the colonial insults, responses became located, and continue to thrive, within village or area localities. (Colonial borders prevented traditional responses to political and socio-economic rupture – migration to new pastures. Possible colonial migration – labor – caused gender and other social tensions.) Since then, the memorialized social experiences/responses to invasion or cultural challenge could only be used from localized fragmented bases. Some of the similarly localized resistance to Western medicine erupts occasionally in regional or national *"mchape"* episodes or coded political resistance.[4]

For the colonialists, smallpox, meningitis, plague, and sleeping sickness posed a constant threat to the economic (and political) viability of the early colonial state (Vaughan 1991). It responded by spending more on European health, at the expense of the Africans: Western medicine became, and remains, *mankhwala achizungu* (European medicine), a phrase laden with racial and class overtones. The discourse from this era of *mankhwala achizungu* (European medicine) and *mankhwala achikuda* (African medicine) or *mtela wachiboyi* (servants' medicine) is still current. Where Africans could access Western medicine the standards were often so bad that "Africans of the better type [sic] flatly refused to enter the hospital" (Thomas 1930).

Unlike Shaw's (1995:1–27) Kenya, minimal "colonial hybridity" resulted in Malawi; the colonial governance was paternalistic, intended to "objectify and subjectify" (Fanon 1970:59–99) the colonized. Colonial responses to epidemics were more "governance" than "medical," using smallpox police to enforce vaccination – eliciting resistance, "evasion [and] concealment" of cases (Bevan-Pritchard 1930). Lepers were isolated (King and King 1992:81). These public health campaigns "pathologized," "objectified," and alienated Africans. Associated "Christian" discourse regarded African beliefs and practices as "ignorant" and immoral (Vaughan 1991:52).

I argue that, in rural and peri-urban areas, given the cultural segregation (McCracken 1998:247–269), the conflict between Christianity and Western medicine on one hand and African Traditional Religion (ATR) and traditional medicine on the other was resolved by the development or adoption of cultural dualities rather than hybridities or cultural subjugation. Many core cultural beliefs, now embedded in village localities, were not significantly challenged by colonial or Christian assaults; they had been placed out of the colonial gaze. This invisibility often gave the impression of, and

was mistaken for, indigenous practices dying out under the overwhelming and inhibitory nature of colonial governance. Dualism enabled many Maravi to survive colonialism without experiencing "dissolution or fragmentation" (Fanon 1970:7 and 77),[5] a more common experience among the educated elite who, unlike the more culturally secure villagers, had to confront the cultural dichotomy head-on.

The nationalist struggles from c. 1912 through to 1964 could be viewed against this background. Some educated Africans, many Christian, were not necessarily in favor of a return to African traditional beliefs and practices; they were after economic and political power (Shepperson and Price 1958; Rotberg 1966). Some nationalist politicians wanted to reduce the power of the chiefs further, in the interests of "modernity" (Chisiza 1961), a conflict that remains unresolved. Postcolonially, politicians still recognize chiefs as guardians of the land (Kishindo 1994:57–66), a recognition tinged with envy. The educated nationalist elite mobilized rural masses, playing to the latter's cultural, economic, and political expectations, but without conceding a postcolonial "cultural renaissance."[6] The "elites" used class, just as the whites had used race before them.

Comaroff's (1983) contention that biomedicine's epistemology is [to an extent] a "cultural construct" has some resonances with how politicians, colonial or postcolonial, view traditional and orthodox medicine, particularly when she argues that in time of illness our helplessness leads to loss of control and alienation (1983:57). This submission to helplessness, which can be politically or otherwise exploited, is a universal phenomenon, found in European welfare states and Malawi extended family contexts.

This helplessness needs salvation, in the form of the cultural constructs of traditional medicine and the extended family in Malawi and the welfare/health systems in Europe. Both are political and economic. Seen in this light, European attempts at re-culturing Africans and postcolonial promises, "renaissance" or otherwise, both without alternative and adequate social welfare and economic provisions, are relevant and promoted disharmony. The colonial environment was not conducive to critical debates about cultural dichotomies. Intercultural conflict produces persistent tension, subjugation, or compromise in the form of hybridity or duality. The coexistence of, and acceptance of, Western medicine should not be seen as its conquest over traditional medicine (cf. Peltzer 1986). Vaccination campaigns, often seen as Western medical successes, may succeed not because "Western medicine has conquered" but merely because it "replaced" previous variolation. And, if yaws and leprosy treatments in the 1920s brought the "injection" culture to Malawi, penicillin (for syphilis) consolidated it. Injections were later to contribute to the spread of HIV. Yet even the magic and potency of *jekisoni* (injection) could not abolish the duality (Feierman et al. 1992:268); Africans, after all, had their own potent scarification culture.

We would submit that from the colonial experience arose some hybridity and considerable duality, leaving significant parts of Maravi and Yao traditional medical culture unscathed (cf. Chanock 1972:429–441). Given the postcolonial issues of class, the urban versus rural dichotomy, and "neo-colonization via globalization," this continuing resistance is relevant to the HIV/AIDS discourse (Lwanda 1999). This is particularly true where traditional medicine provides the bulk of services to the majority of the population.

Aspects of Colonial Western Medicine, Education and Traditional Culture in Malawi

We have already noted African resistance to Western culture and (rationed) medicine. Western medical repression is revealed by "the concerns of the state and the ruling class in society, both with their own safety and with the reproduction of the labor force" (Kandawire 1979; Lwanda 1996:19–37). Until the early 1920s, the medical service was designed primarily to care for government officials (Baker 1975:301). Even after 1945, available resources were not applied universally, despite African protests; most Africans continued to rely on traditional medicine (Ndibwani et al. 1998). A number of factors were responsible. First, many of the qualified medical staff were devoted to the "care of the small and scattered European population"

(Baker 1975:301), a self-preservation imperative partly arising from the initial failure to settle in the "malarious" territory (White 1989; A. Ross 1996). Second, racism contributed to "European-only" hospitals, which survived until 1972 (Mkandawire 1997). Third, preventive medicine was ignored (Baker 1975:301). Given its marginal utility, only some aspects of Western medicine's rituals of history taking, diagnosis, and treatment could be syncretized. Importantly, it lacked the *sing'anga's* psychosocial, communal, and religious elements. The colonial preventive medicine on show confirmed features of African causality in their hut destruction (smallpox) and isolation (leprosy). Fourth, many rural villagers were unable to access Western medical services and remained secure in their faith in traditional medicine. Fifth, primary education, in its Malawi setting, was/is dominated by traditional village culture. The introduction of universal primary education, in 1994, in the context of inadequate resources, has compounded this dynamic, making primary schools more "dependent" on village resources and culture. Sixth, racism and the favoring of "elite" African workers encouraged the *mankhwala achizungu/ achiboyi* (European and [African] traditional medicine) duality. Yet, despite its universal unavailability, Western medical agents and the state continued to attempt to abolish aspects of traditional medicine.

The postcolonial HIV/AIDS debates, which pathologized females, had colonial precedents.[7] Sexually transmitted diseases (STDs) were noted, "among both Europeans and Africans," to be a "problem" from 1896. The arena of STDs generated a multifaceted conflict involving gender (male chauvinism), tradition, Christianity, and European concepts of African sexuality that was to produce a longrunning debate, dominated by views, then current in Europe, about Africans' supposed "primitive, uncontrolled and excessive sexuality" (Vaughan 1991:19–23 and 129–154), variously blamed on African "primitive customs and sexuality" or the ravages of colonization and industrialization on Africans. However, both African traditionalists and colonialists saw African female sexuality as one of the main problems. Then, as now, traditionalists saw the loss of traditional control over women as contributing to their increased sexuality. During World War II the colonial authorities, aware of the recreational needs of their soldiers, treated African cases of STDs vigorously and with sympathy but blamed "prostitutes" for the diseases. Females were forcibly examined and treated. In the 1980s, women were forced to have HIV tests and in the 1990s prostitutes were arrested by the Muluzi administration.

Yet little in the role of ordinary rural women had, or has, changed (I. Phiri 1997). Traditional birth attendants, initiation rite organizers, and other key females resiliently guard traditional practices during periods of rapid change (cf. Kamwendo and Kamowa 1999:165–175). I argue that these traditions are guarded assiduously by women as (i) gender power roles and (ii) defensive mechanisms against forces of change and male gender. This dynamic affecting women continues, firmly rooted in localities. It partly explains the persistence of some traditions, for example initiation rites, which, while empowering specific women, are hazardous to women in general.

Arguably, while appropriating some accessible, useful, and colorful aspects of Western medicine, addressing new threats and diseases and spawning peripheral hybridities in the process, traditional medicine, at its core, did not change fundamentally during the colonial period. And colonialism can be viewed as a brief, if significant, assault on some indigenous cultures (Falola 1996).

Postcolonial Ambiguities

The postcolonial phase is dominated by the ambiguous figure of Dr. Banda (Lwanda 1993; Mphande 1996). By 1961, once the Christian Democratic Party (CDP) with its sizeable rural Catholic constituency was obliterated, Malawi was, effectively, a one-party state (Short 1974). The CDP was potentially an independent politico-religious power with rural penetration which – unlike the more co-optable Protestant urban elites – was an obstacle to the cultural hegemony Banda desired. Next, the 1964 Cabinet Crisis (CC) pitted the "elderly, conservative Banda, with rural support," against the ideological, younger ministers; an unequal conflict between a Chewa imperial "messiah" and an ill-defined concept of modernity. Banda

won. Two aspects of the CC are relevant here. First, realizing Malawi's poverty, Banda continued the colonial rural medical neglect and promoted better (or private) medicine for elites (cf. Short 1974). Second, his culture of dictatorship drove discussions of contentious medical, cultural, or political matters underground, perpetuating the "political duality" of the colonial era and bringing corrupted "village culture" and preventive taboos to the national stage.[8] Culture was his "legitimizing tool" (Lwanda 1993; Forster 1994). His "creation myths" included the attribution of his plans and achievements to his "Gwelo [colonial prison] dreams" in line with African traditional religion and medicine (Chimombo 1989). Coincidentally, *Gwelo* in Chewa means "source"! To survive politically in this "taboo-laden" regime, many "otherwise Christian or Muslim" politicians "justifiably" resorted to *kukwima*. Banda, the *bwana mkubwa* (governor-general), allegedly "built more prisons than hospitals" (Mapanje, pers. comm. 1993) and, like the colonialists, did not encourage African Western-trained doctors. By 1992, only 25 out of 175 sent for medical training had returned (King and King 1992). Clinical officers delivered the bulk of Western medical services.

Banda's cultural ambiguity contributed to the resurgence of postcolonial traditional medicine. It marginalized African medical doctors and privileged a "localized" traditional medicine which avoided direct engagement/confrontation with his regime, perpetuating the cultural duality and neglect of rural health needs. Concepts of *mankhwala achizungu/achiboyi* persisted. Later, only *achikulire* (the elites) could afford expensive anti-HIV/AIDS drugs. Interestingly, Kamuzu Academy, Banda's educational legacy, where students were "crammed with Latin, Ancient Greek [...and] you will not spot a single black teacher" (McGreal 1992), provides many College of Medicine (COM) students, begging the question as to how the COM graduates will handle the cultural dichotomy. That some drank *mchape* in 1995 (written personal communication 1995) indicates desperation or an established duality.

In the ambiguous cultural climate sketched above, the new disease HIV/AIDS arrived and found the epidemic control measures, both traditional and biomedical, wanting. In "puritanical" Malawi, discussions of sex were taboo, although sex, with discretion, was one of the few forms of politically *safe* entertainments in urban areas (Mapanje 1981).

The History of HIV/AIDS in Malawi

If the origins of HIV/AIDS are still mysterious (Karlen 1995), its arrival in Malawi via the international road trade routes from the east–west (Zaire/Kenya) and east–south (Kenya/South Africa) networks could be mapped out (Orubuloye et al. 1994) – if we accept the Zaire/Uganda African entry point. The 2 percent prevalence rate among antenatal patients at Queen Elizabeth Hospital in 1985 (Taha et al. 1998) and the work of L'Herminez et al. (1992) suggest that HIV may have arrived in Malawi around 1977. Oral Malawi discourses state that "HIV/AIDS is new" to Malawi: *kwabwela Edzi* (AIDS has arrived). A phenomenological observation of *imfa kuthamanga* (increase in [unexplained] deaths) occurred among urban young Malawians in the early 1980s. The first hospital cases of HIV/AIDS, described in 1985 (Cheesbrough 1986), followed an increased incidence of Kaposi's sarcoma, an HIV-associated skin cancer. An early high-profile HIV/AIDS case involved a beauty queen deemed "presumably infected abroad" (Wangel 1995:22). The phenomenological observations were later to be confirmed by rising HIV-positive rates at Blantyre antenatal clinics: 2.0 percent (1985), 8.2 percent (1987), 18.6 percent (1989) (Taha et al. 1998). In the rural areas a similar *kuthamanga* of deaths, usually following a "slimming disease," had been noted, and initially blamed on *tsempho* or *mdulo* illnesses (Kumpolota, oral interview July 18, 2000).

As elsewhere, HIV/AIDS was initially blamed on "high risk" groups. The Malawi elite resorted to traditional culture, actual or remembered: in precolonial Maravi culture "adultery was the fault most severely punished" (Stannus 1910:299). Malawians claimed that AIDS was an "American" family planning plot. Family planning was anathema to both Banda and traditional male culture (Malawi National Family Planning Strategy [NFPS] 1994:2–4). HIV arrived at a time when Banda's

"peaceful state" could not accommodate dissent, even by a disease. Public sexual prudery, with strict censorship and dress codes, contrasted with the MCP culture's female sexual exploitation (Mkamanga 2000) which contributed to the spread of HIV. For different reasons, both traditional and Western medical spheres delayed in responding to the epidemic. Public health officials sent out signals which ignored realities, for example, cultural attitudes and the cost of condoms; by 1997 only 21 percent of females had ever used condoms (Namate and Kornfield 1997). Using Western HIV prevention strategies insured that condoms rapidly became linked to "the deprivation of pleasure," forced family planning, Western values, and, paradoxically, promiscuity.

Traditional practitioners in Malawi lacked the (precolonial) ability, from their localized bases, to observe the magnitude and extent of the HIV epidemic; like the scientists, they required time to understand the epidemic. As the young, educated, potential wage earners died, jealousy and witchcraft were often cited. Both traditional and Western medicine had noted that women succumbed at much younger ages (personal observations 1985–95). Research later confirmed that 85 percent of AIDS patients between the ages of 15 and 19 were female; beyond the age of 30 "men predominate" (King and King 1992:163).

One of the first national responses was choosing a local name for AIDS. Traditionally, STDs have encompassing communal aspects, mirroring the "inherent" transgressive element of some sexual activity, thus *mdulo* diseases (Drake 1976). The name chosen, *Edzi*, an onomatopoeic Chewaizing of "AIDS," ignored traditional health promotion concepts. *Magawagawa* ("something shared") (Moyo 1986) and *chiwerewere* (promiscuity) had briefly been popular and invoked "communicability via promiscuity." However, Western-trained health workers lost the opportunity to communicate with their rural compatriots by merely translating AIDS onomatopoeically, as is commonly done with foreign words, perpetuating the "non-communicative" cultural duality. The HIV virus became *kachirombo ka Edzi* (the wee AIDS beast). In Malawi, concepts of the causality of AIDS meant that AIDS was now, unwittingly, a "curable disease": remove the

wee beast (however originated) and the disease
is cured! While the germ theory is significantly
recognized, the singular *kachirombo* encouraged
some patients and traditional doctors to believe
in the "curative removability" of *kachirombo*, a
belief still current (Lwanda 2000). The continued minority use of *chiwerewere* suggests an
understanding of the STD nature of HIV.

Contextually, the choice of (the meaningless) *Edzi*, the vague epidemiological and treatment options, the family planning suspicions,
and the "omnipotent" Banda government's
repeated "there is no HIV cure" led to HIV/
AIDS being named the "government disease"
(*matenda a boma*) (Kanjo 2000, pers. comm.).
This concept persists and recalls the earlier
"superior European" medicine *mankhwala
achizungu* debates: "How can there be no
cure [from the superior European medicine/
government?] This is a family planning
plot!" (Kanjo 2000, pers. comm; cf. Schoffeleers
1999).

The association between shingles and AIDS
was another feature that lent itself to the traditional causality theory. The phenomenological
establishment of an association between the
heralding shingles, the "slimming phase,"
and deterioration into death quickly evoked
sorcery: some who got shingles did not die.
But there was a socio-economic issue here. In
1994, the period between shingles and "terminal" AIDS varied from a few months to ten
years depending on nutritional status and
other variables. Those likely to die early were
the HIV-positive youth with poor nutritional
or "healthy lifestyle" prospects! Obesity, "as
of old," became a sign of good health and
"slimness" indicative of disease. Shingles,
with its "hot" blisters, became the harbinger
of AIDS, a time to seek medical help. As Western medicine was palliative, many resorted to
traditional medicine. Shingles, though resonat-
ing with leprosy in its "heat," did not, in rural
areas, fan the HIV "segregationist" discourse
of urban areas, perhaps suggesting that HIV/
AIDS taboos were yet to emerge. As with leprosy, in life HIV/AIDS victims received good
community care.

Between 1985 and 1993, medical discourse
emphasized the mystery of, and lack of cure
for, HIV/AIDS (*MNACP Manual* 1989) and a
strong religious lobby considered "immoral-

ity" and God's resultant "wrath" responsible
for the epidemic (Catholic Church 1991). Some
Christians, although decrying HIV promoting
cultural practices, approved "conservative" or
formative aspects of African Traditional Religion (ATR) (Catholic Church:51–53).

The finding of a 2 percent HIV-positive rate
among 200 pregnant women in a May/June
1985 USAID-funded survey (Chiphangwi et
al. 1988) galvanized health workers and
donors, culminating in October 1985 in a committee to "ensure that blood for transfusion
was safe." Soon there were HIV screening facilities at Queen Elizabeth Hospital (December
1985) and Lilongwe Central Hospital (February 1986), funded by German aid. The
Germans' generosity ensured that HIV seropositivity figures came out of Malawi, and these
justified donor HIV funding (Wangel 1995:24).

This funding enabled the establishment of a
National AIDS Secretariat responsible to
Hetherwick Ntaba, the permanent secretary
for the Ministry of Health (MOH) and Banda's
personal physician. Ntaba approved all Malawian staff at the Secretariat and at WHO's
regional office, ensuring that all Secretariat activities were visible to the Office of the President. Yet it took until 1987 before the MOH
formulated the first national AIDS campaign
program and four years before the National
AIDS Committee (NAC) was set up in 1989.

The NAC was handicapped from the start;
Ntaba and his superiors controlled and politicized decision making. Local staff, politically
excluded and denied access to donor funds,
were reluctant to input ideas (cf. Liomba, in
Wangel 1995:26).[9] AIDS research was not encouraged and expatriate researchers only fared
better when the "statistics for funding" imperative intervened. This imperative sub-
verted the government's apathy, as did the
deaths from AIDS of civil servants and politicians between 1985 and 1988, the Malawi
Army's Mozambique involvement, the German
test results, the WHO/donors' impetus, the
increased HIV/AIDS burden on hospitals, the
political impact of the escalating rural funerals,
and, as in colonial times, the ruling elite's self-
interest, including the paranoia about Banda
being exposed to HIV by his servants.

The NAC was not, initially, a vibrant body.
The donors' (WHO, USAID, UNICEF, and

EEC) promises of funding forced a change of pace (Wangel 1995:27). The NAC's 1989–93 medium-term plan for the "prevention and control of AIDS in Malawi" (MOH 1988) was "the basis of requests to donors for assistance." The state and individuals realized that the HIV problem could be exploited to secure scarce foreign exchange for research and service provision. The diversion of fridges and video machines, intended for HIV work, from UNICEF to civil servants and MCP officials between 1988 and 1989 is a metaphor for this individual corruption of the HIV problem for personal gain (cf. *kuba mankhwala* – stealing medicine – taboo in Maravi culture). Further, the Malawi "seminar culture" ensured that local workers obtained better income through attendance at donor-funded seminars than through their own jobs.[10] At state level, money meant for AIDS work was sometimes diverted to national coffers to cover foreign exchange shortages. From 1988 the government abused donated test kits – commandeering an entire shipment in 1991 (Wangel 1995:30–32). The 2,000 "state house" staff were tested annually when there were insufficient kits for blood transfusion work in hospitals and the government was minimizing the AIDS problem. This was reminiscent of the colonial "Europeans-only hospitals" and good care for "elite" African workers.

Dr. Liomba's arrival raised the NAC's profile and some media discussion of HIV in Malawi ensued. His appointment coincided with the 1989–91 impetus for political and economic change. Family planning NGOs, like Banja la Mtsogolo (BLM), began to assume a higher profile, and government publications increased their coverage of HIV/AIDS. An exponential increase in research on HIV in Malawi is noticeable from 1988–9 (MOH 1991 and CSR 1999).

Meanwhile, the donor-initiated monitoring had shown rising HIV-positive rates: 21.9 percent (1990) and 31.6 percent in 1993. By 1993 some rural areas had HIV-positive rates of 12 percent (Chilongozi et al. 1996). Beginning in 1990, urban and rural surveys demonstrated that people "were generally aware of the AIDS problem but lacked specific knowledge of causation" (Kishindo 1990). Among school teenagers, only 67.1 percent could be graded as "moderately knowledgeable" (Msapato et al.

1990). Significantly, "prostitution," which is viewed as a "female occupation" in Malawi, was identified as the major "transmitter." Thus, the earlier female HIV/AIDS presentation and mortality and low female social status compounded the cultural stigmatization of women.

Some traditional practitioners, instinctively reacting – as all medical people do – to a new disease, either sought to "cure" the disease by removing *kachirombo* or resorted to witch finding, neo-taboo formulation, and other "marginal" activities. The more Western practitioners condemned these traditional approaches, the more biomedicine's own helplessness, at least from the rural perspectives, was exposed (personal observations 1994). In their "helplessness" both camps seemed to scapegoat culture.

Cultural Practices Usable in HIV/AIDS Prevention

In Malawi, the spread of HIV is largely via heterosexual sex. Many cultural forms normal to rural Malawians are considered problematic by "Westerners," yet many promote good health in the context of rural Malawi (Mwale 1977; Peltzer 1986). Despite the extensive polygamy discourse, monogamy dominates; only 20 percent of marriages are polygamous according to the Demographic Health Survey of 1992. Traditionalists argue that practices like *lobola* (bride price) ensured that extra- and premarital sexual practices were minimized, and men "valued" women. Initiation ceremonies like *chinamwali* and *nsondo* were "a healthy form of health promotion" and minimized premarital sexual experimentation. Elders "controlled society" and taboos "enforced" fidelity: *kutsekereza* could "ensure a spouse's fidelity" during one's absence! Taboos on illegitimate children minimized premarital sex; an unmarried girl in labor "could not deliver" unless she named the father!

Cultural Practices Conducive to the Spread of HIV

Initiation ceremonies have been the main targets of criticisms, blamed for promoting early sex between boys and girls and between men and young girls (Chaima 1994) and for early marriages and divorces (Chiwaya n.d.). Some initiation ceremonies involve a *fisi* (a man tasked with anonymously deflowering virgins). Women's weak societal position and practices that remove choice from them compound the problem. Men refusing to use condoms (Namate and Kornfield 1997) force women into unprotected sexual practices. The use of vaginal tighteners causes STD, facilitating vaginal injuries. Other macho cultural practices (Kamwendo et al. 1999; Tembo and Phiri 1993) privilege males. This male dominance extends to exposing powerful elite women to STDs through the sexual behavior of their menfolk, who have mistresses; thus "high socio-economic status is, in Malawi, a risk factor for HIV-1 infection" (Dallabetta et al. 1991).

Other practices that are considered normal can spread HIV by legitimizing high-risk behavior. These include: *nthena* (widower given wife's younger sister); *chokolo* (widow inherited by man's brother); *m'bvade* (unmarried female's postnatal abstinence is concluded by surrogate sex); the use of *fisi* (surrogate) in male infertility; and the belief that STDs, including HIV, can be prevented with charms and "vaccines."

The Role of Government

In failing to take note of these and many other cultural attitudes, beliefs, and social conditions conducive to the spread of HIV, both postcolonial (i.e., the Banda and Muluzi) administrations can be accused of negligence. At the very least, the social conditions of pervasive poverty dictated a reappraisal of the "condoms" approach. The Muluzi government's own Policy Analysis Initiative (PAI) in 1999 admitted that the rich/poor dichotomy, with an "inbuilt power" to abuse the already skewed gender balance, was not addressed.

If there was neglect by default, a case for the state's active "cultural" contribution to the spread of HIV/AIDS can be made, beginning with the failure to promote health education from 1963 onwards. Dr. Banda banned family planning until 1982, and then only allowed "child spacing," preceding the later "distaste" for condoms. By 1994 only 43 percent of the 756 state health facilities provided family

planning services, as did only 11 percent of the 1,169 Mother and Child outreach services. Inadequate finance and resources were blamed (NFPS 1994–1998 April 1994). The NFPS, informed by the high maternal and child morbidity rates, placed reduction of the "natural population growth rate" above "the reduction of communicable diseases." The half-hearted and under-resourced attempts to bring traditional birth attendants into the national system were not consolidated. The postcolonial failure to empower and utilize village health committees, as "democratic" "motivating factors" in mobilizing rural people in "social change" (Tembo and Phiri 1993), was to privilege the dominant hold of traditional medicine in villages.

Then there was the MCP culture of massive and frequent rallies, Banda's nationwide tours, independence celebrations, Youth Week, Mothers' Day Celebrations, Kamuzu Day, and other events. All involved bussing men and women to these venues where "women were sexually exploited by the MCP men" (Mkamanga 2000). The Banda regime can be faulted for its cynical neglect of duty of care; even though "20–40% of all in-patients had HIV related illnesses" (Lwanda 1995), the government was still minimizing the problem, leaving the population dependent on inadequate hospital services and traditional practitioners. The first substantive AIDS promise from Dr. Banda's regime came just before the 1993 national referendum on democracy.

Two major events illustrate the state's "negligence." First was a 500-strong battalion of the Malawi Army, mostly single men replaced every six months, fighting in Mozambique between 1985 and 1993 in defense of the Nacala railway line. For "recreation" they visited sex workers in Malawi and Mozambique (Nkosi 1999). From 1990, many AIDS deaths occurred in army barracks. Yet until 1996, when some army personnel vandalized the *Daily Times* offices (for publishing this obvious fact), the subject of how the war in Mozambique spread HIV remained taboo.

Another HIV/AIDS story which brought the medico-cultural and socio-economic strands together was the decision by South Africa, in 1988, to repatriate existing Malawi migrant workers and stop recruiting more. TEBA (The

Employment Bureau of Africa) had been important to the economic life of Malawi. Many roadside small traders, shopkeepers, tailors, and bar owners were former migrant workers, and by rural standards they had high incomes. Thus they were favored by both prostitutes (in South Africa and Malawi) and poor women in Malawi, making them vectors and victims of HIV. When testing began in 1985 and 1986, the HIV-positive rate was highest in Malawian workers (Chirwa 1988), and the South Africans classed Malawi as a high-risk country. In February 1988, the repatriation of Malawian workers began, and finished within two years. This hurt Malawi's rural areas economically, highlighting Packard's analysis which saw AIDS, like TB, as being facilitated by the poverty, malnutrition, and other socio-economic disadvantages related to capitalism (1989). In colonial and post-colonial Malawi, migrant workers were an economic tool of the state, tolerated in health, but an embarrassment in adverse circumstances.

Donors can be blamed for colluding with the Malawi state. Foreign NGOs and some donors placed family planning highest on their priority list and did not want this, or their restricted research projects, jeopardized. They turned a blind eye to the state-house abuse of scarce HIV-testing reagents. The WHO regional and local officers were weak and deferred to Banda's "temperament" (King 2000:34–35), shelving their concerns in order not to upset the regime. The donors' promotion of "condoms and personal human rights" in a "communal culture" was "tantamount to counseling free idiosyncratic and irresponsible sexual choices in a communal culture," leaving people free to contract or spread HIV (King and King 2000:34).

By 1991 the HIV/AIDS health promotion discourse was still palliative. The Catholic bishops' challenge to Banda in 1992 (Lwanda 1993) cited health as one of the areas for inequality between rich and poor. Their critique of the Banda regime undermined one of its public health legitimizing constructs: a land of "milk and honey" (*mkaka ndi uchi*) where people were better fed, dressed, educated, and lived in "houses that did not leak when it rained." AIDS and its sequelae, including

worsening poverty and unequal provision of services, exposed this myth. Banda's fall interrupted the second NAC medium-term plan for the period 1993–8.

However, despite their earlier stance – and manifesto – the UDF's promises did not translate into immediate action. Apart from liberalizing research rules, there was insignificant government activity until 1999, when donors provided increased funding. Yet the UDF 1994 manifesto had set AIDS as a high priority. It had good reason, as by 1995 HIV/AIDS-related illnesses accounted for one-third of all admissions to hospital (Lwanda 1994) and the prevalence rate (Kaluwa et al. 1995) among pregnant women ranged from "5% in rural Thonje to 33% in Blantyre with a median rate of 16%." For most of 1994–5 there was a shortage of reagents for blood testing (personal observation 1995). Yet in the first two years of its administration, while emphasizing the alleviation of poverty, apart from one high-profile "HIV awareness walk" by Muluzi, there were no similar high-profile HIV public statements until after 1997. The HIV burden in the meantime was compounding rural poverty, leaving traditional practitioners to formulate their own solutions. The NAC suffered "planning and budgetary" problems, and by April 1995 the "unpaid" Liomba had resigned and returned to the university. The apathy, seminar culture, and "muddling through" started by MCP continued under UDF. Their health ministers missed the opportunity to mobilize youth through schools, the media, etc., as their manifesto had promised. The burden of work on HIV fell on NGOs; mission and state hospitals "blundered through" with few resources. Kakhongwe (1997) identified 73 international and local organizations dealing with HIV/AIDS, largely funded by Action-AID, ODA, UNDP, UNICEF, USAID, and WHO. The Malawi government's contribution was not quantified.

Despite his initial minimal action on AIDS, Muluzi also contributed to a resurgence of traditional medicine by maintaining a similar ambiguous stance. He actively promoted private Western medical provision, claiming that the government could not provide all the services, and his administration did not tighten trading standards legislation, leaving markets full of fake medicines and various neo-traditional practitioners (Lwanda 2000).

However, as with the previous regimes, it was self-interest that roused the Muluzi government from its apathy and forced it to admit that it had a "national problem." Between 1994 and 1998 the UDF lost over twenty of its MPs and senior activists, most, allegedly, to HIV/AIDS. The elites initially used scarce government money for treatment in South Africa. By 1995, South African clinics had adopted a policy of "HIV-positive patient repatriation," because few Malawians could afford the anti-retroviral therapy. Meanwhile, the 1999 Sentinel Survey report (National Aids Control Programme [NACP] 1999) concluded that the estimated crude national HIV prevalence rate was 8.8% (2.2% among the under 15s, 16.4% among the 15–49 age group and 1.1% for those over 50). Among pregnant women, rates varied from 2.9% at Kamboni in Kasungu to 35.5% in Mulanje Mission Hospital. Then the Vice President's policy initiative document (Tsoka 1999:107) admitted: "Despite the severity of the HIV/AIDS epidemic, the response from the Government and the community is not commensurate with the seriousness of the problem." Given the post-Banda donor goodwill and the frantic accumulation, corruption, and misuse of government resources by the elite (Chirwa and Kanyongolo 2000), this was an understatement.

The main immediate initiative, in conjunction with the WHO, was elite centered: the reduction of the cost of Combivir to K10,000 monthly, making it "affordable to high income patients required for Malawi's manpower needs" but not the rural or urban poor. The deficiency of the "condom approach" was shown by the fact that BLM, the biggest family planning NGO, distributed only 612,866 condoms in 1996–7. Malawi has a population of 10 million.

One event encapsulating the cultural, political, and economic aspects of the HIV/AIDS story in Malawi was the *mchape* incident. In 1994, Goodson Chisupe, an ordinary villager, claimed to be able to prevent or cure AIDS with a herbal drink whose formula had been given to him in a dream. People (estimated to be up to 500,000), rich and poor, rural and urban, flocked to his Liwonde village to drink

mchape. When Western white doctors and African medical personnel declared Chisupe a fraud, some African medical personnel demanded "respect for African notions of illness and healing." Chisupe's simple action set in motion a series of events which highlighted the desperation and poverty of the sick in Malawi, exposed the shortcomings of the Western medical establishment, and showed that many still believed in "traditional" remedies. It also demonstrated the intimate relationship between governance, culture, legitimacy, and communal health. In the rural areas the many "AIDS funerals" and the care of orphans had led to a resurgence of the "traditional communal spirit," a spirit at variance with the "personal poverty alleviation" (Lwanda 1996) of the elites.

We would view this *mchape* in terms of those transitional phenomena that arise in public spheres at times of transitions, disruptions, and uncertainties. They seek to address "new threats using old wisdom." In the ontological and epistemological context between Western medicine, traditional medicine, and real life, the *mchapes*, while marginal, are symbolic and heraldic.

They could also be seen as testing the position of traditional practitioners within the legal framework of Malawi. The Medical Practitioners and Dentists Act of 1987 does not prohibit the practice of "any African system of medicine," provided the practice is safe. The *mchapes* attract the gaze of the state but are not the only ones filling a massive unmet need. In 1997, the Malawi Vision 2020 Project (1997:36) suggested that traditional practitioners be more involved and integrated into the health care system to improve rural health care, a call previously heard (Msonthi 1982; Msukwa 1981). Until 1981, health campaigns had concentrated on eradicating "poverty, ignorance and disease," without an epistemological exposition of this slogan and without a formal trans-cultural health policy being formulated. It is not surprising that, as Maluwa-Banda (2000) shows, secondary students, while having "adequate knowledge about the basic facts about AIDS, the transmission of HIV and how they can protect themselves from being infected," still harbor some "misconceptions." Friends were cited as the major influence on the decision to have sex and the school was identified as the preferred source on sexuality. As we have already seen, many schools are "village culture based," and these misconceptions may reflect attitudes carried over from socialization in village schools. Work in progress suggests that these attitudes are a reflection of the cultural duality that informs attitudes to medical issues (Lwanda 2002).

Conclusion

Ambiguity and parallel duality do not disturb the meta-construction of social order in the Malawi context; the apertures of identity are permanently open for people to move in and out without disadvantaging the power brokers of each side. But, while avoiding conflict, such a construction is static and inefficient; to produce motion the two need to engage each other in full epistemological cultural dialogue. Culture, as Mazrui states, "provides lenses for perception and cognition, motives for behaviour, a basis for an identity, and modes of communication."

In the case of HIV then, from the foregoing historical perspective alone, given the issues of class, culture, and socio-economic disparity, one would predict that the site of significant cultural change and effect needs to be the localized cores of traditional practices at village level which had been impenetrable to authorities both colonial and postcolonial.

Yet history also hints at the constancy, resilience, or "conservative nature" of these societal traditions: a conservatism assured by various mechanisms that "permit while resisting change" at localized and indeed national level. In the current environment, where the population, largely rural and subsisting at socio-economic modes sometimes reminiscent of precolonial levels, is under cultural attack in the HIV discourse, the power brokers of tradition may consider themselves at risk. There will thus be an accelerated process of transmission of cultural knowledge from one generation to the next. As argued, in the case of women, at such times, cultural values are even more assiduously guarded. The falling life expectancy also contributes to earlier generational cultural transmission (M. Lwanda, pers. comm. 2000).

If, in traditional medicine, as we have suggested, change is inspired by new and hostile challenges and occurs after experience and survival, we can predict that, given the localized nature, each entity structures its own response. In precolonial days a response would have been possible over national or territorial areas. In the current era, given the use of electronic media by traditional culture, via popular music, more widespread but still fragmented responses may be possible (Lwanda 1999). When, for example, McAulife (1994) suggests that there is no evidence to suggest risk behavior reduction even after people have recognized HIV, she may be missing the point: are these people at "stage one of recognition" in their Western mode or simply following their traditional mode? If the latter, their behavior will appear risky to the Western observer but logical from whatever traditional point of view is informing their behavior. And behavior change is difficult where the socio-economic environment is inappropriate to that change.

From this historical model, to be effective, health promotion measures against HIV will have to first take note of the socio-economic and cultural reality of life in Malawi and then tackle each localized practice separately. For example: If a *fisi* is to act as a surrogate "husband" to a woman whose own husband is infertile, he should be HIV-tested first, and the practice would then continue at reduced HIV risk. The same concepts are being suggested for initiation *afisi* and the other high-risk cultural practices. Engagement with these practices would be on the understanding that while one could/could not, in the short term, change these customs, one would make them safe. This has been done in the West for homosexuals. Explaining the infective or epidemic aspect to the traditional culture practitioners may be possible and is necessary. But a precondition would be the understanding that in some of these residual practices lie residual communal gender, hierarchical power roles, and age-old cosmological beliefs. These cosmologies, we noted, have mounted responses in pre-, colonial, and postcolonial times of famine and epidemics, during the colonial "subjugation," and in encounters with Christianity. A response to the HIV epidemic from African traditional medicine should be expected. The HIV epidemic has now lasted a generation. We would contend that this is long enough for traditional culture to begin to respond. However, some of the "localized" responses that are emerging, like advocating sex with virgins or under-age girls, are, from the moral and Western medical viewpoint, clearly pathological and need to be dislodged before they become firmly – and locally – embedded. They are examples of the exploitation and corruption of culture by the powerful, who may influence some localities. In the fight against HIV/AIDS, prevailing social constructs and realities, particularly localized ones, should therefore be noted in any theories of how to deal with the epidemic.

ACKNOWLEDGMENTS

My grateful thanks to Paul Nugent, Kenneth King, Jack Thompson, Patrick O'Malley, Jack Mapanje, and Chipo Kanjo. A full version of the "History of HIV in Malawi" is in preparation.

NOTES

1. A traditional Chewa/Ngoni song warning of impending strife.
2. Nyamakazi (rheumatism) = Any painful disorder of joints, muscles or connective tissue.
3. Humanness or the concept of humanity as made up of the five essentials of form or *thupi*, spirit or *mzimu*, community or *mudzi*, integrity or *chilungamo*, and productivity or *nchito*. Humanization occurs via social nurture, *maleledwe*.
4. *Mchape* = "the cleanser," a herbal drink used by witch-finders, healers, or opportunists. See, for example, Malawi National Archive (MNA): NS1/23/2.
5. Mental illnesses resulting from cultural alienation/maladjustment.
6. Apart from a few, like Nyerere's proletarian *ujamaa* project, most of the postcolonial renaissance projects, including Thambo Mbeki's, are elite grounded.
7. See, e.g., MNA S1/471/29 and MNA S1/101/38 for some of the debates.
8. In 1969, rumors, possibly due to political discontent, blamed Banda's regime for ritual killings in Chilobwe, "selling the blood of victims to South Africa for loans."
9. See S. Carr and M. MacLachlan in *Malawi Journal of Social Science* 16:1–8, for a discussion of the "double demotivation hypothesis" in relation to Malawi.
10. See S. Carr and M. MacLachlan in *Malawi Journal of Social Science* 16:1–8.

Part II

AIDS In Africa: Regional Perspectives

Introduction to Part II

It is difficult to comprehend the whys of HIV/AIDS without a knowledge of its patterns across sub-Saharan Africa, and the direction of change over time. The next section provides overviews of AIDS as it has spread over the past 20 years. Departing from earlier geographic accounts of dispersion that focused on the virus seemingly devoid of human host (Brown 1995), these regional perspectives incorporate not only rates and patterns of transmission, but brief synopses of social and economic factors creating conditions for risks differentiated along gender as well as class lines. Oppong and Kalipeni's chapter discusses in broader strokes than Lwanda's the colonial social scientific propensity to characterize Africans as simple and simply promiscuous. Subsequent attempts by some social scientists and biomedical researchers to get a handle on AIDS have often perpetuated these characterizations rather than intervening in them, establishing a pattern of interpretation that is difficult to interrupt and potentially deleterious in its impact. Kalipeni, Craddock, and Ghosh's chapter on eastern and southern Africa tracks the spread of AIDS from the early "AIDS belt" countries of east Africa such as Uganda, Kenya, and Tanzania, to Malawi, South Africa, Zambia, and other southern African countries that now are characterized by the highest rates of AIDS in the world. After providing an overview of rates and demographic patterns, Kalipeni, Craddock, and Ghosh discuss the primary reasons for such highly successful transmission, including male and female migration patterns, the 'Sugar Daddy' phenomenon, and differential effects of poverty on men and women.

Oppong and Agyei-Mensah's chapter focuses attention upon the three west African countries of Nigeria, Senegal, and Ghana as examples of countries that are geographically proximate yet highly differentiated in both the rates and trajectories of AIDS. Whereas Senegal has managed to forestall a major epidemic through government outreach and prevention, Ghana and Nigeria are witnessing an alarming increase in their rates of transmission. Oppong and Agyei-Mensah explore the reasons for this pattern, touching upon the impacts of civil war, migration, military presence, circumcision, and the influence of Islam. Their conclusion is that reasons behind different rates of transmission are not monolithic but rather multivalent, with some factors such as religious-based cultural practices staying relatively constant while others such as war or famine pertain at particular moments in time. The heightened vulnerability to HIV resulting from famine or war and subsequent rise in AIDS rates nonetheless remain as a more enduring testament to hardship.

Chapter 3

Perceptions and Misperceptions of AIDS in Africa

Joseph R. Oppong and Ezekiel Kalipeni

Introduction

HIV/AIDS, easily the greatest disease problem the world has faced in our times, continues its march around the world. According to UNAIDS, as of December 2002, 42 million people worldwide had HIV, the virus that causes AIDS. With close to 70 percent of the global total of HIV-positive people, sub-Saharan Africa bears the brunt of the havoc and destruction that HIV/AIDS has left in its trail. An estimated 13.7 million Africans have already died from the epidemic, which is quickly erasing the hard-earned gains in life expectancy in some countries. In southern Africa, where life expectancy at birth rose from 44 years in the early 1950s to 59 in the early 1990s, it is expected to fall back to just 45 between 2005 and 2010 because of AIDS. While both men and women are at risk, recent research suggests that between 12 and 13 African women are currently infected for every ten African men. Infected women infect their children in turn, although new evidence indicates that HIV impairs women's fertility. Ninety percent of the world's mother-to-child transmission in 1999 occurred in Africa.

Data compiled by UNAIDS suggests that HIV/AIDS in Africa has reached epidemic proportions, particularly in the so-called AIDS epicenter in central and southern Africa where up to 25 percent of the urban population may be infected. Rates of infection are assumed to be even higher for certain sectors of society such as commercial sex workers, pregnant women in urban areas, and truck drivers. As Good (1995) points out, the "long wave" character of the AIDS epidemic will continue to spiral out of control in many African countries. While it is currently understood that there is not just one epidemic but multiple local and sometimes national epidemics with different characteristics and patterns, many approaches to the study of the factors that facilitate the transmission of the disease have been largely simplistic overgeneralizations. Indeed, as Nicoll and Brown (1994) point out, the images of Africa conjured in Western minds and perpetuated by the biased media have been those of an oversimplified exotic place variously depicted as a game park or an apocalyptic vision of famine and civil war. Recent ominous accounts by notable journalists such as Kaplan (1994) have tended to perpetuate such stereotypes.

In the medical and epidemiological arena, the different pattern of AIDS infection exhibited by African countries has resulted in a plethora of research which, as Packard and Epstein (1991) note, resembles earlier narrow-minded colonial efforts to understand the epidemiological patterns of TB and syphilis. Indeed, current research on the AIDS epidemic in Africa majors on explaining Africa's unique epidemiological patterns. Explanations invariably blame peculiarities of African sexuality and reproduction customs, traditions, and behaviors but neglect significant factors such as the colonial historical context, poverty, dependency, and underdevelopment (Packard and Epstein 1991).

In this chapter we confront some viewpoints that have guided recent AIDS research in Africa, focusing particularly on those works that overgeneralize, are ethnocentric, and somehow misrepresent Africa through cultural stereotyping. We argue that such viewpoints contribute little to understanding AIDS epidemics in Africa and encourage a premature narrowing of research questions, as happened during the colonial era in the cases of tuberculosis (TB) and syphilis (see, for example, Fendell 1963; Packard 1987; Packard and Epstein 1991). For the purpose of this chapter, we divide these works into four major categories – Overgeneralization, African Sexual Behavior, Patriarchy, Marriage, and Kinship, and finally, Urban Sexuality. We conclude by suggesting new directions for explanation of Africa's AIDS epidemics.

The Overgeneralization Syndrome

Overgeneralization frequently characterizes research on Africa (Ofori-Amoah 1995). Studies based on specific national or people groups assume an African or sub-Saharan African title when it comes to publication of results. Thus, a study on AIDS in Uganda with a special focus on the Rakai District or Buganda region is called *AIDS in Africa* (Barnett and Blaikie 1992). Moreover, despite the rich cultural mosaic and differences in geographical, economic, and historical experiences, Africa is portrayed as culturally homogenous. For example, Rushing (1995) portrays a sex-positive African culture, which sees sex as a

recreation activity, and thus "guides women into prostitution more easily than Western culture does" (1995:73–74), as a major causal factor of AIDS in Africa. While generalizing results is a critical step for theory development in the search for universalism in social science (Nachimas and Nachimas 1981), loose generalizations are inappropriate.

Another example of inappropriate generalization is the African urban hierarchical diffusion thesis which argues that, like the West, the spread of HIV/AIDS in sub-Saharan Africa follows a hierarchical diffusion pattern, spreading from the most urban to the more rural areas (Caldwell 1995; Gould 1993). Oppong (1997) argued that this urban diffusion thesis might be more mythical than fact in some places, primarily because it is an artifact of the data collection process. Geographical variations in availability and quality of health care services, which usually favor urban centers, generate spatial variations in the quality of AIDS data (Smallman-Raynor and Cliff 1991). Completeness of reporting is likely to be higher in major towns, the foci of most AIDS testing and treatment facilities. Shortage of biomedical care and modern laboratory facilities in rural areas likely produces significant underreporting. Moreover, because rural residents are only likely to be diagnosed when they visit urban health facilities, this is bound to inflate the urban AIDS statistics.

Through creating the impression that Africans are homogeneously promiscuous and discussing Africa as though it were one country, not some fifty nations with hundreds of different ethnic groups and cultures, Rushing (1995) epitomizes the overgeneralization syndrome in African AIDS research. This work ignores the reality that Western, Islamic, and sometimes traditional cultural influences may all operate simultaneously within the same locality, a fact that Mazrui (1986) calls Africa's *triple heritage*. Several quotations will illustrate Rushing's rather careless overgeneralizations:

> In contrast to Americans, who usually view sex morally and think that people who have multiple partners (even if unmarried) are immoral and unfaithful, most Africans do not judge sexual behavior in such terms at all. They experience little guilt about sex, and they enter into sex

more casually and have more sexual partners than Westerners do (1995:62)

Most African societies are sex-positive.... Premarital sex for females is accepted. (1995:65)

In sum, for females as well as males, fairly permissive...sexual attitudes are found generally across sub-Saharan Africa. (1995:66)

For most of Africa social norms permit and even encourage sex with multiple partners. Polygamous sexual relations are thus widespread for the married no less than the unmarried. This is the hallmark of a sex-positive culture. It also facilitates the spread of HIV. (1995:66)

Rushing advances four main factors that contribute to the proliferation of the AIDS epidemic in Africa. First, poor nutrition and infectious diseases such as malaria, malnutrition, tuberculosis, or trypanosomiasis in the African environment ultimately compromise the immune system and increase susceptibility to HIV infection. Second, blood transfusions and injections are often used in a range of therapeutic settings in which adequate sterilization procedures are usually lacking. Lack of blood-screening facilities for HIV and other sexually transmitted diseases as well as the shortage of disposable hypodermics ultimately results in the reuse of needles without proper sterilization and increases the risk of HIV infection. Third, the widespread nature of STDs such as syphilis[1] and gonorrhea which, purportedly, rank among the top five diseases in some African countries among persons seeking treatment at clinics is a major factor. Finally, and most important, is the omnipresent polygamous behavior among all African societies whom he interchangeably refers to as "tribes" in spite of his acknowledgment that the term "tribe" was introduced by European colonialists who used it pejoratively because Africans were considered "backward" and "primitive." Citing ethnographic studies such as Radcliffe-Brown (1950) and Southall (1961), Rushing concludes that having multiple sexual partners is a universal cultural practice in many African societies, that such behavior is culturally determined and considered normal and appropriate by Africans, and that it facilitates the spread of HIV/AIDS. Rushing thus invokes the behavioral paradigm to account for the widespread nature of the HIV/AIDS epidemic in Africa. It is this kind

of rush to find a cause, "the sexual life of the natives," and to prescribe an immediate solution, "modification of sexual behavior," that obscures the real risk factors, namely, the historical, social, political, and economic contexts within which such risk behaviors are played out.

Once the central factor in the proliferation of HIV/AIDS in Africa is identified as promiscuous behavior, Rushing tries to rationalize it through the cross-cultural framework. The central idea in this framework is that "behavior patterns that exist in one society but not in others or in varying degrees in different societies are the result of differences in the way societies structure and give meaning to behavior." In the context of African societies, exotic or almost primitive marriage, sexual, and kinship arrangements are highlighted as the culprits for the proliferation of AIDS in both rural and urban settings. Paradoxically, the discourse in the paper reads like Africa was a monocultural society to be contrasted with another monocultural society called America. It should be common knowledge that both Africa and North America are in themselves multicultural rather than monocultural societies, as noted earlier, and that the application of the cross-cultural perspective must fairly treat the many cultural differences that exist among and within African groups if it is to be a meaningful paradigm in the etiology of HIV/AIDS in Africa. This is a glaring weakness of the entire discourse in Rushing's paper. Next, we discuss marriage/kinship patterns and sexual relations and the unfortunate stereotypical aspects of African societies as a sexually craved people.

Sexual Behavior Paradigm

Initial work such as Caldwell, Caldwell, and Quiggin (1989), Rushton and Bogaert (1989), Caldwell (1995), and Rushing (1995) constructed theories based on the eccentricities of African sexuality and in the case of Rushton and Bogaert outright racial determinism. Gould (1993) traces the origins of the AIDS epidemic to African monkeys and argues that initial denial by African leaders in several countries escalated its spread. The two books by Gould (1993) and Shannon, Pyle, and Bashshur

(1991), both of which are conjectural in orientation, indirectly influenced the representations of Africa as a "diseased continent" with little hard evidence about the spread of AIDS to the rest of the world.

Current knowledge confirms that sexual behavior, the primary target of AIDS prevention efforts worldwide, is deeply embedded in individual desires, social and cultural relationships, and environmental processes (UNAIDS 1999b). Because sex takes place in context, sociocultural factors surrounding the individuals must be considered in designing prevention interventions. Besides, larger issues of structural and environmental determinants play a significant role in sexual behavior (Sweat 1995). Thus, giving information alone is not sufficient to induce behavioral change among most individuals.

Overemphasis on individual behavioral change through information dissemination has undermined the need and capacity of research to understand the complexity of HIV transmission and control (UNAIDS 1999b). Focus on the individual psychological process ignores the interactive relationship of behavior in its social, cultural, and economic dimensions and thus misses the opportunity to fully understand crucial determinants of sexual behavior. As Aggleton (1996) points out, motivations for sex are complicated, unclear, and may not be thought through in advance. Societal norms, religious criteria, and gender – power relations infuse meaning into sexual behavior and facilitate or impede both positive and negative changes. In short, determinants of sexual behavior should be seen as a function not only of individual and social but of structural and environmental factors as well (Caraël 1997; Sweat 1995; Tawil 1995).

Patriarchy, Marriage and Kinship

Rushing and many other researchers (see, for example, Hrdy 1987; Brokensha 1987; Green 1988; Shannon and Pyle 1989) blame the "exotic" nature of marriage and kinship systems prevalent in traditional African society for the African AIDS crisis. These works usually discuss polygyny, patrilineage, the culture of sexual permissiveness, and gender stratification at great length and attempt to

show that the sex-positive nature of traditional society, which has been grafted onto contemporary urban society, accounts for widespread prostitution and AIDS. Proliferations of sexually transmitted diseases and AIDS in both urban and rural settings are thus products of deeply ingrained promiscuous sexual behavior.

These studies blame multi-partner sexual relations typified by polygamy as a major factor in Africa's AIDS crisis. Based on the fact that an estimated 30–50 percent of African marriages (3–5 percent elsewhere in the world) are polygamous, they conclude that multiple wives increase the spread of STDs and AIDS in a population and account for the balanced rate between males and females. While this argument may sound appealing, the evidence does not support it. If indeed polygamy were such a potent means of spreading HIV, the Islamic societies of Northern Africa should exhibit larger than usual HIV rates since polygamy is the normative form of marriage in these societies. Yet evidence suggests otherwise. In North Africa and the Middle East HIV is spreading, but more slowly than elsewhere in the world (Tastemain and Coles 1993). Oppong (1998b), examining the geography of AIDS in Ghana, showed that the region with the least polygyny, Eastern Region, had the highest AIDS rate while the region with the highest polygyny, Northern Region (44 percent) had the least AIDS rate. The reason is that polygamy is not synonymous with promiscuity. Senegal, where 93 percent of the population is Muslim and polygamy is the norm, provides an excellent example. While nearly half of all married Senegalese women are in polygynous unions, they rarely have partners besides their husband. In a 1997 Dakar study reported by UNAIDS (1999b), 99 percent of married women said they had not had sex with anyone except their husband in the preceding 12 months. Besides, sex before marriage is traditionally uncommon for Senegalese women. Thus, while poly-partner sexual activity may be an important vehicle for spreading HIV, the context of this poly-partner relationship, whether a closed polygamous unit or unstable liaisons with multiple partners, is the critical determining factor.

In short, polygamy does not automatically produce rapid transmission of sexually transmitted diseases; it all depends on marital norms. Furthermore, the often-cited 30–50 percent prevalence rate of polygamy in Africa may be an exaggeration. Recent data from censuses and the Demographic and Health Surveys (DHS) of the mid-1980s and early 1990s indicate much lower rates of polygamous unions in most African countries. For example, in most southern and east African countries, marriage for women is universal but mostly monogamous. In Malawi census data show that only 20 percent of men over 40 years have more than one wife (World Bank 1992a). In the DHS data only 9 percent of men reported having more than one wife and 20 percent of women reported being in polygamous unions (Malawi National Statistical Office 1994). In a number of African countries such as Ghana, Malawi, Zambia, Namibia, and Botswana, the proportion of husbands in a polygamous union is around 10–15 percent among those below age 30 and about 40 percent for those over age 50 (Ghana Statistical Service 1989; Malawi National Statistical Office 1994; Gaisie 1993; Lesetedi 1989; Katjiuanjo 1993). Younger men and women are more likely to be in monogamous unions than polygamous ones (Bledsoe 1990a). Paradoxically, HIV/AIDS rates are much lower among the most polygamous age group, those over 50 years, in comparison to the less polygamous group, those below age 40.

In typical traditional society, women in polygamous unions were expected to be faithful to their husbands, and husbands were expected to be faithful to their wives, since failure to do so would result in tragedy of one sort or another such as the husband or child dying. For example, among the Chewa of central Malawi, Zambia, and parts of Mozambique, there is a disease called *tsempho* which has been discussed at great length in ethnographic studies (Hodgson 1913:129–131; Rangeley 1948:34–44; Williamson 1956; Marwick 1965:66–68). *Tsempho*, a potentially fatal wasting disease, is attributed to promiscuous sexual relationships or to the indulging of sexual intercourse by spouses during prohibited periods. The disease, which affects men and women as well as young children, is purportedly caused by another's social transgression. Thus, wives and husbands were forewarned of the dangers of promiscuity. Variations of the *tsempho* sexual taboo exist among other ethnic groups of central, southern, and eastern Africa such as the Bemba, Luapula, Tonga, Ndembu, etc. (Richards 1956; Cunnison 1959; Colson 1958, 1960; Colson and Gluckman 1961; Maxwell 1983; Gibbs 1988; Ouma 1996). In other words, traditional societies were not predominantly promiscuous or sex-positive as Rushing and others would like us to believe.

Underlying polygamy and promiscuity, the patrilineal kinship system is blamed as one of the major etiological factors in the African pattern of HIV/AIDS. It is argued that patriarchy gives men the incentive to acquire as many wives as possible because of the value of children as economic assets, and, as such, promotes polygamous behavior outside of marriage. Interestingly, matrilineal descent systems are quite common in Africa, especially central Africa and parts of west Africa such as Ghana. Often men have to move to the wife's village, sometimes in a subservient position. In these societies women have been known to rise to positions of power in society and generally enjoy some autonomy in comparison to women in patrilineal societies (Chilivumbo 1975). In both patrilineal and matrilineal societies premarital sex is taken very seriously. Although rules of chastity differ radically, in patrilineal societies (such as the Tumbuka, Ngonde, Sukwa, and Ngoni of central Africa) stress is laid on a girl's chastity before marriage. In the orthodox form of chastity rules, the girl's virginity on the eve of a wedding determines the value of bridewealth (Southall 1961; Chilivumbo 1975). Among the Bemba and Chewa (matrilineal groups) girls go through *Chisungu* or *Chinamwali*, a puberty rite that initiates them through the symbols of life and death in order to give social form and meaning to their sexuality (Richards 1956; Yoshida 1993; Helitzer-Allen 1994). One of the worst things that could happen to a girl in Bemba traditional society was to bear a child before she had been initiated, a sign that premarital sex was not condoned. Such a child was considered a creature of ill-omen and both the father and mother could be banished.

In short, several social and religious sanctions impact sexual behavior in both patrilineal and matrilineal societies. Sex is not merely a transaction or an ordinary activity in which men are expected to give women money and gifts as an expression of affection, respect, and gratitude for sexual favors. Sex is never considered as a form of recreation as Rushing claims; it is much more than this, a sacred undertaking in most traditional societies. Premarital sex, pregnancy out of wedlock, homosexuality, and other forms of sexual deviance are considered to be abhorrent behaviors and are rarely encouraged. Thus, to argue, as Rushing does, that Americans usually view sex morally and think that having multiple partners constitutes immorality and unfaithfulness, while most Africans do not judge sexual behavior in such terms and have a positive-sex culture, is indeed to go against reality.

If anything, it could be argued that Americans are more sex-positive than Africans are. In the United States and Europe, commercials on TV and billboards often utilize semi-nude if not completely nude models. In the United States and other Western nations, business in pornographic movies, sexually explicit TV programs, and pornographic magazines is lucrative and vigorous. If indeed most Americans were morally upright as far as matters of sex are concerned, such activities would have been banned long ago. The French scientist Luc Montagnier, who was the first to isolate HIV, supports the theory that a mycoplasma, a bacterium-like organism, is the trigger that turns a slow-growing population of AIDS viruses into killers. Montagnier believes that the explosion of *sexual activity* (our emphasis) in the United States during the 1970s fostered the spread of a hardy, drug-resistant strain of the mycoplasma and that the AIDS epidemic began when the mycoplasma got together with HIV, which had been dormant in Africa (Ungeheuer 1993).

Homosexuality and AIDS in Africa – the myth of the bisexual African homosexual

An excellent example of the bias that characterizes these works is Rushing's treatment of homosexuality in Africa. Beginning with

Western notions about causal factors of HIV/AIDS, specifically its homosexual beginnings in North America, Rushing sets out to uncover homosexuality in Africa. Postulating a genetic component to homosexuality as factual, although "medical experts believe that in certain African countries, such as Kenya, homosexuality is uncommon" (1995:84), the component is probably as common among Africans as other populations. "But gay subcultures are not as prevalent... anthropological and historical research shows that gay subcultures do not exist in nonliterate societies, such as the tribal societies of Africa. In most African societies homosexuals are severely ostracized." However, since Rushing's paradigm requires finding homosexuality as a common practice, despite the evidence, he creates a mythical bisexual homosexual:

> It is understandable, therefore, that African homosexuals would take great care to conceal their homosexual orientation, just as American homosexuals did... Designated open places for gays (bars, discos, bathhouses), not to speak of gay marriages, are virtually or entirely non-existent in most African countries today. Men have sex with other men in more clandestine settings. But African men are obliged by their kinship unit to marry, sometimes to more than one woman, and to produce many children. As a result, men who engage in homosexual liaisons are apt to be bisexual.

On the flawed assumption that homosexuality is a universal phenomenon, Rushing looks across the continent to find homosexual populations, gay bathhouses, and other elements of a homosexual cultural landscape. Failing to find it, instead of rejecting the thesis of homosexuality as a major source of HIV/AIDS infection, Rushing concludes that African homosexuality must be carefully concealed. This mythical African homosexual, Rushing's creation, must be under extreme social pressure to conceal his identity because society frowns on homosexuality and promotes heterosexual marriage. Thus the mythical African homosexual, to conceal his true identity, will marry because African culture expects men to marry. The mythical African male homosexual is bisexual and will be a major source for spreading AIDS! They will have homosexual relations in urban centers and heterosexual activity with their spouses in rural areas, creating a high-risk, poly-partner, poly-sexual environment. An entire theory about the spread of AIDS is established without a shred of evidence. Perhaps Rushing can provide some hard data to support this theory: How many homosexuals are there in each African country? What proportion of men in each African country is homosexual, married to women, and thus involved in bisexual, poly-partner sexual relationships?

Urban Sexuality and AIDS

Urban sexuality has been blamed for Africa's AIDS crisis. Rural–urban differentials in AIDS rates have been attributed to high rates of STDs in urban areas, rapid urbanization amidst deeply ingrained polygamous behavior, and the partial erosion of traditional cultures in the urban setting, including those for regulating sexual relations and practices. Central to the proliferation of AIDS in urban areas is the widespread nature of prostitution which, supposedly, has become one of the four main roles to emerge for women in urban Africa alongside being housewives, sellers of cooked food, and brewers of illegal liquor. Opportunities for women are considered to be better in urban than rural areas and such opportunities include sexual strategies for gaining access to economic resources from men.

An excellent but unbelievable example of the far-fetched stereotypical assertions of these works is Rushing's assertion of a normative acceptance that makes trading in sex as acceptable as trading in other services and that African cultures simply guide women into prostitution much more easily than Western culture does. Rushing seems to indicate that virtually all women in Africa trade in sex both within and outside marriage for economic gain and that most Africans experience little guilt about sex, and that they enter into sex more casually and have more sexual partners than Westerners do.

While it cannot be denied that prostitution exists in Africa, Rushing's explanations are simplistic and smack of the earlier "dressed native" and "sexually craved native" colonial explanations of tuberculosis and syphilis in

Africa. It typifies the lack of cultural understanding that pervades intellectual discourse on the African condition. In explaining the different pattern of TB among Africans, medical experts reflected wider stereotypical perceptions about Africans, which were current in European colonial society. Africans were perceived as "primitive" and in the process of making difficult adjustments to conditions of a "civilized" industrial world. Thus, Africans were susceptible to TB because they had not adjusted to the conditions of a civilized industrial society, symbolized by their incomplete adoption of Western clothing and their failure to observe proper dietary and sanitary laws (Packard 1987). Nothing about the low wages and inadequate housing policies of employers and government officials came into the discourse and the prescribed control measures focused naturally on education rather than social and economic reform (Packard and Epstein 1991). The pattern of syphilis infection among Africans was also attributed to the immoral behavior of Africans, to the neglect of other avenues of transmission. In parts of eastern Africa there was an outbreak of non-venereal syphilis during the early years of colonial rule. Non-venereal syphilis, also known as endemic syphilis, is similar to venereal syphilis but is spread through bodily contact in warm climates. Thus syphilis was misdiagnosed and a theory was readily constructed to explain its extraordinary rate of spread, based on assumptions about the extreme sexuality of Africans (Packard and Epstein 1991). Rushing's current study fits nicely into the preexisting assumptions about African sexuality and disease, that is, the "sexual-positive culture" paradigm. As Packard and Epstein (1991) note, the point is not that the sexual behaviors Rushing highlights do not occur or that they are insignificant in promoting the proliferation of AIDS transmissions, but rather that this kind of study myopically promotes one single paradigm which suggests that Africans frequently have multiple sexual partners to the exclusion of the broader patterns of everyday sexual activity which in many cases are both less exotic and more monogamous in character. In the following section we offer a more inclusive paradigm that looks at the social, historical, and economic contexts of sexuality, promiscuity, and the proliferation of AIDS/HIV. In a similar vein to that proposed by Packard and Epstein (1991) and Craddock (1996), other equally important factors in the etiology of AIDS, such as the political economy, the role of background infections and malnutrition, and needle use, also need to be given their proper place in the proliferation of AIDS within the African context.

Towards a Reformulation

We have argued that Rushing's work clearly has several major problems. It suffers from a common pitfall in cross-national research, namely, ethnocentricity. Rushing simply looks at African culture through an American lens. It is full of overgeneralizations in its conclusions and creates the false impression that Africans are homogenously sex-positive and promiscuous. Consequently, it is the sexual life of Africans that is responsible for the HIV/AIDS problem in Africa. This conclusion is simply not supported by the facts, nor is it logical. If there is a unified, coherent, African cultural approach to sexuality and reproduction that increases the likelihood of the transmission of HIV/AIDS, why is there such a varied patchwork of prevalence and infection rates across the continent (Hunt 1996)? Such shallow and sometimes simplistic explanations frustrate serious efforts to explore other avenues of HIV/AIDS transmission since once they have been accepted, they shape the course of subsequent research by privileging or marginalizing certain lines of inquiry (Packard and Epstein 1991).

Moreover, such simplistic explanations lead to simplistic and unworkable solutions. If HIV/AIDS is not spread through homogenous promiscuity of all Africans but through the sexual practices of selected high-risk groups and unsanitary medical practices in biomedical facilities, condom distribution to the general population, while useful, is not the solution. That would be similar to recent attempts to reduce fertility through distribution of contraceptives to women who have no desire to reduce fertility. As long as the socioeconomic conditions that make it desirable to have many children (for example, high infant mortality rates and cultural values that mandate large family sizes to assure future security and agricultural labor), contraceptives, even if distributed freely, will have little impact on birth rates. Similarly, appropriate solutions to the African HIV/AIDS crisis must be based on appropriate explanations of the problem.

We suggest that more plausible explanations of the HIV/AIDS epidemic in Africa may be found in the migrant labor thesis (Hunt 1996; Bassett and Mhloyi 1991; Jochelson, Mothibeli, and Leger 1991) which provides a social, historical, and economic context for urban sexuality, and unsafe medical practices. The migrant labor thesis asserts that the establishment of wage labor on the continent, particularly in eastern, central, and southern Africa, to support the mining, agricultural plantations, and other economic activities of the colonialists, created a situation where migrant labor, mostly young men, was contracted for long-term work (1–3 years). Because families were not encouraged to accompany the laborer, farming and traditional activities, such as raising, feeding, and educating children, became the responsibility of women (without their husbands) in rural areas. The women's limited ability to increase the productivity of the land led to declining fertility of the land and ultimately, absolute shortage of food and malnutrition. When agricultural production becomes untenable as a means of survival, such women often migrate to the city where some engage in one of the very few options open to them: prostitution, an activity that, with a morbid irony, serves as their only lifeline to economic survival in the short term at the same time as posing an enormous risk of curtailing their survival in the long term (Craddock 2000).

Male migrant workers, away from their families for long periods of time, use alcoholism and frequent visits to prostitutes to deal with their loneliness and boredom. For men and women in eastern, central, and southern Africa, these long separations lead to breakdown in the stability of the family, divorce, and a definitive increase in the numbers of sexual partners for both men and women. Thus, the relatively high number of sexual partners is not the result of a longstanding cultural attribute of Africans or an innate craving by Africans for more sex, or promiscuity, but is directly a consequence of the economic and labor markets. Women definitely do not turn to prostitution because African culture encourages prostitution more easily than Western culture does, as Rushing argues they do. As Craddock (1996) shows, women living in households where there is chronic undernutrition, who are most nutritionally at risk, are the ones most likely to seek other options, including prostitution, for survival.

Epidemics of gonorrhea and syphilis in eastern, central, and southern Africa in the 1960s and 1970s, the migrant labor thesis points out, resulted from this migrant labor system. Since the transmission of HIV/AIDS is assisted by previously untreated sexually transmitted diseases, the previous epidemics of sexually transmitted diseases in this area increase the likelihood of transmission. In other words, the population in eastern, central, and southern Africa is predisposed to sexually transmitted diseases and HIV/AIDS because not only are they socially structured to be vulnerable to the disease itself, but previous vulnerability increases present vulnerability (Hunt 1996).

It is important to note that the migrant labor thesis does not overgeneralize for the entire continent, as Rushing does. It also allows a ready amplification for the spread of sexually transmitted diseases in the so-called AIDS belt of Africa, which could also be applied to west Africa. When migrant workers (male or female) are too ill to work, they return home to be cared for by family, which also means that the disease that caused the illness returns with them to the labor reserve. Thus, HIV/AIDS and other diseases are transmitted into the rural network, where previously unexposed populations fall prey and provide fertile grounds for the explosive growth of epidemics.

In west Africa similar patterns of labor migration prevailed, mostly centered on the export cropping zones of Côte d'Ivoire and Ghana (Stock 1995). Prior to 1960, Ghana received more migrants than any other west African country, primarily those seeking to work on cocoa plantations. The steady decline of the Ghanaian economy and the relative political and economic stability of Côte d'Ivoire pushed Côte d'Ivoire to the top after 1960. Some 1.4 million people, about one-fifth of the Ivoirian population, was of foreign nationality by the late 1960s, with an extremely high concentration in Abidjan, the national capital, where the ratio was one-third. As Ghana's economic crisis deepened after 1970, increasing numbers of Ghanaians left for other countries, particularly Nigeria and Côte d'Ivoire. A very important factor is the urban focus of migrant labor in west Africa. Over half of Côte d'Ivoire's immigrants live in cities, particularly Abidjan, compared to only one-third of indigenous Ivoirian citizens (Stock 1995). This high concentration of migrant labor, particularly in Abidjan, may be an important explanatory factor for the high HIV/AIDS rate in this city, also known as the *sexual crossroads of Africa* (Gould 1993). According to Gould, 24 percent of Abidjan's prostitutes tested for other diseases were positive for HIV-1 by 1987, but the figure was 50 percent by 1989. In the city hospital, HIV-infected patients came from over twenty countries, and in one of them, Niger, all 25 men diagnosed with AIDS in Niamey had lived for many months, even years, usually in Côte d'Ivoire (1993:84).

Several writers explain Ghana's HIV/AIDS pattern with reference to migrant workers, particularly prostitutes in neighboring Côte d'Ivoire and specifically Abidjan (Agadzi 1989; Decosas et al. 1995). Unlike other parts of Africa, AIDS in Ghana strikes twice as many females as it does males. According to Agadzi (1989), AIDS was imported into Ghana primarily by female prostitutes in neighboring Côte d'Ivoire (Agadzi 1989). Decosas et al. (1995) observe that more than half of all professional prostitutes in Abidjan are Ghanaian, many from the Krobo tribe in the Eastern Region of Ghana. Moreover, "80% of those who are still working as prostitutes in Abidjan are infected with HIV" (Decosas et al. 1995:827). Accordingly, the female:male ratio of AIDS patients in the Eastern Region, home of the Krobo tribe, is

5:1 compared to the national rate of 2:1. Decosas et al. explain this in terms of female prostitutes infected with HIV who return to Ghana for treatment.

Another important source of the spread of HIV/AIDS is unsafe medical practices. In fact, unsafe medical practices and medical carelessness may be far more important than sexual activity in explaining the geography of HIV/ AIDS in Africa (Minkin 1991). Unfortunately, studies like Rushing's have been so dominant and influential that priorities for HIV/AIDS control have largely focused on sexual activity. In the United States and elsewhere, needle sharing is a major source of infection, particularly among intravenous drug users. Gould and Wallace (1994) report that by March 1992, needle sharing by drug addicts accounted for approximately 23–29 percent of reported AIDS cases in the United States. While needle sharing through intravenous drug use is currently not a problem in Africa, needle sharing through repeated use of unsterilized needles and syringes for injections to cure various ailments such as malaria is. This is particularly true for those who have to rely on itinerant drug vendors, drug peddlers, and bush doctors for medical supplies and most of their health care needs. Blood tests such as those for malaria and sexually transmitted diseases constitute a potential source of HIV infection. If not properly sterilized, contaminated syringes used for blood tests could result in large outbreaks of HIV and related bloodborne diseases. Yet, amazingly, multiple use of syringes and needles is quite standard practice, particularly in rural areas. For example, in Zaire, five needles were used to inject up to 400 patients daily at a mission hospital. The needles were rinsed in water and sterilized once a day (Seale 1986). Moreover, the demand for injectable medications is high throughout Africa (Alubo 1994; Minkin 1991). Thus, such unsafe medical practices, combined with the migrant labor sexual practices necessitated by the political economy thesis, account for the geography of AIDS in Africa, not some homogenous craving for sex among all Africans.

Conclusion

The issue is not that HIV does not spread through poly-partner sexual activity, whether as polygamy or simply multiple-partner sexual activity within or outside a marriage relationship. Wherever poly-partner sexual activity is practiced, whether in Africa, Australia, or the United States, participants are at an increased risk of getting the HIV virus. What is at stake is whether Africans are poly-sexual by nature, and whether African culture (if we can think about one homogenous African culture) promotes and rewards poly-sexual behavior. Is being promiscuous and poly-sexual an African culture trait or is poly-partner sexual activity a survival response dictated and enhanced by a vicious political economic system engendered by colonialism and globalization? Our approach to solving the problem hinges critically on our answer to this question.

We have argued that this view is erroneous, based on ethnocentrism, and that it overgeneralizes. It fails to explain the geographical variations in the incidence of HIV/AIDS across the continent. The simplistic solutions that result from such explanations, which advise on behavior modification and condom distribution, may provide little help to the rural women who out of necessity are unable to turn away paying customers who refuse to use condoms. They do not reach rural residents who get HIV while getting injections from an itinerant drug vendor (IDV) or a bush doctor, the only source of health care, to cure malaria. They do not protect the many people privileged to receive services in urban health facilities who face unsterile procedures, including injections, blood tests, and transfusions, daily. Moreover, it fails to stop the spread of HIV.

Why do such ridiculous explanations as Rushing's persist? Obviously, there is an urgent need to find quick answers that can be easily translated into programs. After all, it is a lot easier to distribute condoms in urban Africa than to change the socio-political and economic contexts that condition the spread of HIV. Nevertheless, any interventions that fail to address the broader issues of African social

and economic life, not merely the sexual promiscuity of Africans, are bound to fail.

NOTE

1. It is important to emphasize that recent careful
reexamination of the medical evidence on syphilis in
east Africa revealed that what was considered an
epidemic of venereal syphilis, transmitted sexually,
was simply endemic syphilis which is transmitted
through bodily contact in warm climates (Dawson
1983). Thus syphilis is not always a sexually transmitted disease and the presence of syphilis in a
population should not be taken as evidence of promiscuity as Rushing does.

Chapter 4

Mapping the AIDS Pandemic in Eastern and Southern Africa: A Critical Overview

Ezekiel Kalipeni, Susan Craddock, and Jayati Ghosh

Introduction

The specter of HIV/AIDS in sub-Saharan Africa continues to get worse rather than better, a fact that generated much discussion in the latest international AIDS conference in Durban, South Africa. As with many broad-based conferences, the results of the high-level talks in Durban produced few innovative recommendations: they stressed more research into the underlying factors of HIV transmission, and more effective prevention programs. While these suggestions seem self-evident, their implementation is fraught with the complexities of a syndrome embedded within international and regionalized social economies, cultural codes of meaning, sexual networks, and interpersonal power dynamics. This chapter seeks to highlight some of these complexities within a broad-based overview of the current patterns of HIV and AIDS in eastern and southern Africa, prevention programs already in place, and prevention strategies that might be considered in the future.

In this chapter we use data from various sources, the most important being the *Human Development Report* produced by the United Nations Development Program and *Country Epidemiological Fact Sheet on HIV/AIDS and Sexually Transmitted Diseases* by UNAIDS. Other sources include *Country Health Statistics Report* by the Center for International Health Information in the United States and, wherever available, specific national health statistics. The data need to be used with caution. Most data on country-wide rates of HIV/AIDS, for example, are extrapolated from small study samples, usually of pregnant women seeking prenatal care or those with STDs seeking clinical care. How representative these samples are is questionable, yet it is the only data available for most southern African countries.

There are numerous problems with data on HIV and AIDS. Due to gaps in diagnosis, underreporting, and reporting delays, officially reported AIDS and other diseases represent only a portion of all cases in any country. For countries in southern and eastern Africa, the reporting of HIV/AIDS cases depends in part on the availability of clinics for testing and treatment, and on the political sensitivities surrounding the syndrome. For example, Oppong

(1998a) notes that some African governments may conceal the real dimensions of the AIDS problem out of a sense of shame and concern that the real figures would drive investors and tourists away. Although national data may not accurately reflect the current situation of health and disease, they can, nevertheless, be used to offer insights into general trends such as regional cross-country variations. Recently, small but well-conducted sample surveys have begun to yield important statistics enabling cross-country comparisons. An example of these surveys is the Demographic and Health Surveys of the late 1980s and the 1990s.

Geographic Patterns

What the data show is that sub-Saharan Africa is currently thought to have fully two-thirds of the total world number of people living with HIV. Yet within this overall statistic lies significant variations in levels of infection across the continent (see Figure 4.1). Southern Africa continues to be the part of the continent worst affected by HIV. A 2001 UNAIDS report indicates that by the end of 1999, there were an estimated 4.2 million South Africans living with HIV and AIDS. In Botswana the proportion of adults living with HIV has more than doubled over the past five years, to the point that it now has the highest infection rate in the world, at 38.8 percent (UNAIDS 2003:17). In 1998, an average of 43 percent of pregnant women tested in major urban centers such as Francistown were HIV positive. In Zimbabwe, infection was estimated at one in five adults in 1996, and one in four by 1999. In Harare, 32 percent of pregnant women were already infected in 1995. In Beit Bridge, a city in South Africa, the proportion of HIV-positive pregnant women shot up from 32 percent in 1995 to 59 percent in 1996, and in Free, North Cape, Mpumalanga, Northern and North West States, infection rates among the same population sector rose from less than 1 percent in 1990 to 21 percent in 1998 (UNAIDS 2003). Although levels in cities were slightly higher than in rural areas, the difference was not great. In one town near the South African border with a large population of migrant workers, seven pregnant

women in ten tested HIV positive in 1995 (UNAIDS and WHO 1999).

East Africa was one of the first areas to suffer a massive regional epidemic. By the end of 1999 the number of people living with HIV/AIDS in Kenya reached 210,000, and there were 820,000 for Uganda, 400,000 for Rwanda and 360,000 for Burundi. Kenya's estimated adult rate for PLWAs at the end of 1999 approached 14 percent, while Uganda, Burundi, and Rwanda's estimates reached 8.3, 11.32, and 11.2 percent, respectively The cumulative number of deaths from AIDS in these countries for 1999 alone reached 369,000 (UNAIDS 2000a). Uganda was among the first to respond with open and concerted efforts to prevent the spread of the virus. For Uganda, this seems to be paying off. All three of the surveillance sites for which figures are now available show infection levels of between 5 and 9 percent, representing a decrease of about one-fifth compared with 1996 (UNAIDS and WHO 1999).

In comparison, west Africa has seen its rates of infection stabilize at much lower levels than in east and southern Africa. However, some of the most populous countries in west Africa are the exception to this rule. For example, the National AIDS Program estimates that 2.2 million people are currently living with HIV in Nigeria, a country whose response to the epidemic needs strengthening (for a fuller discussion of the AIDS/HIV situation in west Africa see Chapter 5 by Joseph Oppong and Samuel Agyei-Mensah in this volume).

From a geographic point of view, throughout southern and sub-Saharan Africa in general, urban areas have been hit hardest by the epidemic in comparison to rural areas (see Gordon 1996; also see Figure 4.2). For example, estimates compiled from blood donors, women coming to antenatal clinics, and people undergoing testing when applying for life insurance reveal that well over 30 percent of the adult population in the major urban areas of Blantrye and Lilongwe, Malawi, may have been infected by the virus (Miotti et al. 1992). This could be explained by a number of factors. Cities sometimes lack the capability to absorb workers displaced from impoverished rural areas and migrating to urban centers in search of employment; un- or

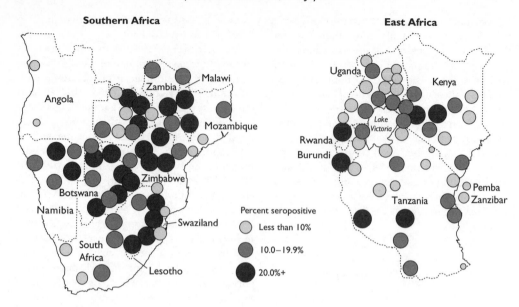

Figure 4.1 *African HIV-1 seroprevalence for lower-risk urban populations in east and southern Africa*
Source: Adapted from U.S. Bureau of the Census, Population Division, International Programs Center, 1999. HIV/AIDS Surveillance Data Base, February 1999. Washington, DC: U.S. Bureau of the Census.

underemployment in turn increases the vulnerability of migrants, especially women, if they are forced to turn to commercial sex work in attempts to gain adequate incomes (Schoepf 2000; Craddock 2000). There is also a greater chance for unscrutinized behavior among migrant populations away from home, families, and the often more confining moral systems characterizing rural life.

While urban areas lead in rates of infection, the disease is spreading rapidly in rural areas, propelled by rural–urban linkages, lower levels of knowledge about HIV in rural areas, and disrupted sexual economies caused by conditions of migration and employment. While highly complex in cause and pattern, rural–urban migration in Burundi, Rwanda, Kenya, and Uganda may in part be explained by the declining contribution of the agricultural sector to GDP since 1980: Burundi from 62 to 58 percent, Rwanda from 50 to 39 percent, Kenya from 33 to 29 percent, and Uganda from 72 to 44 percent (World Bank 1999).[1] Yet most migrants retain links to their rural villages, creating both circular movements and a two-way flow of people that help facilitate the

HIV/AIDS exchange. In addition, in southern Africa, rural areas have from colonial times traditionally sent thousands of its young men to the mines of South Africa to work on two- to three-year contract arrangements. In the case of Malawian workers, migrants spend a week or so in the cities having a "good time" before going back to their home villages in the countryside (Kalipeni 1995), or during the course of their contract they turn to commercial sex workers servicing the mines (cf. Campbell this volume). It is estimated that nearly half of the mine workers returning to rural areas after a work stint in South Africa are infecting their wives and other women (Gould 1993). Indeed, the rapid diffusion of the disease in this region has been ascribed to a high level of "sexual mobility" – to such factors as men's premarital and extramarital sexual activity during frequent work-related absences from home, institutionalized commercial sex work in the towns, the lack of other economic opportunities for divorcees and widows, and polygyny and related postpartum sexual abstinence for wives, but not for husbands (Campbell 1997; Caraël 1996; Chilivumbo 1975). As a result, recent data from southern

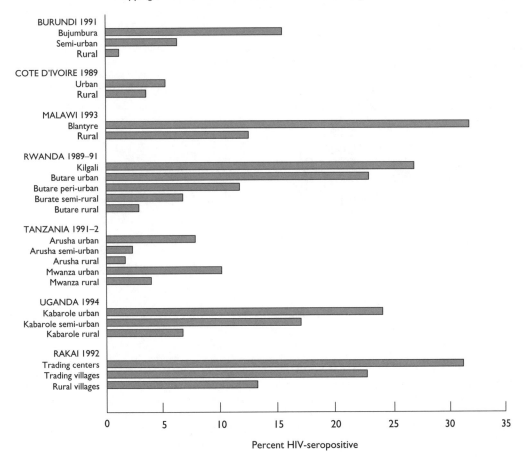

Figure 4.2 *Urban–rural differentials in HIV infection*
Source: U.S. Bureau of the Census.

Africa show that rural–urban differentials have begun to disappear (see Figure 4.3).

Neglected Routes of Transmission

Gender and age have become foci of AIDS researchers for the ominous implications indicated by recent trends in data. The majority of AIDS cases are in the 20–49 age group, with the lowest rates in the 5–14 age range. The 0–4 age group shows significantly higher numbers of infection, an indication that infants are being infected either in the womb before birth or while being taken care of by infected mothers (see Figure 4.4). One interesting trend in the data is that women appear to be exposed to the disease at earlier ages than men. For example, there is a preponderance of females in the age range 15–24 while men are slightly more predominant in the age groups above 30 years. The "Sugar Daddy" phenomenon can be invoked here as a plausible explanation for the age/sex mismatch. Researchers elsewhere in Africa frequently reveal that older men in particular are looking toward schoolgirls for sexual exchange. As these men begin to realize the real and quite personal danger of intercourse with their usual "girlfriends," they entice young girls 10–15 years of age into sexual relationships, hoping that this age range may be relatively free of infection. The age/sex disparities shown in Figure 4.4 seem to support this assertion. Throughout the world, the ratio of female to

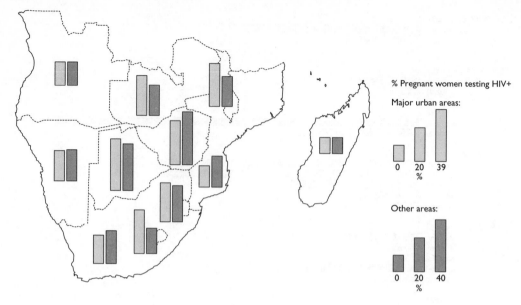

Figure 4.3 *Differentials between urban and rural HIV infection rates for pregnant women in southern Africa*
Source: Authors; data from UNAIDS 2000.

male cases is rising, but women in sub-Saharan Africa are at greatest risk, and show the highest seroprevalence. Reasons for this are not entirely understood, but stem from the convergence of inequitable systems of gender politics and resource allocation, domestic violence, lower rates of education, higher risk of un- and underemployment,[2] rape as a weapon of war, and disproportionate impact of structural adjustment programs, as will be further discussed below (cf. Lurie, Ackeroyd, and Kelby this volume; Schoepf et al 2000).

One of the groups at highest risk in many countries is young people between 15 and 24, where the majority of new infections are concentrated. In one study in Zambia, over 12 percent of the 15- and 16-year-olds seen at antenatal clinics were already infected with HIV (UNAIDS and WHO 1999). Girls appear to be especially vulnerable to infection, but Uganda has recently shown encouraging evidence that in some city sites infection rates have halved among teenage girls since 1990. Even there, however, the rates remain unacceptably high, with up to one pregnant teenager in ten testing HIV positive. That rate is six times higher than in boys of the same age (UNAIDS and WHO 1999).

In South Africa, infection rates of pregnant women less than 20 years old rose from less than 2 percent in 1991 to 20 percent by 1996 (UNAIDS 2001a). In Botswana the infection rate stood at 28 percent for the same group in 1997. Sometimes, young people know of the risks of unprotected sex but feel AIDS could not possibly happen to them. In Malawi, most young men and women know how HIV is transmitted and how it can be prevented. When asked, however, many said they felt invulnerable to the virus. Some 90 percent of teenage boys said they were at no risk or at minimal risk of infection, even though nearly half of them reported at least one casual sex partner over the last year, and condom use was low (Bandawe n.d.).

Men having sex with men is a phenomenon that is either denied in most regions, or about which nothing is known (National Research Council 1996). AIDS in sub-Saharan Africa is considered to be overwhelmingly heterosexual in its transmission, but this perception might be obfuscating sexual exchanges that include males having sex with other men even if the term "homosexuality," as understood in the U.S. or Europe, is unknown. Finally, another route of transmission occurs between mother

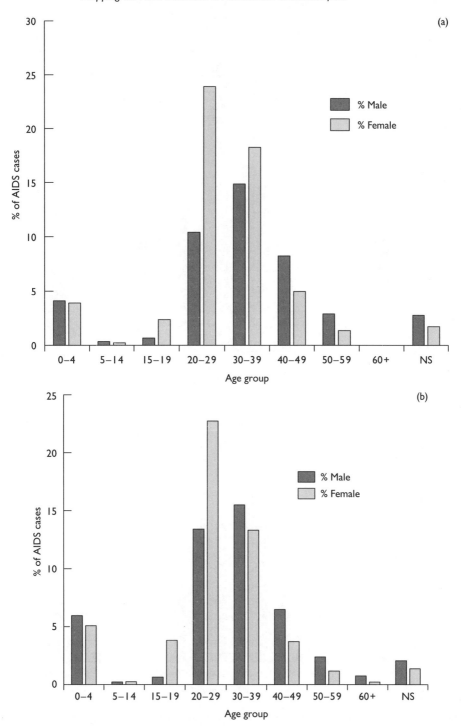

Figure 4.4 *Age/sex distribution of HIV/AIDS in selected countries. (a) Reported AIDS cases for Lesotho, 1999; (b) Reported AIDS cases for South Africa, 1999*
Source: Authors; data from UNAIDS 2000.

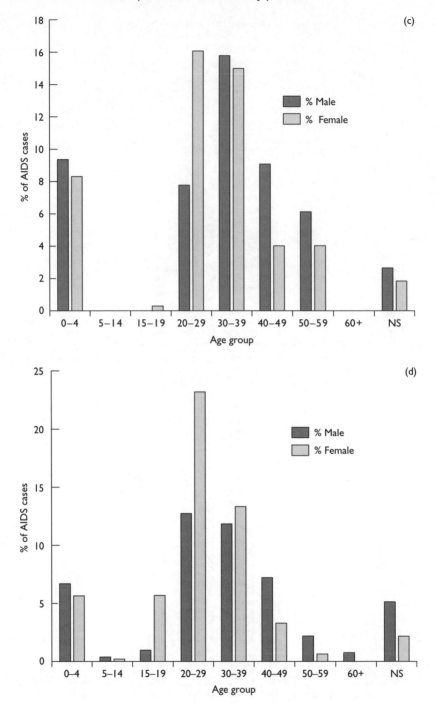

Figure 4.4 *cont'd (c) Reported AIDS cases for Botswana, 1999; (d) Reported AIDS cases for Swaziland, 1999*

and child, with HIV being passed to the infant either during the birth process, or during breastfeeding.

Broader Contexts

Most east African countries recognized the problem of AIDS and instituted some form of prevention program by the mid- or late 1980s (Serwadda et al. 1994). With some degree of variation, these programs have been characterized as targeting behavioral change through educational outreach and increased condom availability. Educational outreach has meant, for most countries, making their constituencies more aware of AIDS as a serious problem, and increasing levels of knowledge about how HIV can and cannot be transmitted. Making condoms more available has usually meant both subsidization and distribution. These strategies, while constituting a necessary first step in AIDS prevention, have proven to be of limited value in diminishing transmission of HIV in most regions. The reasons for this are too many to cover comprehensively in this chapter, but the final section attempts to tease out some of the primary factors.

One of the problems inherent in educational outreach is that greater awareness of AIDS does not necessarily mean the ability to change risky behaviors. Outreach campaigns are based implicitly on the notion of rational behavior, that is, that with new knowledge comes automatic adjustment in social or sexual practices. This approach elides the broader context of power relations, economic necessity, and resource limitations within which HIV transmission occurs. It is little wonder, then, that knowledge of AIDS and its transmission routes is rarely a predictor of less risky behavior in studies that have examined this association (National Research Council 1996). Condom use, for example, has increased considerably in some regions, but not in others. The reasons behind the failure of most countries to raise condom usage encapsulate some of the problems inherent in current prevention strategies.

Whether men or women use condoms in their sexual exchanges depends on a number of factors that are slowly being illuminated (Treichler 1992a; NSC 1996; Miles 1993). One factor is the power dynamics within which sexual exchange takes place. As in most societies, women in east and southern African countries by and large are not considered of equal status to men socially, nor does equity tend to characterize women's personal relationships with men. Where sexual exchange is concerned, this impacts women in two primary ways. First, it means that women cannot always dictate the terms of sex because they do not have the social capital to do so. Purported beliefs in some regions that men by nature must have sex frequently (Caldwell and Caldwell 1993) combine with social hierarchies to create sexual exchanges whose terms are established more by men than by women. Second, it means that women are not always in the economic position to say no to partners who will not assent to using condoms. Whether in a marriage that the woman relies upon for financial reasons, or in commercial sexual exchanges, the longer-term and contingent possibility of HIV infection becomes subordinated to the more acute short-term necessities of economic survival.

Second, condom use is embedded in varied cultural structures of meaning that impinge upon its widespread acceptance. Some studies have determined, for example, that both men and women perceive condoms as impeding sexual pleasure (Msapato et al. 1990), or that in precluding the ejaculation of semen into the vagina, condoms disrupt the underlying value of sexual exchange. As described by Philip Setel in his study of AIDS in northern Tanzania, sex for young men was like a market transaction where taking a man's semen was part of the woman's bargain. Using a condom in this context "was like getting cheated in a deal" (Setel 1996:1175). Finally, condoms are seen in many regions of east Africa as symbols of promiscuity. Asking one's partner to use a condom is thus tantamount to accusations or admissions of sexual promiscuity (NSC 1996).

A better assessment of how condoms might be made more acceptable is in part contingent upon better awareness of sexual behaviors and their many regional differences. This hinges, inter alia, upon better understandings of primary relationships and their different configurations under particular circumstances, and the highly variable conditions, definitions, and circumstances in which commercial sexual exchange takes place.

One of the difficulties of gaining better information about sexual behaviors in different regions of east and southern Africa centers around the definition of concepts such as marriage (NSC 1996). Not only do many regions practice some form of polygyny, but long-term and recent social economic changes have fostered new forms of relationships that may or may not be defined as marriage (Setel 1996). Establishing sexual relationships outside of marriage is relatively common in many areas of east and southern Africa, for example. These relationships may be casual and short term, they may be with commercial sex workers, or they may be stable and enduring (Ndinya-Achola et al. 1997; NSC 1996; Akeroyd 1997). These relationships tend to be more common with men, yet are not unknown to women. In one study undertaken in Nairobi, for example, last sex was with a commercial sex worker or casual partner for 26 percent of those men living with a spouse (Ndinya-Achola et al. 1997:506). Two or more partners during the past year were also reported for 82 percent of the men surveyed, and 25 percent of the women. Migration patterns add to the chances that men will establish second families in their place of work, or that women left behind will seek other relationships in their husband's absence. Many studies are also finding that adolescents of both sexes become sexually active early, sometimes by 13 or 14 (Helitzer-Allen 1994), and have had several partners by the time they enter into marriage. These examples simply serve to enforce greater recognition of a growing diversity of sexual unions evolving in response to changing social economic landscapes, and that asking study participants about their marital status is not necessarily a predictor of vulnerability to HIV.

Many studies on AIDS in sub-Saharan Africa focus on the role of commercial sex workers (CSWs) in transmitting HIV, yet few bother to problematize the meaning of that term or to analyze why women enter into commercial sexual exchanges. In regions of east and southern Africa, women may enter into relationships with men for various financial reasons, and with broadly discrepant results in terms of

their risk for HIV. Full-time CSWs work usually in cities or in peri-urban truck stops, but even here their work takes various forms and entails varying degrees of risk. In one study based in Nairobi, HIV seropositivity was found in 66 percent of CSWs of low socio-economic status, but in 31 percent of those of higher socio-economic status (Kreiss et al. 1986). Most CSWs working in African cities face extremely high risk of acquiring HIV, but more studies need to elucidate why some are at higher risk than others, and under what circumstances condoms may become a possible and even acceptable part of sexual exchange. Recent studies have suggested, for example, that women identifying themselves as sex workers might have greater leverage in negotiating condom use than those who do not identify as sex workers but who use sex exchanges as strategies for survival (Schoepf 2001).

Many women who do not consider themselves CSWs engage in other forms of sexual relationships that incorporate some form of financial exchange. These may come in the form of teenaged girls servicing businessmen in return for school fees or gifts (the Sugar Daddies mentioned above), longer-term relationships in which money or gifts are occasionally bestowed, or infrequent paid sexual exchanges to supplement incomes earned from trading or other occupations (NSC 1996). All of these relationships may be considered commercial to the extent that financial gain is involved, yet they are widely divergent in their form, duration, nature, and risk. As long as "prostitution" and "commercial sex workers" remain undefined and undifferentiated terms in research on AIDS, little understanding will come of the reasons why women engage in different forms of sexual exchange, the conditions under which these exchanges take place, or of the kinds of interventions needed.

Finally, we assert that effective prevention programs cannot be established until there is better understanding of *why* women enter into commercial sexual exchanges that might increase their risk of HIV. In many areas of east and southern Africa, underemployment is a problem for both men and women, a factor that puts into motion a number of contingencies underlying HIV risk. Men tend more frequently than women to migrate in search of jobs in both east and southern Africa (NSC 1996), while women often have few income-earning opportunities available to them if they are not financially supported by their husbands. For those women with little formal education, prostitution or infrequent commercial sexual exchange can be the only way to make a viable living. In this case, expanding employment opportunities makes a more effective AIDS prevention strategy than simply trying to make conditions less risky once women have already entered into commercial sexual exchanges.

Strategies for the Future

Current prevention strategies have increased knowledge about HIV and AIDS in many African countries, but they have not made an overall difference in rate of transmission. More effective prevention strategies will need to address those underlying causes of HIV and AIDS that are rooted in inequitable gender relations, lack of employment opportunities for both men and women, and cultural meanings surrounding forms and functions of sexual exchange. But it also means disrupting current institutional practices at the international level that are negatively impacting national economies and local livelihoods. There is not enough time to adequately address international-scale relationships to HIV transmission in this chapter, so two examples will have to suffice. First, IMF-dictated structural adjustment policies almost certainly have a negative effect on AIDS in sub-Saharan Africa.

As the economies of poor southern African countries such as Malawi, Zambia, and Angola failed in the 1980s, financial and technical assistance from multilateral organizations such as the World Bank was conditioned by the World Bank's structural adjustment programs (SAPs). The SAPs were initiated to promote greater economic efficiency and economic growth to make sub-Saharan economies more competitive in today's global economy (Aryeetey-Attoh 1997; Asthana 1994). As Aryeetey-Attoh (1997) notes, candidates for structural adjustment were those with budget deficits, balance-of-payment problems, high inflationary rates, ineffective state bureaucracies, inefficient agricultural and industrial production sectors, overvalued currencies, and inefficient credit institutions. SAPs have a number of features which have negatively affected the position of the urban poor, women and children, but major features include trade liberalization, government expenditure reduction, devaluation of currencies, reduction of controls over foreign currency, and trade union restrictions.

Evidence indicates that the deleterious effects of SAPs on health and social services throughout Africa have been far reaching. Living conditions for urban and rural populations have deteriorated, the educational infrastructure has crumbled, and the health care services are in dire straits (Potts 1995; Lensink 1996; Lurie et al. 1995; Tevera 1997). For example, Lensink (1996) notes that with respect to Africa the number of people between the ages of 6 and 23 who received education decreased during the 1980s and the number of people per doctor and per nurse increased significantly. Generally, adjustment programs have had dramatic negative effects on quality of care, health service utilization due to the imposition of user fees, search for alternative sources of health care, changes in mortality and morbidity, and nutritional status. Others have analyzed these issues for various regions (Schoepf et al. 2000, Lurie et al. this volume), but we will briefly discuss them here in terms of southern Africa.

Decreased expenditure on health care is one outcome of SAPs that has hit southern African countries hard. Tevera (1997) clearly demonstrates that in the course of the 1980s government funding for the health sector in Zimbabwe became inadequate for the provision of basic health services, and even more so for the support of community-based health care (Tevera 1997). Zimbabwe is one of the few countries in southern Africa that managed to increase government health expenditure in real terms during the 1980s (Chabot et al. 1995). However, this policy of consistent real increases in public financing of health services could not be sustained under the conditions of the structural adjustment programs that started in 1991. As a result, real per capita public expenditure on health dropped by a total of 35 percent between 1991 and 1994 (Chisvo and Munro 1994).

Tevera (1997) notes that the health sector in Zimbabwe has suffered from across-the-board cuts in government expenditures since 1991 and that these cuts have reversed the upward trend in expenditure that had occurred since independence. The end result of the cuts in Zimbabwe's health care expenditure was a 10 percent decline in the number of nurses per person employed by the Ministry of Health and Child Welfare between 1991 and 1992, from more than 9 per 10,000 to just over 8 per 10,000 population. By mid-1992 about 800 health workers had been retrenched and 400 nursing posts had been abolished. This was followed by a substantial decline in the public funding of drugs and the imposition of user fees as part of cost-recovery. The stringent implementation of fee collection together with the requirement of advance payment, particularly for maternity care, has already had a deterrent effect in terms of utilization of government services in Zimbabwe (Tevera 1997). Drugs are in short supply and their costs have increased sharply and are beyond the reach of most of the low-income earners. Perhaps the most tragic consequence in Zimbabwe is a steady increase in deaths from diseases (for example, easily treatable infant diseases and TB) that in the past had been brought under control. This is in large part because of the indirect effects of structural adjustment on nutrition, unhealthy living conditions, and poverty. Similar narratives can be told for health care delivery systems in Botswana, Malawi, Zambia, Zaire, Angola, and Mozambique (see, for example, McPake 1993).

In Zambia poverty is now a major national problem where it is estimated that as much as 42 percent of the urban population lives below the poverty line (Kalumba 1990). The price of basic commodities, such as chicken, has increased more than tenfold during the past decade, whereas in the same period wages only doubled. Studies suggest that the consumption pattern in poor households is changing from relatively protein- and energy-rich food toward less expensive, bulkier foods, with a decreasing number of meals per day (Streefland et al. 1995).

This process of impoverishment hits women harder than men, in particular because SAPs reinforce an already existing process of mar-

ginalization of women's production. Where SAPs lead to an increase in production, they stimulate the production of cash crops for export – such as cotton, cocoa, tea, and coffee – often to the detriment of household consumption (Streefland et al. 1995). The increase in cash crop production, usually controlled by men, also leads to increase in workloads for female family members. Further, women must bear the brunt of the social consequences of adjustment measures. Since they are also responsible for social and health aspects within the family, it is they who must cope with the increased burden of disease and hunger. In short, structural adjustment programs have had a disproportionate impact on increasing their workload while often yielding very few benefits health-wise and economically.

There is growing evidence of the impact of structural adjustment on the health of mothers and infants. Costello et al. (1994) argues that most of the child mortality rates presented in World Bank tables should be viewed with suspicion, as such data are based on extrapolation rather than direct measurements. Directly measured estimates for Zambia show a rise in infant mortality from 176 to 190 per thousand live births in the period between 1975 and 1992. As already indicated above, the Zambia Demographic and Health Survey data confirm this finding. In Zimbabwe, infant and child mortality exhibited a downward trend throughout the early and mid-1980s. The infant mortality rate declined from between 120 and 150 per thousand live births before 1980 to 61 by 1990, whereas the child mortality rate (children one to five years of age) declined from around 40 to 22 per thousand during the same period (Chabot et al. 1995). However, as UNICEF (1994, 1996) data indicate, evidence is accumulating that both indicators began to rise in the late 1980s and 1990s. In addition to economic decline, deteriorating health services, and drought, the impact of HIV/AIDS is suspected to have contributed significantly to these observed changes in infant, childhood, and maternal mortality rates in countries such as Zimbabwe, Zambia, Botswana, and Malawi. These views have been held widely and forcefully enough to cause the World Bank members at recent meetings to list debt forgiveness among future actions. However, there is great need for continued criticism of these policies and the institutions such as the IMF and the World Bank that prioritize loan repayment before people's lives.

The decision by the World Health Organization to encourage women in sub-Saharan countries not to breastfeed their babies in order to curtail mother-to-child HIV transmission shows a similar lack of political morality. Although represented as a difficult choice between HIV transmission and increased dysentery from bottle feeding, the WHO failed to mention that they might have brought their considerable political weight to bear upon pharmaceutical companies to donate AZT and other life-saving drugs as a humanitarian gesture in the face of overburdened health care systems and widespread poverty. Interference in the lives of poor African women and their children is apparently more expedient than interfering in the profit motives of corporate giants. Though the pricing policies of multinational pharmaceutical giants have recently been contested (see Craddock this volume), the issue of pharmaceutical profit versus people's lives remains trenchant. In summary, prevention strategies need to get beyond the rhetoric of "more research" and "more education" to hit hard at the international, national, and local economic contingencies feeding the flames of the AIDS epidemic.

NOTES

1. The reasons for rural to urban migration are of course much more complicated and varied than a depreciating agricultural sector. For more thorough overviews of the connections between rural poverty, migration, and risk of HIV/AIDS, see Schoepf et al. 2000; Farmer et al. 1996; Lurie this volume).

2. In Burundi, Kenya, Rwanda, and Uganda female labor force participation rates ranged between 46 and 50 percent (World Bank 1999). Female illiteracy in Burundi is nearly 78 percent, in Kenya 30 percent, Rwanda 48 percent, and Uganda 50 percent (World Bank 1999).

Chapter 5

HIV/AIDS in West Africa: The Case of Senegal, Ghana, and Nigeria

Joseph R. Oppong and Samuel Agyei-Mensah

Introduction

With 83 percent of the world's total AIDS deaths and 87 percent of its HIV-infected children, sub-Saharan Africa is the worst-affected region for the dreaded disease (UNAIDS 2000a). Nevertheless, the devastation of HIV/AIDS is not uniform throughout the region. Scattered throughout the continent and even in the countries of relatively low HIV prevalence are districts, villages, or ethnic groups coping with high levels of infection that may be several times the national average (Decosas and Adrien 1999). Compared to eastern and southern Africa, west Africa has suffered less, but the situation is changing rapidly. Côte d'Ivoire is among the 15 worst-affected countries in the world, and in Nigeria, by far the most populous country in sub-Saharan Africa, about 5 percent of adults aged between 15 and 49 are now living with HIV. Apart from Senegal, which has shown some decrease, the epidemic continues to rise in Nigeria, Côte d'Ivoire, Ghana, and other west African countries.

This chapter examines the magnitude and geography of the disease in west Africa by highlighting the puzzling inter- and intra-country differences. It raises and attempts to address several research questions: What are the principal features of the HIV/AIDS pandemic in west Africa and how do they vary spatially? What are the most distinctive recent trends? What factors underlie these patterns? We argue that the spatial patterns of HIV/AIDS in west Africa probably reflect the spatial distribution of vulnerable social groups and societal destructuring through gender-segregated labor migration. The chapter begins with a description of the patterns of HIV/AIDS in west Africa, followed by specific case studies from Nigeria, Senegal, and Ghana. The third part attempts an explanation of the observed patterns.

Patterns of HIV/AIDS in West Africa

Why west Africa has such low HIV/AIDS rates compared to eastern and southern Africa is not fully understood. An often-cited reason is the dominance of a different strain of the virus, HIV-2, which does not transmit as easily as HIV-1, the virus responsible for AIDS in the rest of Africa. Moreover, infection with HIV-2 is less likely to cause AIDS. HIV-1 has at least ten genetic subtypes and the five major subtypes are labeled A, B, C, D, and E. The predominant subtype in Europe and North America is type B, but A and C predominate in Africa, and the latter is supposed to be a more aggressive virus that is easier to transmit (Decosas and Adrien 1999). HIV-1 group O viruses have also been identified in west Africa, although in very low rates (0.3 percent) (Peeters et al. 1996, 1997). Subtypes I and J, initially considered rare, have also been identified in west Africa (Montavon et al. 1999).

Although west Africa has an unusually high number of reported HIV-2 cases compared to HIV-1, significant variations exist between countries. Senegal and Guinea-Bissau have consistently shown higher HIV-2 prevalence rates (Smallman-Raynor et al. 1992; Decosas and Adrien 1999). In sharp contrast, Ghana exhibits a higher preponderance of HIV-1 cases (Brandful et al. 1997). Analysis of sentinel surveillance data shows that in 1999, 92.8 percent of Ghana's HIV infections were attributable to HIV-1, with only 2.8 percent being HIV-2, and 4.5 percent due to both (Ghana National AIDS Control Program 2000). Throughout west Africa, the highest rates of HIV-2 infection have been reported consistently among those groups considered at heightened risk for HIV-1 infection, namely commercial sex workers (CSW) and sexually transmitted disease (STD) patients (Smallman-Raynor et al. 1992).

While heterosexual transmission predominates, west Africa's HIV pandemic comprises of mini-epidemics, each with its own characteristics in terms of trends in HIV prevalence, those affected, and the HIV-related opportunistic diseases observed. Considerable variations exist between and within countries. Countries with adult HIV prevalence rates of between 5 and 9 percent include Burkina Faso, Togo, Cameroon, and Nigeria (UNAIDS and ECA 2000). The 1999 survey on HIV/Syphilis in Nigeria places the national average of HIV infection at 5.4 percent, up from a 1990 average of 1.8 percent. Cameroon currently has a rate of 7.73 percent, Ghana 3.6 percent, while Benin and Niger currently stand at 2.45 and 1.35 percent respectively (UNAIDS and ECA 2000). Beyond the national level, significant variations also exist within the major cities. Rural HIV often remains silent and invisible because of poor health infrastructure, restricted access to

health facilities, and inadequate testing and surveillance. It is fueled by poverty, food insecurity, gender inequality, migration, war, and civil conflict and accelerated by migration, trade, the movement of refugees, and strengthened rural–urban linkages (Kalipeni and Oppong 1998).

With an adult rate of almost 11 percent in 2000, Côte d'Ivoire has the most serious and perhaps most studied epidemic in west Africa. HIV-1 seroprevalence among antenatal women ranged between 11 and 14 percent in 1998. While the rate in Abidjan and major urban areas was 16 percent, outside major urban areas it ranged from 6 to 13 percent in 1997 (Diallo et al. 1997). HIV occurs more frequently in younger females. Seven percent of antenatal clinic attendees less than 20 years of age tested in 1997 were HIV positive and among those 20–24 years old, it was 12 percent. CSWs are particularly vulnerable. In a 1995 study of 1209 CSWs, 80 percent were HIV positive (Ghys et al. 1995). Infection was associated with a longer duration of sex work, a lower price per intercourse, and being an immigrant.

Commercial sex, sexually transmitted diseases, and condom neglect are critical factors that fuel Côte d'Ivoire's HIV epidemic (Sassan-Morokro et al. 1996) and spread it to neighboring countries (Decosas et al. 1995; Anarfi 1990). Sexually transmitted diseases are common in pregnant women and, by implication, in the general society (Diallo et al. 1997). Commercial sex work (CSW) by women from Ghana and other neighboring countries is widespread, particularly in Abidjan, and most of the female commercial sex workers are HIV positive (Ghys et al. 1995). Moreover, unnecessary and excessive blood transfusion of poorly screened blood may be contributory factors (Lackritz et al. 1993). The burden on the health system is overwhelming. In 1997, AIDS patients occupied 41 percent of all hospital beds in Abidjan and AIDS-related costs absorbed 11 percent of the total public health budget (UNAIDS and ECA 2000).

With an adult rate of 7.73 percent, Cameroon is west Africa's second most affected country (UNAIDS and ECA 2000). HIV prevalence among antenatal women tested in the major urban areas was 4–5 percent in 1996 but outside of the major urban areas, it was 8 percent. Among sex workers tested in the major urban areas, nearly 30 percent were positive in 1993 for both HIV-1 and HIV-2, but in 1995 it had fallen to 17 percent. In Yaoundé, the national capital, HIV prevalence among STD clinic patients was 16 percent in 1996. Outside the major urban areas, it ranged from 8 to 9 percent. Between 15 and 17 percent of truck drivers and 15 percent of military personnel tested are HIV positive (UNAIDS 2000c).

Burkina Faso is west Africa's third most affected country, with a prevalence rate of 6.44 percent. It is one of the world's poorest countries and ranks 171 out of 174 countries on the Human Development Index. A study of two large cities in Burkina Faso, Bobo-Dioulosso and Ouagadougou, in 1994 revealed an overall HIV seroprevalence of 58.2 percent among female sex workers, 18.6 percent among truck drivers, and 8 percent among pregnant women (Lankoande et al. 1998; Meda et al. 1998). Although most had heard of the disease, 41 percent of pregnant women, 40 percent of truck drivers, and 61 percent of female sex workers did not consider themselves at risk for HIV. Condom use among them was low: 0.1, 18, and 42 percent for pregnant women, truck drivers, and sex workers respectively. A 1996 study of pregnant women in Bobo-Dioulosso revealed a 10 percent seroprevalence rate (Meda et al. 1999).

Benin has a population of 5.7 million of whom 2.45 percent are living with HIV, up from 0.32 percent in 1990 (UNAIDS and ECA 2000). According to the latest figures, the epidemic is spreading quickly to rural areas. HIV prevalence among antenatal women tested in the major urban areas increased from no evidence of infection in 1986–7 to 4 percent in 1998. In 1998, HIV prevalence ranged from 3 to 6 percent. HIV prevalence among sex workers tested in Cotonou and other towns increased from 5 percent in 1987 to 54 percent in 1996 but outside the major urban areas it was 47 percent (UNAIDS 2000d).

Due to political instability and war, HIV/AIDS figures for Liberia and Sierra Leone are unreliable. In fact, scant information on HIV prevalence is available for Liberia. In Monrovia, 4 percent of antenatal clinic women tested positive for HIV in 1992 and 1993. In 1996 and 1997, HIV testing at various sites found no evidence of HIV infection among antenatal clinic attendees. In 1998, however, from an unspecified site, 10 percent of antenatal clinic attendees were found to be HIV positive. According to UNAIDS (2000e), there is no information available on HIV prevalence among sex workers. In 1993, 8 percent of male STD clinic patients attending one site in Monrovia tested positive for HIV. However, the military have been identified as a major source of spread (Pan African News Agency 1998), and young female Liberian refugees who have fled to Côte d'Ivoire and who have resorted to commercial sex for survival are particularly vulnerable.

Similarly, little information on HIV prevalence is available for Sierra Leone. Two percent of antenatal clinic women in a non-specified region tested positive for HIV-1 in 1992. A 1995 sero-survey conducted among sex workers in Freetown found that 27 percent tested positive for HIV-1. Prevalence among STD clinic patients tested in Freetown was about 3 percent between 1988 and 1992 (UNAIDS 2000f).

From this brief review, sexually transmitted diseases, commercial sex workers, truck drivers, and women who provide sex for material benefits on a short-term basis fuel the HIV/AIDS crisis in west Africa. Other important factors include cultural practices such as circumcision and effectiveness of political leadership in the fight against the disease. For a more detailed examination of these factors that appear to be driving the epidemic, and the dynamics accounting for the subtle differences between countries in the sub-region, we present a closer look at three countries that span the spectrum of rapid growth, stable low, and stable medium respectively – Nigeria, Senegal, and Ghana.

HIV/AIDS in Nigeria

Fueled by years of neglect and lack of committed political leadership, HIV/AIDS is quickly becoming a major health issue in Nigeria. According to Professor Ibironke Akinsete, Chairman of the National Action Committee on AIDS in Nigeria, a 1999 survey estimated that 5.4 percent of the adult population or

2.6 million people were infected and that 4.9 million Nigerian adults will be carrying the AIDS virus by 2003 (Akinsete 2000; Oyo 1999). Women in their twenties have the highest rate of HIV infection. Significant geographical variations exist in Nigeria. Prevalence in pregnant women ranged from 0.5 percent in the northeastern state of Yobe to 21 percent in Otukpo, a town in the north central state of Benue, with little difference between urban and rural areas. Benue, where HIV prevalence rose from 2.3 percent in 1995 to 16.8 percent in 1999, is the worst-affected state (Akinsete 2000).

While there are zonal variations, HIV is prevalent in all six geopolitical zones and HIV hotspots exist within every zone where rates are increasing. HIV prevalence in the 20–24 age group ranges from 4.2 percent in the Southwest zone to 9.7 percent in the North Central zone which includes Abuja, the national capital. Among young adults aged between 15 and 19, HIV prevalence ranges from 2.8 percent in the Northeast zone to 8.4 percent in the North Central zone. Hotspots include Akwa Ibom, Benue, Ebony, Kaduna, Lagos, and Tariba. High mobility among Nigeria's population is expected to rapidly spread the high prevalence within the hotspots to other areas as well (Falobi 1999)

Nigeria's HIV/AIDS epidemic is reducing life expectancy and increasing the disease burden and number of orphaned children. According to the 1999 HIV syphilis sentinel seroprevalence survey (Akinsete 2000), disease and death caused by HIV/AIDS will inhibit the development of the country and make individual families and communities poorer. In Nigeria AIDS is not a disease of the poor but afflicts both the poor and the rich. A majority of the cases were HIV-1, but there were also cases of HIV-2 and a mixture of the two strains mainly in border-states. Also, three subtypes of HIV-1 (C, G, and A1) have been identified in the country but there is disagreement on their relative occurrence.

Until Obasanjo became president, Nigeria lacked the political leadership necessary to confront the AIDS crisis. The first National Conference on AIDS in Nigeria was held in Abuja between December 15 and 18, 1998, although AIDS was first identified in the country in 1985.

Organized and sponsored by the Federal Ministry of Health and the Petroleum Trust Fund (PTF), a quasi-autonomous federal agency set up in 1993 to administer proceeds from Nigeria's oil sales, this was the first major government response to the AIDS epidemic in Nigeria. Previously, government activities had been restricted to the severely underfunded National AIDS/STDs Control Program (NASCP), which was established in 1987 (Akinsete 2000). The three-day conference was attended by many participants from government agencies and institutions, but not only was the Head of State, General Abdulsalami Abubakar, absent, but he did not send an address or personal representative. Besides the gap in leadership, the conference revealed that a significant percentage of blood and blood products were transfused without screening in almost all hospitals nationwide (Akinsete 2000; Chikwem et al. 1997; Foundation for Democracy in Africa 2000; Odujinrin and Adegoke 1995).

The threat of a major HIV explosion in Nigeria is high, for several reasons. Knowledge about HIV is very low. Female adolescents are more afraid of unwanted pregnancy than getting AIDS (Ogara et al. 1998). Due to increasing poverty and high rates of inflation – the naira was only 6 percent of its 1985 value in 1996 – the number of commercial sex workers and people who exchange sex for material benefits is increasing (Gill and Aliyu 1992). Poverty is also a major factor in the explosion of female sex work at oil exploration locations (Faleyimu et al. 1999). Orubuloye (1992) describes the deeply rooted sexual networking between long-distance truck drivers and roadside hawkers as a major source of the spread of HIV. Orubuloye et al. (1992) reveal that sexual networking is extensive in most of the country and promotes a slowly increasing epidemic. Moreover, a high level of premarital and extramarital sexual activity exists, usually occasioned by the need for material or economic assistance, particularly among the younger wives in polygamous marriages. In addition to all of these, sex education is still opposed in some parts of the country, and stigma and discrimination against people with AIDS are widespread (Akinsete 2000). Untreated sexually transmitted diseases, a major factor in the spread of HIV, are wide-spread (Decosas 1996). A community survey of genital tract infection reported by Brabin and colleagues found that among 158 girls aged 17–19 years in a rural area, 44 percent had a current genital tract infection, although fewer than 3 percent had ever sought treatment (Brabin et al. 1994). Besides, young girls who have little education or vocational training or capital often have few survival choices but to have sex with older men (Decosas 1996).

Addressing the current leadership gap in AIDS in Nigeria is critical to stem further spread and devastation. President Obasanjo's leadership is promising so far. Supporting this commitment with resources to facilitate research and programming may enable Nigeria to postpone or prevent a major disaster. The supplementary budget allocation for AIDS control for 1999, which exceeded the total budget for AIDS from 1996–8 (UNAIDS 2000j), is a good beginning, but more is required. Since Nigerian males generally resent using condoms, introducing the female condom very quickly should be a high priority. Without some major radical programs, Nigeria faces a major epidemic with widespread disastrous consequences.

HIV/AIDS in Senegal

Senegal has been widely proclaimed as a model AIDS success story. With a per capita income of U.S. $530 a year, and life expectancy of only 52 years, Senegal is among the world's poorer countries, and not much different from other west African countries. Some 57 percent of adult men and 77 percent of women are illiterate. Government spending on health from public funds is around U.S. $1 per capita, and at least 40 percent of spending on health comes out of family budgets. In the 1980s and early 1990s, an economic downturn and devaluation of the currency under economic restructuring led to the collapse of much of the government-run infrastructure in health. The number of medical consultations fell by eight percent between 1978 and 1986, even though the population grew by 28 percent over the same period.

In a very fascinating way, religious practices are a major factor in Senegal's HIV/AIDS suc-cess. About 93 percent of the population is Muslim and 5 percent is Christian. In add-ition to Muslim and Christian religious leaders actively promoting fidelity and family and sexual norms that reduce HIV transmission, various religious traditions and practices limit its rapid spread in Senegal (Oppong 1998b). First, circumcision is universally practiced, producing a reduced risk of transmission of HIV from men (UNAIDS 1999e). Second, in accordance with Islamic tradition, alcohol consumption is uncommon, reducing the associated risk of casual sex and thereby HIV transmission.

Polygamy is common in Senegal but prom-iscuity is not. Polygamy is the norm in Islam, but promiscuity is stringently punished to promote stable poly-partner fidelity. While nearly half of all married women are in polygamous unions, they rarely have partners other than their husband. In a 1997 Dakar study reported by UNAIDS (1999f), 99 percent of married women said they had not had sex with anyone except their husband in the preceding 12 months. Among men, the figure was 88 per-cent. Besides, sex before marriage is tradition-ally uncommon for Senegalese women. In the Dakar behavioral study, 68 percent of women but only 10 percent of men said they had not had sex before marriage. Moreover, Senegalese women tend to be relatively old at first mar-riage compared to women in other countries in Africa. While half of all women are married by age 20, half of men remain unmarried by age 31. Paradoxically, then, while poly-partner sexual activity may be the norm, Senegalese may not be as vulnerable as those in other countries that frown on polygamy but accept a long series of monogamous sexual liaisons.

Intriguingly, while commercial sex is legal in Senegal, an aggressive war against STDs appears to have limited the spread of HIV. Ever since prostitution was legalized in 1969, registered sex workers have been required to have regular health checks, and are treated for curable STDs if necessary. This system of registration provided a framework for ap-proaching sex workers with educational and health campaigns. Moreover, to prevent STD spread in the general population, a national STD control program was established and STD care was integrated into regular primary health services. A massive program of training health workers in the management of STDs produced improved quality of care compared with a baseline study before training. Provision of correct advice about future prevention as well as about partner notification rose dramatically (UNAIDS 1999e).

When AIDS was first detected in Senegal, preventive interventions centering on the promotion of condom use with clients were immediately put in place. Many sex workers began to join support groups to safeguard their health in the face of AIDS. Over thirty such groups have been established. Members attend talks, films, and other information sessions about HIV and AIDS, usually around five times a year. They also act as outreach educators for women who work in the sex trade but who have not joined support groups. There are also renewed efforts to reach populations that may be regular suppliers or consumers of casual sex, whether or not in exchange for money. These include mobile populations such as migrant workers and transport workers. Locations where casual sex may take place, such as weekly markets, are also targeted for more active prevention efforts.

Government leadership, exemplified by rapid, decisive actions and unqualified support, has been a major factor in Senegal's success. When the first six cases of AIDS were reported in 1986, a national AIDS program was immediately set up, and steps were quickly taken to protect the population from exposure to the virus. For example, a system for screening every blood unit for transfusion for HIV antibodies had been established in all ten regions of the country by 1987. While politicians in some other countries ignored the threat of AIDS and some vehemently denied its existence in their countries (Gould 1993), the Senegalese government aggressively waged war against the disease. It invested close to U.S. $20 million in AIDS prevention programs between 1992 and 1996 and tackled obstacles to program success (UNAIDS 1999e). For example, an excise tax that quadrupled the price of condoms was dropped to help condom promotion campaigns. Consistent political support for the leadership of the national AIDS program has also contributed to a successful response.

While religion is a major fact of life in Senegal, conflict with religious leaders over AIDS prevention campaigns, a problem that paralyzes and cripples prevention efforts in some countries, does not exist. Religious leaders are actively involved in AIDS prevention efforts. As early as 1989, a conservative Islamic organization, Jamra, approached the national AIDS program to discuss HIV prevention strategies. Although initially rather hostile to condom promotion and some other aspects of AIDS prevention, the group became an important partner in a dialogue between public health officials and religious leaders. Subsequently, educational materials were designed to meet the needs of religious leaders. Training sessions about HIV were organized for Imams and teachers of Arabic, and brochures were produced to help them disseminate information. AIDS became a regular topic in Friday sermons in mosques throughout Senegal, and senior religious figures addressed the issue on television and radio. The moral support for AIDS prevention given by religious leaders allowed secular and health authorities to work productively in providing education and specific HIV prevention services.

Senegal's effort at preventing the disease among young people has been spectacular. Although sexual activity starts relatively late in Senegal, an effort was made to introduce sex education early. By 1992, sex education was part of the curriculum in both primary and secondary schools. In addition, an effort was made to reach young people who were not in school, mostly through youth groups. Through religious and community organizations, parents were actively encouraged to assume responsibility for protecting their children's sexual health by providing full information and support for safe behavior.

AIDS awareness campaigns have clearly been a tremendous success in Senegal. UNAIDS (1999e) reports that condom use rose from virtually nothing before the AIDS epidemic to 67 percent among men having casual sex in 1997. Moreover, in repeat cross-sectional surveys in 1997 and 1998, over 95 percent of secondary school pupils and 99 percent of sex workers knew about AIDS and could name at least two correct ways of preventing it. High proportions also knew about more complex issues such as asymptomatic infection. Four out of five students and close to 70 percent of sex workers knew that someone who looks per-fectly healthy could transmit HIV. HIV counts from 1989 to 1996 for pregnant women in Dakar have remained quite level with no upward trend, while the prevalence of various STDs among sex workers fell sharply from 1991 to 1996 (Ross et al. 1999).

In short, Senegal's success is attributable, among other things, to cultural practices – cir-cumcision, fidelity in polygamous relations – and effective political leadership that trans-lated into early decisive and comprehensive action to prevent an AIDS crisis.

HIV/AIDS in Ghana

HIV/AIDS is becoming a serious problem in Ghana where the number of AIDS cases reported has been increasing in the past five years. From a low figure of 42 AIDS cases in 1986, the number of reported cases stood at 41,229 at the end of September 2000. Out of this number, 25,753 are females and 15,476 are males. Sentinel surveillance data suggests that about 380,000 persons were already infected in 1998. HIV prevalence in the 15–49 age group in Ghana, which rose from 2.7 per-cent in 1994 to 4.0 percent in 1998, is now estimated to be 4.6 percent and is expected to increase to 6.4 percent in 2004, 8.2 percent in 2009, and 9.5 percent in 2014 (Ghana National AIDS Control Program (GNACP) 1999). More than 90,000 Ghanaians have died from AIDS since the early 1980s, and an estimated 120,000 children have become orphans. The number is expected to increase to 160,000 in the next five years.

The demographic pattern of the epidemic in Ghana is quite distinct (Oppong 1998b; Deco-sas et al. 1995). Unlike many African countries that exhibited a higher or equal male–female ratio at the beginning of the epidemic, typical of Pattern 2, a heterosexually transmitted epi-demic, the pattern in Ghana was about 5 females to 1 male. However, this has changed and a gradual convergence to a 1:1 female–male ratio is imminent. While 83 percent of reported cases in 1986 were female, in 1998 it was only 58 percent. Thus Ghana's current pattern resembles the typical sub-Saharan Africa pattern with females comprising 55 per-cent (Agyei–Mensah 2001).

Young people have become more vulner-able, especially young females (Addai 1999). For example, at the end of 1998, whereas about 2.8 percent of total national AIDS cases were reported among females aged 15 to 19, for males in that age group it was only 0.7 per-cent (Ghana National AIDS Control Program 1999). Evidence from sentinel surveillance data also provides disturbing information about the age patterns. The sentinel site at Agomanya in the rural Krobo area recorded 11.9 percent of infections for 1999 coming from the 15–19 age group. This is the highest, followed by the 25–29 age group with 11.4 percent. In the Ada-braka site in the Greater Accra region, the 15–19 age group recorded the highest percentage of HIV infections with a percentage of 5.2. Similarly high percentages for the 15–19 age group were also visible at the sites at Bolga-tanga (2.2 percent) and Wa (5.2 percent) in the Northern region (Ghana National AIDS Con-trol Program 2000). Ankomah (1998) attributes this vulnerability of young females to their inability to negotiate condom use in premarital sexual exchange relationships. It is important to note that these are not commercial sex workers.

Unique geographical patterns also charac-terize Ghana's epidemic. The brunt of the epi-demic has been in the rural, not the urban areas (Oppong 1998b). HIV prevalence in 1998 was highest in the rural Eastern region with a rate of 7.8 per 100,000, followed by the Ashanti region with a rate of 5.8, Upper west with 1.3, and Northern 0.8. Greater Accra, the most urbanized region (83 percent urbaniza-tion) including the Accra Metropolitan area, had only 2.4 (Ghana National AIDS Control Program 1999). Thus, the Eastern region (only 28 percent urban) has consistently shown a higher incidence of HIV cases and, interest-ingly, the Ashanti region (about 33 percent urban) has the highest number of reported cases of AIDS. Moreover, the spatial pattern of HIV/AIDS is changing as well. During the initial stages of the epidemic in Ghana, the disease was concentrated in the Eastern region but moved to the Ashanti region in the 1990s. In 1998, the Upper East region was quickly emerging as a hotspot, a startling fact given it had no cases at all until recently (Neequaye et al. 1997).

Efforts to explain these unique spatial patterns abound (Oppong 1998b; Decosas et al. 1995; Bedele 1993; Anarfi 1990). The initially high number of cases in the Eastern region is attributed to the return migration of female commercial sex workers from neighboring west African countries, especially Côte d'Ivoire. Anarfi (1990) has shown that many of these women came from the Eastern region, particularly from the Krobo ethnic group who constitute the majority of Ghanaian commercial sex workers in Abidjan, Côte d'Ivoire (Neequaye et al. 1997; Addai 1999; Anarfi et al. 1997; Decosas 1996). Relatively high rates among Krobo women have been attributed to cultural factors, including lack of opportunities for women in a patrilineal inheritance society that prevents females from inheriting land and compels them to migrate and survive by selling sex (Bedele 1983; Decosas et al. 1995; Decosas 1996).

The escalating number of cases in Ashanti should be seen in the context of migration patterns of the Ashantis to both African and western European countries during Ghana's recent economic crisis which precipitated the adoption of structural adjustment. Economic necessity produced risky sexual behavior, including commercial sex work among these economic refugees. Besides, Ashanti region has a chronic shortage of biomedical health services. This translates into limited treatment of sexually transmitted diseases, particularly genital ulcerating diseases, known to facilitate HIV spread. Many people also likely use unsafe medical services, such as multiple injections for different people without sterilization, provided by poorly trained or untrained health-care providers such as itinerant drug vendors (IDVs) (Oppong and Williamson 1996).

In fact, iatrogenic spread has been raised as a major source of concern (Francois 1992; Addo-Yobo and Lovel 1991, 1992). Francois (1992) identifies inadequate facilities for blood screening, and improper use of needles and syringes, as important avenues of spread. The study warns that the poverty and ignorance of patients and health workers put them at risk and that patients should be educated to protest against improper use of needles and blood transfusion. Similarly, Addo-Yobo and

Lovel (1991) conclude that 20 percent of blood transfusions in three hospitals in the Ashanti region were unnecessary and avoidable. Arguably, the situation in the Ashanti region is not much different from the rest of the country. Morover, across the country, HIV, STDs, hepatitis, and other diseases continue to be misdiagnosed (Stauffer 1999) and mistreated.

Several hotspots of HIV are emerging. Generally, the port city of Tema, the mining town of Obuasi, and the border towns of Bole and Hamile in northern Ghana are seen as special risk areas. The spread of AIDS in Tema can be understood within the framework of its historical past, port status, unemployment, and low wages. Even though Tema is an industrialized town, most residents are un-or underemployed and thus have no regular income. This has produced many residents who sell sex for cash. Tema experiences a lot of recurrent migration because a considerable proportion of workers and seamen, separated from their families for long periods, engage in temporary sexual liaisons that increase the risk of HIV spread (Akoto 2000).

The increase in northern Ghana probably reflects cross-border movements to Burkina Faso as a result of the depressed economic activities in Ghana. Evidence from sentinel sites in the region supports this view. For the country as a whole, between 1994 and 1998, the highest rate was recorded in Agomanya in Eastern region with a prevalence rate of 10 percent. This was followed by Hamile, a border town in Upper West region, with a rate of about 4.7 percent. Bole, another border town in the Northern region, follows next with a rate of 4.1 percent. The lowest rate was recorded in Nalerigu in the Northern region with a prevalence rate of 1 percent (Ghana National AIDS Control Program 1995). Recent years have seen an increase in the number of reported cases in the region, especially in the border towns of Bole and Hamile. Despite the predominance of Islam, it appears that harsh economic conditions in the area and in Ghana in general have produced increased migration, particularly of young girls to Burkina Faso to practice prostitution while providing laundry services to miners.

A feature of the age/sex distribution we observed earlier in Ghana was the higher percentage of females aged 15–19 who have been infected as compared to males. While this has something to do with the fact that females enter into sex at relatively much younger ages than men do, it also reflects other factors. In Ghana age at menarche has declined from a median of about 14.5 years to around 13 years in the past three decades due to improvements in diet, personal hygiene, health delivery, education, and general welfare. Within the same period, the median age at first marriage has increased from about 17.5 years to 19.1 years in 1998. This has extended the period between physical maturation and the period of marriage, creating a biosocial gap. Median age at first sexual intercourse, however, was reported to be 17.6 years for females in the 1998 Ghana Demographic Health Survey. Thus there is a gap of 1.5 years between period of initiation into sex and age at marriage. It is within this period that some females have been infected (Awusabo–Asare 2000).

While high levels of HIV/AIDS awareness (over 90 percent) prevail throughout the country, over 70 percent did not consider themselves or their families to be at risk of HIV infection. People seemed to perceive AIDS as a problem that affected "other people." The fact that the initial cases were associated with those who "had traveled outside the country" seems to contribute to the idea that those who do not travel to other countries are not at risk. In summary, Ghana has a relatively low and quite localized problem but immediate comprehensive and aggressive intervention is urgent. Effort should be targeted particularly at vulnerable young females in economically deprived regions of the country, especially those adjacent to high HIV-prevalence countries such as Burkina Faso, Togo, and Côte d'Ivoire, to prevent a major disaster.

Discussion

International prostitution is a major factor in the spread of the disease in west Africa. Reports of Senegalese and Guinea Bissauan commercial sex workers (CSWs) in Gambia, Togolese CSWs in Côte d'Ivoire, and Ghanaian CSWs in Benin, Côte d'Ivoire, and Senegal are examples (Smallman-Raynor et al. 1992; Decosas 1996). The initial pattern of HIV/AIDS concentration in

Ghana accords well with returning CSWs in neighboring west African countries who had previously lived in Côte d'Ivoire and Nigeria. Most of these people were females, thus accounting for the high initial female–male sex ratio.

Why do more women than men have HIV in west Africa? Biological differences make women more vulnerable to HIV infection than men. First, a larger mucosal surface increases exposure. Microlesions, which can occur during intercourse, may be entry points for the virus. This makes very young women even more vulnerable in this respect. Coerced sex increases the risk of microlesions. Second, there is more virus in sperm than in vaginal secretions. As with STDs, women are at least four times more vulnerable to infection because of the presence of untreated STDs, a major risk factor for HIV. Besides, financial or material dependence on men means that women cannot control when, with whom, and in what circumstances they have sex (UNAIDS 1999f). In the present difficult economic circumstances, many women have to exchange sex for material favors, for daily survival, in a semi-formal relationship. For some women, this may be the only way of providing for themselves and their children. While men are seeking younger partners, women are expected to have relations with or marry older men, who can support them, and are more likely to be infected.

The effect of civil wars and the military/police

Relatively little attention has been paid to the effects of civil wars on the geography of HIV/AIDS in west Africa. Recent evidence suggests that this may be an important factor in explaining the scourge of the disease, particularly in Liberia and Nigeria. The volatile mix of refugees, soldiers, desperate women with children, and the chaos associated with war facilitate the spread of HIV/AIDS. Chaos incubates disease. During the civil war that engulfed the country for nearly ten years, most Liberians fled to Ghana, Nigeria, and Côte d'Ivoire. The difficulty in adjustment and economic survival forced some of the women into commercial sex work, producing high rates among these refugees. It is not certain whether the deadly virus was contracted before or after migration. Sexual exploitation is frequently an element of persecution, particularly for refugee women, and may be part of the experience with border officials and other people in the host region. Besides, rape is widespread in many refugee camps (Kalipeni and Oppong 1998).

Military personnel have an elevated risk of exposure to sexually transmitted diseases, including HIV/AIDS. Posted far away from their families and social controls, usually with no other means for sexual gratification, soldiers on deployment regularly have sexual contacts with commercial sex workers and the local population (UNAIDS 1998e). Between 30,000 and 50,000 Nigerian soldiers were engaged in peacekeeping, beginning in 1991 in Liberia and Guinea, and lately in Sierra Leone. West African soldiers, for example, fathered some 25,000 children during peacekeeping missions in Liberia between 1990 and 1998 (Pan African News Agency 1998).

In Liberia, for example, a 1998 epidemiology report showed that the highest incidence of AIDS and sexually transmitted diseases was in Grand Bassa County some 90 kilometers (55 miles) southeast of Monrovia. The county was host to the Ugandan contingent of the "expanded" west African peacekeeping force in 1994. Grand Gedeh and Maryland counties, which border Côte d'Ivoire, may have higher rates, but health authorities have been unable to screen people in these areas because of a lack of resources and the poor state of roads. Infection rates are expected to rise as more refugees return from neighboring countries where many young girls with non-marketable skills who sought refuge there engaged in commercial sex work as a matter of survival.

On the role of the police force, recent studies in Ghana have shown that AIDS-related illnesses are among the leading causes of death among junior police officers, who make up 75 percent of the force. Among the risk factors identified are frequent transfers of police personnel, which create situations where the police have to live without their families for long periods, providing opportunities for entry into other relationships. The uniforms and the power the security forces wield in society probably attract many females (*Daily Graphic of Ghana*, March 4, 2000).

Cultural factors

One reason often cited for west Africa's low rates of HIV is the widespread practice of male circumcision, a practice that is almost completely absent among the ethnic groups of Africa's main AIDS belt (Caldwell and Caldwell 1996; Buve et al. 2000; Gray et al. 2000; Serwadda et al. 2000; Taljaard et al. 2000). Lack of circumcision either directly facilitates HIV transmission or facilitates it by rendering chancroid genital ulcerative diseases more likely. Caldwell (1995) attributes southern Sudan's considerably higher seroprevalence rates to the absence of circumcision among the predominantly non-Muslim population. Moses et al. (1990, 2000) observed similar findings among countries in west Africa. Their study shows that the major areas of non-circumcision of males in parts of Côte d'Ivoire and Ghana are associated with higher levels of HIV prevalence than elsewhere in west Africa.

Previous research suggests that Muslim Africa has generally lower HIV/AIDS rates than the rest of Africa, although underreporting may be a problem (Gould 1993; Caldwell 1995). Studies in Senegal and Côte d'Ivoire show that even where Muslims and non-Muslims live side by side, Muslims usually have less than half the rate of non-Muslims. Islamic cultural practices may restrict the spread of HIV in two main ways – strict sanctions against promiscuity and the widespread practice of circumcision. First, circumcision is a method of induction into Islam. While not mentioned in the Quran, it was adopted by Mohammed, is considered a duty, and neglecting it is punishable. Muslims consider the uncircumcised as unbelievers and unclean, and require the worshipper to be ritually clean (Tritton 1962).

How is circumcision a protective factor for HIV/AIDS? A 1993 study from the Arkansas Cancer Research Center (Weiss 1993) indicates that special skin cells that provide immunity, the epidermal Langerhans cells, are deficient in the human prepuce. When the foreskin is present, there is an unprotected area at the inner surface devoid of these special cells. Furthermore, the folds over the glans allow a moist, warm area to incubate and encourage organism growth. The circumcised penis, on the other hand, develops a thicker, tougher skin over the glans that is more resistant to disease than a prepuce-surrounded glans penis (Weiss and Weiss 1994). These conditions probably account for the increased vulnerability of the natural penis. While circumcision is not an absolute protection, it lessens the risk of contracting the virus.

Second, while permitting polygamy, Islam frowns on promiscuity. Two penalties are prescribed in the event of adultery. One penalty assigns one hundred strokes to be given to both parties. The other penalty, which mentions women only, says they are to be kept in houses until they die or be stoned to death. If a husband charges his wife with adultery he may kill her without being liable to retaliation (Tritton 1962). The relatives of the guilty woman kill her, drowning being the usual form of punishment. Because promiscuity is severely punished, fidelity is usually the social norm. Thus, these practices of Islam, circumcision and fidelity, can limit the spread of HIV/AIDS and probably contribute to the low prevalence rate in northern Ghana, Senegal, Niger, and Mali, areas with high rates of people professing Islam (Oppong 1998b).

In contrast, Christianity promotes monogamy, but the message of grace and forgiveness appears to have been misconstrued as a license for promiscuity. For a Christian, salvation is not based on deeds but on faith and belief. People are not saved by what they do, even though that is important, but by what they believe. Moreover, those who sin, commit adultery, for example, can be forgiven by God and presumably by society, if they confess their sin and repent. Sin in the form of extramarital sexual activity is not punishable by death, at least not in this life. Thus, the absence of an immediate harsh or drastic retribution for sexual impropriety may produce more acts of infidelity in Christianity than in Islam. Paradoxically, while poly-partner sexual activity is the norm in Islam, participants may not be as vulnerable as those involved in commercial sex work or a long series of monogamous sexual liaisons. Between Christianity and Islam, other religions usually have sexual practices that combine elements of the two – polygamy, serial monogamy, circumcision,

and commercial sex work – and consequently, comparable or higher rates.

Postpartum sexual abstinence for females has been identified as a factor that facilitates the spread of HIV in west Africa (Awusabo-Asare and Anarfi 1997; Cleland et al. 1999). Women are expected to abstain from sex for some time to ensure survival of the child and mother, but men are not. This health benefit, however, appears to be offset by the increased probability that husbands will seek extramarital partners without using condoms, or actually enter polygamy, increasing the risk of HIV. While the general consensus is early resumption of sex with suitable methods of postpartum contraception, attitudes toward such socially constructed practices as postpartum sexual abstinence need to be changed by intensive education of both men and women (Awusabo-Asare and Anarfi 1997).

Economic restructuring and HIV/AIDS

Preventing the spread of HIV in the context of economic reform is an extremely difficult task. Reduction of government expenditure on health and social services, a common requirement of economic reform packages, may undermine prevention efforts and increase rates of HIV infection, in several ways. According to UNAIDS (2000k), effective prevention measures include access to condoms, prophylaxis and treatment of opportunistic infections, including STDs, sex education at school and beyond, access to voluntary counseling and testing, counseling and support for pregnant women and efforts to prevent mother-to-child transmission, promotion of safe injection practices and blood safety, and access to safe drug-injecting equipment. Because these measures require increased, not decreased, government expenditure, economic restructuring makes it extremely difficult to accomplish these goals, in several ways. First, reduced government funding for diagnosis and treatment of STDs increases the risk of transmitting HIV (UNAIDS 1999e). Reduced funding for blood screening, and poor hygienic practices in clinics (for example, inadequate or no sterilization of equipment), may also spread HIV in health care facilities.

Second, intensified economic recessions and increasing inequality and poverty rates, usually associated with economic restructuring, compound the problem. In Ghana, frequently cited as an example of successful economic restructuring, poverty appears to have increased considerably throughout the country. In 1997, more than 6.5 million (about 30 percent) Ghanaians lived in absolute poverty, and the poverty of 1.8 million people (about 10 percent of the total population) was described as hard-core (World Bank 1997b). The proportion of the population classified as poor increased from 43 percent in 1981 to 54 percent in 1986 and 55 percent in 1997. In fact, poverty in the national capital, Accra, tripled from only 7 percent in 1988 to 21 percent in 1992 (World Bank 1995). Poor people engage in more risky behavior and lack access to health care resources that would lower their risk of contracting HIV. Throughout west Africa, women appear to be hardest hit by the increased poverty, producing increased marginalization and making them more vulnerable to HIV. Erosion of women's real incomes and increasing poverty intensify gender inequality and weaken women's ability to negotiate sexual relations and practices.

Third, economic restructuring programs, through their focus on increasing incentives for greater trade openness, promote an export-oriented pattern of economic growth and improved rural–urban spatial interaction and migrant labor patterns that enhance the spread of HIV.

Caring for AIDS patients in the context of health sector reform – autonomy of management for hospitals and introduction of user fees – is a major problem throughout west Africa. A short course of zidovudine given during the peripartum period reduced vertical transmission by 38 percent in Burkina Faso and Côte d'Ivoire women despite breastfeeding (Dabis et al. 1999), but unfortunately, that treatment is not widely available. Most patients are admitted to the hospitals in very poor clinical conditions and usually total depletion of their economic resources. Because they are unable to pay for hospitalization, the costs are supported by the hospitals whose budgets are already deficient and stretched. In Burkina Faso, a presidential decree (May

1991) states that hospitalization for AIDS and tuberculosis patients is free for third to fifth categories of room conditions in the public hospitals. However, because of budgetary constraints and other problems, enforcing this decree is nearly impossible. Similarly, medications to treat tuberculosis and other opportunistic infectious diseases are rare in Nigeria. While Glaxo-Wellcome and Roche Nigeria Ltd market antiretrovirals, only the affluent can afford them (Emah 1998). In Ghana, the Korle Bu Teaching Hospital has started treating opportunistic infections of HIV/AIDS with herbal medicine due to the dearth of antiretrovirals (*Daily Graphic of Ghana*, December 7, 2000).

Conclusion

West Africa has much lower HIV/AIDS rates than eastern and southern Africa, but considerable variations exist within the region. Societal destructuring due particularly to economic crisis and reform, civil strife, and gender-segregated labor migration appear to be important contributory factors. A combination of cultural and other factors make young females particularly vulnerable throughout the region. Sexually transmitted diseases are common and, where they remain untreated, usually due to expenditure cutbacks associated with economic restructuring, exacerbate the spread of HIV. Political leadership appears to be a major determinant of the severity of the HIV/AIDS crisis in each country. When it is present and effective, as in the case of Senegal, rates are much lower and stable; when it is missing or ineffective, as was the case in Nigeria, prospects are dismal. Political instability and civil war fuels the spread of AIDS through general chaos and the activities of the military.

Misidentifying the agents of the spread of HIV in west Africa is easy – commercial sex workers, truck drivers, young females providing sexual services in exchange for material survival. Addressing the real culprit is not. The real culprit, though, is an economic and social context that condemns some people to risky behaviors that make them victims of disease. It is time to look beyond the behavior that spreads the disease to the context that motivates and rewards such behavior. Whether west Africa can avoid the current AIDS crisis in southern Africa depends on how quickly and effectively we respond to the challenge of modifying the context that facilitates the spread of HIV/AIDS.

Part III

Beyond Epidemiology: Understanding the Issues in Social Terms

Introduction to Part III

"The social" is an encompassing phrase and we have capitalized on that breadth in our third section to signal our theoretical understanding of HIV/AIDS as a phenomenon whose complex embeddedness in the social demands multiple points of analytical entry within that term. Accordingly, we have subdivided the section into three categories that, though inevitably somewhat arbitrary, nonetheless encapsulate some of the more important optics of analysis for understanding the multiple and regionally varied contexts underlying transmission, experience, and local understanding of AIDS. The first section focuses on gendered vulnerabilities, while the second looks at sexualities and their critical importance to understanding identity, sexual practices, and interventions; the third section focuses on the effects of poverty, war, and migration on HIV transmission and interpretation. The arbitrariness of these sections comes from the fact that all of these optics – gender, poverty, migration, war, sexuality – in reality are inextricably connected to each other. To understand one requires understanding its relation to others, and for this reason many of the chapters contained in one section could easily have been placed in another.

Over the past several years there has been increasing recognition that gender constitutes a major fault-line of HIV vulnerability (Baylies and Bujra 2001; Akeroyd 1997; Schoepf 1992a). Adequately explaining the reasons behind gender's significance is more difficult, however, as it requires the elucidation of structural factors as well as those areas of everyday life such as sexual exchanges and domestic practice that are tricky for researchers to gain access to and more likely to change over short periods of time. The chapters included in this section illustrate the spectrum of analysis necessary to gaining better understandings of gender as it plays out in transmission, vulnerability, and prevention. "Gender" does not simply mean a focus on women and women's vulnerability, even though one salient question explored by Akeroyd and Schoepf is why women are at higher risk of HIV in much of Africa. Schoepf explores this question through a poignant ethnography of a young woman and the confluence of political, cultural, and personal factors placing her in a position of risk and ultimate exposure to HIV. Akeroyd directs attention to domestic violence and rape as an underexplored arena of analysis for women that, like everywhere in the world, resists intervention by hiding behind cultural and legal barriers. Clearly, coerced sex in any situation is an indication of larger structural inequities mapped onto gender subordination, and these both need to be addressed for effective intervention in AIDS.

Increased attention to women's vulnerability has also meant a corresponding focus on women's responsibility in risk intervention, which as Akeroyd and others (Obbo 1993a) argue is misguided given women's relative powerlessness in determining the conditions of sexual exchange. More focus in future needs to be turned to men in the drive toward higher rates of condom use. Mbugua turns to another underexplored issue, that of adolescents, their sexual practices, and understandings of risk. As she argues, adolescents are critical to intervention because they are highly sexually active and more liable to sexual experimentation that can place them at risk for HIV. Many adults living with AIDS today probably acquired HIV in their teens. In her appraisal of high school girls in and outside of Nairobi, Mbugua highlights the fracture points of mother–daughter relations, social change, and gender expectations.

The focus on gender has raised awareness of the importance of sexuality as a related but separate sphere of analysis. Like gender, sexuality is a multivalent and slippery construction contingent upon a broad range of factors, including regional political economies, social ideologies, and national movements. As the chapters in this section suggest, they also cover a wide arena of political interventions. For Susser and Stein, women's sexuality is shaped by and in turn shapes localized gender politics and discourses of customary practice, and as such is highly influential in determining whether women possess the political leverage required for adopting the female condom. In Campbell's investigation of South African mineworkers, constructions of masculine sexuality, emerging in part from the serious dangers inherent to mine work, play a key role in perpetuating risky sexual practices. Phillips problematizes the pat understanding of African AIDS as overwhelmingly heterosexual by asking how heterosexuality can even be understood without corresponding analyses of homosexuality. Indeed, homosexuality has either been made invisible or vilified within community and national arenas. The active demonization of homosexuality as a "white" pathology by some African leaders, such as Zimbabwe's Mugabe, is representative of the discursive postcolonial politics surrounding issues of sexuality. These actions also drive gay and lesbian movements underground and disturb the complacency of naming African AIDS as heterosexual.

Finally, the effects of war, poverty, and mobility have been devastating for significant populations within sub-Saharan Africa. The protracted warfare characterizing several regions of Africa in the past or present is being recognized as having profound impacts on rates of HIV/AIDS through destruction of local economies, loss of life, and refugee movements. Lyons' chapter takes war into consideration in her exploration of whether Uganda's rates of AIDS really have been reduced, and if so, whether they will continue their downward trajectory. Her incisive look at the "risky milieu" of forced migration, refugee camps, and economic insecurity stand as counterpoints to her observations of increased awareness of AIDS and a corresponding rise in condom use. We need more studies like Lyons' that trace effects of regional warfare on HIV transmission. We also need better elucidation of the degree and nature of international involvement in many of these regional conflicts, not only for analytical accuracy but as a further strategy for contravening prevailing attitudes that AIDS in Africa is "not our problem."[1]

The other three chapters in this section tackle in different ways the causes and effects of poverty on HIV. Lurie et al.'s piece takes a critical look at the role of Structural Adjustment Programs (SAPs) in further immiserating the poor in affected African countries, and consequently suggests the culpability of SAPs and their governing institution, the IMF, in contributing to AIDS. This piece is one of the first to critically assess the contributions of high-level international financial institutions to AIDS in Africa; there is now a growing movement in and outside of academic research calling for reform of high-level institutions such as the International Monetary Fund (IMF), World Bank, and World Trade Organization (WTO),[2] and for the World Bank in particular to implement debt relief programs to countries hard hit by AIDS. Without this relief, say critics, crippling debt payments leave African governments effectively unable to intervene in HIV transmission and treatment because they lack the funds for rebuilding economies and health care systems. Zulu et al.'s piece traces the effects of increasing poverty on an underexplored population, slum dwellers in major urban areas. Focusing on slums in Nairobi, Zulu, Ezeh, and Dodoo paint a poignant portrayal of individuals struggling to survive, many having migrated from rural areas when agriculture no longer provided a viable living. Yet within slums, they face lack of sanitation and running water, undernutrition, and higher HIV vulnerability. Rugalema offers an incisive ethnography of two populations, a village in Bukoba district, Tanzania, and agro-estate workers in Kenya. Beginning with a brief political economy of vulnerability for each area and its populations, Rugalema then ascertains personal interpretations of AIDS and risk, a move that proves critical to effective interventions given the degree to which understandings of the same epidemic differ. As Rugalema comments, the virus is the same in each location, but different socio-economic environments produce different epidemics.

One area needing further investigation within a social context is the relationship between religion and AIDS. Religions are highly varied and sometimes hybrid across sub-Saharan Africa, and the influence of religious beliefs and policies on sexual practices can be significant. Muslim traditions of fidelity and circumcision are touched upon by Oppong and Agyei-Mensah, but Islam takes somewhat different forms in different regions. Indigenous religions often encompass medical practices as well as influencing social and sexual conduct. The Christian church has played a complex role in the AIDS problematic, sometimes coming out against condoms as vehicles of sexual promiscuity, but most recently publicly calling for establishment of religious structures to carry out advocacy for and intervention into AIDS, urging African governments to withhold debt service payments to the World Bank, challenging pharmaceuticals to lower drug prices, and asking G-8 governments to contribute to the Global Fund (African Religious Leaders 2002). Actions such as these are not only highly commendable but also exemplify the growing recognition that meaningful interventions will only occur with religious, civil, governmental, NGO, and corporate collaborations.

NOTES

1.   Of course, the other side of this would be to explore the effects of international neglect of some regional conflicts such as the recent genocide in Rwanda. See Schoepf this volume.
2.   The protests during meetings of the World Bank and WTO in Davos, Seattle, and Genoa were not about AIDS specifically, but about the unfairness of upholding debt payments and maintaining inequitable trading policies, respectively. See Dommen 2002; Soros 2002.

Gendered Vulnerabilities
Chapter 6

Coercion, Constraints, and "Cultural Entrapments": A Further Look at Gendered and Occupational Factors Pertinent to the Transmission of HIV in Africa

Anne V. Akeroyd

Introduction

The AIDS pandemic combines the basic elements of sexuality, blood, morality, illness, and death, of violence, stigma, rejection, and despair, of compassion, hope, and courage. Responses to it raise questions about the understanding and interpretation of illness, behaviors, taboos, beliefs, gender relations; individual versus group interests; human rights; the cultural contexts of behaviors and beliefs and individual responses and motivations, as well as an understanding of national and international socio-economic and political contexts. Waldby (1996:9) contends that the management of an epidemic cannot be a politically neutral matter but always reflects power relationships and the defense of a particular social order. This is shown by one of the earliest analyses of African policy issues by Nzioka (1994:168), who argues that in Kenya the class framework, political reasons, the patriarchal society, and dominant sexual beliefs based on male chauvinism led to a concentration of medical surveillance mainly on the victims of deprivation and ignored the political elites,

and that the behavior and silences of the elites served to confirm the association of HIV/AIDS with the lower classes and members of disadvantaged social categories.

The assumption that *risk groups* exist still occurs in epidemiological, biomedical, and public health papers, but in anthropological and sociological literature the emphasis is on *risk behaviors*, not group membership, and the concept of *risk situations* has also been introduced. New and more complex understandings of the structural, institutional, and cultural contexts of sexual relationships (facilitated by the expansion of qualitative research studies) and the more recent emphasis on *vulnerability* rather than risk analysis have helped explain why people can remain personally vulnerable to HIV despite their knowledge of HIV/AIDS educational messages. The identification of human rights as the basis of vulnerability to HIV has also opened a new way of thinking about empowerment, albeit a demanding and problematical one.

The content of HIV/AIDS discourses has also changed, from control or exclusion to rights and empowerment (Seidel 1993) in line with changing approaches to HIV prevention. Reid (1994) pointed out that the dominant discourses (of epidemiology, public health, biomedicine, and education [IEC]) which focus on core groups and epicenters use metaphors of distancing (not metaphors of spread which include the speaker as well as others) and they result in blame and denial. Mobilization in affected communities, on the other hand, creates new discourses of inclusion, empowerment, and processes which reflect the complexity of the reality of the epidemic. We know much less, though, about African indigenous AIDS discourses, but Whyte (1997:10) gives a brief account of these from Uganda which she contrasts with "the national 'enlightened' discourse of 'living positively with AIDS'."

In Africa the prime mode of transmission is through heterosexual contact, with minor parts played by homosexual contact, mother–child transmission, blood transfusions, and injecting drug use. One manifestation of the vested interests in managing AIDS is the lack of attention paid to risky behavior in male-to-male sexual relationships; little is known about its effects, partly because of the denial, shame, and stigma surrounding homosexuality in much of Africa. From the outset the sex ratio of HIV/AIDS cases was almost equal, but in the younger age groups (under 25 years) infections in women increasingly outnumber those in men. The emphasis on heterosexual transmission, the impact on maternal and child mortality, the sharp increase in HIV infections and AIDS cases in African women and girls, and the growing burden they faced in caring for others placed women, and children and adolescents, at the center of research and interventions from the mid-1990s.

Numerous publications by international organizations, governments, non-governmental organizations (NGOs), academics, and activists and personal testimonies have documented the disadvantaged situation of African women and the personal, structural, cultural, and contextual factors which rendered them vulnerable to HIV. They highlighted the reasons why Africans were often powerless to protect themselves from harmful sexual activities and relationships; the problems they faced in coping with the consequences of their own HIV infection and AIDS; and their growing burden of caring for the sick and the orphaned.[1] As the deleterious impacts of the African epidemic were further exacerbated by debt, economic recession, and structural adjustment programs (which were not gender-neutral) the economic underpinnings of women's vulnerability became obvious. An additional complication for African women is their legal status; even in countries where they now have de jure adult status they may still be disadvantaged in respect of custom and of some citizenship rights, matters which may be crucial for relations with their husbands and husbands' kin and for the way HIV/AIDS impacts upon them.

Though the wider sociocultural and socioeconomic contexts of HIV/AIDS are well recognized, many studies and preventative approaches are premised on the KAP (Knowledge, Attitudes, Practices) model, which takes an individualistic perspective and emphasizes the protection of self, not of others. Messages such as the ABC refrain – "Abstain!," "Be Faithful!," "Use Condoms!," and similar slogans like "Protect yourself," "Love carefully," "Zero grazing" – reinforce this. However, many individuals, and especially young women, may be powerless to control the sexual behaviors of their partners or are unable, for reasons of economics or customary norms for example, to resist engaging in sexual interactions even though these might put them at risk of infection. In more recent programs, mainly those of NGOs, communities and women's groups have become actively involved in directly addressing issues of gender relations, vulnerability, and empowerment.

The salience of gender relations for the transmission of HIV was brought out by the sociological and anthropological qualitative studies that situated the sexual act, personal relations, and economic strategies in the wider political, social, economic, and cultural contexts. The emphasis on the situation of women has become the more vital as the toll the epidemic has inflicted on them escalates; but the shortcomings of an approach which puts upon the weaker partner in sexual interactions the onus of self-protection and of preventing the transmission of HIV are now only too clear. From the late 1990s, then, international attention began to be paid to the position of men and their involvement in, if not the whole responsibility for, the transmission of the virus, and also to the specific sociocultural and other factors that predispose some categories of men to engage in risky behaviors and render them vulnerable to HIV.

Another issue that has come to the fore is gender-related violence and sexual abuse directed against women and children and its involvement in the transmission of HIV. For other reasons, in the late 1990s gender-related violence had become a matter of widespread concern in several African countries (as well as elsewhere), especially in relation to human and women's rights and the health of women and children. Developments in medical, political, and legal arenas have begun to address the problem in many countries, and it is also an international political issue, no longer just the concern of feminists and other women activists.

* * * * *

This chapter focuses on three themes: vulnerability, risk, and gender in occupational contexts; the gendered culture of violence; and the new gender agenda, the responsibilities of men. It concludes by briefly discussing change and "cultural entrapments" (Mhloyi 1995).

Vulnerability, Risk and Gender in Occupational Contexts

HIV infection occurs in all social and economic classes but much research concentrated on specific disadvantaged and deprived communities. Early reports (Piot and Caraël 1988; Ainsworth and Over 1994), however, stressed the impact on elites, the urban educated ruling classes, the bureaucrats, technocrats, and businessmen, and even clerical workers, and regarded them as being particularly at risk. Ryder et al. (1990), for example, demonstrated differences in infection rates between managerial staff and manual workers and between women employees and wives. However, little solid information was available and there is still little specific research on the real elites (see Nzioka 1994 for one explanation). Those studies rarely involved social scientists; occupations of respondents and participants might be mentioned but their implications were rarely discussed; explanations for statistical associations were sparse; and the investigators

used inference and assumption rather than investigation and evidence for their conclusions. The likely accuracy of the responses went unquestioned, few or no indications were given of possible socio-economic biases in the sample population, and the studies were rarely set in the wider socio-economic context. There is little consistency in class attributions between studies (early or recent) and there are problems in interpretation, and comparison with other studies is therefore difficult. The clustering of several occupations under a generic category in survey results may mask the possibility that some jobs may present more risks than others in a particular organizational setting or locality and may also obscure important gender differences between categories of workers. For example, "nurse" referred to nursing officers, nurse assistants and attendants, midwives, laboratory workers, and other staff in a study of occupational risks among Tanzanian health-care workers (Gumodoka et al. 1997; and in the Masaka District study army personnel, police, drivers, and office workers were all categorized as "other salaried workers" (Nunn et al. 1994).

Snippets about occupational issues and about certain categories of workers can be gleaned from reports, notoriously for the truckers and prostitutes who have been singled out for epidemiological, public health, and educational attention and interventions, but detailed information about the occupational associations and risks of HIV infection and AIDS is still lacking, as it is about class associations. Even when studies are concerned with workers in a specific industrial or other organizational setting, they rarely investigate the HIV-related risks that these locations or job categories pose or facilitate (but for one example see C. Campbell 1997; C. Campbell and Williams 1999). There are obvious high-risk jobs such as those involving exposure to blood products or to sex work, but London (1998), for example, suggests that in South Africa there are limited possibilities for infection directly linked to other occupations and work-related activities and that therefore many workers are infected through sexual relationships in their private lives, which also seems to be the basic assumption of workplace IEC activities. A similar assumption appears in studies of risks and HIV infection among health care workers: Wilkinson and Gilks (1998:500) assert that "HIV infection among hospital workers is not associated with occupational exposure to HIV," citing a study of hospital workers in Kinshasha, Zaire, published in 1986. None of the questions on possible risk factors in Siziya and Hakim's study (1996 figure l) referred to occupational risks, even though the study was a cross-sectional multicenter study on the risk of occupational exposure to HIV.

Sexual liaisons are not the only association between the workplace and HIV and AIDS: stress is another. This is partly the result of the work environment, staff shortages arising out of HIV-related matters, etc. Workplace counselors may suffer greater stress (Baggaley et al. 1996). A study of Zambian primary school teachers (two-thirds of them women, the ratio in the profession) who had trained as counselors found that stress was occasioned by the problems facing their pupils (poverty, HIV-related illness and deaths of parents, sexual abuse, violence in the home, teenage pregnancy, etc.), the deaths of pupils and teachers, and the impact of HIV/AIDS on the teachers' lives (Baggaley et al. 1999). Stress and burnout is something with which the medical profession, especially nurses, have to cope, as must other careworkers and paid or unpaid helpers in hospices, orphanages, etc.

There are additional problems in respect of women: the gender as well as the class biases need investigation. However, it is not only researchers who exhibit gender-blindness. Obbo (1993a) found that in Uganda when Ganda women died, their deaths might not be overtly recognized as worthy of report to outsiders. Even in villages where more women than men had died, reference was made only to the deaths of men; and while people talked of attending funerals of farmers (men), women who were cultivators were rarely referred to by their occupation, although other female occupations such as teacher were mentioned in connection with the deceased.

Risk and occupational categories

As a first step to aid thinking about the nature of the risks and vulnerabilities that particular occupations or economic sectors present we need to distinguish between occupations, work settings, and statuses in relation to the aspects of risk that they present. Then the gendered aspects can be explored.

A. Occupations and tasks in which the risk of HIV transmission is inherent/integral

- Occupations that put workers into direct contact with blood and other bodily fluids and in which the risk of injury is ever-present, such as medical work and occupations allied to medicine in the formal (modern) and informal (traditional) sectors, dentists, and morticians. In Africa the risks in this sector are exacerbated by such factors as: the shortages of equipment and of prophylactic medicines for treating those exposed to needlestick injuries; the preference of patients (and perhaps of health workers and traditional healers) for injections rather than pills; the ever-increasing proportion of HIV-infected patients occupying hospital beds, many of whom are not clearly identifiable using the clinical definition alone; heavy workloads; and the increasing proportion of HIV-infected staff.

- Occupations involving the unmediated provision of sexual services – sex work or prostitution. Much epidemiological work has concentrated on these workers, as have many of the discussions about the pressures facing women, especially poor women, which push them into professional sex work or into sexual exchanges which involve the exchange of money or goods for sex.

B. Occupations in which danger and accidents are integral to the work and expose workers to blood and to medical risks of transmission

- Occupations in which work is dangerous and accidents are not uncommon and which present dangers of exposure to blood and bodily fluids, or involve the need for blood transfusions, injections, or operations after accidents, such as military service, mining and industrial jobs, road haulage and other driving work, police, and prison. (There are associated roles which similarly carry a risk (often high) of accidents – being a car driver or passenger.)

C. Occupations that require the separation of workers from their families or regular sexual partners and expose them to sexual opportunities and temptations

- Occupations that involve migrant workers and commuters (short- or long-term), especially those forced to live in single-sex settings, either on a seasonal basis or because of local recruitment problems or industry policies (as in the southern African mining industries and the fishing industry in Namibia), or which involve regular travel and stays away from home (seafarers, military personnel, airline crews, professional sportsmen, truck drivers, workers on large-scale development projects, labor migrants); and occupations which require periodic changes of location or postings away from home (such as expatriate African and Western professionals, civil servants such as medical, veterinary agricultural, administrative personnel, and the armed services.).

D. Occupations in which workers may be expected to offer sexual services or may be coerced into sexual acts

- Sexualized occupations in the leisure/entertainment/tourist industry, such as hotel, night-club, and bar workers, escorts, beach boys, and other work roles in settings in which sexual services are presumed by clients to be on offer or to be negotiable, especially jobs in which there are pressures on the workers to conform to clients' expectations.
- Occupations that have a standardized expectation that access to sex or display of "virility" is part of the job, a perk, or a necessary display. Politicians, diplomats, businessmen, sportsmen, and other, especially, powerful and/or rich men may be offered entertainment and access to sex workers/hostesses as a means to or reward for clinching a deal or be expected to maintain an entourage of women (especially young and beautiful ones) as symbols of their wealth and power.
- Occupations and activities that expose the incumbents to sexual harassment and violence, in which subordinates and peers, and those in captivity, must submit to har-

assment, demands for sexual favors, or rape (heterosexual and homosexual) in order to retain a job, gain advancement, acquire economic favors, provisions, loans, and so on. The perpetrators are usually men and boys – policemen, military and other security personnel, and prison officers; work superordinates (employers, managers) or fellow employees, teachers and university staff, fellow school pupils or university students; fellow prisoners (who may commit rape from choice or at the instigation of prison officers); suppliers of goods; providers of lodgings, etc. The victims are usually but not exclusively women and girls – school pupils and university students; employees; nurses; businesswomen and entrepreneurs; especially secretaries; prisoners; women caught up in riots or civilians in war-torn countries, and women in refugee camps, etc.

Gendered vulnerabilities and occupational risks for women

Both women and men work in risky settings and occupations, though the gender distribution in work and occupations varies between countries and over time. Some occupations may predispose men to engage in risky sexual activities and put themselves at risk should they fail to use condoms. But too often it is their female partners within and outwith the workplace who are at the greater risk of infection. Men are generally far less likely to have sexual intercourse forced on them than are women, but in some roles and locations they may face the risk of rape or less-than-willing voluntary homosexual acts (in prisons, military camps, mining industry hostels, labor camps, war zones, etc.). In some cases homosexual acts will be imposed as a form of social control and degradation, notoriously in prisons, or be the result of (or be attributed to) boredom or to the lack of readily available heterosexual opportunities.

Discussion about the problems faced by women in relation to sexual practices has usually focused either on the domestic domain, on relationships with husbands, lovers, and casual partners, or on commercial sex workers. We know much less about the occupational and class issues in respect of women. What might be the risk factors, the sexual pressures and opportunities facing women in work environments? Are there specific risks and vulnerabilities for women associated with particular occupations and locations, other than those associated with commercial sex work?

The main occupations in which women are likely to face direct occupation-related risks are in the medical sector, as doctors, nurses, midwives, or other health-care workers, though there are few discussions of this (but see Siziya et al. 1996; Siziya and Hakim 1996). There is little discussion of HIV infection and AIDS among female elites, and women in managerial, bureaucratic, and other white-collar occupations. Even when women do achieve professional status it is their sexual identity rather than their professional abilities that is foregrounded in interactions with male colleagues (as in N'Galy et al. 1988; Siziya et al. 1996; Siziya and Hakim 1996). It is often assumed that professional women, such as women politicians in southern Africa, "because they operate in a male-dominated environment, must be sexually immoral, must have 'rubbed the right shoulders,' or worse still 'slept their way up'" (Geisler 1995:571). Comments about the general assumption that employers, managers and other superiors, or co-workers force or coerce women into sexual relationships, as in Uganda (Sebunya 1995), on a Zambian commercial farm (Bond and Dover 1997:386), and in South Africa (London 1998:587) are additional evidence of the sexualization of work environments and of the harassment faced by women therein. London (1998:576–577) drew attention to the paradox that health promotion activities take place in the public workplace yet sexual relations between employees occur in the private domain and are not regarded as anyone else's business; and noted that training programs in South Africa do raise issues of violence and sexual harassment, and that gender relations between workers may be related to imbalances in power. London might perhaps have underestimated the coercive context of work relationships: they may arise directly out of the structural contexts of the workplace environment and involve sexual relations, voluntary or coerced, between co-workers both at work

as well as outwith the workplace or other establishment. Business women, entrepreneurs, and traders may perforce use sexual ploys and engage in sexual exchanges to obtain commercial and financial favors or supplies of goods as they have done in Zaire (Schoepf 1992a; J. MacGaffey 1986), Ghana (Ankomah and Ford 1994:132; Anarfi et al. 1997) and Zambia (Mwale and Burnard 1992). Zambian women fish sellers have been encouraged to group themselves into co-operatives to protect themselves against unscrupulous traders; and female itinerant traders in Ghana may be further put at risk by their need to find accommodation in settings where staying in hotels is not a common practice for ordinary people (Anarfi et al. 1997).

The sexual exploitation of women workers is not uncommon. They may be faced with sexualized occupational risks, be pressured to engage in sexual relations, or have to proffer sexual favors. Such sexual exchanges provide some evidence of particular occupational risks for women. There are structural causes for women's and girls' vulnerability in occupational sectors; but their vulnerability can also be linked to the widespread generalized sexual harassment and assault in the wider society as well. Furthermore, their vulnerability may also be rooted in, or exacerbated by, customs and laws which render African women subordinate to men in everyday gender relations.

The Gendered Culture of Violence

The vulnerability of women is increased by the extent to which they are subjected, not only to male control, but also to violence against the person and to a gendered culture of violence. Violence done to women's bodies through cultural modifications to the genitals from various forms of circumcision or the use of intravaginal substances to "dry" and "tighten" the vagina prior to sexual intercourse, for example, may cause damage to tissues and facilitate the transmission of HIV. Cultural practices affecting the genitals are not, however, the only forms of violence to the body that may facilitate the transmission of HIV. Young girls are also at increased risk through sexual intercourse because of the immaturity of their genital tract;

and physical and sexual violence also has major impacts on the physical and mental health of women and children (G. Gordon and Kanstrup 1992; Heise and Elias 1995; Heise et al. 1994; Kisekka 1990; Kornblit 1994; Tlou 1990; Turshen 1991; and Raikes 1989 who also pointed out the threat to women posed by HIV/AIDS). Women's susceptibility to HIV infection needs to be set in the context of health, sexuality, and reproduction (see Akeroyd 1996:43–50; Bond and Dover 1997; McNamara, n.d.).[2]

Gender-related violence is increasingly being implicated in the transmission of HIV through coercive sexual encounters (P. Gordon and Crehan, n.d; Maman et al. 2000; Mehrotra et al. 1999). Piot (1999) called it "a particularly insidious aspect of the AIDS epidemic." This may occur in sexual encounters between spouses and other sexual partners involving unprotected, rough, or forced sex, or through rape by relatives and acquaintances, strangers, government officials, military and political party personnel. A useful distinction here is given by Ampofu (1993b) – *interpersonal violence* between sexual partners who may or may not be members of a domestic unit and *institutional violence* against women which is sanctioned or even prescribed by the state.

Numerous armed conflicts, wars and the disasters arising out of political crises, destabilization, and drought have created millions of refugees and displaced people. Battlegrounds and peacekeeping zones are classic examples of "risk situations": the vulnerability of women and girls in war zones is an international phenomenon (see Bennett et al. 1995). The attitudes of military personnel, inculcated by formal training or part of the informally learned military culture and reinforced by peer pressure – a willingness to accept risk, to be aggressive and to feel a sense of prestige vis-à-vis civilians and especially women – "may increase the likelihood of soldiers engaging in anonymous, purchased or even coercive sex" (UNAIDS 1998e:3). (Similar pressures and attitudes may also occur in other paramilitary and dangerous occupations (see Campbell this volume; C. Campbell and Williams 1999 on the southern African mining industry).) A workshop on women in the aftermath of civil war in west Africa identified nine forms of explicit violence against women and fourteen forms of

implicit violence (Turshen 1999a:125–126). Sexual assaults and rape by military personnel during liberation struggles, civil wars, and ethnic conflicts have been reported from many countries, including Sierra Leone, Namibia, South Africa, the Democratic Republic of the Congo, Rwanda, and Mozambique. A report on repression in Kenya since 1991 found that hundreds of Somali women had been raped in refugee camps in 1992–3, many by members of the Kenyan security forces, and women prisoners had been abused by police and by male prisoners who were sometimes encouraged to rape and given access to the women's cells (Amnesty International 1995). Internal political and civil conflicts, too, may engender sexual violence – rape and other forms of sexual assault have been deployed against suspected opponents of the Mugabe regime in Zimbabwe. Refugee camps may not provide a safe haven. In an overview of the problems of refugee women in relation to HIV, Long (1998:87–88) identified "a refugee women's sexual subculture," and discussed why they are unable to negotiate sexual relations and why their experiences (both prior to and in the camps) may also have long-lasting consequences for their postwar sexual relations. Most people at risk in these settings are women, but men are not immune though documentation of men's experiences of sexual assault in African conflicts is scanty.

It is not only extreme events that create risk situations for women. Beatings, sexual harassment, and sexual assaults are facts of life for many women; and the abuse of children, boys as well as girls, especially of street children, is a growing cause for concern in many countries. In the domestic domain, the workplace, on the streets, in rural areas, towns, schools and universities, prisons, and elsewhere women and girls face sexual harassment, abuse, or rape, a manifestation of what Hubbard (1991) terms the "culture of rape," violence which may also culminate in murder as Rude's (1999) account of gendered domestic homicide in Zambia shows. The culture of gender-related violence has had particularly tragic implications for South Africa which belatedly came to terms with the need to take concerted action against HIV/AIDS across racial, political, and sectoral divides. Geisler (1997:92) drew attention to the revival of virginity testing for young girls in Kwazulu, intended as a solution to teenage pregnancy by stopping girls from indulging in sex, in a country where rape statistics are among the highest in the world. Rapes of young girls and even of babies in the belief that sex with a virgin will cure AIDS have recently appalled South Africans.

Women are not necessarily any safer in their homes. Fears about the transmission of HIV may have exacerbated domestic dangers; in Uganda, for example, domestic violence increased because of fears about HIV transmission (Kisekka 1990:45–46). Women's inability to refuse their husband's demands for sexual intercourse or to negotiate the use of condoms and their vulnerability to domestic violence impact severely on their ability to protect themselves and to practice forms of "safer sex," as Kesby's action research project with Zimbabwean women demonstrates (this volume). Disparities in the ages of spouses may also encourage compliance and passivity in women. In Setswana culture, for example, the ideal gap is at least ten years (Mandevu 1995); it is also considerable in Tanzania, and Mgalla et al. (1998:9) also suggest that a similar age difference may occur between non-marital sexual partners thereby giving men easier access to young girls – certainly "sugar daddies" are both older and richer and/or more powerful than their partners ("sugar mummies" are a rarer phenomenon). Even consensual relationships may involve rough or violent sex; violent and coercive practices were so common in adolescent Xhosa girls' sexual experiences in South Africa that some of them perceived these as an expression of love (Wood et al. 1998).

Rape and other forms of sexual assault and forced sex have not only been under-discussed and under-researched in relation to HIV/AIDS; they were rarely included among the "risk factors" investigated by biomedical researchers whose focus on "promiscuity" and "paid sex," in conjunction with their normative model (and often Western-based assumptions) about conjugal and sexual relations, seems to have precluded attention to them. Van der Straten et al. (1995) did investigate coerced sex in an epidemiological study in Rwanda; and Meursing (1997:201) mentions it very briefly in the context of non-marital sexual relationships in Matabeleland, Zimbabwe. These are, of course, very difficult issues to investigate, especially in the KAP surveys, and much of what we now know has been the result of qualitative research and longer-term studies. There is now much greater awareness of their salience in HIV/AIDS research, as are other aspects of violence against women and the sexual abuse of children.

Violence against women, too often regarded as an individual and private matter, has become a major concern for women's groups, and has been taken up by newspapers, international agencies, the courts, the medical profession, and governments in a number of countries. Some campaigns (or individual campaigners) oppose all use of violence by men against women. Others take a more tempered view, like some of the campaigns in Kenya: they may urge action against the excessive use of violence which they see as a distortion of the "normal" state of affairs, a consequence of other societal changes which have jeopardized the position of men and left them with nothing other than their power over women which they then exercise to excess. Ms Muragu of the Federation of Women Lawyers in Kenya said that "custom" was simply being used as an excuse and attributed an increase of 50 percent in reports to the police of cases of wife-beating to the effects of economic decline (Gough 1998).

There are initiatives by communities, women's groups, and NGOs, for example in Tanzania and Zambia (Baylies and Bujra 2000; Tanzania Gender Networking Programme 1997:58–61), and in Harare, Zimbabwe where the Musasa Project has confronted violence against women for over a decade and has developed various strategies, including discussions of violence into health education talks on HIV/AIDS (Njovana and Watts 1996; Watts et al. 1998). In Uganda, Action AIDS's innovative Stepping Stones Training and Adaptation Project recorded a decline in domestic violence after its first workshop which discussed violence and other gender issues (Reeves 1998).[3] A guardian scheme was set up in primary schools in Mwanza, Tanzania in 1996 to protect adolescent girls against sexual violence and harassment as part of a project to develop interventions to reduce the transmission of HIV and STDs (Mgalla et al. 1998). Though sexual abuse by teachers, fellow pupils, and village men was less hidden and abuse by teachers might have been made less easy, a complication was that the women teachers were opposed to any sexual activity among the girls and were reluctant to give advice on contraception. The evaluators suggested that a much broader scheme, of which a guardian program would be only one component, was needed effectively to address the issue of adolescent sexuality.

Violence against women is also high on the agenda of international agencies and some national governments. Female Genital Mutilation (FGM) has been the subject of campaigns in a number of countries; female circumcision is now outlawed in some African states, and in 1997 the WHO Regional Office for Africa launched a Regional Plan of Action to Accelerate the Elimination of Female Genital Mutilation. A worldwide campaign on nonconsensual sex in marriage organized by a London-based NGO, CHANGE, included Uganda in the first set of country reports (CHANGE 1999; Odida 1999). The UN General Assembly adopted the Declaration against Violence against Women in 1993. UNIFEM has established a Trust Fund in Support of Actions to Eliminate Violence against Women, and launched regional Campaigns to Eliminate Violence Against Women in 1998 with the support of ten UN agencies. The matter has also been discussed in other United Nations fora, and other international organizations such as the World Health Organization and the Commonwealth Secretariat have also addressed the issue in various ways, including violence against women.[4]

Rape and other forms of sexual violence are manifestations of the exertion of power over the powerless. At one extreme are war-rape and other forms of violence; at the other is the refusal of an HIV-infected man to use a condom to protect his uninfected partner, a finding not uncommon in studies of discordant couples. Violence against women is linked to the subordinate legal, social, and economic position of women, and to cultural assumptions about relations between men and women; but it also reflects the general level of violence in the wider society. The tide is now running strongly against male violence – but to challenge its acceptability strikes at conceptions of masculinity and the structure of gender relations.

The new gender agenda: the responsibilities of men

The recognition that it is men who spread the epidemic to women was underemphasized until the late 1990s. Women were the focus of attention from moralists and policymakers alike, and AIDS prevention strategies were aimed at them even when they were intended to alter men's behavior. That women cannot be expected to control the sexual behavior of men, and if the epidemic is to be controlled men must be directly addressed, has become a major theme for the new millennium. Behavior change must be initiated by the powerful, not cajoled or negotiated by the powerless. Men must shoulder the responsibility for preventing the transmission of HIV, for protecting their own health and lives as well as those of their female partners. The 2000 World AIDS Campaign focused on men and boys for five main reasons: "Men's health is important but receives inadequate attention; ... Men's behavior puts them at risk of HIV"; ... Men's behavior puts women at risk of HIV; ... Unprotected sex between men endangers both men and women; ... Men need to give greater consideration to SIDS as it affects the family" (UNAIDS 2000l).

"HIV transmission – men are the solution," wrote Obbo (1993a): but the implications of, and the modes of implementing, the calls for men to take on the responsibility for the sexual health and the lives of themselves and of their women partners and thereby, too, of their children have yet to be fully worked out. Another difficulty in transferring the onus to men is finding ways of getting prevention messages to them. Messages targeted at women are usually in places which they attend in their roles as mothers and homemakers, such as family planning and prenatal clinics. Men have been mainly targeted as workers, not in their familial roles; C.A. Campbell (1995) argued that new ways of targeting and addressing men are needed, ones that do not simply reinforce traditional stereotypes of gender roles and masculine identity. One example of this comes from Lesotho where football teams passed on prevention messages. Workplace approaches have been used in Zimbabwe, though, with good effect (Williams and Ray 1993), and there and elsewhere they have become even more necessary as infections and death rates rise. Other communicative initiatives began to be developed in the 1990s as the problem of children's (especially adolescents') sexual behavior began to rise high on the agenda. Innovative approaches have been developed to address those age groups, tackling issues of sexual knowledge, gender relations, masculinity, male violence, etc., and often involving peer educators. Some of the most interesting and accessible ones are magazines which are available in print and online, and programs in schools which may also involve peer educators.

The problem of communication between partners remains the major stumbling block. "The crucial challenge for HIV control in the workplace is to extend negotiations on wages and working conditions in the boardroom to negotiations on sexual relations and the right to say no in the bedroom" (London 1998:578). The notion of communication and negotiation stressed in preventive health-care models is too often based on a Western (and idealistic) model of gender relations and of the partners' ability to communicate sexual needs and desires. Kesby's (2000a) work in Zimbabwe shows how many personal and cultural barriers have first to be overcome before people there will readily talk about unsafe sex. (There are also difficulties in promoting safer sex practices in societies in which local beliefs and practices act as cultural entrapments, for example running counter to calls to use condoms, where children are strongly desired by both men and women, men express a strong desire for "flesh-on-flesh" intercourse and/or a preference for "dry sex" and women have other fears about condoms, and regular intercourse is believed to be necessary for the bodily health of men and women, and often for a fetus.)

The missing element in most of the HIV/AIDS literature and approaches in Africa (as elsewhere) has been about heterosexual and homosexual male behaviors, about concepts of masculinity and male sexuality. There are many references in the African HIV/AIDS literature to men's sexual behavior, their multiple liaisons and the like, occasional references to their need (as well as desire) for regular sexual intercourse to ensure good health, and evidence of a particular expression of masculinity in sexual and physical violence directed against women. There are still too few, let alone very detailed, studies of the contextual constraints on and cultural entrapments affecting male behavior. Information can be gathered from qualitative studies such as Bond and Dover's (1997) account of "the trouble with condoms" in their study of prevention interventions in rural Zambia, Bawah et al.'s (1999) on family planning in northern Ghana, and Meekers and Calvès's (1997) account of adolescents' premarital sexual unions in Yaoundé, Cameroon. Some projects, such as one in Botswana aimed at getting men to talk about sex (Gaelesiwe 1999), are explicitly aimed at discovering information about men, sex, and the construction of masculinity. Other discussions and details of anti-violence groups, projects, and websites in Africa (and elsewhere) are in a special issue of *Development* on "Violence Against Women and the Culture of Masculinity" (*Development* 2001).

The issue of violence and heterosexual masculinity in South Africa began to receive attention from the end of the 1980s (C. Campbell 1992; Vogelman and Eagle 1991); but there was little information about contemporary gay men and other men who engage in same-sex relations. Gevisser (1998) discusses the denial of past realities of Zimbabwean societies, and the silencing or pathologizing of African homosexualities by scholars. In Zimbabwe, the silence may be partly attributed to the vested interests of political and church elites in asserting an indigenous homophobia. This lacuna is now being actively redressed; for example, on same-sex relationships, sexual practices, and sexual identities, gay and lesbian, in Zimbabwe and South Africa see Gevisser (1998) and Gevisser and Cameron (1994). Kiama (1998) referred to studies by AMREF (African Medical Research Foundation) among Kenyan truck drivers which found homosexual activity between older men and boys; but a study of Kenyan adolescents at truck stops (Nzyuko et al. 1997) seems not to have explored that possibility – it implied that the boys' sexual relationships were only with female prostitutes. The Kenyan Parliament recognized that men in certain occupations or social categories who faced lengthy separations from their regular sexual partners were at risk, but a Ministry of Health spokesman commented that homosexual transmission is negligible "and should not take up our resources and time," and, explaining the lack of targeting of men who have sex with men, the UNAIDS Resident Advisor said, "Homosexuals are not easily accessible. They will need to come out of the closet if they are to get any attention" (Kiama 1998). In South Africa, gay men with hemophilia were infected early through blood transfusions. At the level of the state and formal rights, South Africa presents a very different picture from other African countries; but at the level of interpersonal relations, especially among black citizens, the matter looks very different and intolerance and homophobia are common. In South Africa black and white gay men as well as whites are involved in AIDS education and prevention; but it is clear, too, that there are men who have sex with men without identifying themselves as homosexuals, whether from choice or for situational reasons in the tourist trade, in prisons, or under the conditions of labor migrancy, and these men too need to be addressed in education and prevention measures. Many gay men, too, may have married for social and personal reasons: fear, stigma, shame, or overt persecution of homosexuals, as in Zimbabwe, discourages openness and also makes it difficult to know the extent to which male bisexuality may put women at risk.

Sexuality must be set within the wider social context of gender relations, as Dixon-Mueller's (1993) framework demonstrates. Moore (1994:140) identifies some of these outcomes, commenting that gendered aspects of violence in South Africa needs to be put into "the context of the development of multiplex and multilayered discourses on masculinity and femininity." One important aspect of the wider context is that in southern Africa (and elsewhere) there is an intensifying tendency

for adults to refuse to marry, women so they can keep control over themselves and their children, and men because they cannot afford marriage. This trend will have a variety of consequences for cross-sex gender relations as well as for same-sex relations.

The HIV-infected status and the "risky" sexual behaviors of men have been linked to factors such as mobility, marginalization, relative or absolute wealth, power, the naturalness and uncontrollability of the male sexual drive, susceptibility to temptation and the like; and the men are often depicted as selfish, irresponsible, chauvinistic, ruthless, unconstrained by their social position or taking advantage of it. Their "victims" are women although, judging by the tone of some accounts, the victims sometimes seem rather to be other men who subsequently become infected, and it is then the women who are "culpable." Such views are, of course, linked to assumptions about femininity and masculinity, and they often take an essentialist approach to gender." Such assumptions, gender ideologies, and gender relations are beginning to be explored but are still not foregrounded in the HIV/AIDS literature; an "in-depth understanding of why and how men come to act as they do sexually is absent" (Wood et al. 1998:240). The summary report of a session on male sexuality in the 12th World Conference on AIDS in 1998 commented that "[i]t is surprising how researchers working in the field of gender studies, have not analyzed more systematically the links between masculinity construction and the risk of AIDS."[5]

There are still too few detailed studies of the cultural entrapments and contextual constraints on male behavior in Africa, and how men, masculinities, and male sexualities are constructed, and though the output is growing it cannot yet match the corpus of work on African women. An important early contribution was Shire's (1994) autobiographical account of the representations of masculinities in Zimbabwe. That there are masculinities, too, needs to be recognized, though the debate on these has barely begun in relation to southern Africa; Morrell (1998) used interdisciplinary work on masculinities and insights from men's studies to identify a range of masculinities in the South African past. There are even fewer studies which concentrate these questions in relation to HIV/AIDS. Another early example is Setel (1996) who linked historical changes in society and the import of these for the impact of AIDS in a study of the Chagga in the Kilimanjaro region of Tanzania, showing how the changes were "part of the gradual emergence of a sad paradox of productive and reproductive adulthood. AIDS in Kilimanjaro served to encode local sentiment about the moral value of young adult lifestyles – particularly those associated with the market and with urban spaces" (Setel 1996:1169).

There is now explicit recognition that "the global epidemic is driven by men" (Foreman 1998a; Foreman 1998b:3; Gaelesiwe 1999), even though women are contracting AIDS at a faster rate because of their physiological susceptibility and because men have a greater number of sexual partners (Foreman 1998b:5). But caution has been advocated in assigning "blame"; recognizing that male behavior puts women at risk "does not mean that men are 'responsible' for the AIDS epidemic" (Foreman 1998b:4) but they must accept more responsibility for sexual and reproductive health matters. Involving men in HIV prevention is essential if the epidemic is to be contained. That, however, will "require a considerable scaling up of existing efforts, and, in the absence of new resources, some re-orientation of existing gender-sensitive programmes and interventions, many of which work with women alone" (Rivers and Aggleton 1999).

> Work is needed to transform existing agendas of prevention, health promotion and development so as to make them more sensitive to gender and sexuality as principles structuring the lives of both women and men, and influencing HIV-related vulnerabilities in ways which could not easily be imagined only a decade or so ago. (Rivers and Aggleton 1999).

Paradoxically, though, as Baylies and Bujra point out, bringing African men into the equation is essential if adults and children are to survive; but men "may have good reason to fear that the empowerment of women in respect of sexuality and sexual relations could have an impact on other aspects of gendered (power); understandably then, men are torn between their desire for life and the loss of

their control over women" (Baylies and Bujra 1995:214). As in development studies, then, where it has been found that initiatives benefiting women may be perceived as being at the expense of men, so too in HIV/AIDS research this issue must be confronted. Emphasis needs to be shifted to the powerful, to the men who face "de-powerment" (to coin a phrase) or, if the issue can be constructed in non-zero-sum terms, who must be "re-powered." The empowerment of women, problematical though that may be, is still on the agenda: Mhloyi, for example, calls for measures to improve women's socio-economic position in the long term and, immediately, "to empower them with the knowledge and courage needed to encourage and demand safer sex" (Mhloyi 1995:18). However, in an interesting reversal, she also advocates the *empowerment of men*, arguing that: "Their roles must be redefined to promote the idea that responsible sex, to protect their loved ones and their sexual partners, is an enhancement of manhood" (Mhloyi 1995:18–19). That is a challenging agenda for the new millennium.

Conclusion: Change, Constraints and Cultural Entrapments

Throughout the 1990s the primary focus of studies was women (in this field, as in others, "gender" was synonymous with "women") and the emphasis was on ways of reducing women's vulnerability and of empowering them, even though it was recognized that the solution might depend on long-term structural changes. Gender relations are now recognized as a key factor in vulnerability to HIV and the impact of HIV/AIDS on women and their families; but they also constrain men. Therefore, as Baylies and Bujra (2000:176) say, it is "not gendered difference but gendered inequality that puts both men and women at risk" and "[t]he challenge is to devise interventions which, whilst recognising gender inequity, essentialise neither 'men' nor 'women'" (Baylies and Bujra 2000:1). A decade ago Schoepf explained why women "resort to sexual 'survival strategies' at a time when these have turned into their opposite, becoming strategies of death" (Schoepf 1992a:276); now it is also clear that "causal unprotected sex as an assertion of masculinity is in practice a death wish and lack of protection in marriage can bring about mutual demise" (Baylies and Bujra 2000:xii).

The new agenda is a daunting one for men: it calls not only for change, but directly addresses the need to enrol them as the initiators of change so as to protect not only women but also themselves and to share out the burdens of the epidemic in a more equitable way. But it must be remembered that willingness to adopt changes in sexual behavior by individual men or specific categories of men is not the whole solution. Attention has been paid *to* men and to the recognition *by* men of their role in the transmission of HIV and of their own vulnerability; but to create the necessary changes in behavior it is not enough to recognize only the problem *of* men; it is also necessary to understand the problems *for* men, the structural, ideological, and other constraints and cultural entrapments which make men as well as their partners vulnerable to HIV.

Much of the earlier work (and standardized epidemiological survey type and KAP studies) emphasized the problems of inducing change in respect of sexual behavior and in particular the use of condoms. "Culture" and "custom" were constantly invoked as showing how difficult it would be to alter behavior and much effort has been devoted to finding out how far this had been taking place. While much earlier work referring to "African culture" (i.e., sexual practices) drawn on by non-social scientists or produced by some social scientists at the behest of the biomedical researchers was resoundingly criticized by other social scientists, we cannot ignore aspects of culture and the taken-for-granted aspects of everyday life. Culture and behavior are not static – they have long been, and are being, challenged and changed in Africa. For example, much of what passes in central Africa as tradition and custom in the domain of marriage and customary law and the associated controls over women is actually the product of the colonial period, developed by an alliance of European colonial administrators and African elders who for different reasons wished to bring African women back under the control of men (Chanock 1985). Fierce resistance was then, and still is, put up to changes which

would alleviate the lot of women; men seem to feel much less attachment to traditions which might hamper their activities other perhaps than those that hinder their control over women and the young.

There is, however, also ambivalence about some efforts at inducing change in gender relations. The Gender and AIDS Group in Tanzania and Zambia found that older people displayed ambivalence, and sometimes fear and hatred for the young, and commonly blamed unruly young people for the epidemic; so that while concern and compassion were manifest in attempts aimed at empowering and protecting young women, these measures could also become attempts at controlling and repressing them (Baylies and Bujra 2000:1). Campaigns such as those of Kenyan women seek to challenge male violence, but with an awareness of how deeply entrenched it is (Gough 1998; Nation Correspondent 1999). Given the extent to which the physical, economic (and psychological) power of men over women is taken for granted by both sexes, and even regarded as acceptable by a considerable proportion of women in many African countries, we can understand challenges to male violence by women's groups which do not necessarily seek (or, perhaps, at least initially?) to outlaw totally that culturally sanctioned form of behavior. The relationship of women to custom is, indeed, problematical: an account of female initiation in southern Africa "shows women's agency in the making of 'traditions' that might be interpreted as confirming and deepening women's subordination to men" (Geisler 1997:92).

For Cohen and Reid (1996) "the object of policy is to understand [culture] and to try and work with the forces which are changing norms, values and behaviors"; and they go on to suggest that as both men and women "are dying unnecessarily," then "[w]here there are only gainers and no losers from social and cultural change then surely there can be hope and something for policy makers and programmes to work with?"

An approach from gender and development might help here, the distinction between women's practical needs and strategic interests: "[N]eeds point in the direction of satisfying choices, while interests refer to expanding control over the interpretation of needs and the conditions of choice" (Kabeer 1994:300). Help with daily practical needs can have transformatory or redistributive effects which will facilitate the satisfying of [long-term] strategic gender interests which "entail challenge to the structural basis of women's disempowerment" (Kabeer 1994:301). In some of the participatory community-based programs, such as the Stepping Stones project, which go beyond the narrow provision of HIV/AIDS education to discuss gender relations and other issues like domestic violence, I think we can see a middle-level community-based tactical program which answers some of the daily practical needs by changing some aspects of gender relations between men and women and facilitating women's empowerment, but which in the long run may or should help toward meeting strategic interests of both women and men.

But what of *"cultural entrapments"*? I have taken this term from Mhloyi (1995:18–19): "To reorder the social system, the men who control it also need empowerment. They must be intellectually and emotionally released from the cultural entrapments that require women to be submissive". However, she also argues for some degree of compulsion to speed matters:

> Governments would prefer to wait for voluntary change, but it is imperative that laws prohibiting these formerly sanctioned cultural practices be instituted and enforced immediately. Such legislation would reduce the helplessness of people who are frightened of breaking ancestral and spiritual tradition but fearful of infection. Granted these laws would be unpopular, but Africa cannot afford political popularity at the expense of its people's lives. (Mhloyi 1995:17)

The notion of "cultural entrapment" is an interesting one, though it was not developed by Mhloyi. "Constraints," a term resonant of duress, of forces outwith the control of the individual, is consonant with the controls imposed by structural and institutional forces. "Cultural entrapments" resonates with challenges to forms of behavior understood as entrenched custom which privately and publicly raise women's and men's, and governments', awareness of the issues, and which can help to change not only the climate of opinion but also

laws and ultimately (some) individual behaviors. Entrapment has connotations of struggle and the possibilities of escape or release from the trappings of culture; whereas earlier accounts of culture and tradition, stressing control and constraints on choices and behavior, made culture seem much more like a straitjacket from which individuals could not free themselves, even to save their lives.

ACKNOWLEDGMENTS

This is a revised version of the paper presented to the Symposium on "HIV/AIDS in Africa; Reviewing the Past: Understanding the Present and Charting the Future," Champaign, Illinois, July 14–17, 1999. I am grateful to the editors for their invitation to the Symposium and for their comments on an earlier version; to the publisher's editor for help in pruning the text and incorporating some last-minute changes; and to Philippe Serres, formerly Action AIDS' Stepping Stones Project Officer in London, for providing copies of the evaluation materials for its Ugandan trial. The chapter also draws on material first published in the Occasional Paper Series of the Centre of African Studies, University of Edinburgh.

NOTES

1. See, inter alia, Abrahamsen 1997; Akeroyd 1996, 1997; Bassett and Mhloyi, 1991; Baylies and Bujra 2000, 1995; Kisekka 1990; Mandevu 1995; Mwale and Burnard 1992; Obbo 1993a; Reid 1995; Schoepf 2001, 1992a; Ulin 1992. For electronic materials see the UNIFEM Gender and HIV/AIDS Web Portal [<http://www.genderandaids.org/>]; the ELDIS Gender and HIV/AIDS Dossier [<http://www.eldis.org/gender/dossiers>]; the BRIDGE Cutting Edge Pack Gender and HIV/AIDS (2002) [<http://www.ids.ac.uk/bridge/reports_gend_CEP.html>] and the Siyanda database [<http://www.siyanda.org>].
2. Akeroyd (1996) is actually a later and much expanded version of Akeroyd (1997).
3. The Stepping Stones materials are now used worldwide; see the Strategies For Hope website [<http://www.talcuk.org/stratshope/index.html>].

4. Websites on these and other initiatives are now legion: see, e.g., UNIFEM, "Africa Campaign to Eliminate Violence Against Women: A life free of violence: key to sustainable human development in Africa." Electronic document. <http://www.undp.org/unifem/campaign/violence/africa_htm>; World Health Organization, 2003: *World Report on Violence and Health.* <http://www5.who.int/violence_injury_-prevention/main.cfm? p = 0000000682>; INSTRAW database on *Gender Aspects of Conflict and Peace.* <http://www. un-instraw.org/en/research/gacp/ index.html>; End Violence Against Women Information and Resource database [<http://www. endvaw. org/index.htm>]; The First South African Conference on Gender-based Violence and Health, held in 2002 <http://www.mrc.ac.za/conference/ genderviolence.htm>.

5. XII World Conference on AIDS, Track D: Social and Behavioral Sciences, Summary of Monday, June 29, 1998. Electronic document. <http:// www.aids98.ch/archive/30_UESDAY/300698_sum-marysession_trackd .html>

Chapter 7

Strategies for Prevention of Sexual Transmission of HIV/AIDS Among Adolescents: The Case of High School Students in Kenya

Njeri Mbugua

Introduction

The discussion in this chapter is based on findings from research conducted in 1996 among high school students in Kenya. The study aimed to determine the knowledge, attitudes, practices, and beliefs of high school students regarding sex and HIV/AIDS. Based on the findings, the study postulates several strategies aimed at slowing sexual transmission of HIV/AIDS among adolescents.

Unlike most parts of the developed world where the main modes of HIV transmission are through homosexual contacts or infected drug needles, HIV transmission in sub-Saharan Africa is primarily through *heterosexual* contacts. In Kenya, heterosexual transmission of HIV accounts for about 74 percent of all AIDS cases, followed by perinatal transmission (23 percent) and blood transfusion (3–5 percent) (Republic of Kenya 1991).

The study focuses on the prevention of sexual transmission of HIV among *adolescents* for four reasons:

1. Adolescents comprise the most sexually active age group. Statistics indicate that worldwide, the majority of those infected with HIV are aged between 20 and 45 years. When we factor in the slow rate of progression from HIV infection to AIDS, a period of about 5–10 years, it is highly likely that many of these adults were infected with HIV during their teens (Panos Dossier 1990; Berer and Ray 1993).

2. Adolescence is characterized by experimentation with, and initiation into, risky behavioral practices, including sex, alcohol, and drugs. Thus adolescents are at greater risk of contracting HIV than other age groups.

3. Despite being sexually active and adventurous, most (African) adolescents are not knowledgeable about sex and contraceptives (Boohene et al. 1991; Ajayi et al. 1991; Lema and Hassan 1994; Kiragu 1991; Njau 1993; Okumu et al. 1994; Maina 1995).

4. Sub-Saharan Africa is characterized by a young population. In Kenya, the age group 10–19 years comprises over 25 percent of the country's total population and is

the fastest-growing segment (Kenya Demographic Health Survey 1993 [National Council for Population and Development 1993]). Since adolescents' sexual behavior will determine the future level of HIV infection, it is crucial to protect the current generation from contracting HIV in order to ensure healthy future generations.

The study focuses on prevention of sexual transmission of HIV among adolescent *girls* because gender-disaggregated HIV/AIDS prevalence data indicates that the rate of infection among younger women is higher than among males – the number of AIDS cases among girls aged 15–19 years is more than double that of boys of the same age group (Republic of Kenya 1991). One explanation is that adolescent girls engage in sexual intercourse with older men as opposed to boys their own age because of the financial favors these older men (referred to as Sugar Daddies) offer (Njau 1993; Balmer 1994). Because of their age and economic affluence, Sugar Daddies engage in sexual intercourse with numerous partners and are therefore likely to be exposed to HIV. They choose young girls because they believe them to be sexually inexperienced and therefore less likely to be exposed to HIV (Barnett and Piers 1992).

The study focuses on *high school* girls for three main reasons. Firstly, education is important and every effort must be made to ensure that girls attain an education. Research shows that investment in female education enables women to improve their lives, that of their families and the country as a whole. Indeed, education empowers girls socially, economically, psychologically, and health-wise by providing them with tools to improve themselves as well as their environments (Azikiwe 1992; King 1990).

Secondly, the majority of girls are disadvantaged at all levels of education in terms of access, participation, completion, and performance (Republic of Kenya 1991).

Thirdly, in-school girls are overlooked in research and funding. Indeed, the majority of studies on adolescent girls conducted in sub-Saharan Africa dwell on the problems of pregnant teenagers (Khasiani 1985; Kiragu 1991; Njau 1993). Many resources are directed at

helping these "troubled youth," oftentimes at the expense of in-school girls who cope with society's expectations.

Knowing that girls are disadvantaged in school and that they are sexual prey for older (infected) men, this study seeks to find ways in which in-school girls can be protected from contracting sexually transmitted diseases or becoming pregnant. This will not only save the girls' lives, but also enable them to complete their education. While the study focuses primarily on in-school girls, who are more disadvantaged than boys of their age, it also includes information from high school boys since their inclusion is important in any research dealing with adolescent sexuality.

Methodology

This study employed several research methods, including: a) survey, b) focus group discussions, c) interviews with key informants, and d) observation. A cross-sectional study design was used, which captured the students' knowledge, attitudes, beliefs, and practices at the time of the study.

The survey

High school education in Kenya lasts for four years. The average age of students in their first year is 14 years (17 years in their fourth year). There are only a few mixed (co-education) high schools in Kenya, the majority being single sex schools. The target population in this study was high school students in their fourth year of study (commonly referred to as fourth form, and equivalent to 12th grade in the US education system). These students were selected because they had almost completed their high school education and therefore knew what the school taught about sexuality and AIDS. These students also were considered mature enough to assess their own views and feelings about sex, and how these had changed through the four years of high school education. This was also the best age to discover the determinants of sexual abstinence from those who were not yet sexually active.

The survey was conducted in randomly selected schools located in Nairobi and Nakuru districts, chosen because they have a relatively heterogeneous ethnic population. Nairobi is the country's capital city and has a high rate of HIV infection, and represents an urban district. Nakuru district is a rural farming district situated about 100 miles from Nairobi. It has a few small towns (Nakuru town, Gilgil, Njoro, and Molo). Surrounding these towns are rural farming areas which have low HIV infection rates. Since Nakuru district was chosen to represent a rural district, none of the schools in the principal towns was included in the survey.

All the fourth form students in the selected schools were included in the survey, yielding a total of 725 respondents. However, of these, ten provided incomplete data and another four had extremely contradictory information. Consequently, these 14 were excluded from the analysis. Of the 711 students included in this report, 534 (75 percent) are girls and 177 (25 percent) boys. There are fewer males than females since only the males in mixed schools were included in the survey. The percentage of respondents from schools in Nairobi (55 percent) was slightly greater than that from Nakuru (45 percent). A total of 267 (38 percent) were from rural areas and 443 (62 percent) from urban areas. It is noteworthy that Kenyan students often attend schools located far away from their home district. Thus, despite being situated in a rural area, a school could still comprise a majority of students from urban areas.

The survey instrument

The study utilized a self-administered questionnaire. Many of the questions were adapted from existing surveys on sex and HIV/AIDS conducted in various parts of Africa as well as the USA, and modified to fit the Kenyan cultural and linguistic setting. A self-administered questionnaire was used because the research dealt with very sensitive and personal issues (e.g., sexuality, substance usage) which most people have great difficulty discussing face-to-face due to fear of incriminating themselves or because of cultural barriers. For example, most Kenyans consider it vulgar, offensive, and culturally inappropriate to mention words associated with human sexuality (such as the genitals or the sexual act). Thus, to gather data on the sexual knowledge, atti-

tudes, beliefs, and practices of adolescent students without mentioning these "offensive" words necessitated the use of a self-administered questionnaire. Through this medium, students could read these terms and write about them yet avoid the cultural embarrassment of verbalizing them. In addition, the study took into consideration the fact that during a face-to-face interview respondents may conceal some information to save face, especially when the interviewee is involved in socially unacceptable behavior such as premarital sex or substance usage. A self-administered questionnaire gives "distance" between the interviewee and interviewer, thereby reducing the former's need to conceal any "incriminating" behavior.

The students took an average of one and a half hours to complete the questionnaire, and were then given an opportunity to ask questions. A few (mostly boys) asked questions verbally while most wrote down their questions. The main questions asked about HIV/AIDS included: a) origin, b) cure, and c) prevention of the disease, with stress on whether condoms were efficacious in preventing the transmission of HIV. The main questions asked on dating and sex included: a) ideal age to start dating/having sex, b) how to discern the right partner, and c) the best methods to use to perform/enjoy sexual intercourse. The fact that these questions were raised in *each and every* school surveyed apprised me of their prominence. Indeed, the students' responses (in the questionnaire) indicated that these were the issues they wanted addressed in regard to HIV/AIDS and sex. I answered all the questions to the best of my ability, and advised students who suspected they had a sexually transmitted disease to seek medical help.

Focus group discussions

I formed three focus groups each comprising 10–11 girls, two in Nairobi and one in Nakuru. I used these groups to pre-test the questionnaire, gather qualitative information, and interpret findings from the survey. The focus groups met once a week for a month. Though each session was scheduled for 90 minutes, most of the sessions took more than two hours.

During these discussions, I (as the facilitator) took the role of an uninformed outsider. I encouraged the girls to share their personal experiences and opinions on a wide range of issues, including academic life, sex, HIV/AIDS, relationships with their peers, teachers, and parents. The focus groups were extremely useful in bringing out members' experiences and viewpoints. The qualitative data from the focus groups supplemented the (quantitative) survey data with contextual information.

I tape-recorded the sessions. I also requested the discussants to take five minutes at the end of each session to write down what they considered important from that day's discussion. Once at home, I immediately transcribed the recordings and read through the students' notes. I combined their notes with mine, and made a summary of the key issues raised during the particular session. In this way, I was able to keep accurate notes of every meeting. In each subsequent meeting, I began by reading to the focus group participants the summaries of the previous meeting. I then invited them to comment on the accuracy of my summaries. They responded by either reiterating their statements or clarifying some viewpoints. This process helped us review the issues discussed in the previous session. It also provided a smooth continuation of (and transition into new) discussions from week to week.

Research Findings

HIV / AIDS

The study found that all the respondents had read or heard something about AIDS and that the majority 462 (65.4 percent) learned about HIV/AIDS between ages 12 and 15 years (Table 7.1).

Asked at what age young people should be taught about AIDS, 60 percent stated it should be taught between 10 and 13 years. The focus group discussants explained that they preferred AIDS be introduced to young people at this age because learning about such a fatal disease before this age (under10 years) could be very overwhelming and scary. One girl from focus group #3 (Nakuru) narrated her experience:

I was told about AIDS when I was 9 years old by my *big sis* [older sister]. From then on, I kept thinking everyone I met had AIDS. This made me scared to the point I did not want to shake hands[1] with people, and worse still, to travel in a *matatu* [public transport] in case I got scratched by someone with AIDS and became infected. To be honest, even now when I know I can't get AIDS this easily, that fear is still in me.[2]

The discussants added that age ten was ideal because this was the age most of them had become sexually aware of themselves and would have desired to be given a talk on sex as well as AIDS.

Frequency of HIV / AIDS messages

Asked when they last read or heard something about AIDS, 52 percent stated that it was less than a month before the survey. Given that youth are constantly exposed to sexual temptations, it is worrisome to find that 48 percent had not read or heard anything about HIV/AIDS in the month prior to the survey.

Discussing the frequency with which adolescents should be taught about AIDS, the focus group discussants stated that AIDS information should not be a one-time lesson but should be taught frequently, for two reasons: Firstly, most youth need to keep learning about AIDS until they fully comprehend it. If they are given only one talk, some would not understand it while others might forget the lesson. Secondly, throughout their lives adolescents are bombarded by various information, misinformation, and myths regarding HIV/AIDS. Consequently, they need constant accurate information to counteract false messages.

Content of HIV / AIDS information

The study sought to find out how knowledgeable respondents assessed themselves to be regarding AIDS, and what they wanted to learn about it. It is important to identify what they want to know, otherwise AIDS educators may lose students' interest by concentrating on material that students already know a great deal about and failing to cover the topics that students want to learn about.

Table 7.1   *Initial age at which respondents learned about HIV/AIDS*

Age	Frequency	Percentage
5–8	16	2.3
9–11	102	14.4
12–15	462	65.4
16–18	122	17.2
19–21	5	0.7

Note: Missing = 4. Two of these four respondents indicated that they could not remember the age at which they first learned about HIV/AIDS.

Table 7.2   *Preferred AIDS subjects by gender*

Desired AIDS content	Girls N = 534 %	Boys N = 177 %
Origin	92	91
Symptoms	91	90
Prevention	65	64
Cure	66	40
All of the above	13	12

The majority of respondents wanted to be taught about AIDS' origin, symptoms, prevention, and cure (Table 7.2), and AIDS communicators must address these topics when talking to youth about AIDS.

Asked how knowledgeable they judged themselves to be (vis-à-vis HIV/AIDS), 40 percent stated that they knew a great deal about AIDS, 58 percent that they knew only a little, and 3 percent thought they knew extremely little. Since each school surveyed reported that someone had talked to the students about AIDS, I sought to find the reasons for this difference. From the focus group discussions, I gathered five possible reasons.

Firstly, before learning about AIDS in school, some students had learned about it from other sources such as the media, peers, community-based programs, or religious-based programs. Such students found it easier to understand and retain the additional AIDS information they learned in school, and comprised the majority of students who assessed themselves as knowing a lot about AIDS. This finding highlights the fact that adolescents in school do not begin at the same (AIDS) knowledge level. Secondly, some schools had invited several people to speak about AIDS, including social workers, medical professionals, people with AIDS (PWAs), and the clergy. Students in these schools reported being

knowledgeable about AIDS because they had learned about varying aspects of AIDS from these speakers. Thirdly, most of the students who claimed to be knowledgeable about AIDS had been taught about it using various methods (videos, plays, books). More students in these schools assessed themselves to be knowledgeable about AIDS than in schools where only one method (mainly a lecture) had been used.[3] Fourthly, students felt confused when AIDS talks given by professionals differed from the general (street) knowledge they were constantly receiving, and did not know whether to believe the speakers. Perhaps their confusion made such students report that they were not knowledgeable about AIDS. Fifthly and closely related to the fourth reason, some discussants stated that they felt they knew little about AIDS when their questions remained unanswered.

When the respondents were asked to name three main sources from which they got most of their HIV/AIDS information, their choices in descending order were: 1) radio, 2) teachers, and 3) magazines. This finding is similar to that of Maina (1995), who conducted a study among 12–19-year-old Kenyan in-school and out-of-school youth. She found that adolescents got most of their information about STDs and HIV/AIDS from the radio, television, and teachers. That teachers were the

Table 7.3 *Socializing agents with whom respondents have discussed HIV/AIDS by gender*

Socializing agent	Girls N = 534 %	Boys N = 177 %
Same-sex peers	81	70
Teachers	76	67
Parents	70	44
Sisters	69	44
Brothers	59	61*
Relatives	59	47
Girl/boyfriend	49	57*
Religious leaders	44	33
Sex partner	24	48*

* Indicates variables in which boys outnumber girls.

second most cited source highlights their crucial role in disseminating AIDS information to youth.

Table 7.3 lists the significant socializing agents with whom respondents discussed HIV/AIDS. The majority of students (81 percent of girls and 70 percent of boys) had talked to their peers about AIDS, which highlights the importance of peer education in disseminating AIDS information. Table 7.3 also shows that more girls than boys had talked about AIDS to all the socializing agents mentioned other than their sexual partners, boyfriends, and brothers (highlighted by the asterisk). This is a reflection of African traditional culture whereby members of the opposite sex rarely discuss sex with each other. Indeed, the focus group respondents revealed that the relatives with whom most girls discussed AIDS were same-sex relatives such as aunts and female cousins.

Though teachers were cited as one of the commonest sources of HIV/AIDS information, respondents indicated that they discussed AIDS mostly with their peers. This implies that they received most of their information from teachers (and other sources) and discussed it among themselves. Many of the teachers expressed discomfort in teaching students about sex and AIDS. They traced this to African traditional practices which bar elders from talking to youth about sex except under certain conditions[4] which a classroom situation does not foster.

Similarly, most parents stated that they felt uneasy discussing AIDS or any sexual matters with their children. This does not mean that parents do not talk to their children about AIDS. On the contrary, 70 percent of girls and 44 percent of boys stated that they had talked with their parents about HIV/AIDS. However, findings from both the survey and focus group discussions show that most parents were not the initial or main source of HIV information for their children. These findings are similar to those in many sub-Saharan countries such as Nigeria (Owuamanam 1983); Zimbabwe (Wilson et al. 1989; Pitts and Jackson 1993); Burundi, Ghana, Liberia (Gage and Meekers 1994); and Zambia (Pillai and Benefo 1995).

Effective teaching approaches

Apart from the above-mentioned sources, respondents indicated that they had received information about AIDS from presentations by several non-governmental organizations. Asked what methods used by these organizations they considered effective in teaching about AIDS, the respondents listed four: a) use of plays or short skits depicting adolescent dating behaviors and how these lead to HIV infection; b) use of films/documentaries depicting the stories of individuals whose lives have been affected by AIDS; c) use of visuals (drawings, pictures) showing how the virus is transmitted; and d) talks about HIV/AIDS from individuals with AIDS, or those who were knowledgeable about AIDS such as medical people.

HIV blood testing

Seventy percent of the respondents had heard about HIV blood testing; 16 percent had never heard of such a test and 5 percent were unsure

– which implies that they had not. It is unfortunate that 30 percent of Kenya's educated youth do not know that an HIV blood test exists. But even when respondents knew about HIV testing, about half were doubtful as to whether the test is accurate. Specifically, 40 percent of the respondents stated that they were not sure whether the test was accurate and 9 percent thought it was not accurate. With this attitude toward HIV blood tests, it is not surprising to find that only 20 percent had ever taken a test.

During a discussion about HIV testing with members of focus group #3 (Nakuru), one girl aired the following sentiment which captures the fatalistic attitude held by most students with whom I discussed HIV blood testing.

> I have heard of people like that [who claim they do not have AIDS but in fact they do]...but what is worse is that HIV tests for some people come out positive, only to be tested later and it shows that they were actually negative. Why go through such an ordeal...and torture yourself? At least with malaria, one can take Malariaquin in case of doubt...But what can you take if suspected of having HIV unless your own life?

The most widely used test for HIV infection is known as ELISA (enzyme-linked immunosorbent assay). ELISA does not directly detect HIV in the blood but reveals HIV antibodies. Most people show antibody response to HIV long before they develop symptoms of infection. However, since it can take many months for people who have been exposed to HIV to develop antibodies, it is recommended that tests be taken six months (or longer) from the date of possible exposure. A positive test result (seropositive) means that someone has developed antibodies and is therefore highly likely to be infected with HIV. Only on very rare occasions do people test positive yet do not become infected with HIV. An example occurs when fetuses that receive antibodies from their infected mothers do not become infected with the virus itself.

Those who receive a seropositive ELISA test and need further confirmation can use the Western blot test (commonly referred to as PCR – polymerase chain reaction). This is an expensive but sure test for it detects the virus itself.

Respondents' HIV status

Asked whether they had AIDS, most students (52 percent) were not sure and 44 percent stated they did not. Only 1.3 percent (7 girls and 2 boys) stated that they were HIV-positive. Since only 20 percent of the respondents had ever taken an HIV blood test, this implies that the majority of respondents were not sure whether they were HIV-positive or not. Most of the respondents guessed their HIV status – most likely based on their sexual behavior and their health. Similarly, the majority of respondents were unsure or did not know their friends' and sexual partners' HIV status. Very few respondents (8 percent) stated that their friends had AIDS.

Asked whether they could detect whether someone had AIDS merely by looking at them, only 38 percent of the respondents stated that they could not. The majority indicated that they could detect PWAs by looking for such physical symptoms as hair loss, skin rashes, and sickly demeanor. As long as students use physical manifestations to determine whether people have AIDS, they are at risk of contracting the virus if they have sex with healthy-looking PWAs.

I asked the focus group discussants whether they had ever asked their partner (or a potential partner) about their HIV status. I gathered that it was difficult for them to ask a partner whether he had AIDS and therefore they relied on their gut feelings or looked for physical symptoms. The following narrative from a member of focus group #2 (from Nairobi) captures the above sentiments well. She stated:

> Most of us know that you can't tell whether someone has AIDS by looking at them. Yet when it comes to, like, my boyfriend, I can't ask him whether he has AIDS or not. I have to go with my gut feeling. If I feel deep down that he is sick, well, I'll be suspicious and start looking at his physical appearance, like whether he has a rash, is losing weight, and things like that. But, to be honest, by this point, I'll already be thinking of *booting* [leaving] him.

Sex

Age at which they first learn about sex
The majority of respondents learned about sex between the ages of 12 and 14 (Table 7.4). The

Table 7.4 *Age at which respondents initially learned about sex*

Age	Frequency	Percentage
5–8	49	6.9
9–11	148	20.8
12–14	331	46.6
15–16	129	18.1
17–19	27	3.8

Missing = 27.

three commonest sources of information were peers (35 percent), teachers (26 percent), and parents (12 percent). A study investigating communication networks of adolescent girls in rural Malawi for sexually transmitted disease prevention messages found that 75 percent learned about sex from their best friends, with parents being conspicuously absent in the sexual education of their children (Helitzer-Allen 1994). Similarly, studies conducted in Zambia (Pillai and Benefo 1995) and Zimbabwe (Bassett and Sherman 1994) found that most of the adolescents' sex information was from friends and the media (romance novels, movies, and magazines). Focus group discussants stated that most parents tried to talk to them about sex when it was too late as they had already learned about it from other sources.

Asked whether sex talks with parents were helpful, most focus group discussants stated that they were not, as they comprised lengthy lectures and warnings against associating with boys. The girls referred to these talks by the *Sheng* word *msomo* – which means "lengthy lecture" (usually against something). As a result of these *msomos*, most girls stated that they had poor relationships with their mothers. The following narrative from a member of focus group #3 (Nakuru) sums up most discussants' experiences and sentiments towards their mothers:

I could stay in the house and do all the cleaning the entire week, but if I ask to go out on a Saturday afternoon to watch a movie or just visit with my friends, my mother turns against me like I have asked for the impossible. She gives these *msomos* about what happens to girls who run away from home, who open their legs to men, who get pregnant, who do not listen to their parents, etc. She forgets all that I have done the whole week and says that all I do is just want to

go out, out, out … I really get mad for she never appreciates my efforts.

This reveals how Kenyan parents control their teenage children by restricting their movements. This is akin to the curfew system enforced by parents in the West. However, while in the West teenagers may go out as long as they return at a specified time, in most African homes teenagers (especially girls) are not permitted to leave home unless accompanied by other members of the family or chaperoned by an adult. Some parents go to the extent of forbidding their daughters to receive any visitors.

Sexual activity

Findings indicate that 79.7 percent of boys and 23.2 percent of girls were sexually active. More respondents from rural areas were sexually active than from urban areas. Asked what factors led them to begin having sexual intercourse, most sexually active girls (52.8 percent) stated that their first sexual encounter was motivated by love for their boyfriend. This percentage was four times that of boys (13.2 percent) who cited love for their girlfriends as the motivation for their initial sexual encounter. The majority of boys (74.4 percent) stated that their first sexual encounter was motivated by the need to experiment and experience sex for themselves.

Another gender difference pertained to sex for money. While none of the boys claimed that they had sex for money, 4 percent of the girls stated that they did. This finding highlights the plight of young poor girls who turn to sex to meet their financial needs. In the course of discussions, the girls stated that some girls they knew had sex for money to enable them to pay school fees.[5] This is *survival sex* without which the girls could not afford

Njeri Mbugua

Table 7.5 *Relative likelihood of respondents from poor economic backgrounds being sexually active*

Independent variable	Percentage virgin	Percentage non-virgin	OR		95% CI
Been suspended from school for non-payment of fees:					
Females	51.2	30.1	2.433*	1.611	3.673
Males	23.2	76.8	0.763	0.366	1.588

* $p < 0.01$, one-tailed test.

school fees and would therefore be expelled. In this AIDS era, sex is a very high and risky price to pay for education.

However, not all girls who have sex for money are from low-income families. Indeed, the focus group discussants pointed out that some of the girls who had sex for money did so because they yearned for a lifestyle which they could not otherwise afford.

Sexual activity and poor economic status

The study sought to discover whether there is an association between sexual activity and disruption of studies[6] for financial reasons. Most Kenyans value education very highly and, therefore, having one's studies disrupted for financial reasons (mainly inability to pay school fees) implies dire financial need. Two hundred and sixty-five respondents (37 percent) stated that their studies had been disrupted for financial reasons. That only 37 percent of high school students in their final academic year have had their studies disrupted for financial reasons may be explained by the fact that high school education in Kenya is expensive, and the majority of the poor cannot afford it. Thus, by the fourth year of high school, the majority of poor students have dropped out of school.

Table 7.5 indicates that females who have been suspended from school for non-payment of school fees are roughly two and a half (2.433) times more likely to be sexually active than those who haven't. This comparison is statistically significant (Pearson chi-square $p < 0.0005$). However, among males, we find no statistically significant difference in sexual activity between those who have been suspended from school for non-payment of school fees and those who haven't (Pearson chi-square $p = 0.468$). This gender difference may be due to the fact that females who

are suspended from school for lack of school fees are likely to turn to sex for money. In Kenya, it is rare for men to have sex for money, which may explain why males with school fees problems are not likely to turn to sex for money.

Sexual activity and parental monitoring

As mentioned earlier, most Kenyan parents restrict their children's movements in a bid to ensure that they remain sexually abstinent. The study hypothesized that *students whose parents are overly strict are likely to be sexually abstinent*. Test findings are shown in Table 7.6.

Contrary to the hypothesis, strict parental monitoring does not prevent adolescent females being sexually active. Indeed, females whose parents are overly strict are three times more likely to be sexually active than those whose parents are not. This difference is statistically significant (Pearson chi-square $p < 0.0005$). The 95 percent Confidence Interval for the odds ratio extends from 1.915 to 5.426, so the hypothesis that the odds are the same is rejected. Similar findings were found by Kiragu (1991), who conducted a similar study among high school students in Nakuru district.

The above conclusion is supported by notes from focus group members who stated that the more parents restrict their movements, the more they are tempted to defy their authority. This is especially true when parents not only restrict the girls' movements but also constantly scold, nag and lecture them on how evil boys are.

Unlike the counteractive effect on females, parental monitoring lowered the odds of boys being sexually active. Table 7.6 shows that boys with very restrictive mothers are 0.733 times less likely to be sexually active, and those whose fathers were strict were 0.655 times less likely to be sexually active than

Table 7.6   *Relative likelihood of respondents with strict parents being sexually abstinent*

Independent variable	Percentage virgin	Percentage non-virgin	OR		CI
Mother is overly strict					
Females	75.9	49.3	3.235*	2.004	5.220
Males	57.1	64.5	0.733	0.324	1.658
Father is overly strict					
Females	51.4	36.0	3.224*	1.915	5.426
Males	71.8	45.5	0.655	0.272	1.575

* $p < 0.01$, one-tailed test.

those whose parents were not strict. These comparisons are substantively but not statistically significant (Pearson chi-square $p > 0.4$). Parental monitoring of males may have the desired effect because, on the whole, parents do not unduly subject their sons to the harsh restrictions imposed on their daughters. Consequently, males may not have the impetus to rebel against their parents as females do.

Sexual activity and risky behaviors

The study tested whether there is an association between sexual activity and such risky behaviors as using alcohol, smoking cigarettes, taking drugs, frequenting discos, and associating with people with these behaviors. The test results indicate that all these behaviors significantly increase the odds of high school students being sexually active (Table 7.7).

Sexual activity and alcohol

Table 7.7 reveals that females who take alcohol are nearly three times (2.723) more likely to be sexually active than those who do not. This is statistically significant (Pearson chi-square $p < 0.0005$). Similarly, males who take alcohol are nearly three and a half times (3.451) more likely to be sexually active than those who do not. This comparison is also statistically significant (Pearson chi-square $p = 0.004$). Therefore, we accept the hypothesis that adolescents who drink alcohol are likely to be sexually active. A 95 percent Confidence Interval for the odds ratios of both cigarette smoking and use of alcohol does not include the null hypothesis of no difference. Consequently, we accept our hypothesis that substance use is positively associated with sexual activity. This test finding is not surprising, seeing that

alcohol (and other substance) abuse affects people's risk assessment process. Substance use coupled with impulsive sexual desire can reduce the ability to make responsible decisions. Other studies conducted in Kenya show similar results (Acuda 1982; Dhadphale et al. 1982; Kiragu 1991). The linkages of these problem behaviors were stronger for girls than boys, a pattern that is consistent with the notion that these activities represent a more deviant behavior for girls.

Sexual activity and smoking

Test findings indicate that females who smoke cigarettes are three times (3.229) more likely to be sexually active compared to those who do not. This comparison is statistically significant (Pearson chi-square $p = 0.009$). Among males, those who smoke are roughly nine and a half times (9.459) more likely to be sexually active than those who do not. This comparison is also statistically significant (Pearson chi-square $p = 0.006$). The fact that smoking cigarettes highly increases the odds of high school students being sexually active is an important finding in the fight against sexual transmission of HIV. This is because for the most part in Kenya, there is less stigma attached to smoking than to drinking alcohol (especially among males). Indeed, the focus group discussants stated that among males, smoking is a symbol of adult status. To exert this status, most males smoke in the open – concealing it only from their parents and teachers. Since most youth are willing to admit that they smoke (but may conceal other drug habits), smoking can be used as a means of detecting those who are most likely to be sexually active.

Several studies have found an association between cigarette smoking and early onset of

Table 7.7 *Relative likelihood of respondents using substances being sexually active*

Delinquent behavior	Percentage non-virgin	Percentage virgin	OR		CI
Smoking cigarettes					
Females	8.9	2.9	3.229	1.388	7.512*
Males	21.3	2.8	9.459	1.245	71.901*
Drinking alcohol					
Females	37.1	17.8	2.723	1.747	4.243*
Males	49.6	22.2	3.451	1.472	8.092*
Abuse drugs**					
Females	0.8	1.2	0.659	0.076	5.690*
Males	9.9	–	N/A	–	–
Frequents disco					
Females	46.0	23.2	2.821	1.851	4.298*
Males	66.0	27.8	5.038	2.245	11.304*

* $p < 0.01$, one-tailed test.
** An odds ratio for drug use is not possible given a cell frequency of 0 for reported use among virgin males, and is not meaningful among females due to the small numbers.

sexual behavior (Rosenbaum and Kandel 1990; Gillmore et al. 1992). According to these researchers, negative adolescent behaviors such as cigarette smoking can be associated with risky sexual behavior because they are manifestations of a common underlying syndrome of problem behaviors.

Sexual activity and discos

Table 7.7 shows that females who frequent discos are nearly three times (2.821) more likely to be sexually active than those who do not. Males who frequent discos are five times (5.038) more likely to be sexually active than those who do not. Both these comparisons are statistically significant (Pearson chi-square $p < 0.0005$). A 95 percent Confidence Interval for the ratios does not include the null hypothesis of no difference. Therefore, we accept the hypothesis that frequenting discos is (positively) associated with sexual activity.

Controlling for locality, we find that students from urban areas who frequent discos are three times (3.069) more likely to be sexually active than those who do not. Students from rural areas who frequent discos are seven times (7.217) more likely to be sexually active than those who do not. Both these comparisons are statistically significant (Pearson chi-square $p < 0.0005$). A 95 percent Confidence Interval for the ratios does not include the null hypothesis of no difference.

The above findings indicate that the odds of rural adolescents who frequent discos being sexually active are greater than for urban adolescents, confirming the opinion of focus group discussants that most discos in rural areas – held during holidays, especially Christmas, New Year, weddings, circumcision rites – are opportunities for youth to be sexually active. They explained that during such functions, boys' goal is to have sex. In addition, the rural disco environment – poor lighting, loud music, availability of alcohol, and absence of adult supervision – may explain why students in rural areas who frequent discos are more likely to be sexually active than those in urban areas.

Impact of associating with delinquent friends

The study tested the influence on adolescents' sexual activity of associating with friends involved in risky behaviors such as smoking, drinking, taking drugs, and being sexually active. The findings indicate that association with delinquent peers increases the odds of youth being sexually active, and that the odds of being sexually active are highest for those who associate with sexually active peers (Table 7.8).

Sexual activity and associating with peers who are sexually active

Table 7.8 indicates that females who associate with sexually active peers are roughly 15 times (14.887) more likely to be sexually active than

Table 7.8   *Relative likelihood of respondents involved in delinquent behavior being sexually active*

Peer risky behavior	Percentage non-virgin	Percentage virgin	OR		CI
Friends smoke					
Females	20.4	14.2	1.545	0.890	2.680*
Males	54.0	34.4	2.238	0.996	5.028*
Friends drink alcohol					
Females	51.4	36.0	1.879	1.215	2.907*
Males	71.8	45.5	3.051	1.386	6.716*
Friends abuse drugs					
Females	7.9	3.8	2.173	0.915	5.163*
Males	24.2	20.0	1.277	0.477	3.417*
Friends frequent disco					
Females	68.1	46.9	2.426	1.550	3.797*
Males	79.2	56.3	2.967	1.311	6.716*
Friends are sexually active					
Females	64.9	11.1	14.887	8.434	26.72
Males	35.1	88.9	14.267	5.432	37.467

* $p < 0.01$, one-tailed test.

females who do not have such associations. Similarly, males whose friends are sexually active are 14 times (14.267) more likely to be sexually active than those whose friends are not sexually active. Both these comparisons are statistically significant (Pearson chi-square $p <$ 0.0005). The odds ratios range from 5.432 to 37.467, so at 95 percent Confidence Interval we reject the null hypothesis of no difference.

Associating with sexually active peers increases the odds of being sexually active so highly because it has a direct impact on the respondents' sexual behaviors. The other variables impact sexual behavior indirectly. For example, associating with peers who frequent discos may influence a girl to frequent discos which in turn predisposes her to sexual activity.

Condoms

The majority of sexually active students (68 percent) relied on condoms as their chief method of birth control. But even among these students, the rate of consistent condom use was as low as 2.1 percent for girls and 10.7 percent for boys. The main reason given was that the respondents, or their sex partners, did not like using condoms. Specifically, 32 percent of boys and 4.2 percent of girls stated that they did not like using condoms, and 3.4 percent of girls and 5.7 percent of boys stated that their sex partners did not like using condoms. Other reasons given against condom use included embarrass-

ment, spontaneity, and use of other birth control methods. Specifically, 45 percent of the students indicated that they would be too embarrassed to purchase or use a condom.

Seventy-seven (sexually active) boys and 12 girls wrote (in the questionnaire) that sex was more enjoyable for them and their partners without a condom. They stated that condoms made sex feel "unnatural." The narratives below express some of the respondents' sentiments towards condoms. The last two sentiments were expressed by girls and all the others by boys:

Condoms are cumbersome, time taking and make people so nervous that you don't enjoy sex. How do you insert a condom when a girl you have been *tuning* [courting] all night suddenly melts in your arms and says "yes"? You do not look for a condom, no you look for your zip and do it [sexual intercourse] before she changes her mind. But you have to do it [sex] well, so that she gives you *bone* [sex] another time. If you use a condom, it's a guarantee both of you will not enjoy it, and that will be the end 'cos she won't do it with you ever again.

Using a condom is like taking a shower with a raincoat, or eating a sweet with a wrapper, you miss the joy of it. You feel nothing, and worst of all, you feel uncomfortable.

I would like to use a condom but most times I end up having sex with a girl when I have gotten drunk. I am drunk, she is drunk, and it [condom] is the last thing I am thinking of at that crucial time.

A condom is useful only when in doubt of the sex partner, but why sleep with someone you are in doubt with unless you are a *pro*?[prostitute]

A condom is cold, and uncomfortable. When I have sex, I want the real thing, warm and human, not rubbery.

With these negative perceptions, it is not surprising that the rate of condom usage among sexually active high school students is very low. People who think that condoms are embarrassing or reduce sexual pleasure are unlikely to use them.

During focus group discussions, the girls stated that most sexually active youth use condoms as contraceptives rather than as prophylaxis (against HIV or other STDs), with most girls using condoms during the initial sexual encounters with a partner. Once they established an ongoing sexual relationship, they resorted to other contraceptive devices such as the pill. This suggests that youth use condoms as a temporal precaution until they gain the trust of their sexual partner. Secondly, the discussants stated that some girls who relied on the rhythm birth control method used condoms during their "unsafe" days.

The focus group participants also identified alcohol use as an influence against condom usage. They stated that most girls get drunk at parties and are taken advantage of sexually. In a drunken state, they are not able to resist sex, or to ask the sex partner to use a condom. The role of alcohol in limiting condom usage was also expressed by boys, as reflected by the third narrative regarding condoms discussed earlier.

Monogamy

Discussions with focus group members revealed that most girls were disillusioned with males because most (teenage or adult males) were sexually unfaithful to their partner. In all three focus group discussions, the girls were unanimous that Kenyan males are "polygamous in nature" – unfaithful to their girlfriend(s). They wondered whether it was worthwhile heeding the AIDS warnings to remain sexually abstinent or monogamous if they eventually might marry an unfaithful man.

Policy Options/Recommendations

Based on the above findings, this study makes the following recommendations.

Family socialization strategies

1. Sex talks should be given early in life: This study recommends that parents talk to their children at an early age – preferably before they turn age ten. After age ten, most children have already heard about dating, sex, contraceptives, and AIDS from other sources. Some have already become sexually experienced and therefore do not benefit greatly from such talks. It is equally important for other AIDS awareness and prevention programs to address children during early childhood, for failure to control the epidemic at an early stage will result in far more damaging and costly consequences in the future.

2. Communication not condemnation: Based on the discussions with focus group members, this study recommends that parents give factual talks about sex, and also listen to their children's opinions. This can help them give useful counsel without alienating their daughters. As noted earlier, most girls complained that their mothers never listened to them but instead gave them *msomos* (constant lectures and threats against pregnancy) which caused the girls to rebel or feel resentful against their mothers.

3. Parents give sex talks to both boys and girls: Findings indicated that most parents constantly lecture their daughters on the dangers of sex, but rarely do the same with their sons. This gives the covert message that it is tolerable for boys but not girls to be sexually adventurous. If the youth are to change their sexual behavior, there is a need for parents (and other sex educators) to socialize boys to be honorable in their dealings with girls. Both males and females should be taught to assume equal responsibility in sexual decision-making.

4. Fidelity as a good norm: There is need to train (both boys and girls) to be sexually faithful to their partners. Simple as this seems, this is a very crucial recommendation because *dogging* (unfaithfulness to partners) and premarital sex – behaviors that would have shocked previous generations – are slowly becoming accepted as a norm by Kenyan youth. There is therefore an urgent need to socialize youth to value fidelity before and within marriage.

5. Adults act as responsible role models: As stated above, the study findings indicated that adolescents perceive most adults (especially males) as sexually unfaithful. If youth are to value fidelity, and boys to behave honorably toward girls, there is a need for adults to be good role models.

6. "Relax" parental monitoring: Since the test findings indicated that being overly strict in regulating adolescent movements (such as forbidding girls to socialize with boys or their peers) increased the likelihood of adolescents becoming sexually active, this study recommends that parents "relax" these extreme measures. It recommends that parents give their daughters some latitude to have healthy fun with their friends instead of maintaining stringent rules which eventually defeat the ultimate purpose of protecting them.

Educational strategies

7. School teachers should give sex/AIDS education: Since students showed a trust and willingness to learn from their teachers, this study recommends that schools make the most of this opportunity and give sex education in schools. They could address such topics as AIDS' origin, symptoms, cure, transmission, blood testing. These were topics that respondents knew little about, or wanted to know about.

8. Give candid and practical sex lessons: If adolescents are to benefit from safer-sex messages, there is a need for teachers to give candid sex education, talk about condoms and give practical demonstrations of their usage. This will ensure that AIDS education goes beyond mere dissemination of information to development of practical skills that can empower youth to make (and more importantly execute) responsible decisions. Without it, the current trend of premarital sexual behavior is likely to continue, with the negative consequences of unwanted pregnancies and sexually transmitted diseases.

9. Train school teachers: It is imperative that teachers be at ease when teaching about sexual intercourse and practical contraceptive usage (such as demonstration of condom use) because these are sensitive and embarrassing topics for teenagers. This calls for teachers to be trained to teach about human sexuality. They must be both effective communicators and knowledgeable about sex/AIDS if students are to learn without undue discomfort.

10. AIDS educators address all questions asked: AIDS educators should answer all questions asked – despite the nature of the questions. In so doing, they will give adolescents accurate information to counter the misconceptions and "rumors" that surround them. Failure to answer the questions is perceived as lack of knowledge on the part of the speakers, or an attempt to conceal the truth about AIDS.

11. Teach sex/AIDS to same-sex students: Most students discussed sex/AIDS with members of their own sex (whether peers or relatives), and girls were uncomfortable in the presence of boys during sex talks. Consequently, the study recommends that effort be made to separate boys and girls when teaching these topics. This applies mainly to mixed schools but can also be applicable when teaching out-of-school youth.

12. Sex education be given frequently using varied methods: Since findings show that students in the same school varied in their knowledge regarding HIV/AIDS, this study recommends giving students repeated AIDS training sessions using varying teaching methods. Four approaches identified by the students as being effective in teaching about AIDS included: a) plays/short skits; b) lectures on HIV/AIDS from PWAs and others knowledgeable about AIDS; c) visual media; d) print media.

13. Empower adolescents to implement safer-sex practices: There is a need to help youth develop a sense of self-efficacy in regard to safer-sex practices. Adolescents can be given practical demonstrations of how to protect themselves from AIDS through role playing. For example, students can be encouraged to participate in resistance training. Specifically, they can role-play negotiation of safer sex with potential sex partners. In enacting scenes that depict real-life situations – such as how to resist sexual advances, how to insist on condom use, how to purchase condoms without embarrassment, how to handle condoms effectively – youth learn how to use safer-sex methods and, more importantly, how to resist sex. This is especially important for most African girls who as a result of gender socialization are unable to communicate with their sexual partners. Play acting would give such girls the skills necessary to talk to their partners. Play-acting exercises would also help them retain the safer-sex information they have been taught.[7]

14. Meet education costs of disadvantaged girls: Since test findings indicated a significant and positive association between inability to pay school fees and increase in likelihood of females being sexually active, this study recommends that girls from poor economic backgrounds be assisted to pay school fees. As shown in the study, some girls were determined to excel in school following payment of their school fees by a concerned teacher. Without such an influence, they might have turned to sex for money.

Youth-oriented strategies

15. Train peer counselors: Since adolescents are easily influenced by their peer group, trained peer counselors can have a positive influence on their fellow youth in a way that adults may not. Peer counselors can serve as both role models (influencing positive behavior) and sex educators (disseminating accurate sex and AIDS information).

16. Provision of teenage recreation activities: There is a need for youth (especially rural youth) to be provided with entertainment opportunities where they can have fun without being exposed to sexual dangers. Three such activities are: a) daytime alcohol-free discos, which can be held under adult supervision; b) athletic activities, an ideal entertainment because they provide fun, have low budgetary requirements, and are a healthy means through which youth can vent their robust energy; and c) formation of social clubs.[8] Youth can be encouraged to join (or form new) social clubs.

17. Enforce laws barring adolescents from participating in risky social activities: There is a need to bar youth from participating in adult entertainment or engaging in substance abuse. This entails enforcing age-limit laws that prohibit teenagers from night clubs, make it illegal for youth to purchase cigarettes and alcohol, and expel students from school if they participate in such activities.

Contraceptive-oriented strategies

This study emphasizes that sexual abstinence is the best and safest strategy against HIV infection and unwanted pregnancy. However, it also notes that despite all efforts to discourage adolescents from sexual activity there always will be the "hard core" who do not heed such warnings. Since these students are sexually active and intend to continue being so, they require different HIV prevention strategies from the majority of high school girls who are not sexually active. The immediate strategy is to influence them to practice safer sex, that is, influence them to use condoms and to be monogamous. Consequently, I recommend:

18. Teach adolescents to perceive condoms as prophylactic: Since most sexually active respondents stated that they used condoms as birth control measures, they should be socialized to use them as prophylaxis against STDs. Using condoms as prophylaxis calls for consistent condom use even when adolescents are on oral (or other) contraceptives – whether they trust their sex partners or not.

19. Development of school–service links: Since the manifest function of education is to disseminate academic knowledge to students, teachers can give only a limited amount of sex and AIDS information. To supplement their input, this study recommends that schools develop links with health or social services (such as family planning clinics) which can mediate between schools and students. Professional workers from these services can visit schools, teach students about sex/AIDS and make known the services they have available. In turn, students can visit these services to learn more about sex/AIDS, and if necessary to be given contraceptives and counseling.[9] Such visits could continue after school hours, or even after students complete their high school education. Since the study findings showed that students were willing to learn about sex/AIDS from knowledgeable professionals, developing such links to services could be an effective strategy for preventing sexual transmission of HIV among high school students.

Conclusion

The study has shown that there is a need to focus on adolescents because they are becoming sexually active at an earlier age. Since adolescence is characterized by experimentation and adventure, they are at a greater risk of contracting HIV/AIDS than other age groups. But compared to adolescent boys, adolescent girls face even greater risks. Not only are they disadvantaged at all levels of education in terms of access, participation, completion, and performance, they are also twice as likely to contract HIV compared to boys of their age. Since in-school girls comprise the future (women) leaders, there is a dire need to ensure that they do not initiate sexual intercourse, or practice unsafe sex, thereby having their lives cut short by sexually transmitted diseases. Indeed, as sub-Saharan Africa suffers from the HIV/AIDS epidemic, there is great need to protect all youth from initiating sexual intercourse, which may change the course of the epidemic.

Using both qualitative and quantitative data, the study has postulated numerous practical AIDS prevention strategies addressing the social, cultural, spiritual, medical, economic, academic, recreational, and sexual lives of in-school adolescents. These practical strategies can be implemented by youth, parents, teachers, religious leaders, secular leaders, and policy makers to change the lives of today's youth in Kenya as well as in other parts of Africa. Some of these strategies have been proposed in other studies but have not been implemented in Kenya. When implemented, I believe they will promote both short- and long-term sustainable changes that will slow down the sexual transmission of HIV among Kenyan high school students in particular, and other youth in general.

Due to insufficient time and finances, this study sampled only two districts in Kenya. Future studies should include schools from all Kenyan districts, conduct more focus group discussions over a longer time period, and form focus groups comprising male students. Instead of the current cross-sectional study design, which captures girls' knowledge, attitudes, beliefs, and behaviors at the time of the study, they should conduct a longitudinal study which would capture the processes that occur in adolescents' lives over time, as well as assess the impact of any programs implemented.

NOTES

1. The majority of Kenyans greet each other by shaking hands, and may also shake hands when parting. To refuse to do so is considered very rude and insulting. Living in such a community can be traumatic for someone who fears contracting HIV through a handshake.
2. The fear of contracting HIV "accidentally" through casual contact such as shaking hands, being pricked by an infected needle, or being scratched by someone with AIDS was repeated by several students. Educators need to emphasize that to a large extent AIDS is transmitted in ways that people can control if they assume responsibility for their own behaviors.
3. Most of the schools where more than one approach to learning about AIDS was used were

urban schools (in Nairobi). The fact that some rural schools did not have electricity, and that some were not easily accessible (especially during rainy weather), may explain why these schools did not have such varied means of AIDS education as those in urban areas.

4. These conditions include circumcision rites and premarital counseling.

5. A student wrote in her questionnaire, "I take this opportunity to thank Mr. Waciuri who paid school fees for me in Form 2 and Form 4. My parents were ready to have me drop out of school because of school fees problems, but Mr. Waciuri talked to them and told them that he would pay the fees. He keeps organizing for my fees to be paid . . . and I am working very hard to make him proud of me . . . and not to waste his money."

6. School disruptions are not the same as dropping out of school. Unlike those who drop out of school, students who cannot afford school fees usually leave for a short period of time. This can be as short as one or two days, or at most a month.

7. Studies conducted in the US among school youth found that role-plays and Question and Answer interventions were the most effective means for communicating about safer-sex practices and preventing the forgetting of information about AIDS (Smith and Katner 1995).

8. Chastity and anti-AIDS clubs have been used in some countries (Rwanda, Malawi, and Zambia) and have been found to be effective against premarital sex. Efforts could be made to help adolescents in Kenya form similar clubs.

9. This would be an extremely useful service. As stated earlier, in the course of my research, several students asked me questions related to their personal health problems which I could not answer. I recommended they visit health clinics for medical checkups and counseling. Most likely such students will not heed my advice due to embarrassment, lack of finances, or lack of knowledge as to which institutions offer counseling services and free (or cheap) checkups. Links with institutions that offer such help would be extremely useful to such adolescents.

Chapter 8

AIDS in Africa: Structure, Agency, and Risk

Brooke Grundfest Schoepf

From the 1970s, research on the status of women in Africa, and especially research on gender relations, has been informed by the understanding of knowledge as power and of the ability of those in power to create and define knowledge. This understanding was culturally shared in many hierarchically organized precolonial societies. Thus understanding of the relationship between knowledge and power long antedated Michel Foucault, whom it is fashionable to cite as the source of this insight. Medical knowledge was integral to the exercise of political power and the maintenance of control by rulers. Knowledge of AIDS in Africa is about power: the power to name and define; the power to know; the power to attract funds; the power to act to reduce risks of becoming infected with HIV (Schoepf 1992a).

My earlier chapter discussed AIDS as a series of stories about power and resource control; about women and men; youth and elders; about bio-power and its opposites; about the congeries of beliefs and the institutions that have shaped claims to knowledge of AIDS. This chapter examines some of those claims in the light of African women's knowledge of AIDS. It looks at AIDS through the lens of

gender to show how gender inequality and the status of women are central to the epidemic spread of HIV.

As in the earlier chapter, I draw primarily on field research with the CONNAISSIDA Project in Kinshasa from 1985 to 1990. I also include some literature review and field notes from visits to seven other African countries in the context of international AIDS prevention consultancies from 1990 through 1997. Epidemiological data are from reports published by members of the international biomedical research group working in Kinshasa, Projet Sida, unless otherwise noted.

Formed from the French words *connaisance* (knowledge) and *Sida* (AIDS), CONNAISSIDA means "knowledge of AIDS." The CONNAISSIDA Project was one of the first in Africa to use ethnography, rather than survey research, to understand locally constructed meanings of AIDS. In addition, we experimented with a participatory community-based action-research prevention methodology (Schoepf, Walu, Rukarangira et al. 1991; Schoepf 1992b, 1993).[1] From this we learned much about what people knew and what they could do to protect themselves, their friends, and their families from HIV.

Social Epidemiology of AIDS in Kinshasa

Other contributors to this book provide updates on the spread of HIV and AIDS across the continent, where an estimated 80 to 90 percent of HIV infection is transmitted during heterosexual intercourse. Women with multiple partners are at high risk when men refuse to use condoms. Poor sex workers are the most vulnerable. A small sample of sex workers in Kinshasa's central entertainment district tested in 1985 found 27 percent to be infected. Only 8 out of 85 women reported regular condom use (Mann et al. 1988). In 1988/89, a wider survey of 1,233 sex workers in Kinshasa that included many very poor sex workers found 35 percent seroprevalence. Thirty-six percent of poorer prostitutes working from their homes or in hotels, but only 24 percent of street prostitutes, were infected (Nzila et al. 1991). The latter were younger, better educated, and more knowledgeable about AIDS. They reported fewer clients and higher fees. They were more likely to perceive themselves to be at risk, and three times as likely to use condoms with clients. These "elite" sex workers also had fewer sexually transmitted infections (STIs), which increase risk of acquiring HIV by three to five times. Investigators reported that despite relatively good knowledge of AIDS and STIs, regular condom use was low, reported by only 12 percent of the entire sample. The project opened a clinic in Matonge, a popular entertainment district, offering free diagnosis, treatment, and condoms, along with sustained prevention counseling. Condom use rose significantly, while seroprevalence fell. The relatively lower rates of STIs in Kinshasa compared with other central and east African cities may help to explain why the HIV rate has remained lower, too (Laga et al. 1994).

Programs in other countries also have been quite successful when they offer free treatment of STIs and provide sex workers with empowering education and counseling (Ngugi et al. 1996; Steen et al. 2000). In Senegal, where prostitution was legalized in 1969, and registered women were treated for STIs and provided with condoms without charge, HIV prevalence has remained low. Such interventions should be generalized to all cities, market towns, truck stops, and army bases, with sex workers engaged as outreach workers. The rationale for targeting sex workers was that as these "core transmitters" would transmit HIV to more than one other person, targeted prevention would be cost-effective, yielding "more bang for the buck." However, this strategy contributed to stigma and denial of risk.

By the time epidemiologists studied HIV prevalence in Kinshasa, commercial sex workers were not the only women at risk. Significant prevalence was found among all cohorts of sexually active girls and women, married and unmarried. A 1984–5 population-based survey found HIV in 5 percent of blood samples taken from 5,099 healthy residents of all ages. The rate in girls 15 to 19 was double the general rate and more than twice as high as among boys of the same age. Prevalence in young women aged 20 to 29 years was more than double the general rate, and they were nearly three times more infected than men in their age groups. Most men become infected at later ages (data in Quinn et al. 1986). The sample included many single women who by no stretch of the imagination could be called prostitutes. Young women who have not yet found a marriage partner may have sex with older men, contributing to the high rate, but many are already married. By 1990 adolescent women in Rakai District, Uganda, aged 15–19 years were five times more likely than males of the same age to be HIV positive (Konde-Lule et al. 1997). Similar findings are reported from Ndola, Zambia, and Kisumu, Kenya (Glynn et al. 2001).

In 1986, seroprevalence among 6,000 women delivering at the public Mama Yemo Hospital was 5.7 percent, and reached 8 percent among mothers attending a well-baby clinic nearby. Among 2,574 women at two private hospitals, the rate was 6.7 percent. Women at the latter hospitals tended to be in less advanced stages of disease, however, and fewer of their infants became infected (Ryder et al. 1989). Clearly, women are not protected by marriage. In a sample of 1,458 pregnant women seen in Kigali, Rwanda, in 1988, 86 percent had been married for an average of 8 years. Two-thirds reported a single lifetime partner, yet 25 percent were HIV positive. Overall prevalence was somewhat higher: 32 percent, while among women age 19 to 24 years, the rate was 38 percent (Allen et al. 1991:1660).

Seroprevalence among male managers in two large Kinshasa enterprises studied in 1987 was 4.6 to 6.8 percent. Rates among their wives were lower, 3.3 to 5.7 percent; the highest levels were found in the younger women. While some might have become infected before marriage, this and other studies of married women have found that the greatest risk factor for women is an infected spouse. Seroprevalence among women employees age 20–29 was higher still: 16.7 percent of young female hospital workers and 11.1 percent of female textile factory workers tested positive in 1987 (N'Galy et al. 1988). Most were single and few could ask their partners to use condoms. Our early research identified numerous social and cultural constraints surrounding the use of condoms in casual, as well as in committed couples. Issues include trust, ideas of "normal" sexuality, gender relations, and desire for children. Projet Sida experimented with counseling "discordant couples" in which only one partner was HIV positive. The health workers' labor-intensive efforts were most successful in promoting consistent condom use when the infected partner was female (Kamenga et al. 1991). Apparently, many men are more likely to protect themselves than to worry about their spouses or outside partners.

Focus on prostitution as a risk factor continues to cloud researchers' perspectives. A recent study in South Africa found that while 80 percent of prostitutes serving a mining camp were HIV positive, only 30 percent of their male clients were infected. In a township fifteen miles from the mine, however, 60 percent of a sample of women aged 20–30 years tested seropositive. They had not engaged in prostitution, and about half reported fewer than three lifetime partners (Gilgen cited in Epstein 2002). Epstein reports that the authors of the study were "surprised" by their findings. This suggests that the investigators had failed to read articles by Lindan and colleagues (1991) from Kigali, or Schoepf (1991b, 1992b,1993).[2] The South Africans "discovered" that while miners might use condoms with prostitutes, they do not use them with long-term partners, where issues of "trust" and fidelity intervene. CONNAISSIDA reported similar findings from Kinshasa. In 1987 many women not engaged in sex work, but who had had several partners

over the years, stated that they would feel highly insulted if a man proposed to use a condom (Schoepf 1988), a finding replicated elsewhere across the continent. Additional constraints are situated in the cosmology of sex and reproduction, another reason for devising ways to open dialogue among committed partners (Schoepf 1988, 1992b).

Prevention of HIV encounters many obstacles, economic, sociocultural, and institutional. Other chapters of this book discuss some of these. The case study that follows connects the epidemic in Kinshasa to local and global political economy, and illustrates relationships between policies and AIDS. I go on to give some examples of problem solving by community groups (also see Schoepf, Walu, Rukarangira et al. 1991; Schoepf 1993).

Ethnography:
Listening to Voices of People at Risk

The use of narratives is a way to examine the interrelations between macro-level conditions, structures, and processes, and the lived experience of individuals and social groups. This quintessentially feminist research strategy can capture the interplay of "structure and agency." It allows researchers to document the struggles of individuals and groups to affect their life circumstances. It also shows how their efforts may be constrained by conditions that they are powerless to overcome (Marks 1987; Schoepf and Mariotti 1975; Schoepf 1978, 1988, 1992a, 1998). Nsanga's story is replicable across the continent.

"Kobeta libanga" means breaking stones

There is a broad avenue in central Kinshasa where women sit by the roadside hammering on big stones to break them into smaller pieces used in house-building. Used metaphorically in everyday life, *kobeta libanga* is the work that women do to support their families.

In 1987 Nsanga was 26 and very poor. She lived with her two children and a younger sister in a small room, one of eight rooms grouped around a communal courtyard. The families living in the compound shared a water tap, a latrine, and a roofless bathing stall. The electric company disconnected the hookup, because the landlord failed to pay the bill for six months. The women cooked on charcoal braziers made by local artisans. When money for charcoal ran out, they reverted to the village method, setting their pots on three stones over fires of scrap wood and cardboard scavenged by the children. They also washed dishes and clothes outside and left them there to dry.

Sanitation in most of Kinshasa was dilapidated or absent. Nsanga and her friends knew their neighborhood was unhealthy. Waste ran into open drains. Flies, cockroaches, and mosquitoes were ubiquitous. In the dry season, dust containing fecal matter blew about and settled on water containers and food. In the rainy season, latrines sometimes overflowed into the courtyards. Beautiful Kinshasa ("Kin la Belle") of the 1960s had become Kin la Poubelle (the garbage can) in popular discourse. Malaria, gastrointestinal disorders, malnutrition, and persistent coughs were common. Many mothers, without money for adequate food and medicines, had lost at least one young child to illness.

Nsanga hadn't always been the head of her household. She grew up in a village, and married Lelo, a schoolteacher, when she was 18. She joined him in Kinshasa, where even on his meager salary, and despite galloping inflation, Nsanga managed to feed her family two meals a day. But soon their lives began to change. In 1983 the international financial institutions (IFIs) instituted a series of "economic recovery" measures designed to reduce Zaire's public expenditures so that its corrupt government, which had borrowed heavily in the 1970s, could make payments on its foreign debt. The government removed price controls, and sharply cut social service budgets, raising user fees for health services and education. Neither health nor education had been free in Zaire prior to strategic adjustment programs (SAPs). Ironically, only higher education, from which the poor were blocked by lack of access to secondary education, offered free tuition and a small stipend. Private schools and clinics mushroomed in the 1980s as the quality of public services declined.

In 1984, as an additional way to cut expenses, the government fired more than 80,000 teachers and health workers, further reducing poor people's access. The term used, *assainissement*, is unintentionally ironic; it means "cleaning up" and, by extension, making healthy. Bringing health to the budget, this housecleaning also brought malnutrition, illness, and worry to low-paid government employees, their families, and those whom they formerly served. Retrenched civil servants and their families no longer had access to free health care. Not only high-level officials, but thousands of non-existent "ghost workers" (*fantômes*), whom a housecleaning might have been expected to sweep from the payroll, remained in place. The

phantoms were a boon to needy administrators who collected their pay packets. Although Zaire (now Congo again) has long been viewed as a worst-case scenario, many of the processes of corruption – some linking internal and external actors – came to be found in other countries as the crisis deepened. Mobutu's Zaire was a harbinger of Africa's crisis – with all its attendant processes – rather than an exception.

Without a powerful patron to intercede for him, Lelo lost his job. The family lost his income, health insurance, and the subsidized rice allotted to government employees. After six fruitless months waiting in offices in an attempt to obtain another position, Lelo's morale fell. He began to drink, selling off household goods to pay for beer and then for *lotoko*, a cheap but potent home-distilled alcohol. Nsanga berated him for wasting money; their relationship deteriorated. Often drunk and despondent, Lelo beat his wife and eight-year-old son.

Nsanga tried many things to earn money. Like most poor women in Kinshasa, she had had only a few years of formal schooling. She lacked well-connected friends or family who could help her find a job cleaning offices. Forced into the "informal" economic sector, Nsanga prepared meals for the men who worked in her neighborhood. She also sold food, such as dried fish, when she could walk several miles across town to obtain such items cheaply. Meanwhile, prices climbed with each successive currency devaluation, unemployment rose, and real wages fell sharply. Even men still working had little money to spend and many skipped the noon meal. Week by week, Nsanga had fewer customers; she faced heightened competition from other women attempting to sell similar goods. Her best efforts at petty trade brought in only pennies at a time. She grew vegetables in a vacant lot, but soldiers stole her crop. Nsanga was forced to find something else that would provide money food and rent.

One day early in 1986, Nsanga returned home from hawking mangoes to discover that Lelo had left. Stunned, because she had performed the duties of a "good, faithful wife," Nsanga rationalized his abandonment: "Good riddance! At least he won't beat me any more, and besides, now there is one less mouth to feed." Then Nsanga said that Lelo was angry because "Just now I could provide him with only one meal a day." This situation was actually the rule in poor households. Where women are responsible for feeding the family, lack of food may be taken as a sign that they are at fault.

When Nsanga's children ate the food she had intended to sell, she went into debt to the landlord. She begged her elder brother for a loan, but he had a large family and no savings to lend, despite his steady job on the docks. Wage freezes and sharply rising prices made it difficult for workers to stretch their incomes to the end of the month. Insulted by her brother's failure to "understand" and to help her, Nsanga ceased visiting his family. The breach of relations with her only relative in the city left her alone and vulnerable. Asked why she didn't return to her parents' village, Nsanga responded:

> That's unthinkable! My relatives there are old and very poor, they barely scrape by. They would expect gifts from the city, but they would not be able to help me clear land and build a house. Where would I get food for the children to tide us over until next year's harvest? Go to the village? Impossible! Something might happen to my children . . .

That was Nsanga's oblique way of alluding to her fear of witchcraft, which in many urban areas became more acute as the crisis wore on.

Desperate for cash, and without money to start a business, exchanging sex for subsistence appeared to be Nsanga's only recourse. In the first year of this new strategy Nsanga thought she was lucky. She became the second, but unrecognized, wife of a government official who paid her rent and provided regular support. In Zaire, and elsewhere in Africa where the national language is French, a woman in this relationship is called a *deuxieme bureau*, or second office. The relationship is a common one, particularly among men of means, in the absence of official polygyny. In anglophone west Africa, she is an "outside wife"; in Swahili, her house is the *nyumba ndogo*, or "little house." The men are generally called "husbands," but the degree to which families and friends recognize the relationship varies, as does the extent to which women in such relationships are faithful to their partners. In a socially recognized relationship the woman's family concurs in the relationship and receives a gift. In Nsanga's case, her brother had not received a gift.

Even without family recognition, adult women are perceived to need regular sexual relations "for their health," and no opprobrium attaches to a woman in such a relationship. She is certainly NOT a prostitute, and in the 1980s, a "husband" would not think of proposing to use condoms with his *bureau* (Schoepf 1988). In fact, children are often desired in such relationships. Women hope that children will provide long-term stability, while men generally desire many offspring as a proud marker of virility and status. One expected perquisite of the relationship is access to capital and other resources with which to start a business (Schoepf 1978; MacGaffey 1986; Schoepf and Walu 1991). Nevertheless, these relationships may be relatively short-lived.

With a small gift from her new "husband" to start her off, Nsanga again sold cooked food to the men in her neighborhood. She also had occasional partners, "spare tires" to whom she turned for money in an emergency, for example, to buy medicine when one of her children became sick. But then she got pregnant. Shortly thereafter, this "husband" told her that because of inflation, his salary could not stretch farther, and he left. This was a sign of hard times, since men of means usually recognized the children they had with their *bureaux* and provided some support (Schoepf 1978).

Nsanga's business (an example of what the development literature terms a "microenterprise") was not enough to support her and the children. She began to take on more sexual partners. The going rate for a "quickie" in her poor neighborhood was 50 cents. On a good day she might find two or three partners, but she worked only about two days out of three, for a total of $20–25 per month. By comparison, the average salary for a hospital nurse at the time was about $30 per month. Between her small business and her sex work, Nsanga and her children lived precariously, never quite sure of making ends meet.

Nsanga's children were healthy, and her own health was good, except for a persistent cough and a few bouts of itching and vaginal discharge. Nsanga did not consult a doctor or the nurse who had a private "clinic" on the next street. "I treated myself with pink pills from the local medicine shop. The vendor assured me they were a 'strong anti-biotic.' They looked like the ones I found in my husband's pocket some years before. Maybe he had the disease then?" In 1988, Nsanga had abdominal pains for several months, but without money to consult a doctor, she again self-medicated. "What else could I do? The European nuns at the [neighborhood] clinic do not treat those diseases. They call them 'immorality' or 'shame' sickness. If you go to the hospital they charge you more than you can make in a month."

Around the time of the baby's birth, Nsanga was sick a lot. The new baby was sickly and died before her second birthday, following prolonged fever, diarrhea, and skin rashes. Nsanga believed it was because semen from so many men spoiled her milk. She blamed herself for ignoring the traditional abstinence period following the baby's birth. "But," she asked me rhetorically, "what else could I do?"

In former times many societies required women to practice "postpartum abstinence" while they were breastfeeding, for as much as two years. It served as a means of birth spacing that prolonged the average period of protection from conception conferred by lactational amenorrhea by an average of four months (Romaniuk 1967).

In polygynous families, husbands could have sex with other wives. Christian missionaries attempted to do away with both polygyny and postpartum abstinence. The consequences of their preachments and heavy male labor migration were more closely spaced births, shortened periods of breastfeeding, and recourse by men to extramarital partners. Nevertheless, many Christians, especially in rural areas, continue to practice postpartum abstinence out of fear that semen will harm the nursing infant.

In 1987 the government and media began to acknowledge publicly the threat of AIDS. A leaflet warned men against visiting prostitutes. Most of Nsanga's clients, however, were neighborhood men who came to her each month. As her friends or "husbands," they did not label her a prostitute. Nor was Nsanga stigmatized as a "bad woman." On the contrary, as a mother fallen on hard times through no fault of her own, she was admired for trying her best to "break stones" (*kobeta libanga*) in order to meet family obligations. In the presence of HIV, however, this survival strategy had become a death strategy.

In 1989 Nsanga had diarrhea and grew very thin. She believed that people whispered about her. Indeed, several neighbors said they were sure that she had AIDS. "But then," Nsanga reasoned, "people say this about everyone who loses weight, even when it is just from hunger and worry. All these people who are dying nowadays, are they really all dying from AIDS?" Similar defensiveness was expressed by many other women. Denial was a stratagem for coping with situations women saw no way to change.

Nsanga grew very sick in 1990 and was cared for by her younger sister. She died of what Kinois referred to as a "long and painful illness" in 1991. Her neighbors believed that she had become infected during the time that she used sex with several partners as a survival strategy. Scrutiny of the time frame casts doubt on this assumption, however, for until the end of 1986, Nsanga had had sex with only one partner – her husband. Given the long incubation period between infection with HIV and manifestation of AIDS disease, he was more likely to have been the source of her infection than were subsequent partners.

Nsanga's neighbors assumed that she had been infected as a result of her "promiscuity." While the government's public health advice warned men to avoid "prostitutes," it was silent about the possible risks to steady partners from those already infected. Many women were disarmed by official advice that assured them that faithfulness to a single partner would protect them from AIDS. Such advice about marital fidelity was still being given across Africa well into the 1990s, especially by churches.

The temptation for poor families to betroth or marry off their girls is very strong. As knowledge of AIDS spread, men began to seek out young girls because they believed them less likely to be infected. Rumors reverberated around the continent, sometimes spread by "traditional healers" (THs), to the effect that men could rid themselves of AIDS (or "bad blood") by having sex with a virgin. This is another example of earlier ideas about sexually transmitted diseases and contagion adopted into response to HIV/AIDS. Many other popular beliefs conflict with the knowledge put forth by public health officials. Failure to identify and address these in practical ways has retarded prevention (Schoepf 1991b, 1992b).

Women in groups

Leaders of a Baptist churchwomen's club in another poor Kinshasa neighborhood understood the predicament to which Nsanga's position leads. They sought to protect themselves and other women in their congregation from a similar fate (field notes 1987). When they learned of our workshops with sex workers in the neighborhood, the women deacons invited CONNAISSIDA to hold workshops in their church. They viewed AIDS as a problem for married women who could not control the extramarital activities of their husbands. Despite a homily by their pastor who assured them that fidelity to their spouses would protect them, the women knew that this was untrue. They requested prevention workshops for their husbands so that they, too, could become concerned about the risks to which some of them exposed their wives and children.

The women also pointed to abandonment, divorce, and widowhood, and especially to a child's medical expenses, as circumstances forcing women without other resources into commercial sex work. They told of widows stripped of any assets remaining by the husbands' relatives. Sex was also part of the expected exchange in various forms of patron–client relationships. They reported widespread

sexual harassment of women in formal employment. Women in Kinshasa, and everywhere
that I went subsequently, worried about their
daughters. Their own experience led them to
fear the worst. They told of male teachers who
preyed on schoolgirls, especially as deepening
crisis left parents with less money to pay school
fees and bribe poorly paid teachers to give children passing grades. They noted that girls were
the first to be withdrawn from school. Without
education young women have little to offer on a
crowded job market. They observed many poor
girls forced into selling sex to help their families
survive. They sought a micro-credit scheme to
enable women to fend for their families.
Women's experiential knowledge was more accurate than the epidemiologists' and demog-
raphers' models of projected AIDS spread at
the time.

Avoidance, denial, and notions of propriety
combine with poverty and gender inequality
to increase young women's vulnerability. For
many adolescent women, however, desire
does not enter in; they are socialized for submission to the desires of men, and frequently
coerced into sex. Abusive or not, immaturity of
the adolescent reproductive tract renders the
girls especially vulnerable. Many are infected
at first intercourse, when rupture of the hymen
creates a portal of entry for the HIV.

Young men readily take up condoms when
adults allow them to gain access to free supplies (field notes: Kinshasa 1987–90; Lusaka,
Zambia 1990; Dar es Salaam and rural
Pemba, Tanzania, 1991; Kampala, Mbale
town, and rural Rakai District, Uganda, 1992).
Whether or not "traditional" sexual mores
allowed a period of premarital sexual experimentation, today many adults consider this
illegitimate. Many elders continued to refuse
adolescents (and women) access to condoms
because they believe it would promote "immorality." "Abstinence only" ideology makes
it difficult to promote condoms to sexually
active youth who otherwise might also prevent
accidental pregnancies. Delayed onset of
sexual activity unaccompanied by condoms
simply postpones onset of HIV infection in
women, rather than reducing the risk if the
partner is infected.

Even in a male-dominated society, women
in groups are not totally without power. Al-

though parents, especially fathers, are reluctant to think of their daughters as sexually
active, role-plays enacted in a workshop demonstrated participants' detailed awareness of
the dangers they faced. In a workshop they
organized with other university students,
young women were able to address male
peers with respect to postponing sex. They
did it in terms of preventing pregnancies that
would cut short their studies, and reminded
them that educated women can contribute
more effectively to household budgets. Together they decided that anyone should use
condoms if they could not abstain.

It was on the basis of pregnancy prevention
that a number of women were able to address
husbands on the subject. Rather than voicing
suspicions about the men's extramarital sex,
the women spoke of the prohibitive costs of
raising and educating the children they already had. Even when they knew that they
were at risk, husbands were more able to
accede to such reasoning than to implied accusations of unfaithfulness.

Personal identity, self-worth confirmed by
others, and social power are at stake for men.
Cultural constructions of masculinity contribute to the spread of HIV. Linkages between sex
and trade are evident from epidemiology and
ethnography (MacGaffey 1986; Schoepf et al.
1988a, 1988b; Schoepf, Walu, Rukarangira et al.
1991; Schoepf and Walu 1991). My field notes
from the 1970s and informants in the 1980s
also identified linkages between sex and politics that became institutionalized during the
first 25 years of the Mobutu regime (Schoepf
2002, and my forthcoming book).

Reproductive and sexual health

Most African women are greatly concerned
about reproductive and sexual health: their
social status and security depends on producing healthy children, as does their own sense
of self-worth. Most men also desire numerous
progeny and may be pressured by parental
families to produce many descendants. This
means that couples who have not reached
their desired family size will reject condoms,
even when one spouse is HIV positive.

A nurse in the churchwomen's group suggested a way to overcome this constraint.

Couples can use condoms for birth spacing. Then when they want to conceive, they can have intercourse without condoms until the woman has conceived. The solution is not perfect, but at least it diminishes risk. She also suggested a way around the cosmological significance of semen in "growing the fetus" (see Schoepf 1992b). Teaching people about the timing of ovulation in the menstrual cycle could further shorten the exposure period. At present, many believe that conception occurs directly following menstruation (another old belief). Students who have incorporated this misunderstanding into their use of the "rhythm" method of contraception are often surprised by unwanted pregnancies, but refused to use contraception because being prepared for sex was seen as a marker of "immorality" (field notes, Lubumbashi and Kinshasa, from 1974). Many studies find that fertile women's births generally exceed their notions of an ideal family size. Small but growing numbers of women and men began to use biomedical contraceptive methods in some countries in the late 1970s and 1980s, and still more did in the 1990s.[3]

"Classic" sexually transmitted infections, which often led to reproductive health problems in the past, have become epidemic, with an estimated 65 million new cases each year in sub-Saharan Africa. Women, and especially adolescents, are more vulnerable than men for both biological and social reasons (Duncan et al. 1990). Not only does their presence substantially increase risk of acquiring HIV from an infected sex partner. They also lead to sterility in both women and men, and to reproductive failures and serious congenital health problems in newborns. Many women may not experience symptoms in early stages of infection, or may not be aware that discharge, itching, or burning *are* STI symptoms.[4]

A number of Africanist historians have argued that colonial medical and administrative authors greatly exaggerated the prevalence of STIs in Africa, especially syphilis, which they confused with yaws. However, Romaniuk, who studied female infertility in Equateur Region and northern Kasai in the 1950s, found that in some communities, 50 percent of women had no children. He believed that high rates of untreated gonorrhea were the principal cause, consequent upon social dislocations of the colonial period, with its forced labor drafts and military conscription. As the area was one of intensive recruitment into the military prior to independence, it was plausible to suggest that the men brought home STIs to the villages after sex with prostitutes at the army camps. He reported that: "I was literally assailed by women asking for medicine against sterility" (Romaniuk 1967:296). Men, however, frequently accused women of provoking abortions. Given the high prevalence of STIs, Romaniuk believed that these were more likely miscarriages and spontaneous abortions.[5] Marie appears to have been one such victim.

Marie's ordeal

I was born in Equateur Region in 1940. When I was 15 my father married me to a much older man to whom he owed a large debt. He already had two wives, but neither of them was giving him children. The eldest one was past the age. Her daughters were already having children. The younger one kept losing her babies and the old man wanted to send her away, but she was a good worker. So he asked my father for me. I had just started showing red and my breasts stood out straight. For a whole year my mother-in-law kept shaking her head when she saw me washing my [menstrual] cloths. Then I became pregnant. When it began showing, the [husband's] family was very happy. There was great rejoicing. But when my time came, the baby was dead. My mother-in-law told me it was my fault, that I had been careless. It wasn't true. My father's sister had taught me what to do [after sex]. I had to wipe my man and myself, and wash with certain herbs to purify myself. So they took me to a healer and he, too, was sure that I had committed some fault. He scared me, so I did all the things he said. I washed with the herbs he gave me and drank some of the water. Then I brewed beer for my husband's ancestors. I got pregnant again, so I prepared beer and food for additional sacrifices. But still I lost the child. They took me to a different healer. It was even more frightening this time. The nganga accused me of adultery, but it wasn't true. He said I would have to drink something to prove it. If I was lying, the medicine would kill me. My father believed me, and my mother said that even if I survived the poison drink, the husband's family would accuse me of witchcraft, of doing something to abort the child. She told me that my father was too poor and could not afford to repay his debt to the old man, so I would have to run away. Then the parents would give him my younger sister. In Boende town and Lisala (urban settlements on the Congo River) my condition became known. I was called *ndumba*, "the empty one." Nobody else wanted to marry me, so I did this [sex work]. What else could I do? (Field notes and translation by Noella M. Ngirabakunzi, Kinshasa, April 1989)

Pickering (1993) cautions that the hard-luck stories told by many women in prostitution are "just-so stories" fabricated to arouse researchers' sympathy, or to justify themselves in their eyes. This may be the case for the women her assistants came to know in The Gambia. Most were from Senegal, where, as I noted above, free STI treatment was available from 1969 and a culture of protection evolved. It was also true of a number of stylish young women in Kinshasa who turned tricks while waiting to catch a well-to-do husband. But not all women with multiple partners (FPM or *femmes à partenaires multiples*, a descriptor we invented in the project, intended to lessen stigma) enjoyed the "elite" status of these women. The majority were very poor and at high risk for STIs, including HIV/AIDS (Nzila et al. 1991). In 1987 CONNAISSIDA researchers observed the hand-to-mouth existence of women in two compounds of sex workers in a working-class neighborhood (field notes 1987). In 1990 Dr. Walu and her colleagues found sex workers in the port of Matadi to be a mixed group, including many very poor women as well as some long-distance traders. Most were not using condoms and could not afford STI treatment (letter, August 25, 1990).

Women's symptoms are often subtle and many men do not notify their partners. Thus women may not know when they are infected. Women are heavily stigmatized if their STI affliction becomes known. When they suspect an infection, shame or lack of money may prevent women and girls from seeking treatment, especially at public health services. Often even the private care available is inadequate, prohibitively expensive, or undignified and lacking in confidentiality. Where health services primarily target married women or mothers, where such services are unable to provide private examining spaces, or where nurses are rude, many at-risk women and girls are discouraged from seeking care. The observations of Dr. Christine Minja-Trupin in Mwanza, Tanzania, echo ours from Kinshasa:

The most difficult aspect of health worker training is the psychosocial one. Many are not comfortable talking about sex. Or making visual, let alone hands-on examinations. They generally have little experience using condoms themselves, are inept teaching condom use, and have no idea how to teach negotiation with a partner. What is still worse, many health workers share the stigmatizing attitudes of lay people toward people with STDs. (Interview, Dar es Salaam, October 1991)

The AMREF's Mwanza project provided laboratory diagnosis and treatment, as did Projet SIDA in Kinshasa (Laga et al. 1994) and a few others connected with HIV/STI research. Although user fees can be an even greater deterrent to successful STI treatment than discourteous reception, most health facilities do not offer free care. Introduction of user fees in a Nairobi research clinic in 1988 was found to cause declines in attendance by both women and men: 65 percent fewer women and 40 percent fewer men sought care. When fees were removed, rates rose again, but many fewer men used the services (Moses et al. 1992). The regional health officer at USAID, an agency that promoted the fees policy, maintained that the study was deficient (interview, Boston, February 1993).

Where biomedical treatment is unaffordable or unfriendly, people who recognize the symptoms of an STI self-medicate or seek advice from medicine sellers or folk ("traditional") practitioners. Both types of care are likely to be inadequate. Lack of biomedical treatment can leave a substantial pool of STIs in a population, and may lead to drug-resistant organisms, and to further spread of infection with both classical STIs and HIV. An unknown, but possibly underestimated, percentage of HIV infections may have been spread by unsafe injection practices. Both biomedical health services and "informal" practitioners (a congeries of "injection doctors," poorly trained nurses' aides, and "traditional healers") who provide services to the poor without medical supervision, routinely have employed unsterilized, possibly contaminated, needles and syringes (field notes, Lubumbashi, Kinshasa, and rural eastern DRC from 1975). The most frequent reason for adult consultations of "informal" practitioners is the presence of symptoms that suggest the presence of an STI.

Many rural people, especially, resort to "traditional healers" who claim to cure conditions they believe to be due to sexual "pollution" by women who fail to follow certain prescribed rites, as we saw with Marie. Even so, rural health centers report that STIs are the most frequent reason for adult visits (field notes, Katanga village 1976, Kenya[6] 1977, Liberia 1981, Mali 1984, Pemba 1991, Côte d'Ivoire 1997). Romaniuk (1963), sensitive to the tragedies caused by sterility, recommended that STI treatment be made widely available. He advised considering it a health issue, rather than invoking moralist or Malthusian concerns.

Along with regular condom use, prompt treatment of STIs is an effective HIV prevention strategy. Primary health care in Congo is delivered mainly by religious NGOs, many of which consider STIs shameful and evidence of "immorality," and do not promote condoms. Although USAID has funded some excellent condom social marketing campaigns, its reproductive health projects are designed for married women, and focus exclusively on contraception. They still fail to incorporate STI diagnosis and treatment, and few health workers are comfortable with condom promotion. Early suspicions voiced by African intellectuals that population control is the foremost goal of U.S. health policy in Africa find support in this situation continuing in the face of the AIDS epidemic.

Mvula's hospital visit

Citoyenne Mvula, a participant in a CONNAISSIDA workshop with sex worker colleagues, agreed to try to cajole her clients to use condoms. Later she complained of painful intercourse, itching, and a smelly discharge, and reported that since condoms increased her pain, she had ceased using them. Already apprised of the local NGO health workers' attitudes, Dr. Walu and I drove Mvula to the University Hospital.

She was examined by a physician, who washed his hands under running water with soap I pulled from my purse, as there was none in sight on the sink. As he performed the internal examination, the doctor made a wry face and commented to me (in French) about "these women are so unclean." He used a speculum that had been sitting in a pink liquid which the nurse said was a diluted solution of Dettol, the last of her supply. The hospital charged the equivalent of $15 for the visit (nearly one month's wages for someone with

a low-level government job). The doctor asked Mvula to return the next day to have a sample taken for lab tests that cost as much again. Then she would have to return for a third visit to learn the result.

But since he surmised that the patient would not return, the physician gave her a prescription, telling her (in Lingala) that she needed to take the full prescribed course. To me, he said (in French) that he had made a presumptive diagnosis, guessing that the infection was *Chlamydia trachomitis*. In any event, he said he was prescribing tetracycline, even though it was expensive, because in his experience, so many STDs were resistant to penicillin. Walu translated in a low voice for Mvula, who did not speak French. The physician surmised (correctly) that having transported the patient to the hospital, paying the fee, and making sure that she would be examined despite her lack of appointment, I would also pay $12 for the medication. Mvula said that she had had enough of the place. To her, the one visit was quite daunting. Since the doctor assured us that tetracycline would take care of whatever it was, we did not press her to return for lab work. (Field notes Kinshasa, July 1987)

What the doctor did not take into account was that Mvula would be under pressure to share her antibiotics with her "sisters," the other sex workers with whom she shared accommodations. Actually, we were on the lookout for this, as Dr. Walu had discovered similar sharing of medications when she investigated mothers' action against malaria in 1986. We also discovered that it was common practice for poor women engaged in sex work to use antibiotics as what they believed was "preventive medicine," by opening the capsules and sprinkling the powder on the perineum. Thus when women state that they "use antibiotics," they may not be referring to the same methods that physicians have in mind. Part of the ethnographer's contribution is the ability to draw on past current and field experience, as well as literature review, so as to foresee what otherwise might be misconstrued meanings and the unforeseen, perhaps harmful, assumptions of medical advice and its consequences.

Conclusion

CONNAISSIDA's "political economy and culture" approach is related to methodological advances made in the study of African societies over the past quarter-century, including the search for contextualized understanding of how macro-level political economies affect sociocultural dynamics at the micro level – including the political ecology of disease and social response to epidemics. Because AIDS is propelled by class, age, and gender inequality, it underscores the need for sustainable development to reduce the rapid global spread of HIV. The epidemic is emblematic of the process of capital accumulation that drains resources away from the villages, upward to national ruling classes and outward to world markets.

Women's poverty and gender issues are related to their special vulnerability to AIDS. The story of Nsanga shows the risks taken by a poor urban woman struggling to feed her children, her struggles sharpened by SAP policies. It indicates the impact of neo-liberal policies that mandated the demise of the welfare state and ended the entitlements of urban workers in the 1980s. It provides patent evidence that the informal sector cannot be relied upon to create development imperiled by stagnation in the formal sector.

Nor can the extended family take the place of social welfare institutions. In situations of dire poverty, the limits of "the economy of affection" are quickly reached. Family ties that might once have provided enduring support give way under the combined assault of poverty and disease. People unable to count on family solidarity must accept high degrees of risk, as they struggle to fend for themselves. Many situations lead people to shed their relatives. Marie's story shows how the weight of traditional constructions of female infertility may be compounded by lack of biomedical health services. Unschooled, without capital in money or social relations, she made the most of her body, her only resource. Mvula was in much the same situation. They embody the fate of poor women unable to leave sex work behind as they age.

In much of Africa, economic and cultural factors circumscribe the ability of women, married or single, to refuse sex with a steady partner, even if they suspect he may be infected, or to insist on condom protection. Even in the context of casual sex, the agency of girls and women in condom use is often severely constrained because they need their partners' gifts or financial support. These personal tragedies embody that of Africa, with its legacy of systematic structural and corporeal violence, the political economy and culture of AIDS. The three narratives underscore the need for productive activities that effectively increase women's financial independence and their sense of self-worth. These conditions do not, in themselves, lead to social empowerment in the face of widespread gender inequality. They may, however, provide resources that women can use to protect themselves and their children. In the context of Mobutu's authoritarian state, however, the most feasible route to financial independence for poor women, and many in the middle class, as well, was through sexual patron–client relations with powerful men.

AIDS prevention can stimulate countercurrents of resistance to dominant cultural norms. Gender relations need not be static, and recent scholarship highlights many examples of women's struggles to change their condition. However, these struggles take place in circumstances not of women's making; without external solidarity they may be overwhelmed. Combined with creative mass media productions, community-based empowerment methods can foster realistic risk-assessment and problem-solving spirit that begins to overcome cultural constraints. It means seeing girls and women as whole persons, rather than simply as "either madonnas or whores," as vectors of disease, as wombs for procreation, or as "empty vessels" into which the contents of medical information can be poured. Effective AIDS prevention requires changing the health services available to the poor, especially to poor young women. In the final analysis, however, it means changing the status of women and youth to increase their material independence, their psychological autonomy, and their social power. Powerful and wealthy men can make these changes happen.

Biographies and local-level ethnography have limitations. The stories we collected from working-class and middle-class women did not encompass the political struggles brewing in Mobutu's Zaire. They were not involved in the early pro-democracy movement that began among members of the "political class." Nor do they show how the international system brought the corrupt dictator to power and kept him in place, nor how its lack of enthusiasm undermined the forces pressing for democratic change (Nzongola-Natalaja 2002). We learn nothing from them of the criminalization of the informal economic sector (De Boeck 2000; MacGaffey et al. 1991; MacGaffey and Bazenguissa-Ganga 2000), or its relation to the state and to local and international warlords who profit from trade in minerals and guns. Nor are the episodes of state-sponsored ethnic cleansing or the aftermath of the 1994 genocide in Rwanda foreshadowed in their lives. To capture these processes, which have resulted in millions of deaths in DRC since 1992, we need other analytical studies (see the *Review of African Political Economy*, 93–94, September–December 2002 for analysis and extensive bibliography).

The multiplex crisis of the state has pushed "women's issues" to the rear, yet this chapter indicates that they are basic issues of African social and cultural survival. Community-based ethnographic action-research offers an opportunity to explore a range of issues with people variously situated in society whose intimate lives are affected by them. Broad social issues are at stake in AIDS prevention. Because the impact of AIDS will be so devastating, the complex realities of HIV prevention might be used to initiate far-ranging dialogues about the consequences of persistent inequality. Thus engaged, people may seize the opportunity to "reinvent" culture and restructure social relations. Like most of AIDS prevention and treatment, the work is labor-intensive and costly.

AUTHOR'S NOTE

Acknowledgements and many references found in the bibliography of the earlier chapter are not reprised here.

NOTES

1. While I returned to the U.S. to write an elaborate proposal to seek funding (Schoepf 1986),

Dr. Rukarangira, a public health specialist, and Co-Director of CONNAISSIDA (1985– 8), led a KAP survey in Lubumbashi in 1986–7 using snowball sampling. Funded by my USAID consulting fees, it proved not very informative. It showed that, as we had surmised, those most informed were educated males, but that even among these men, little behavioral change had occurred.

The first offer of funding came from a physician-epidemiologist at the Canadian International Development Agency (CIDA). She wanted to change the methodology from ethnographic action-research to a KAP survey. This despite the presence of another group of researchers already beginning a large, population-based survey funded by USAID. Our group declined the CIDA offer, which, in addition to altering the methodology, would have marginalized me to the status of an "advisor." Perhaps the official believed the research would be less expensive this way (although I worked in CONNAISSIDA for five years without salary, as did Claude Schoepf). She sought to give control of the project to a physician friend, the late Dr. Lurhuma, director of the institute in which we had planned to lodge the project. Through colleagues, I learned that in 1991, the CIDA officer denigrated CONNAISSIDA's ethnographic findings as "merely anecdotal," despite their having been replicated subsequently by other researchers.

2. Articles cited in MEDLINE, with abstracts available online.

3. In the 1980s eight countries of sub-Saharan Africa registered declines of more than one percentage point (15–20 percent) in total completed fertility (World Bank 1997b:6–8, T1.1). Half the rural women surveyed in eastern Zimbabwe were using contraception in 1996–8. This was due to a vigorous outreach program through primary health care centers from 1984, for which I wrote the government position paper stressing women's health, rather than population control (see Schoepf 1983).

4. Left untreated by antibiotics, STDs can lead to pelvic inflammatory disease, and sterility; to cancer, miscarriage, and congenital blindness.

5. Similar histories of gonorrhea were recorded from east Africa in the 1950s and 1960s (see Barton 1991).

6. Family planning training program participants, Kenyatta College, July.

Sexualities
Chapter 9

Culture, Sexuality, and Women's Agency in the Prevention of HIV/AIDS in Southern Africa

Ida Susser and Zena Stein

Introduction

The tragic AIDS epidemic that is presently engulfing southern Africa is based on heterosexual transmission. An estimated 1 in 10 young uninfected women in southern Africa can expect to become infected each year (S. Abdool Karim 2000, pers. comm.) in an epidemic that shows no signs of abating (Joint United Nations Programme on HIV/AIDS and World Health Organization 1999). At a conservative estimate, an effective vaccine could be ten years away.

Successive field studies were carried out by teams of anthropologists, including one or both of the authors at five sites in southern Africa between 1992 and 1999 to explore women's awareness of HIV/AIDS and what they can do in heterosexual negotiations to protect themselves from infection. On the basis of questionnaires, interviews, and open-ended discussions concerning use of the male and female condoms and abstinence, and the circumstances under which each method was regarded as appropriate, we were persuaded of the urgent need for fresh approaches to prevention (Karim et al. 1993).

Here we present some of our observations, which lead us to conclude that with regard to women at least, each community needs to be studied in terms of the local situation, and the preventive measures advised and facilitated for residents must take account of the differences between communities. These differences include employment and access to resources for men and women, level of political awareness, and a related issue – the perception of the boundaries of sexual authority for women and men. HIV/A1DS prevention will be successful only to the degree that the changing needs of women as well as men are recognized and responded to by local, national, and international policy makers (see for example Stein 1990; Schoepf 1992; Farmer et al. 1993; Gupta and Weis 1993; Reid 1997; Parker et al. 2000).

Background

The latest prevalence figures estimated by UNAIDS for the numbers of men and women in sub-Saharan Africa infected with HIV are10.1 million and 12.2 million, respectively (Karim and Karim 1999). These estimates are even higher than those given for 1996, the midyear of our studies. AIDS is the leading cause of death in many of these countries. In the Republic of South Africa, where the statistics are the most complete, annual rates of seropositivity have shown the most alarming and consistent rise year by year, and those among women, the steepest.

As noted above, statistical models based on the quoted rates estimate that at least 1 new infection occurs among every 10 uninfected women each year. By some counts, this is an underestimate: first, infected women, who tend to be less fertile than uninfected women, are underrepresented in prenatal clinics, which is where most cases are first diagnosed: second, direct estimates of recent cases, nowadays based on laboratory studies, have in some areas suggested a 20 percent annual infection rate. Mortality studies, too, are projecting substantial increases in deaths from AIDS, especially, again, among young women. We can assume from these data that the greatest risk of infection in the areas we studied is faced by young women, probably those in the 15- to 25-year-old age group.

Although tests for HIV/AIDS are often not accessible, counseling is rare, and confidentiality is not always maintained, it is also the case that medical treatments for HIV/AIDS are unavailable to most women in southern Africa. When available, treatment generally focuses only on the opportunistic diseases that often accompany infection. Thus, prevention has to be the focus of public health messages. Although breastfeeding is now known to transmit the virus from mother to child, the dilemma involved in discouraging breastfeeding and thus subjecting infants to the risks of fatal gastroenteritis or starvation has yet to be addressed on a community-wide level among poor populations. Nevertheless, preventive messages focusing on "one partner" and "love faithfully," the compromise solution frequently adopted by governments in southern Africa and elsewhere, overlook the realities of life for many.

The broader social context – which includes widespread poverty and unemployment, particularly among women; a history of men's crossing national boundaries in battles for independence or other military actions; social disasters; and the increase in intra-Africa economic exchanges, which are based on colonial patterns of production reinforced by uneven regional investment in the global economy – is heavily incriminated in the spread of HIV/AIDS in Africa. Advice to be monogamous is hardly likely to be heeded in such circumstances (Bond et al. 1997). Polygyny has been the rule in many African societies and is still common in many. In addition, the involuntary migration associated with men's employment away from home, experienced by almost all families in rural and semirural areas, is associated almost inevitably with casual and extramarital encounters, and not only for the men. As a result of all these factors, extramarital sex is frequent among men and widely tolerated, if not enjoyed, by women. This statement is derived from comments made both on formal questionnaires and in focus groups.

There is at least one sad circumstance that favors preventive behavior: as people observe the deaths of family members, infants, and neighbors infected with HIV/AIDS, their awareness of their own risk becomes more firmly internalized. Although this awareness occurs rather late in the epidemic, it is a stimulus for women to take action and search, sometimes desperately, for steps they can take, individually or collectively, to protect themselves and their community. This was certainly a phenomenon we observed during our visits.

Two points emerge from this analysis, and they were validated in our work. First, under the threat of the AIDS epidemic, seeing kin and neighbors succumb and knowing these victims are no different from themselves, women are demanding methods of prevention and are willing to use them. Second, there are approaches that informed communities can develop collectively both to care for those infected and to limit the further spread of infection. The women in communities such as the ones we visited are neither unaware nor passive. They are ready to express their views and ready to mobilize to achieve realistic goals.

Field Sites

The field observations were carried out by the first author (Ida Susser.), joined by Eleanor Preston-Whyte and Quarraisha Karim on the

South African visits, Richard Lee on all the visits in Namibia and Botswana, and Karen Brodkin in Namibia in 1997.

The research at the two sites in Durban, South Africa, was part of a larger community education project dealing with HIV/AIDS, with ongoing evaluation both through questionnaires and through participants' comments about community groups and political avenues of representation for men and women. In 1992, with the participation of Zena Stein, observations were conducted in an agricultural village outside Durban and an informal settlement on the outskirts of Durban. In 1995, Eleanor Preston-Whvte and Ida Susser returned to the informal settlement to follow up on the research of 1992. (The agricultural village could not be revisited at that time because it was the site of intense political violence.) We conducted three public meetings with women who had participated in the original community education efforts.

The research in Namibia was conducted with Richard Lee as part of a larger project that was concerned with training students from the University of Namibia in anthropological research with respect to HIV/AIDS. In 1996 we interviewed informants in the Ovambo-speaking region of Qkavango. In 1997, with Karen Brodkin, we conducted similar interviews and observations in Rundu along the Okavango River. In 1996 and 1999, Richard Lee and Ida Susser conducted interviews along the border between Namibia and Botswana, the home of the Ju/'hoansi, a Bushman people living in the Kahahari Desert. At each site, we were accompanied by translators who were familiar with the area as well as the language.

The research at each of the three sites in Namibia included interviews with health care providers and other institutional representatives, such as church officers, teachers, and representatives of local and international nongovernmental organizations. We also talked with both men and women at public meetings and in their homes. Although our inquiries and discussions on each occasion were informal, when talking with women alone or with mixed groups we did ask questions about their understanding of HIV, what they thought about possibilities of preventing infection, and how they perceived their sexuality in re-

sponse to the risk. We also asked people whether they had seen or used either a male or a female condom.

Although the focus of the research was not use of the female condom, our interviews were open-ended, and as it turned out, the reactions of women respondents frequently brought this method to the forefront of the discussion. Nevertheless, the discussions did not always take the same form, and certainly both the level and the nature of the response differed widely from site to site, a point to which we return in the conclusion.

Agricultural village outside Durban, South Africa (1992)

The first visit was to a rural village, scattered over a series of hills, and was a three-hour bus ride from Durban. It was, in 1992, part of the area designated to the control of the Zulu king. Both men and women went to Durban for work. However, transportation was expensive and difficult, and the common pattern was for men to go to town for the week and return on weekends. Most of the women participated in a communal gardening project three days a week when the irrigation was turned on. Although the women earned some money by selling fruit, vegetables, and old clothes and through child care and domestic work, many relied on men for cash contributions (Karim et al. 1993). At the time of the initial fieldwork, laundry and bathing were done in the river at the bottom of a hot, dusty hill upon which the mud and ashbrick homes were built, and drinking water was carried up by women and children from the same source. In 1991 and 1992 a public works project was instituted that introduced electricity and running water to the village.

Residents were represented at civic council meetings, and in 1992, all civic council members were men. All members of the tribal court were men, and many of these were the same men who represented the village in African National Congress (ANC) regional meetings. Although there were 120 organizations among the approximately 10,000 residents, women did not often speak publicly. Field researchers reported that in 1992 women were not expected to speak up in front of men in this rural community, which was under the control of the largely male-hereditary chiefdoms.

Through answers to our questionnaires and through the public discussions we observed outside one clinic, it became clear that AIDS was associated with witchcraft and with the disease that, according to folklore, a man contracts if he sleeps with another man's partner. At the meetings held by researchers outside the clinic, the women scarcely spoke; the few men on the periphery of the group of women actually attending the clinic were much more vocal than the women. A survey of 200 households in the village indicated that the women did not know how to identify sexually transmitted diseases or the names of any such diseases. In contrast, the men were very well informed.

It appeared difficult, in this setting, to involve women in meetings and for women to negotiate safe sex with men or even to talk about their own health issues (Karim et al. 1993).

Informal settlement on the outskirts of Durban (1992, 1995)

The informal settlement north of Durban consisted of about 5,000 homes inhabited by an estimated 30,000 people. This population had only begun to move to the area after the pass laws that restricted African residence in urban areas were revoked. In 1992 the area had no sanitation, running water, or public services such as garbage collection, roads, or lighting. People walked and drove along winding, dusty, narrow, and precipitous paths. As a result of the efforts of the women's community organization, seven faucets had been built in scattered locations around the settlement. People could collect water for use in their households from these faucets.

Children had to travel to neighboring municipalities to attend school, and educational levels were low. Most residents spoke Zulu; many also spoke some English. Among this large population, still disenfranchised at that time, a vibrant informal economy existed. Bricks were made in the settlement and used to build houses. Although men still had more options for paid employment, women in the

settlement, because of their proximity to the Durban markets and service opportunities, had more ways to support themselves than women in the rural village. Because of these opportunities, women who migrated to the new informal settlements on the periphery of the city were often single heads of households. They found work as household servants or babysitters to support their families. Many also tried to generate cash by making candles, baskets, and clothes and selling them locally or in Durban.

Although the informal settlements lacked electricity, nearby townships were sources of information and television. It is important to note that people in the area did have access to international media. During one informal discussion, a group of young people asked about riots that were occurring in New York City at the time we were talking with them – they had seen coverage of the riots on CNN. They were exposed to a wide variety of topics through the international media. Thus, in general, people in the informal settlements were aware of HIV and other issues.

The researchers made contact with the community through a sewing cooperative organized by and for local women. As noted above, this cooperative had also worked to bring water to the community. They had begun to weave baskets for sale and were concerned with developing ways to tie into the informal economy.

In terms of discussion of sexuality and HIV infection, the women in this cooperative presented a contrast to the women in the rural community. In a 1992 meeting, members of the research team discussed HIV with about 50 women and 3 or 4 men. Even before the meeting started the room was in an uproar – the local community organizer, a woman, had brought in copies of the ANC constitution, newly translated into Zulu. The transition from White domination of South Africa to a multiracial government was about to take place. (In 1994, South Africa held its first multiracial election, and the ANC won by an overwhelming margin.)

Dr. Nkosasana Zuma, who later became the Minister of Health (1994–9), was a member of the research team at the time and the ANC representative from the area. She spoke to the group in Zulu about the importance of HIV and the need for women to protect themselves. Next, a representative from the US foundation that funded the community education research project spoke briefly in English, and then American researchers mentioned the development of the female condom.

At this meeting, the women were very outspoken in front of the men. Women in the audience stood up and argued with the men in the back of the room who claimed that the young girls hanging around the harbor were "asking for it [sex]." The women talked about the lack of economic alternatives that led women to sell sex. One woman explained that a woman who had spent the entire day in Durban unsuccessfully looking for work and returned to the settlement with no money might exchange sex for 10 rand to buy sugar for her children that night. The women did not see these situations as being restricted to a group of "sex workers" or "prostitutes" but rather talked about the sale of sex as one last option available to women whose families were in desperate need of money and food.

The women were explicit about economic needs and said that the best method they could imagine for preventing HIV in the settlement was to provide work for women. They requested that the project consider funding a candle-making factory. They pointed out that since there was no electricity in the settlement, this would be an extremely profitable concern.

When asked if they would use the female condom, the women became enthusiastic. They said that they would definitely use something like that, over which the woman had control. They asked when the female condom might be available and asked that the researchers provide them samples as soon as possible.

Thus only a few miles removed from their previous existence in the rural areas, women's experiences and their perspectives on sexuality – as well as their willingness to speak in public – were dramatically altered.

In 1995 Eleanor Preston-Whyte and Ida Susser returned to the informal settlement with the community liaison person from the l992 project. At the meeting convened by the liaison person, we found that the women were well aware of the threat that HIV infection held for them and their children. When asked who was

most at risk, they immediately replied that it was women; they said that this was because their partners had other women, and they themselves were dependent on men for support. As before, they made the point that if they had jobs, they would be able to refuse sex to men who refused to use condoms. The point was also made, without prompting, that women should be able to avoid unprotected sex with a number of men. "Poverty makes prostitutes of us," they said. The connection between sex, particularly sex with more than one partner, and HIV infection was made again and again. Also repeated was the fact that condom use prevents infection.

Although the women at the meeting demonstrated a knowledge of HIV risk and of the role of male condoms in protection, when we asked if their partners were using male condoms, no woman said yes. When we asked why not, one woman commented, "It is good to have women's groups to help us, but there is no group to support you when you are alone with your husband." Another woman said, "It might be better if we had a female condom," and this comment led to an excited discussion.

The women asked to see a female condom, and when we returned a few days later, we brought a demonstration kit with us. The reaction was immediate and positive. About 25 women had collected in the community hall to meet us, and after the demonstration, they eagerly handled the condoms and jokingly practiced using them with the dildo provided by the liaison person. When we cautioned that men might reject their use, as they did the male condom, the women overrode our hesitation. "We can use it and teach other people to use it. It is better that you bring it quickly and that it is free."

This opened the way for a discussion once again of the problems women faced in the area, the lack of adequate housing and employment being paramount. One woman said, "In these small two-roomed shacks the children can hear everything...maybe it will be difficult to talk about this new kind of condom...What we need is better houses." Another noted, "It will be easy to use the female condom if you are working. You just say to your husband that you must not get pregnant or you lose the job. Even a woman can stay alone with her children if she has a job. So we need jobs." Still another commented. "If we have this new condom, we will get our men to use it...It will help us a lot." Finally, a woman said, "We are mostly relying on our husbands because of unemployment. The only way of leaving them is employment. If we earn money, we have power...If we can wear them, we will be free."

Although they are available in some pharmacies in South Africa, female condoms are extremely expensive, even for relatively wealthy middle-class women. The national AIDS program and the Ministry of Health intended to make them available free through clinic services. However, there was to be a delay of at least three months before female condoms might become available. (Five years later, at the time of writing, the program is still facing barriers to implementation.) When we relayed this information to the women at the meeting they were indignant. "You must tell the minister [of health] to send us female condoms first...We need them here, and we will show they can work," said one. Another said, "Tell the minister to bring the female condom quickly...If it should have come before, we would have limited our families more easily." We ended the meeting by writing a letter to the minister. The women signed their names in an exercise book and spoke into our tape recorder so that "she [the minister] can know that no lies are being told."

Namibia: The Ovambo-speaking region (1996)

In 1996, Richard Lee and Ida Susser visited the University of Namibia in Windhoek to work with Namibian students in sociocultural research on HIV. Two students, a man and a woman from the Ovambo area, then accompanied us to their home region, serving as guides, informants, translators, and, by the end of the project, interviewers and researchers.

In the Ovambo-speaking region, we interviewed hospital administrators, nurses and doctors, church leaders and counselors, and men and women in their homesteads in the communities along the road north. We visited the homestead of one student and he intro-

duced us to his mother, his aunt, his brothers and sisters, and neighbors in the farming area. His father and older brothers were away, working in a town about two days' drive distant. Most of the families in this area relied for cash on the men's work in the towns, particularly Windhoek. The men traveled the 700 km from Windhoek to their homes in minibuses Friday night and returned in the minibuses and public buses that began the drive back to Windhoek Sunday morning and continued all day Sunday.

Families who owned homesteads cultivated the fields surrounding their homes. Men and women who had no land and lived in the shanty areas might find temporary work, often unpaid but providing food and shelter, as laborers on the land. The women, responsible for children and with few options for employment, might also sell home-brewed beer in little shacks along the highway, especially at the major bus stops for the journey down to Windhoek. Such stops were also places where women could exchange sex for money.

The church and the hospital were major institutions that helped to define the treatment of HIV/AIDS in the region. We learned from hospital administrators that many elite members of the Namibian government and their staffs had received medical care for AIDS but that the government kept this information confidential. Nurses at the hospital said that community members did not believe in AIDS because illnesses were not given that name, and the doctors would say someone died of one of the opportunistic diseases, such as diarrhea or tuberculosis.

A pastor in the area told us that people did not believe in AIDS because "no one has died of it." He claimed, "You'll never know if somebody died of AIDS, only maybe after somebody is buried it is a rumor." He added that the church "can't ask what the sickness is, even for your own child...They have codes for sicknesses, one will never find out what the person died of...It is a heterosexual matter, and the church doesn't know how or what to do...It is not discussed because there is not evidence that the person died of AIDS." Like the doctors and nurses, the pastor claimed that people did not talk about AIDS openly or admit to others that they had the disease, even when they might be dying from it.

The pastor also said that he was opposed to the distribution of condoms, which was based on the assumption that people did not practice chastity before marriage and monogamy within it. In his words, "Our church does not support the case of condoms to be used, especially by unmarried persons. They are based on the issue of woman and man – a condom, it's like you get rid of principle and breaking it and giving freedom for people to go around." He would not discuss AIDS with his congregation except in terms of sin and chastity.

Although it was a progressive force for African freedom and a strong supporter of the South West African People's Organization (SWAPO) in the war for African independence, the church in Namibia has developed constraining views of family norms that do not directly correspond to the lives of migrant workers, who have a history of polygamous living on homesteads. Many Namibian ministers, including those we interviewed, have been trained in the United States and reflect some of the fundamentalist moral trends that are strong in certain sectors of the US population. In some ways, for example, in its opposition to the distribution of condoms the church has contributed to the silence about and stigmatization of AIDS. AIDS counselors at the hospital said they believed many religious leaders initially opposed the government's program for the distribution of condoms and made effective prevention difficult. However, as the following cases demonstrate, such ideas were not always expressed by rank-and-file members of church congregations.

In one homestead close to the church grounds, in the midst of harvested fields that resembled a desert because of the overgrazing in the densely populated region, we found women who knew of and talked openly about people with AIDS. Similarly, when we visited a devout church worker and her sister and children in another homestead several miles down the highway, we found women who were concerned and knowledgeable about the AIDS epidemic in their midst.

In the middle of a hot, dusty day we were brought to the first interview by our student, who had gone to a religious school with one of the daughters in this homestead. Inside the compound of mud shacks and shanties made of corrugated iron, we were greeted by a woman carrying a small boy and surrounded by many other children. We began talking to the woman, and she called in her sisters, who then called in their teenaged daughters to join the discussion. Although both of our students were with us, which meant we were two men and two women, the women did not seem reluctant to discuss contraception or AIDS.

Women in this compound were very aware of the issue of AIDS and also knew people with AIDS. To quote one of the women, "People know that there is AIDS and they talk about it. They are not hiding it any more, because they know people are getting it. They know people that have AIDS and they talk to them. People in the community are taking care of AIDS victims." One of the sisters took up the discussion. She said they were all concerned about AIDS: "Women are very open. They talk to each other about AIDS ... Yes, they acknowledge that it is possible they have it. They are very afraid."

These women knew that AIDS was sexually transmitted, and they wanted their husbands to use condoms but they could not insist. "It's different," said one. "There are some women who ask men to use condoms but some women don't say it." Later another said, "A husband will not agree to use condoms with his wife...He says he sleeps around but will use condoms outside, but she can't be sure." They said they were worried that they would get AIDS and die.

Eventually, we showed the women the female condom. They became very animated and said it was what they needed: "We want the female condom today." One woman noted, "It is important that the semen will remain in the woman because men don't like to take the semen out." Another woman said, "You can bring it [the condom] here."

The women asked where female condoms were available and discussed the cost of the condoms at the local pharmacy. They were eager to use female condoms; they said that although they could not say anything to their husbands, they could use anything they chose. They said definitely that it did not matter that the men could see the female condom; if it was theirs, they had the right to use it: "A woman can make her own decision." One woman said, "This will be protective from the woman's side." When we pointed out that we could not provide female condoms and that they were expensive, one woman insisted, like the women in Durban, "Go to the ministry [of health] and tell them to order female condoms...Maybe it's better if we have this report [that we said we were writing] and write them a letter."

We then interviewed a man and his girl-friend in the shanties along the edge of the road, which housed the poorest laborers of the region. The man and the woman said they knew people who had died of AIDS and they knew about the male condom, but they were not willing to talk to us for long.

The next significant interview was with our student's mother and aunt. Since he thought his mother would be more comfortable talking with women, he and Richard Lee went to interview a neighbor while the woman student and Ida Susser stayed to talk with his mother and her sister. Both women were in their 40s. They showed us around the homestead. The small buildings were made of mud with straw roofs and were separated by bamboo screens. Each son and daughter over a certain age had his or her own hut, and the entire compound was surrounded by a bamboo wall. Outside the wall were dried-out fields where cattle grazed. The student's mother showed us the beer she had brewed, alcoholic for adults, non-alcoholic for children, and the enclosed but roofless area where she and her sister cooked in huge iron pots over an open fire, using spoons and other instruments made from local material. Four little children, dusty and dressed in rags, played around our feet as we all sat down on the ground under the trees for the interviews.

However, lest this homestead sound like an unchanged traditional setting, it should be noted that the son who was working with us was a college student (the first in the family), the husband had a civil service job far away, and in the teenaged son's hut, next to his bed, was a pack of condoms. The mother worked as a liaison for the church, helping to identify children with disabilities. The student who was working with us had run away as a teen-

ager to join SWAPO in Angola when the South African army occupied Namibia, returning only after Namibia had won its independence.

In this "traditional" compound in a rural area in the far north of Namibia – where water had to be fetched from a faucet a mile away, most of the food was prepared from subsistence crops, and the utensils in the enclosed patch of sand that served as a kitchen were fashioned from local materials – we found extensive knowledge about AIDS. Both women talked about people they had known who died of AIDS. A couple who lived across the highway had both died recently; the wife had asked her neighbor to visit her so that she could tell her neighbor she had AIDS and that others should know. The two women also told us about a member of their church who had been in the hospital and had written a letter to be read during the Sunday service. He said he was dying of AIDS and he wanted people to know. He did not want to die in secret but wanted to warn other people about the disease. The women told us that everyone thought his girlfriend and her baby must have AIDS and that she had left the district and disappeared. They were also wondering whether her next boyfriend, who now had another girlfriend, might be infected.

As this example demonstrates, people were very aware of the possibility for heterosexual and perinatal transmission of AIDS. Although this awareness sometimes led to stigmatization (which might explain why the girlfriend left the area), people knew very well the mode of transmission. Devout, respectable church-women told us that women had no say in an Ovambo bedroom – they could not ask a man to use a condom or discuss any other sexual issue. However, they were extremely enthusiastic about the female condom, saying that this was something women could use. It would be under their control. They said explicitly that if they used a female condom they would not be inviting a beating, as they would if they dared to ask a man to use a condom.

These cases give a sense of the dynamics between women and men in Ovambo society. They suggest areas for mobilization for the treatment and prevention of HIV infection and demonstrate the significant agency, open-mindedness, concern, and knowledge to be found among women who might at first appear to be most constrained by church and family.

Namibia: Rundu, a Kavango-speaking region (1997)

In July 1997, Richard Lee and Ida Susser returned to Namibia with Karen Brodkin to conduct interviews among the Kavango people, the second largest population in northern Namibia. At Rundu, a regional center on the border between Namibia and Angola, we met with health workers, workers from non-governmental organizations, and the head of the health district (an extremely articulate and knowledgeable nurse trained by the community health movement in South Africa), who took us to talk with some women in a sewing cooperative.

The sewing factory, which employed about 60 women, had been started at the suggestion of Oxfam Canada workers and was now an active concern run by the women themselves. They worked on their sewing machines at the back of a large shop. Their products were displayed in the front of the store, with no division between the seamstresses and the customers.

We walked into the store and started talking to the women at their sewing machines. Since it was an impromptu meeting, rising out of our request to be introduced informally to local women, we did not start by talking about HIV/AIDS. We asked the women about their sewing and the materials they used. They asked us what we did, and we told them we were concerned with AIDS. The women said they knew about HIV/AIDS. They had been told the modes of transmission by non-governmental organization workers. They seemed somewhat bored by the topic.

At the end of the conversation I (Ida Susser) casually mentioned the female condom. One of the women, who had been listening in a desultory way, turned around and said, "Oh! I've seen one of those in the drug store here." Another woman said, "Do you have one, can we see it?" I said I had not brought one with me, but I asked, "Would you use it?" The women said: "Yes, yes, tell us about it." I started to talk about the female condom as one method that women could use, and several women left

their sewing machines and moved closer to listen.

We drove back to our rooms for the demonstration materials. When we returned about an hour later, the women were waiting for us. They left their sewing machines, looked at the books and pictures we had brought, handed the female condom around, and asked us to give them some. They said they were too expensive for them to buy. I said they would have to get their own government to provide them, and that this would be possible only if they mobilized collectively, as they had for the sewing cooperative, to make this a government priority.

These women wanted the condoms and were positive they could use them. They wanted to make a political demand for women's condoms – a reaction almost identical to that of the women in the Durban informal settlement and the women in the Ovambo region. Once again it became clear that given the resources, people would act to protect themselves, even if it meant changing sexual mores. The women in the sewing cooperative were familiar with AIDS. They had seen people die. They knew that they or their friends could easily be next. With appropriate resources and support, they said, they were ready to act.

The Kalahari Desert (Namibia 1996; Botswana 1999): The Ju/'hoansi

Next we visited the Ju/'hoansi of the Kalahari Desert, who were first contacted 30 years ago by Richard Lee. At that time, they were gatherers and hunters living in semi-nomadic band societies, with egalitarian relations between men and women (Leacock and Lee 1982; Lee 1979; Lee 1993). The Ju/'hoansi now live in settled villages around government-supplied water sources. They support their households on a combination of government food supplements, temporary government-sponsored work groups, gathering, and infrequent hunting.

Here, we got a different response. As at our other sites, men and women knew about HIV/ AIDS. They knew people who had died of the disease. However, the Ju/'hoansi women's description of their sexual negotiations differed from those of our other informants. One single woman, expressing the entire group's view, said, "If he won't wear a condom, I won't have sex with him." Another woman, exhibiting autonomy of women described by Eleanor Burke Leacock, Richard Lee, and others (see Leacock and Lee 1982; Lee 1979; Shostak 1981), said, "He can't control me, I will do what I want, and if he doesn't do what I want, I don't have to have sex."

The young Ju/'hoansi men also talked of their relations with Ju/'hoansi women as negotiations with equal agents whose opinions have to be taken into account. In fact, the young men said they hoped that a girl who became a sexual partner would agree to be the man's wife.

Discussion

The five sites we visited offer contrasting opportunities through which women might be helped to protect themselves against HIV infection; no methods are currently in use or playing effective roles. At the first site, a rural village in what is now Natal Kwazulu, South Africa, women were, in 1992, reluctant to discuss HIV infection or contraception and tended to remain silent in the presence of men. They were poorly informed about sexually transmitted diseases in general and about HIV in particular. They had a small role in community organizations, appeared to be subservient to men outside as well as within the home, and were the only group visited that displayed the passive response and disempowered demeanor sometimes ascribed to African women in the literature.

The situation was very different in the urban settlement on the outskirts of Durban. Although they had only recently come from rural areas, the women here were articulate and politicized; they showed no hesitation in speaking up in the presence of men, contradicting the men when moved to do so. They were open and explicit about their experiences with men, equating their bargaining power with their need for money and resources: "Poverty makes prostitutes of us." Jobs would buy them independence. They were familiar with the male condom but were unable to insist that men use it. The female condom was just what they wanted; it would give them the control they sought. How can we demand that the government give us the female condom, they asked.

The women from Rundu, Namibia, also saw the need for political action; they wanted to mobilize and insist on their rights. Namibian women from both Rundu and the Ovambo region, like the women in Durban, did not believe that they could ask a man to use a male condom. Although they were just as emphatic about their wish to protect themselves from HIV/AIDS as the women in Durban, the Namibian women expressed a similar sense of cultural limits in their approach to sexual negotiation.

A complex cultural distinction underlay the demands of the women from Durban and Namibia. In their system of thought, women have rights over their own bodies, as men have over theirs. It is a man's prerogative to use or not use a male condom. However, although women cannot control men's actions in many situations outside the home, within the bedroom a man cannot prevent a woman from making decisions that affect her own body. Hence, when told about the female condom, the women became extremely enthusiastic. They could and would use this device, because it would be within their accepted domain of autonomy.

This point was confirmed independently by an ANC man who visited one of our meetings in 1995 at the informal settlement in Durban. He said, explicitly with reference to the female condom, "If it's in her room and it is her condom, she can use it." Well aware of AIDS, the women wanted desperately to be helped to acquire this single possibility for protection. They knew that they could not control what their men did – seeking other partners when they were away from home, for instance. Men might use the male condom on such occasions, but not with their wives.

It is striking that both the women in the urban setting in Durban and those in the rural sites of northern Namibia knew about AIDS but felt quite unable to preserve a monogamous relationship or to insist that their men use condoms. Yet both groups of women were quite confident that they could and would use the female condom, and they urged us to help them obtain some.

Quite different were the Ju/'hoansi women, who assured us that they would stand no nonsense from their men. Either the men would follow instructions to use condoms or the women would withhold sex. The young Ju/'hoansi men confirmed this view of relations between Ju/'hoansi men and women as negotiations between equals. We must add that although AIDS has certainly hit Ju/'hoansi villages, we have little evidence that the male condom was actually used. In addition, many of the sexual partners of young Ju/'hoansi women today are not Ju/'hoansi men but men from neighboring populations who are working in the Ju/'hoansi region. Ju/'hoansi women may not have the same autonomy in their relations with such partners, who have greater access to work and money than the Ju/'hoansi women or the Ju/'hoansi men.

At least three generalizations can be made from these studies. First, with the exception of those in the South African rural village, our respondents were by no means passive or submissive, and they were well aware of their vulnerability to HIV infection. Second, although they are well aware of the hazards of unprotected sex, women in southern Africa do not have access to methods they believe they could use. Faces brightened at our demonstration of the female condom, and the women responded eagerly to the suggestion that these condoms might be made available to them. Unlike some women in the developed world, but similar to women studied in Mexico, Senegal, and Costa Rica, they saw the female condom as a serious option (Parker et al. 2000). Third, the women understood that in order to obtain this protective device, they would have to take political action, probably by collective organization. They did not expect that women's needs would be recognized or understood by the government.

Conclusions

Contrary to the view of African women as helpless victims, most of the women we spoke to saw themselves as active participants in the search for a way to protect themselves in sexual situations. Nevertheless, their methods of sexual negotiation are shaped by cultural and historical perceptions of the bounds of the human body. Among some groups, the Ju/'hoansi for instance, a woman can insist that a man use a male condom, and she can withhold sex if he refuses. Among other groups, a woman's request that her partner use a male condom is seen as a challenge to his authority. A woman controls her own body, however, and has the right to use a female condom. In our interviews in these various settings, both urban and rural, the women demanded that the female condom be provided to them.

Woman-controlled methods of protection, such as the female condom, are regarded as culturally appropriate among many men and women in southern Africa and are crucial to the future of HIV/AIDS prevention. Since women have been clearly asking for such methods, political and economic concerns, combined with historically powerful patterns of gender discrimination and neglect of women's sexuality, must be considered the main barriers to the development and distribution of methods women can control.

ACKNOWLEDGMENTS

Research at two sites in South Africa in 1991 and 1992 was funded by the International Center for Research on Women and was carried out by Quarraisha Abdool Karim, Nkosasana Zuma, Eleanor Preston-Whyte, Zena Stein, and Ida Susser. The researchers wish to thank the PSC-CUNY Fellowship from the City University of New York and the University of Natal for support and assistance in 1995. Research in Namibia in 1996, 1997, and 1999 was funded by the Forgarty AIDS International Training and Research Program and was carried out by Richard Lee, Pombili Ipinge, Karen Nashua, Maria Nadjua, Karen Brodkin, and Ida Susser. This chapter is reprinted with permission from the *American Journal of Public Health* 90(7), July 2000, pp. 1042–1048.

Chapter 10

Migrancy, Masculine Identities, and AIDS: The Psychosocial Context of HIV Transmission on the South African Gold Mines

Catherine Campbell

Introduction

High levels of HIV infection are characteristic of a range of unstable and/or economically disadvantaged social settings in the southern African region. The life situation of migrant workers in a range of contexts renders them particularly vulnerable to HIV (Hunt 1989). The situation on the South African gold mines is no exception to this general rule (Campbell, 2003). Levels of HIV infection are high amongst mineworkers, with heterosexual sex being the main form of transmission of the virus (Jochelson et al. 1991; Williams and Campbell 1996). The gold mines currently employ about 350,000 male workers, 95 percent of whom are migrants, some from rural areas within South Africa and others from surrounding countries such as Lesotho, Botswana, and Mozambique. The vast majority of these workers are housed in single sex hostels close to their workplaces. In the interests of exploring the psychosocial context of HIV transmission amongst vulnerable migrant communities, this chapter examines the social identities of a sample of underground workers on a gold mine in the Johannesburg area, drawing on detailed interviews with 42 workers. Based on the assumption that social identities play a key role in shaping people's sexual behavior, the chapter illustrates the way in which this group of miners' identities are shaped and constrained by their living and working conditions. It also identifies some of the key interpretative repertoires used by informants in providing an account of their experiences of health, ill-health, HIV, and sexuality.

In the absence of prophylactic drugs or vaccines, HIV interventions on the mines take the form of the treatment of sexually transmitted diseases (which increase the transmission of the virus) and the treatment of diseases such as tuberculosis (which increase mortality and morbidity among HIV positive people) as well as health education programs which aim to change people's sexual behavior. This chapter is informed by a particular interest in the social psychology of health education and behavior change. Some gold mines are putting great effort into developing a range of innovative and creative HIV awareness and educational interventions. Others still rely on traditional information-based awareness programs such as videotapes and lectures, designed to impart information to a passive target audience (Crisp 1996; Macheke 1996). The conceptual underpinning of such information-based educational programs is the ubiquitous KAP (Knowledge – Attitudes – Practices) model. According to the KAP model, health-related behavior is determined by an individual's knowledge and attitudes. Thus if people know that AIDS is a deadly disease, and that using condoms will diminish their chances of getting it, they should be more likely to use condoms. Within this framework, information-based education programs seek to change people's behaviors through providing them with information or knowledge about the dangers of particular kinds of behavior.

Despite the assumption made by the KAP model, research has found that even people with relatively high levels of knowledge about HIV/AIDS often indulge in high-risk sexual behaviors (Campbell and Williams 1996). Information alone has thus not proved sufficient to bring about consistent changes in behavior. If factual knowledge is merely one determinant of behavior, a challenge for those interested in bringing about changes in sexual behavior is to develop understandings of other co-determinants of high-risk HIV-related behaviors and to develop more innovative attempts to bring about behavior change (Mechanic 1990; Kippax and Crawford 1993; Zwi and Cabral 1991).

Critics of the KAP approach have warned of the limitations of reducing sexuality to a series of isolated and quantifiable items of behavior (e.g., whether people use condoms or not; how many sexual encounters a person has per month). They argue that sexuality consists not of isolated items of behavior, but of a complex of actions, emotions, and relationships, "whereby living bodies are incorporated into social relations" (Kippax and Crawford 1993:257), and which are too complex to be apprehended using quantitative research alone. According to Stockdale, "Sexual behavior is inextricably linked with the norms characteristic of the social groups with which we identify. These norms shape the boundaries of permissible behavior and define the limits of deviance" (Stockdale 1995:46).

In this chapter, it will be argued that explanations of why people engage in high-risk behaviors involve an understanding of their social identities and of the social conditions within which such identities are constructed. Thus for example, investigations of a number of heterosexual settings have suggested that the dynamics of condom use or non-use cannot be understood without taking cognizance of a context in which men see their virility as compromised by using condoms, and women are reluctant to insist. Within such a social setting, simply telling people to use condoms will have little effect, because it ignores the broader social context of masculine and feminine identities which makes the negotiation of condom use a far more complex process than KAP-type models would suggest. It is on the basis of the complex psychosocial dynamics of sexuality that qualitative research has been identified as a top priority in understanding the psychosocial context of HIV transmission in Africa (Ankrah 1989; Scott and Mercer 1994).

Methodology: Identities, Repertoires, and Behaviors

The theoretical starting point for the research in this chapter is the sub-discipline of social psychology, and more particularly Social Identity Theory/Self-Categorization Theory (SIT-SCT) in the Tajfel – Turner tradition (Hogg and Abrams 1988; Tajfel 1981; Oakes et al. 1994), which holds that the social self consists of a loose association of *self-categorizations or group memberships*. Theorists in the SIT-SCT tradition have tended to focus much of their attention on the psychological processes underlying group formation, focusing on the cognitive and motivational processes involved in identity formation, while paying relatively less attention to the content of specific identities or the role played by day-to-day life situations in the shaping of identities. However, a more recent development of the theory has focused on the way in which such cognitive and motivational processes are structured within dynamically changing social contexts (Campbell 1995a). It has been suggested that different group memberships are associated with different sets of *recipes for living* and are shaped in the context of particular *life challenges*. Recipes for living consist of (a) sets of behavioral possibilities and constraints; and (b) repertoires of interpretative frameworks through which all behavior and experience are mediated. In this model, identity is never static, but constantly constructed and reconstructed in response to the *life challenges* posed by the relevant social and material worlds. The concept of life challenges highlights the situation-dependent and context-specific nature of social identities. Identities are a socially negotiated and flexible product, constructed in dynamic interaction with those around us.[1]

Miners in the current study categorized themselves in terms of a range of informal *group memberships* including collectivities of underground work – team mates, hostel room-mates, "home-boys" (fellow workers from the same geographical place of origin), as well as rural homestead communities, family groupings, and so on. This chapter will examine the way in which social identities are shaped in response to the *life challenges* of work, leisure, and interpersonal relationships within the particular living and working conditions of the gold mines.

Gender ideology saturates many of the group memberships constituting social identities across a broad range of situations, with gender often serving as an important organizing principle in the process of social identity construction (Campbell 1995b). Against the background of this conceptualization of identity, one of the key issues that emerged in the present study was the way in which the social construction of masculine identities within the dangerous and socially impoverished context of life on the mines presented mineworkers with a particular repertoire of sexual relationships and practices. The argument is developed with reference to data from a recently conducted study into mineworkers' perceptions of health and illness. This study was conducted on a Johannesburg gold mine in early 1995 under the auspices of the Epidemiology Research Unit, and involved semi-structured, open-ended interviews with 42 Zulu-, Xhosa-, and Sotho-speaking underground mineworkers. Interviews were conducted by the author, together with a multilingual team of co-

interviewers. The interviews were on average three hours long, and aimed to elicit informants' life histories with particular focus on their experiences and perceptions of health, healing, sexuality, and HIV/AIDS. This life history approach was chosen because it corresponded with the view of social identity as a resource that people draw on in constructing narratives which provide meaning and a sense of continuity in their lives, and which guide their actions. Eliciting such life history narratives should throw light on the social context in which the social and sexual identities which inform sexual behavior are constructed, and help to draw out the socially negotiated interpretative repertoires which shape and constrain such behavior.

Miners' Perceptions of Health and HIV/AIDS

On the mine where the interviews were conducted, management was making strenuous efforts to educate workers about AIDS with educational videotapes, pamphlets, and posters. Preventive behavior was also promoted through free supplies of condoms. While one cannot generalize on the basis of 42 interviews, it was quite clear that amongst the interviewees in the present study, these information-based programs were having only a limited effect. Each informant reported having seen the mine's educational videotape on HIV/AIDS; each was also aware of the pamphlets and posters, and of the free supply of condoms. Every person said that HIV/AIDS was transmitted during unprotected sex, and that condoms would prevent its transmission. Most people said it was incurable. Beyond these basic facts, however, people's knowledge of HIV/AIDS was patchy, and often contradictory (Macheke and Campbell (1995) provide a more detailed account of inconsistencies and ambiguities in this group of informants' perceptions of HIV/AIDS.) Many said that while they had heard of HIV/AIDS they remained unsure about its existence because they had never seen anyone suffering from it. Certain informants asserted that the disease did not exist, that it existed in countries to the north but not in South Africa, or that it could be cured by traditional healers. They cited the major symptoms of HIV/AIDS as sores on the body, and when asked to estimate the time lapse between infected sexual contact and appearance of sores, informants often answered in the region of two weeks to two months. Most significantly, for all their exposure to the educational materials, in our sample of informants, unprotected sex with multiple sexual partners (frequently commercial sex workers) appeared to be the norm rather than the exception.

In the interviews, informants articulated a notion of health that was more holistic than that of the biomedical model that dominates Western thinking about HIV/AIDS. They characterized health in terms of a harmonious balance between person and environment. The person was conceived of as an interaction of physical, mental, and spiritual/supernatural imperatives. The environment included the living environment, working environment, and social environment. They were comfortably located within a plurality of healing systems, moving between these without tension or sense of contradiction, oscillating between representatives of Western biomedicine (hospitals, clinics, pharmacies, private general practitioners) and traditional healers (diviners, herbalists, and faith healers) (Abdool-Karrim et al. 1994).

Informants took the biomedically biased information they were presented about HIV/AIDS (by people they saw as representatives of the Western biomedical establishment), and interpreted it through a filter of health knowledge and experience in which Western biomedicine plays only a partial role. This filter led certain of the workers we spoke with to treat the claim that HIV/AIDS was incurable with a certain degree of skepticism:

Interviewer: Is there anything that the traditional healers or Western doctors can do to help, once one gets AIDS?

Informant: Black people can heal AIDS. AIDS is centered around sores and black people are really good when it comes to sores.

Interviewer: Can they eliminate it altogether?

Informant: It is possible that they can eliminate the disease altogether if it is detected in its earlier stages.

If HIV/AIDS education programs are to be effective, they must take account of a range of local knowledges and beliefs into which target audiences will insert and evaluate the information that the programs seek to impart. Health education audiences will always engage in an internal debate between the new information presented by the educator (e.g., AIDS is incurable), and their previous information about the topic in question (e.g., AIDS is characterized by sores – and it is well known that traditional healers can deal with such sores even if hospital doctors cannot). Well-planned educational programs need to predict the way in which old information might seek to block the reception of the new messages they seek to impart. Even more importantly, programs that aim to change people's behavior need to be informed by understandings of the way in which behaviors are shaped by socially negotiated identities within particular social contexts – issues that are central to the current research.

Based on the conceptualization of identity outlined above, the analysis of the interviews centered on two issues. The first of these concerned the particular set of working and living conditions that make unprotected sex with multiple partners such a compelling behavioral option – a recipe for living – for this particular group of migrants. The second concerns the interpretative repertoires used by informants in accounting for their experiences of health, healing, sexuality, and HIV/AIDS, since it is these repertoires that form the filter through which workers interpret and respond to health educators' attempts to change their behaviors. It will be argued that miner identities are constructed in a way that makes them particularly vulnerable to HIV infection.

Social Context of Identify Formation: Working and Living Conditions on the Mines

As has already been emphasized, the process of social identity construction is context-dependent and situation-specific. In the interviews, factors such as the general working and living conditions on the mines, the ever-present danger of accidents, and mineworkers' perceived lack of control over their health and well-being repeatedly emerged as important features of the world in which mineworker identities were fashioned. *Living and working conditions on the mines* are dangerous and highly stressful (Leon et al. 1995; Molapo 1995). Firstly, the majority of mineworkers live some distance from their homes and families, in large single sex hostels, with up to 18 people sharing a room. Informants described compound life as dirty and overcrowded, with no space for privacy or quiet. While some facilities exist for wives and families to visit, informants said that these were extremely limited. Opportunities for leisure are few. Some workers spend time in the African townships near to the mines, others avoid them as dangerous places. From the accounts of our informants, drinking and sex appeared to be two of the few diversionary activities easily available on a day-to-day basis.

Even more stressful than life outside of work, however, was the time spent in the mines themselves. While miners' accounts of their working conditions varied widely according to their specific job underground and according to the demands of particular production team leaders (who, some informants commented, sometimes seemed to be more concerned with productivity than with the well-being of the team), there were many common themes. Many men said that they were expected to engage in physically taxing and dangerous work for up to eight hours with infrequent breaks, sometimes with minimal access to food or water, under conditions of tremendous heat, in air that was frequently stale and dusty, and sometimes with unpleasantly noisy machinery.

In talking about the stresses of daily life on the mines, the issue of rock-falls emerged as the central concern of most of the informants. They reported living in daily *fear of fatal, mutilating, or disabling accidents*. This fear is well based. The South African mining industry has long been characterized by an alarming accident rate. Based on the average fatality and reportable injury rates published by the South African Chamber of Mines for the 10-year period 1984–93, an underground worker has a 2.9 percent chance of being killed in a work-related accident and a 42 percent chance of suffering a reportable injury in a 20-year working life (Chamber of Mines 1993).

Informant: Every time you go underground you have to wear a lamp on your head. Once you take on that lamp you know that you are wearing death. Where you are going you are not sure whether you will come back to the surface alive or dead. It is only with luck if you come to the surface still alive because everyday somebody gets injured or dies.

Interviewer: Do you worry about death from accidents, working underground?

Informant: This thought scares us when something has happened – maybe to a person one knows, or even a person one does not know. You might hear that so-and-so has gone (in an accident) and you think: "Eish! our brothers are passing away," that's all. We cannot know, maybe we are also on the way, and we live in hope – and with the knowledge that it will happen to everyone sooner or later. We live for dying, no one lives forever. Every day people lose their arms and legs and we just live in hope.

Many had witnessed accidents in which friends and co-workers had either been killed or injured, or witnessed the dead or injured being brought above the ground after accidents, and the stress and distress caused by such incidents cannot be underestimated. The psychologically disabling effects of being subject to life-threatening or shocking incidents are well documented in the literature on post-traumatic stress, as is the fact that while some individuals are able to make a quick recovery, others suffer the after-effects for varying periods of time after the incident. Members of the latter group were amongst our sample. They reported the classic symptoms of post-traumatic stress disorder following the trauma: social withdrawal, problems in concentrating as well as flashbacks or nightmares in which they relived the shocking

incident. Such flashbacks or nightmares sometimes troubled them for months or even years
after the accident. Several informants talked
about the disturbances at night caused by the
screaming of men suffering nightmares, who
would then be woken up and comforted by
room-mates.

Informants referred to accidents in a fatalistic way.

Informant: The rock can just fall anytime
and we try not to think about
that. A rock can fall and kill
someone while you are working
with them, it has happened to me
before...last week someone in
my team met his fate that way
and we had to pull his corpse
from under the stones.

Interviewer: Are there any religious measures
that people take before starting to
work?

Informant: No one prays or does such things –
because when a rock is going to fall
it just falls anytime and there is
nothing that can be done about it.

Interviewer: Is there any form of traditional
protection that people seek out
to try to protect themselves
against falling rocks?

Informant: There are those that seek help
from traditional healers for protection, but when the rocks fall,
they fall all over, and it does not
matter whether you are protected
or not – they fall on those with
and without the protection.

It is argued that this sense of powerlessness is
an important feature of the contextual back-
drop in which miners' sexual identities are
negotiated. *Self-efficacy* (or the degree to
which a person feels that s/he has control
over important aspects of his or her life) is an
important determinant of health-related behavior. The greater one's sense of self-efficacy,
the more likely one is to engage in health promoting behaviors (Prieur 1990). It was not only
in relation to accidents that informants referred to a sense of powerlessness. In the interviews, they repeatedly articulated their lack of
control in a range of contexts. For example,

virtually every interviewee said he hated
his job, but that he had no choice given his
lack of education, high levels of unemployment, and chronic poverty in his rural place
of origin.

Interviewer: Is your job easy or difficult?

Informant: The work is heavy but I have endured it because I have no education. It's risky – every time I go
down I am not sure if I will come
back. But I have no choice. I am
forced to do it.

Interviewer: Would you say that this is a
source of pride for these men
that they do this dangerous and
difficult job?

Informant: Facing such struggles is not a
source of pride. It is because of
frustration and poverty that men
do this job.

Many commented on their powerlessness to
avoid a range of health problems. Tuberculosis
(TB) was one such problem.[2] One 25-year-old
man said it was inevitable that if he stayed on
the mines for 20 years he would get TB, no
matter how much he tried to avoid it. A 41-
year-old man who looked considerably older
than his years appeared depressed and apa-
thetic. Telling us about his recurrent bouts of
TB, he said he was pessimistic that he would
ever be in good health again.

Interviewer: Given the situation you are
working in, are there any attempts that you make to improve
your health?

Informant: There is nothing that I try because I don't have that privilege.
Where I am living on the mines, I
don't have any choice on how to
conduct my life, it is imposed on
me. Most of my life that I have
spent here has not been so fruitful and when I look ahead, I don't
see myself having a long life.

Interviewer: Why do you say that?

Informant: Because of my ill health and I
don't spend a year without
visiting a hospital.

Interviewer: Do you not feel that this negative
attitude might encourage you

Informant: I care about my life very deeply
but I can really feel that I am
suffering with my health – I feel
that my life won't last for much
longer, and that due to my
working conditions I am prevented from prolonging it.

While people spoke with feeling about
frightening working conditions and poor
living conditions, they had little faith in their
ability to bring about improvements. Complaints to unions or *indunas* seldom bore fruit.
As one man commented wryly in response to a
question about channels for complaint:

Interviewer: Is there any way you can complain
about things you do not like?

Informant: There are several channels for
complaints but we are never considered. So, we just complain for
the sake of complaining.

One informant commented that the risk of
HIV/AIDS appeared minimal compared to
the risks of death underground, and suggested
that this was the reason why many mineworkers did not bother with condoms.

Interviewer: Why is it that men think about
pleasure first before thinking
about their health?

Informant: The dangers and risks of the job
we are doing are such that no one
can afford to be motivated with
life – so the only thing that motivates us is pleasure.

Having pointed to features of the social context within which mineworkers construct their
identities, attention turns to the interpretative
repertoires drawn on by mineworkers in
presenting their health-related life histories. It
is argued that such repertoires shape not only
people's sexual behavior, but also their responses to HIV-education programs that attempt to change sexual behaviors.

Health, Intimacy and Sexuality

Dunbar Moodie has written in detail about the
role of masculinity in shaping South African

mineworkers' general social identities.[3] In
the current study, masculinity emerged as a
master narrative penetrating informants'
accounts of their more specifically health-
related experience and behaviors. In this
section of the chapter, attention is given to
the way in which the social construction of
masculine identities on the gold mines makes
migrant mineworkers especially vulnerable to
HIV infection.

Much has been written about the creative
and innovative way in which mineworkers
have responded to the alienation and danger
of their working lives, constructing personally
meaningful identities despite massive social
constraints.[4] Particularly evident in the interviews was the way in which masculine identities had been shaped and crafted by workers
as a way of dealing with the fears and
struggles of their day-to-day working lives.
Men frequently spoke of their terror as new
workers the first time they entered the "cage"
(lift) that would carry them to their work sites
up to 3 km underground. They recounted how
more experienced workers would encourage
them by urging them to remember that they
were men. A man was someone who had the
responsibility of supporting his family and
hence had no choice but to put up with the
risks and stresses of working underground.
A man was someone who was brave enough
to withstand the rigors of the job.

Interviewer: How did they console you when
you entered the cage?

Informant: They told me that in this situation
you must know that now that
you are on the mines you are a
man and must be able to face
anything without fear.

Interviewer: Is this theme of being a man
common in the mine?

Informant: To be called a man serves to encourage and console you time
and again...You will hear
people saying "a man is a sheep,
he does not cry." I mean this is
the way to encourage or console
you at most times.

Interviewer: Can you explain more about the
metaphor of "a man being a
sheep"?

Informant: ...I can explain it this way: no matter how hard you hit a sheep or slaughter it you will not hear it cry. The animal that can cry is a goat. So, that is a comparison that whatever pain you can inflict on a man you will not see him cry.

Thus the notion of masculinity plays a key role as a coping mechanism whereby men overcome their daily fears of injury and death as well as the exhausting demands of the work. As one informant told us: "We commit ourselves as men because if we don't do it our children will suffer." Another commented:

"You show your manhood by going underground, working in difficult conditions – this shows that you are man enough to accept that if you die you are just dead. Once you go underground you are a man and no longer a child."

Closely intertwined with this notion of masculinity – which brings together the concepts of bravery, fearlessness, and persistence in the face of the demands of underground work – is that of a macho sexuality, which was captured in another informant's comment: "There are two things to being a man: going underground, and going after women." Linked to this masculine identity were the repertoires of insatiable sexuality, the need for multiple sexual partners, and a manly desire for the pleasure of flesh-to-flesh sexual contact. All these are factors that put mineworkers at risk for HIV/AIDS. Ironically the very sense of masculinity that assists men in their day-to-day survival also serves to heighten their exposure to the risks of HIV infection.

Interviewer: Why do you think that men have sex on their minds?

Informant: I think that is the way men were made, that is to always have a desire for a woman.

Interviewer: You have a family that you love and support but on the other hand you behave in a way that can make you vulnerable to diseases. Why should men behave like that?

Informant: The truth is that "a man is a dog" meaning that he does not get satisfied. That is why we come across

such things. Because when a man sees "a dress," meaning a woman, he follows her.

Interviewer: Why do people think about pleasure before they think about their life which is at risk?

Informant: The truth is that we are pushed by desire to have sex with a certain woman. We do not think about AIDS during that time but about it when we are finished. It is a matter of satisfying your body because of someone beautiful. Basically it is the body that has that desire.

Informants made a strong link between sex and masculinity in relation to their general physical and mental health and well-being. Particularly important for health was what was referred to as the maintenance of a balanced supply of blood in the body. Several people commented that sex played a key role in the regulation of a balanced supply of blood and sperm, and that regular sex was essential for the maintenance of a man's good health. A range of possible ill-effects of poorly regulated bodily fluids resulting from prolonged celibacy were mentioned. Informants dwelt the most on mental ill-effects: depression, short-temperedness, violence, and an inability to think clearly. Less frequently mentioned were such physical ill-effects as pimples and obesity. Behavioral ill-effects included recklessness and impulsive behavior. A normally prudent and responsible man who had been celibate for too long might, it was claimed, be unable to control his desire for sex when he encountered a commercial sex worker in the street, even if he did not have a condom with him. Lengthy celibacy might also lead a man to consider homosexual relationships which he would not have considered in other circumstances.[5] Unrequited sexual urges might also lead a man to take unnecessary risks in the African townships near the mines, by seeking out women whose friends or brothers might beat him up or steal his money.

The continued practice of dangerous sexual behaviors by mineworkers must also be located within a context that provides *limited social support and scant opportunities for intimacy*.

Research in both Europe and America has found a significant correlation between level of social support and safe sex. Thus for example gay men in Norway were far less likely to engage in unprotected sexual intercourse if they live in a supportive social environment. In conditions where they felt lonely and isolated, flesh-to-flesh sexual contact came to symbolize a form of emotional intimacy that may have been lacking in other areas of their lives (Prieur 1990). Amongst American adolescents, safe sexual behavior is predicted more by teenagers' perceptions of how much their parents care for them, than by the frequency of health warnings, social class, or parents' health status (Mechanic 1990).

This correlation between social support and risk-taking behavior provides an interesting framework within which to consider the high levels of unsafe sexual behavior practiced amongst mineworkers. Informants spoke at length about the loneliness of being away from their families. They spoke of anxieties that their distant rural wives or girlfriends might be unfaithful; of worries about their children growing up without a father's guidance; of their own guilt about money they might have wasted on drink and commercial sex which they should have sent to their families. These absent families were never far away in their accounts of their lives and their health. Others spoke with dread of fears that they would die underground, and that their bodies might not be returned to their families for proper funeral rites, a particularly frightening prospect in a context where deceased ancestors may often play a pivotal role in people's lives.

While hostel room-mates, underground teammates, and men from the same home village appeared to constitute support systems in certain contexts, informants were adamant that male friends could not make up for the loss of female partners and children within a homely domestic setting. The youngest of our informants (aged 19), also the most sexually active and least interested in condoms, spoke wistfully of his close relationship with his parents in rural Lesotho, and how much he missed them. The 41-year-old interviewee referred to earlier, who had been plagued by recurrent attacks of tuberculosis for five years, ascribed his distance from his wife as one of the main reasons for his poor health.

Informant: There is no one who can help me here and it is quite impossible for me to know all my needs. If I was nearer to my wife, she would take care of me, look after me.

In response to questions regarding their reluctance to use condoms, informants repeatedly reiterated their desire for flesh-to-flesh contact. When asked specifically about the reasons for this desire, informants referred to pleasure, and also to the fact that this was simply something that men needed: "a man must have flesh-to-flesh" was something of a cliché in the interviews. Research findings cited above suggest that another reason for the desire for flesh-to-flesh contact might be the broader social context of general loneliness and reduced opportunities for intimate social relationships. The task of changing mineworkers' sexual behavior, and persuading them to use condoms, for example, cannot be achieved without attention to the broader context of sex and sexuality, including the symbolic role of flesh-to-flesh contact in the face of stresses and loneliness.

In the highly patriarchal rural communities from which many mineworkers originate, one of the main pillars of masculine identity construction is participation in homestead and family leadership (Dunbar Moodie 1994). In the particular context of life on the mines, for many migrants, deprived of such key markers of masculinity on a day-to-day basis, frequent assertion of what are regarded as healthy and manly sexual urges could arguably serve to compensate for reduced opportunities for assertion of masculine identities in other contexts.[6]

Hayes (1992) criticizes the tendency in much health education literature to regard high-risk health-threatening behaviors in a negative light. He suggests that risk-taking is better conceptualized as a "wager," in which social actors weigh up potential losses and gains of those behavioral options available to them. While mineworkers may be aware of the dangers of unprotected sex with multiple partners on the one hand, such behavior may be beneficial at a range of other levels in the stressful and socially impoverished living and working environments of the gold mines.

Implications for Health Interventions

In this chapter, working within an SIT-SCT framework, attention has been given to the way in which social identities are forged in response to the life challenges of the mining context in a manner that makes mineworkers particularly vulnerable to HIV infection. In particular, attention has been paid to the role played by masculine identities in this process. The contexts and identities that give rise to high-risk sexual behaviors will vary from one social context to the next. Thus the applicability of the empirical material presented in this chapter to migrants or other HIV-vulnerable communities in other contexts in sub-Saharan Africa is a matter for empirical investigation. It is our claim, however, that the chapter's broader argument about the role of social identities in the task of shaping people's sexual behaviors, as well as promoting health-related behavior change, has more general applicability.

One of the aims of this Chapter has been to illustrate the argument that high-risk sexual behaviors (such as unprotected sex with multiple partners) are too complex to be changed by simply providing people with health-related information, as traditional health education programs have sought to do. This is because – far from being a matter over which individuals exercise rational control as the KAP framework suggests – sexuality is shaped by a complex process of identity formation nested within the dynamic web of cultural, psychological and social factors (Campbell, 2003).

Against this background, the challenge facing HIV educators is that of designing creative and innovative health education programs that aim to do more than provide information. One successful example of such a program is that of the peer education program developed by Wilson and colleagues in Zimbabwe (Dube and Wilson 1995), based on the fundamental social psychological principle that people are more likely to change their behavior if they perceive that their peers are also committed to behavioral change (Lewin 1958). In the workplace context, peer education is conducted by selected members of the workforce who receive training in basic health-related information, as well as training on how to facilitate discussion and debate in group settings. They are also given free supplies of condoms. Such educators are then sent back into the workforce to raise debates about the issue of HIV as often as possible in informal work and recreational settings in such a way that people are encouraged to debate new health-related information in the light of their old views, opinions, and identities.

The success of this program is consonant with the processes that have been articulated above. In terms of the social identity framework adopted in this chapter such programs succeed in changing sexual behavior because they provide a context in which members of HIV-vulnerable groups are given space to refashion their social and sexual identities in a collective way. In such contexts people play an active role in debating the possibilities of alternative recipes for living, rather than passively listening to information presented by a relatively impersonal source in the style of more traditional health education programs. These processes operate at the group rather than the individual level in changing people's group-linked sense of previously taken-for-granted behavior through the collective renegotiation of social and sexual identities. Such programs provide a context for the transformation of group-linked recipes for living rather than seeking to alter individual behaviors through the provision of information.

In the final instance HIV is a social problem insofar as those with the poorest health experiences the world over are generally those who come from the most disrupted social settings, and are the least constrained or protected by family and community expectations (Mechanic 1990). HIV in South Africa is no exception to this general rule. The current research strongly supports the claim that the most important aspect of slowing down the spread of STDs and HIV infection would be to alter the broader social and material conditions which encourage high-risk sexual practices (Zwi and Bachmayer 1990). However, such changes involve ongoing long-term struggles. Given the lack of HIV drugs and vaccines, and given the speed at which the epidemic is progressing in South Africa,[7] additional short-term strategies are required to deal with HIV, and the challenge for HIV educators remains a strong one.

ACKNOWLEDGMENTS

This paper is reproduced as a chapter in this book by permission of the editors at *Social Science and Medicine*. The paper first appeared in Social Science and Medicine 45(2), pp. 273–281, 1997. The research for this chapter was conducted as part of the South African Epidemiology Research Unit's (ERU) Perceptions of Health Project. The ERU is an independent body which conducts research into the health and safety of mineworkers. Its management committee consists of representatives of the academic and medical establishments, mine management, and the trade unions. Particular thanks to Brian Williams, ERU Director, who set up the Perceptions of Health Project, and conducted many of the interviews reported on in this paper and was extensively involved in discussions of the data. John Carson gave detailed advice on the manuscript. The following people also contributed in various ways to the research process and the ideas presented here: William Beinart, Joy de Beyer, Karen Jochelson, Cecil Macheke, Phampang Manato, Gerhard Mare, Oupa Raymond Matsi, Sello Molefe, Nokuzola Mqoqi, and Jan Stockdale.

NOTES

1. This point has been illustrated in relation to South African mineworkers in the accounts by historians Harries and Moodie of the history of homosexual "mine marriages" on the South African gold mines, which were common prior to the 1970s. They argue that such "marriages" played an important role in consolidating a range of masculine, generational, and rural identities within the hostile urban context, and they illustrate the interactional and socially negotiated nature of their evolution. The system of "mine marriages" had eroded by the 1970s (Harries 1990; Dunbar Moodie 1994).

2. The incidence of tuberculosis on South African gold mines increased from 620 per 100,000 workers per year in 1988 to 1,070 per 100,000 workers per year in 1992 (Packard and Coetzee 1995).

3. Dunbar Moodie (1988, 1994) comments that an aggressive and macho masculinity forms a pillar of identity formation amongst large collectivities of working men in a range of contexts and continents, and is certainly not peculiar to southern Africa, or to mineworkers.

4. Sitas (1985) has written of the "defensive combinations" of rural, urban, and protest identities that mineworkers have creatively integrated in the task of dealing with the day-to-day stresses and indignities of their lives. Dunbar Moodie (1994) speaks of the "integrity" and "character" of such coping mechanisms.

5. While homosexual relationships in the form of "mine marriages" were a common feature of life in the mine hostels until the 1970s, these are no longer common. Dunbar Moodie (1994) provides a fascinating historical account of the way in which the popularity of such interactions arose, flourished, and later declined, this process being shaped by the changing face of the social and economic contexts of people's lives on the mines and in the countryside. Our own informants echoed Moodie's findings, saying that homosexual relationships were not as common as they had been in the past.

6. Campbell (1992) argues that there are a range of ways in which men might seek to compensate for the loss of masculinity as more traditional patriarchal family structures (in which men had a great deal of power over women and children) are eroded. In a study of township men in Natal, where family structures are in a state of rapid transformation, she suggests that involvement in political violence (strongly associated with a macho masculinity in her research findings) might be a compensatory mechanism as the opportunities for the assertion of masculine power within the family are increasingly diminished.

7. To date there are no published epidemiological data regarding HIV rates amongst mineworkers. The only nationwide South African data that currently exist deal with antenatal clinic attendees. According to Kustner (1994), the doubling time of HIV infection in this group is 13 months.

Chapter 11

The Invisible Presence of Homosexuality: Implications for HIV/AIDS and Rights in Southern Africa

Oliver Phillips

It has become commonplace to talk of HIV/AIDS in the context of southern Africa as distinctly "heterosexual," signifying a difference from the "homosexual" spread of HIV/AIDS in western Europe and North America.[1] While much of the transmission of the virus in southern Africa does take place through sex between men and women, there is nevertheless a problem in assuming that this allows us to talk of HIV/AIDS as "heterosexually" transmitted. The highly contentious atmosphere that pervades any discussion of homosexuality in a southern African context should surely alert us to parallel difficulties in assuming that notions of heterosexuality are appropriately employed in this same context. More simply, the inappropriateness of assuming homosexual identity has been recognized through the use of the term "men who have sex with men," referring to behavior that is often not exclusively practiced, and allowing for a variety of cultural constructions of sexual behavior. But there has been little parallel destabilization of the assumed appropriateness of the term "heterosexual," and its suggestion of an exclusive pattern of behavior. This is odd since it is not possible to identify a person or a form of behavior as "heterosexual" without simultaneously identifying what is "homosexual." It is impossible to define either term without implicitly relying on the other. This chapter sets out to consider the manner in which this homosexual/heterosexual binary has been deployed with reference to sexual behavior and identity in southern Africa, and to engage with associated difficulties arising in relation to socio-political rights and the prevention and treatment of HIV/AIDS.

Other chapters in this book make clear the extent to which dying from AIDS has become a result of global economics, as death is mapped onto locations of poverty and distributed through a lack of economic power, rather than carried by a disease that is inevitably insuppressible. The familiarity of this scenario in southern Africa is awful as we become ever more acquainted with its broader social and economic implications.[2] But I want to relate this to recent developments in sexual politics, by discussing the place of the sexual in politics as a whole, and then assessing how these might help or hinder attempts to reduce

HIV infection rates. I shall make disproportionate reference to Zimbabwe, not only because it has been the location of the most vociferous discussion concerning homosexuality, but also because it is one of the southern African countries with which I am most familiar as it has, at different times throughout my life, been my home.

In this chapter, the regional situation will serve to illustrate that definitions of appropriate sexual behavior are indicative of broader social relations of gender and age. It seems trite to state that contests around sex and gender are increasingly important not only in this regard, but also in relation to attempts to prevent and treat HIV/AIDS. I want to make clear how the spread of HIV/AIDS simply emphasizes the importance of extending our understanding of social and economic rights, as well as civil and political rights, to include some (at times indefinable, at times highly defined) understanding of diversity with regard to sexual behavior.

Some observers of Zimbabwe may have been under the impression that sex, and more specifically homosexuality, has taken a position of exaggerated significance in national politics in the seven years since President Mugabe engineered the expulsion of the Gays and Lesbians of Zimbabwe (GALZ) from the Zimbabwe International Book Fair (ZIBF) in August 1995.[3] The importance of sexual orientation appears questionable when measured against the right to life, land, employment, or freedom from torture. Indeed, in a recent interview with a French magazine, Keith Goddard, the administrator of GALZ, might have added to this impression:

Zimbabwe is not the worst place in the world to be gay. Contrary to what one reads in the local press controlled by the State, or in the international press, there are very few arrests of homosexuals and we are not particularly harassed. Gay bashing has become extremely rare. Nothing as serious as the Matthew Shepard case in the United States has ever happened here. (Goddard, K. in *Têtu* (52) p. 58, January 2001)

This is not to refute that the law prohibiting sex between men has led to many attempts at blackmail, which have in turn led to acts of violence, sometimes resulting in death (see Phillips 1997:484); nor is it to deny that some, and in particular Goddard himself, have at some stage found themselves the target of State or police harassment on account of their homosexuality. But what this statement emphasizes is that such difficulties experienced with issues of sexuality and gender are universal, and that the assumption that more industrialized countries (e.g., the U.S.A.) have overcome these difficulties is both false and arrogant. By his own admission, Goddard is able to make this statement because in Zimbabwe the spotlight on sexuality has been usurped by a more pressing preoccupation with the freefall of the economy, the redistribution of land, the new challenge of a sizable opposition party (MDC), and unprecedented levels of political violence (pers. comm.). And yet, the connected questions remain to be asked: Why did sexuality become such a hotly contested national issue in the 1990s, why did this reverberate around the region, and what are the connections to, and implications for strategies for combating, the worst effects of HIV/AIDS?

An attempt to answer these questions makes up the bulk of this discussion, which postulates that these sexual politics reflect the growth of an individual's (particularly a woman's) rights as negotiated through the State, indicating a growing autonomy from lineage, and that this issue is therefore bound to bring about controversy again. This is made all the more likely by the significance of sexuality and gender in managing the spread, prevention, and treatment of HIV/AIDS.

Sex as a Social Marker Throughout the Region

In the 1990s, the sexual activities of people living throughout the southern African region have alternately assumed and been allocated increasing significance as social markers. Unprecedented public discussion has arisen of the proclaimed rights or declaimed immorality of sexual activities between people of the same sex, frequently invoking the boundaries of nationalism and humanity.

In March 1997, the newly formed Gays and Lesbians of Swaziland (GaLeSwa) was refused recognition by the Prime Minister of Swaziland, although there appears to be no existing legal prohibition against homosexual acts. At much the same time, the Rainbow Coalition was founded in Namibia, and President Sam Nujoma proclaimed that homosexuality "should be uprooted totally" from Namibia, calling it "a hideous deviation of decrepit and inhuman sordid behavior" (*Weekly Mail and Guardian* February 14, 1997).

In 1998 the Botswana government, fearful that its legal prohibition of sex between men would be challenged on the grounds of sexual discrimination, passed new legislation that prohibited sex between women; in the same year, an association called Lesbians, Gays, and Bisexuals of Botswana (Legabibo) was formed. In August 1998, the Lesbians, Gays, Bi-Sexual, and Transgender Persons Association (LEGATRA) of Zambia was formed, amid uproar from government and press (see *The Daily Mail of Zambia* September 2, 1998).

It is worth noting that the movements calling explicitly for "lesbian and gay rights" have mushroomed in the region both as a result of governmental derogations of such rights and as a result of individual and collective affirmations of social identities which deliver these rights. The coming to power of the ANC in South Africa provided a singular opportunity for such a delivery as the new South African constitution became the first in the world to explicitly prohibit discrimination on the grounds of sexual orientation. This allowed the National Coalition for Gay and Lesbian Equality (NCGLE) to take legal action leading to the decriminalization of homosexual sex and successfully challenging discrimination against homosexuals in many social and economic domains (De Vos 2000:194–207; and Stychin 1998:52–88).

While Uganda and Kenya have both borne witness to the issuing of statements on homosexuality by their presidents (*East Africa Standard* September 30, 1999), Zimbabwe has attracted the greatest notoriety in this regard, as the threats and statements made by its government speakers and neo-traditionalists[4] have been the most vociferous. Mugabe's comments have frequently been made on international platforms ostensibly convened to affirm human rights, but the most colorful idioms are found in the so-called debates en-

titled "The Evil and Iniquitous Practice of Homosexualism" that took place in Zimbabwe's parliament.

> to support the presence of these people (gays and lesbians) in this country is to be an accomplice in promoting lechery . . . It means, if we support them, we want our nation to be vile. We want out nation to be unchaste. We want our people to be animal-like and immoral in behavior. In cultural terms, what it amounts to is that the homosexuals are like a witch weed in Zimbabwe, which in Shona we call "*bise*." It is therefore supposed to be eradicated. The moment you see it you eradicate it . . .

> The whole body is far more important than any single dispensable part. When your finger starts festering and becomes a danger to the body you cut it off. The moment you come to the conclusion that you cannot cure the finger, you cut it off. The purpose for cutting it off is to preserve the body . . . The homosexuals are the festering finger endangering the body and we chop them off. (Anias Chigwedere MP, *Zimbabwe Parliamentary Debate* September 28, 1995, Hansard pp. 2779–2781)

President Mugabe has made it clear that he believes homosexuals and their advocates should have "no rights whatsoever" and are "behaving worse than pigs and dogs" (*The Herald* August 12, 1995). This latter statement was made in Shona, which gives "dogs" (*imbwa*) a particular idiomatic significance consistent with his reference to homosexuality as a threat to the moral fiber of society. Mugabe proclaimed a return to "traditional" culture, saying "We have our own culture, and we must rededicate ourselves to our traditional values that make us human beings" (*The Citizen* August 12, 1995).

This and many of the comments made by leaders throughout the region refer to pride in a national culture "free" of homosexuality, and rely on notions of *ubuntu* (or *munhu*) which invoke an Africanist conception of humanity and society.[5] While recent colonial and postcolonial definitions of "national culture" are heavily engaged in reinventing notions of "tradition" so that cultural boundaries conform to postcolonial geographical and moral – religious boundaries,[6] a philosophy of "humanness" arising from *ubuntu* is being applied here in a highly instrumental fashion. For implicit in the oft-recurring theme of homosexuality as a "white man's disease" alien to "African tradition" is a confusion between sexual identity (which some might argue is too individualistic to be reconcilable with *ubuntu*) and sexual behavior (the varied possibilities of which appear to be less restrictively defined through the concept of *ubuntu* than through the finite paradigm of the Western homo/heterosexual binary).

Nevertheless, it is also simplistic to claim that "gay" or "lesbian" identities are imposed through an imperialist cultural discourse or economic dominance, for they are actively assumed and proclaimed from below, by those marginalized in local social formations that assume exclusively heterosexual relations. These "new" identities are merged into local histories and contexts, so that they include local social signifiers and practices while simultaneously providing a strategy of access to some benefits of globalization. Thus, they are often used as a means for laying claim to the protection of human rights as enshrined in international treaties, or enabling more effective AIDS/HIV prevention work, or simply buying into an expanding market of Western signifiers of "modern" and bourgeois status. They frequently serve all of these purposes simultaneously, and ultimately provide some agency for those who find themselves structurally disempowered by their gender nonconformity. Whatever the case, as Neville Hoad suggests, it is clear that the cultural imperialism model needs to be nuanced with an acknowledgment that strategies and identities are transformed when deployed from below, and that laying claim to the perceived prestige of things Western can serve to empower people who find themselves vulnerable in the local context. Furthermore, it may only be the privileged, traveling, cosmopolitan intellectual who recognizes these sexualized identities as Western (Hoad 1998:35–36).

It is the educated and privileged President Mugabe who appears more determined than anyone to see these definitions (of homo/heterosexual) as fixed categories between which one cannot slide and yet he claims only one of them (homosexual) as a definitive signifier of cultural imperialism. It is his position of privilege that allows Mugabe to define the homosexual as specifically marginal and par-

ticularly deviant to Zimbabwean culture, and by clothing his disgust in the language of neo-traditional nationalism, he escapes having to explain its unusual ferocity and its source. But more pertinently, his assertion of an African universalism that is specifically and exclusively heterosexual is predicated on the a priori concept of a binary division of hetero/homosexuality. This intellectual notion of "a binary sexuality" fixed within individuals is far from the integrated human potential of the *ubuntu* concept, but is a distinctly western European polarization of individual erotic desire as homo/heterosexual, initially popularized by European sexologists in the late 19th century (Weeks 1989).

Rather than any new activities, it is this categorical fixity of definition and the accompanying promotion of sexual object choice as something that marks the individual irrevocably that has been imported into Zimbabwe and into the region as a whole. Mugabe's assumption of this binary notion, and his colonization by its prejudices, leads him to deprive Zimbabweans of the agency that a more fluid self-definition arising from *ubuntu* might permit. A free-market, highly individualized culture accompanies and requires a far greater fixing of identity in the self than the wide potential of humanity allowed for in the physical, spiritual, and communal harmony that is envisaged through *ubuntu*. Mokgoro derides notions of a categorical definition of *ubuntu* and suggests that "any attempt to define *ubuntu* is merely a simplification of a more expansive, flexible and philosophically accommodative idea" (1998:16). Accommodation is invariably only possible where visibility and interaction can lead to an understanding of something shared, whereas polarization thrives on the isolated discretion of distance and emphatic differentiation such as that promulgated by President Mugabe. HIV/AIDS obliges an unprecedented level of public engagement with sexual behavior, and the visibility that necessarily arises from this may actually produce a familiarity that begets acceptance and undoes differentiation. A practical illustration of this appears in Goddard's account of the funeral of a GALZ member who had died from AIDS-related illnesses.

Before his death, Noah's family had accused GALZ of turning their son into a homosexual and giving him the HIV virus. At times, they refused to let visitors from GALZ Positive see and care for him. Undaunted, GALZ Positive provided a wheelchair and access to a doctor while he was alive. When Noah died, GALZ paid for the coffin. At his funeral, GALZ members fulfilled most of the domestic duties generally assigned to women in this country, including all the cooking, cleaning and serving food.

During the funeral Noah's father, near tears, publicly acknowledged the contributions of Noah's gay friends. He said this had made him realize just how caring gay people could be. Even the church pastor, known for his disapproval of homosexuals, could not help but be impressed by the efforts of GALZ Positive. At the close of the funeral, Noah's clothes were distributed to members of his family: some of the clothes were also given to Noah's "gay family," a profound symbol of acceptance and recognition within Shona culture. (Goddard 2001:1)

Yet it is this same visibility that frequently provokes an antagonistic reaction, as it so directly threatens the proclamation of "tradition" as inherently heterosexual and exclusive of any possibilities beyond such a patriarchal model. Just as developing open discussion of any sexual behavior leads to contestation about its social significance, so increasing denunciations of homosexuality fuel the significance it comes to acquire in defining notions of culture, tradition, and belonging. One incidental result of this is that previously "innocent" behavior comes to be invested with new sexual power. It is tempting to ask whether Michael Gelfand's "normal" Shona men[7] will continue to hold hands so freely in a society increasingly conscious of marking out the boundaries of heterosexuality.

The appearance of self-identified gay men and lesbians in Zimbabwe and throughout the region does certainly contribute to the growth of specifically sexual identities, but the well-publicized and evocative attacks on homosexuals by local politicians and neo-traditionalists and their exhortations on patriots to be exclusively heterosexual have been far more powerful. They have played a significant role in introducing social identities based on a polarized sexual orientation into public discourse throughout southern African states.

The effect of this has been the development of the "sexual subject" in that politicking about its cultural significance has given sexuality a far greater role in the formation of national identities and subjectivity than was previously the case. The language used by Mugabe and the party faithful to describe homosexuality is unambiguous in its juxtaposition of "good Zimbabwean" and "bad homosexual," and in expressing the conviction that homosexuals do not belong in Zimbabwe. Implicit in articulating this exclusion is the suggestion that all "true" Zimbabweans are therefore "heterosexual." This is a strategy echoed by neighboring leaders, albeit less frequently, and it locates a polarized sex at the center of national identity; suddenly heterosexuality is a condition of being Zimbabwean/Namibian/Kenyan, etc., and one is supposed to be able to distinguish a "sexual" relationship from simple physical intimacy. This sexual citizenship is not simply dependent on having a primary relationship with someone of the opposite sex, but demands that you *only ever* desire someone of the opposite sex, and *only ever* have any sexual contact with someone of the opposite sex. Citizenship becomes sexualized as Mugabe, Nujoma et al. confer a far more restrictive notion of sexual behavior on Zimbabweans and Namibians than had previously been stated, and immediately compel Zimbabweans and Namibians to identify as explicitly heterosexual. In doing this, they introduce sex into what had been a virginal subject, as it is arguable that up to that point most Zimbabweans had invested neither their sexual behavior with such national significance nor their national identity with such emphatic sexuality.

This nationalist approach to sexuality serves the purpose of marking cultural insiders and outsiders, and while Mugabe's immediate objective in 1995 appeared to be related to electioneering, the intervening remarks by him and other regional leaders have invariably claimed that homosexuality was "white" and therefore carried the twin implications that white (Western) culture was depraved, and that homosexuals could not be truly Zimbabwean/Namibian/Kenyan. Attacking homosexuality as a white man's disease imported to Africa was a means of highlighting the "decadence" of white settler culture while marking it out as different from, and corrupting to, the purity of true "African culture." Ironically, such a totalized notion of culture (whether "African" or "white") replicates much of the colonial discourse on African sexuality in that it misrepresents Africa as statically monocultural. It also ignores the richness of differing cultural constructions of desire within the region and the world over. The heterogeneity of all different cultures in southern African states, whose physical, social and spiritual borders are so inescapably hostage to their colonial past, is masked in this attempt to consolidate a national identity predicated on the homo/heterosexual binary.

A Partial HIV/AIDS Education

One of the most serious consequences of this imposition of heterosexual identities upon ordinary southern African nationals is that mechanisms and strategies aimed at preventing the spread of HIV/AIDS are fundamentally compromised. The information given about modes of transmission is inevitably partial, as sexual activity between men or between women can rarely be discussed openly and invariably starts from a premise of denial and disengagement. Large-scale governmental campaigns, or campaigns complicit in defining the parameters of sex "in the national interest," fail to acknowledge the possibility of homosexual sex and so exclude it from information on HIV transmission (National Aids Coordination Programme 1998a). Many other organizations that might include homosexual sex in their programs have in the past decided to exclude it for fear of alienating their ordinary service-users who don't like to think that they may be associated or sharing services with such people (Goddard pers. comm.). This has meant that those organizations incorporating information on homosexual sex tended to be small, independent, and marginalized in gaining access to large resources. The information about HIV transmission is therefore inherently incomplete, and this undermines broader attempts to prevent transmission.

In some cases, there has been a shift in that the larger body of HIV/human rights organizations have come to recognize the indivisibility of rights and the inseparability of exclusion and infection. This is evidenced by increasing attempts to target "men who have sex with men" (m/s/m). This term is employed with the good intention of preempting the assumption that the binary of homo/heterosexual accurately fits those cultures not steeped in Western sexological epistemology. Yet its potential is consistently undermined in southern Africa by governmental emphases of precisely that binary, deeply polarized. This is because the broader public culture of compulsory heteronormativity alienates those men who fail to recognize the handy utility of differentiating "homosexuals" from "m/s/m." For those men who do have sex with other men, and might not self-identify as "homosexual" but do still recognize governmental vilification of "homosexuals" as somehow including their behavior, this neat linguistic strategy might be no more than an unhelpful solecism. A simple awareness of one's sexual behavior is enough for governmental disparagement (as vociferous as that quoted earlier) to set in motion denial, fear, and deep-seated insecurity. It is certainly enough to interfere with the efficacy of "safe-sex" campaigns and broader education about transmission of HIV/AIDS. In sum, these attacks on same-sex love seriously compound the already present difficulties of reaching those men who have sex with men, or more significantly those men who have sex with both men and women, in HIV prevention campaigns.

This problem can only be addressed through recognizing that humanity is not inevitably and definitively framed by the homo/heterosexual binary, but that the reality may be more fluid, with people transgressing that neat binary in a variety of ways. Moving beyond the homo/heterosexual binary not only allows us to recognize greater diversity in the locations of sexual practice in social lives, but it may also move us out of the discursive realm of "local/imported." Questions of convention and identity may still arise, but they do not ab initio rely on a restrictive binary derived from a specific cultural source. This raises many complex questions about the relationship between sexual acts and social identities, and also about the development of "tradition," both of which are central to the articulation of gendered power. It is my hope that this brief attempt to consider the rise of such a sexualized social identity as became apparent in southern Africa in the 1990s will sketch out some possibilities for developing an understanding of these complex questions.

An analysis of gender relations provides a "trace" that is very productive in watching the development of both HIV and a more pronounced sexual subjectivity. Gender is central both to the epidemiological pathways along which the virus is transmitted and to the conflict over sexual identities. Tracing gender configurations highlights socially institutionalized relationships of power between men and women, and more specifically, it highlights the role of morality in fracturing "traditional" relationships of lineage, and developing "modern" sexualized individuals whose autonomy is overseen by the State. Diana Jeater's work has shown us how colonial law brought with it a discourse of morality that was very significant in the construction of individual subjects (and particularly of individual subjects in possession of a "sexuality"). These individual subjectivities exist in a tense relationship to lineage, as conceptions of power and desire tend to be subordinated to the greater needs of the lineage and the economics of the family. By focusing on the development of individualized (as opposed to more "communal") subjectivities, we can trace their connection to the increasing significance of sexuality in the formation of identity in southern Africa, and the implications for HIV transmission.

Sex as Morality

To claim that colonial settlers brought any new sexual activities to the region would be to insult the erotic imagination of southern African people, but it is absolutely clear that the settlers did bring new offenses, as the repertoire of activity remained much the same, but acts were newly defined (Phillips 2000:19–30). Which acts constitute sex, and what social implications they carry, are definitions that are always culturally construed and contingent, and the arrival of proselytizing settlers who administered their morality through law, criminal justice, and religious conviction meant

that sexual values and definitions were irrevocably altered (Bullock 1950:40, 50; and more generally see Burke 1996).

While the broader structures of family and gender tend to give shape to the priorities regulating sexual intimacy between people, it would be a mistake to see these as inevitably and universally framed by a hetero/homosexual binary. The possibilities of this in a southern African context are most interestingly illustrated by separate research carried out by Gay (1985:97–116) and Kendall (1998:223–241), who each looked at relationships between women in Lesotho in the 1980s and 1990s respectively. Both found that "lesbian" or lesbian-like behavior was and had been commonplace, and even conventional, but that it was not viewed as "sexual" despite its erotic nature, since it was not viewed as an alternative to heterosexual marriage, which occupies both a sexual and an economic part of the culture. These erotic and romantic relationships between women do not require an individual's autonomy from family, marriage, and kinship. The relationship is seen as quite distinct from (but supplementary to) marriage and so it does not disturb the economic and reproductive implications of marriage. This means that the fixed categories of homo/heterosexual which are so much a part of western European conceptions of sexuality do not reside within individuals, nor even within the relationships between individuals, and sex is far more fluidly negotiated.

Marc Epprecht's research suggests that this fluidity, existing outside of the hetero/homosexual binary, was also prevalent in Southern Rhodesia (1998:197–221). While my research indicates that virtually all the prosecutions for "unnatural offenses" in the most recent 30 years (1965–95) in Zimbabwe involve a white man (Phillips 1997:476–480), Epprecht's research indicates that the objects of colonial policing were quite different. In the first 30 years of settler rule in Southern Rhodesia (1896–1926), 90 percent of prosecutions for "unnatural offences" involved black men, and these men were prosecuted for sexual acts that took place in a predictably varied range of relationships (1998:206–216). Some of these relationships were consensual and some weren't; some were long term and constant, while others were more casual affairs. Many of them remind us that the neat and definitive binary division of homo/heterosexual is not so clearly replicated in reality as it is in ideology. But they do all suggest that the classification of acts of sex between people of the same sex as "unnatural offences" in newly "settled" Southern Rhodesia was a new way of defining and categorizing sex. By declaring specific "acts" to be immoral, the discourse of an abstract morality is being used to regulate sexual behavior, whereas prior to this categorization of acts as "moral" or "immoral" the likely impact on the family was the significant determinant of the acceptability of sexual relations. "Illicit sexual acts were only illicit in so far as the partners disrupted kinship relationships" (Jeater 1993:30–31).

Sexual relations were not simply the business of the individuals directly involved, but structures such as marriage (*roora/lobola*) had an effect on the economic power and social identity of the entire lineage. They were not conceived as erotic acts separate from kin, but were physically and figuratively constitutive of kinship relations. But the introduction of abstract "moral" judgment separated eroticism further from questions of reproductive consequence, into an economy of desire which gave a social value to each confessed act, and each exhorted repression, so that the sum of these values could be represented in the individual. For this "discourse of morality" required the labeling and definition of specific acts of what were declared to be "perversions" residing within the self, rather than a situation where sexual acts were regulated only when they impacted on the broader social context of the reproductive relationships between people. What had been important was consequential physical activity, but the law and the church both introduced categories of projected cognitive desire (homo/heterosexual) to be judged morally as perversion or sin.

Conjuring fantasy and denial, this location of a metaphysical sex residing within the self was accompanied by the more specific production of individual stereotypes of morality which provide the capacity to alternately create or censure individual identities through sex, and more specifically through the binary division of homo/heterosexuality. This is a capacity that has come to be deeply embedded in the discourse around sex in contemporary southern Africa as a whole.

It is this creation of individual subjectivities with the emphasis on the self that is of contemporary significance. It appears in the current notions of criminal liability, and custodial punishment as retribution is exacted through the deprivation of an individual offender's liberty (rather than damages negotiated through families), and rehabilitation is specifically aimed at reforming the self into a better social being. It is also invoked in our understanding of sexual offenses (such as rape) as an offense against the bodily integrity of an individual, rather than an offense against the father, husband, or family of the victim. So the individual legal subject underlies our current understanding of criminal justice, and is also integral to the notion of individual human rights. This emphasis on individual subjectivity provides a thread of continuity between the colonial law's creation of individual subjects bound by their specific proclivities, who are held individually responsible for specific social acts, and the globalization of a notion of human rights which reside in the individual and are often signified through these same proclivities.

Fitting Sex with Gender

The promotion of individual human rights inevitably relies on a notion of personhood and autonomy which conflicts with the proprietorial relations of gender power implicit in a patriarchal and polygynous base, such as that which exists in so much of southern Africa. Sexuality is highly contested in the region because a woman's independence (particularly her sexual autonomy) is habitually subsumed in the interests of lineage. The interests of the clan are seen to incorporate the interests of women – this theme has consistently appeared as the basis on which women have been protected or prosecuted in law (Phillips 2000:25–30). Both women's position and that of homosexual men indicate that the establishment of a sexuality independent of lineage and guardianship disturbs both inter-family and intra-family relations, as well as the highly structured nature of broader gender relations in a society that has a long tradition of polygyny. There are social and economic implications for other members of the family if one does not marry, or if one has sex outside of marital relations, or if one divorces eroticism from reproductive relationships (unless one does this in the shadow of a heterosexual marriage such as Gay and Kendall show). Thus, "lesbian and gay" politics appear to threaten some fundamental structures in any form of arranged marriage, in any payment of *lobola*, in any production of grandchildren, in all the structural and economic implications of heterosexual marriage. Lesbians' accounts of their families' attempts to coerce them into pregnancy affirm this prioritization of reproduction and lineage, over the notion of the autonomous sexual self (Machido 1996:123).

Sexual autonomy has been a constant issue in the historical contests about the position of women both within civil society and in nationalist debates. Early colonial legislation attempted to protect African women from being forced into marriage, by requiring that the women consent and by outlawing the pledging of young girls into marriage (Southern Rhodesia's Native Marriage Ordinance 1901). The insistence on a woman's consent to marriage immediately bestowed on women a measure of potential legal autonomy from the men who were their custodians, as accountability to the State began to usurp accountability to ancestors and lineage (Jeater 1993:81). While this might be the first requirement for recognizing women as recipients of "rights," it cannot be assumed that it will operate to this effect. For it was the Zimbabwean state that during the 1980s carried out random street clear-ups of any women not possessing a marriage certificate or proof of employment (Jacobs and Howard 1987:39–42), and that on numerous occasions during the 1990s facilitated a social atmosphere that led mobs of men to strip women naked in the street for wearing mini-skirts that were "too short" (Phillips 1999:238–244; and Jackson 1993: 25/6).

In all of these cases, the harassment of women was justified with their denunciation as prostitutes or *mahure*, a word frequently used to describe women who display eco-

nomic independence, or most particularly a sexual autonomy. The widespread application of this label to independent women is epitomized by a statement made in the early 1980s by the then Zimbabwean Minister of Home Affairs that the abolition of *lobola* (bridewealth) would "legalize prostitution" as "a woman for whom *lobola* was not paid could easily move to another man" (Seidman 1984:432). While he was merely referring to those women who did not undertake a "customary" marriage, the conflation of lesbian and *hure* (whore) is also completed through this absolute resistance to sexual autonomy. Lesbianism presents a clear challenge in that it implies a recognition that women can (and might choose to) survive without men, let alone without men as their guardian, a "problem" compounded by the lack of *lobola* that a lesbian relationship would bring for the rest of the family, thereby affecting their ability to marry. And yet, a more comprehensive acknowledgment of women's rights requires that their sexual autonomy be recognized and that the possibility of a lesbian relationship be permitted. This is not only because gays and lesbians have come to represent the marginal despised whose acceptance is a litmus test of the extent to which the country is prepared to put the principle of human rights above that of prejudice (however strongly held), but it is primarily because accepting that a woman can choose her partner is a fundamental precondition for her recognition as a fully entitled legal subject. For sexual independence is implicitly connected to broader structures of social and economic power, as well as being anchored in more corporeal discourses (Kesby 1999:27–47).

Sex since HIV/AIDS

A measure of individual autonomy is fundamental to one's accession to rights, to liberties, and, it is argued, to social responsibilities. The importance of individual legal subjectivity both for claiming rights and for being held accountable for one's actions has been emphasized by the challenges presented to all southern Africans with the spread of HIV/AIDS. And it is the very "heterosexual" course of HIV infection in the region that has heightened the awareness of the significance of sex in the constitution of the social body as a whole.

Thus, the silences around the sexual that are so deeply but differently embedded in so many languages have had to be filled with an articulate currency of anatomical terms and definitions of sexual behavior. Where previously, in Shona, certain references to sexual practices and relations were spoken only between men or between women (Shire 1994),[8] there has had to be a concerted attempt to develop language accessible to all. HIV/AIDS has impacted enormously on how much sex is spoken about, and in what manner (Pattman 1995), but the vital need to discuss it is constantly challenging the place of sex in relation to "traditional" gender practices.

> Culturally, female ignorance of sexual matters is considered a sign of purity, and conversely, knowledge of sexual matters and reproductive systems is viewed negatively. The equating of ignorance with innocence may inhibit some women from seeking information that is critical to their well-being (National AIDS Coordination Programme 1998a:5.1)

Women are said to be the section of the population most vulnerable to infection, partly on account of their structural position and consequent powerlessness to negotiate safe sexual practices, and partly on account of the gendered silences around sex; it is these factors that create enormous difficulty in establishing sex/health education classes for women and girls (Misihairambwe 1997). But nevertheless, conceptions of sexuality have been considerably affected by the development of AIDS/ HIV. For this new currency of language not only renders sexual what may not have been considered "sexual" before, but also fixes an unspecified fluidity in the concrete shape of definition. Creating terms and definitions inescapably binds and fixes behavior which might before have been more malleable, removing a potential variety of interpretations, and fitting it into a larger discourse around sex as a whole. The recent growth of the homo/heterosexual binary as a framing device is a clear example of this fixing process.

The Zimbabwe National Aids Coordination Program asserts that premarital abstinence followed by lifelong fidelity to one partner is "the fundamental and most crucial behavior which will guarantee an effective and sustainable solution to the problem of HIV/AIDS" (1998b:57). While condom use is seen as an important intervention, it is clearly seen as secondary to that of abstinence and monogamy. The assumption that abstinence is a realistic strategy is already problematic, but the further assumption that monogamy is a realistic primary strategy is deeply problematic in a traditionally polygynous country. While it might well be strategic to encourage both abstinence and monogamy, it borders on criminal naiveté to configure them as the most realistic bases for prevention. Nevertheless, the discourse around HIV has so far been shaped to emphasize an individual morality constructed around monogamous marriage and the notion of fidelity. This has implied a certain elision of individual responsibility, as safety is portrayed as resting on the "good behavior" and morality of couples joined in marriage. Any notions of individual responsibility or diverse sexual practices are sidelined in attempts to discourage sex outside of marriage, and to rely on historically unconventional relationships of monogamous fidelity. This not only ignores the dangers associated with those (probably married) men who do have sex with other men, but it also ignores the fact that married women are the most vulnerable to infection on account of their inability to negotiate safe sex within their marriage to a husband who very often has other wives or lovers. The responsibility is seen as shared in that it is expected to reside in (presumably monogamous) joint fidelity, rather than impressing on men the individual and personalized methods of ensuring one's own safety and thereby the safety of those with whom one interacts.

In short, in a context where AIDS affects the lives of virtually everyone and the risks of infection are extremely high, preventative policy still relies on a patently false assumption of monogamous morality. This not only prevents the development of a notion of individual responsibility, but it also makes it much harder to educate people that the spread of HIV is not about what you do or who you do it with, but about how you do it. It is possible to have safe sex with thousands of HIV-positive people and not get infected; but it is also possible to have unsafe sex just once and become infected. Emphasizing abstinence and monogamy is incompatible with the promotion of condom usage. It also makes it much more difficult to discuss relationships that involve people who in reality are neither abstinent nor monogamous, and to devise a strategy for enabling women to exercise greater independent control over their own sexuality, fertility, and sexual health.

Despite the dangerousness of this "morality" approach in a predominantly polygynous society, its promotion is not surprising in that it dovetails with attempts to conserve "traditional" gender roles and the importance of lineage within a christianized (officially monogamous) context. It is this "traditional" christianized morality (which is actually far from traditional) that also lies behind the utter omission of any mention of sex between men or between women in this National AIDS Coordination Program. Such a prioritization of morality over reality fundamentally undermines any possibility of educating people about true paths of transmission. A primary strategy for preventing transmission must be to make people aware of routes of transmission, and yet it is precisely this that is being sacrificed on the alter of "morality." As a result, many southern Africans have a partial understanding of HIV transmission that results in a sustained risk of acquiring HIV/AIDS.

This suggests that the notion of individual responsibility (for safe sex or for other issues of health and justice) can only develop where there is a more developed concept of individual rights and subjectivities. This concept of individual responsibility and rights can only develop at the expense of those whose power resides in structures that subordinate individual subjectivities in their claim to represent communal interests. Thus, the call to sexual abstinence outside of monogamous married relationships is a call to a lineage-based morality, rather than the potentially "safer" practice of rooting protection in a notion of individual responsibility that can account for autonomous action and diverse sexual behaviors. The efficacy of an approach of individual responsibility would require an emphasis on individual rights and individual autonomy. To proclaim these would be to challenge both a misleading notion of fidelity (practiced in a sexist manner), and also the "traditional" subordinated position of women under the power of a male guardian. The inability to account for sexual fluidity therefore extends beyond the hetero/homosexual binary to a fundamental inhibition of women's sexual independence. The development of a rights discourse cannot avoid invoking notions of autonomy and so a degree of responsibility for one's self. On the one hand, the establishment of these individual rights and responsibilities presupposes a democratic framework, through which people are able to represent their own interests and account for their own behavior. On the other, the development of these individual rights and responsibilities might be claimed to be a precondition for the operation of an effective democracy.

NOTES

1. Cindy Patton suggests further that this labeling equates heterosexual transmission with "otherness," performing "the final expiative act for a Western heterosexual masculinity that refuses all containment" (1997:279).
2. For more detailed figures see UNAIDS Report, Aids Epidemic Update, December 2001a.
3. For more about this particular event see Dunton and Palmberg (1996).
4. One example of this took place on March 4, 1997, when Michael Mawema convened a meeting at the Kentucky Hotel in Harare. The hotel is owned and managed by the Zimbabwe Council of Churches, and the meeting was publicized with a full-page advertisement in the government-owned *Herald* newspaper (March 3, 1997). Citing the restoration of "traditional justice," Mawema called for the castration and public flogging of sexual offenders, explicitly including homosexuals.
5. For some general discussion of the concept of "unbuntu" as it relates to law and human rights, see Mokgoro (1998).
6. For more on this see Hobsbawm, E. and Ranger, T., eds., 1991 The Invention of Tradition. Cambridge: Canto (C.U.P.); and Vail, Leroy, ed., 1999 The

Creation of Tribalism in Southern Africa. London: University of California Press.

7. Gelfand, M., 1965 The Normal Man: A New Concept of Shona Philosophy. NADA IX (2):78–93.

8. In July 1988, at the trial of ex-President Canaan Banana, the first interpreter had to be replaced as she was not in a position to translate even such clinical terms as "erections" and "semen" (Matyszak, D. 1998, pers. comm.).

Poverty, Migration, War
Chapter 12

Urbanization, Poverty, and Sex: Roots of Risky Sexual Behaviors in Slum Settlements in Nairobi, Kenya

Eliya Msiyaphazi Zulu, F. Nii-Amoo Dodoo, and Alex Chika Ezeh

Introduction

The AIDS epidemic is becoming the most serious health problem facing sub-Saharan Africa. The prevalence of the disease across countries in sub-Saharan Africa, particularly the east/central/southern belt, ranges from 16 to 30 percent, and roughly 70 percent of the world's infected people live on the continent (Caldwell and Caldwell 1993; Goliber 1997; UNAIDS 1998c, 2000a; WHO 1998). Eighty percent of AIDS-related deaths in the world in 1998 occurred in the region, while over 90 percent of all AIDS orphans in the world are found there (National Council for Population and Development et al. 1998). Life expectancy has fallen below 50 years in many countries in the region in the past few years. For instance, Botswana's life expectancy at birth is estimated to have declined from 58 years in 1980 to 46 years in 1998, while that for Kenya declined from 55 years to 51 years over the same period (World Bank 2000a; see also UNAIDS 1998c).

There is general awareness of the fatal consequences of the disease and, more importantly, that behavioral change provides the best opportunity to combat its spread (Cleland and Ferry 1995; Hope 1995; van der Straten et al. 1995). For example, the Kenyan government promotes premarital abstinence, commitment to one partner, and condom use to stem the spread of HIV in the country (Government of Kenya 1999), but behavior on the continent largely continues to be risky, with individuals initiating sexual activity early, retaining multiple sexual partners, and being reluctant to use condoms even in sexual encounters with prostitutes (Ampofo 1993a, 1995; Bertrand and Bakutuvwidi 1991; Blanc and Way 1998; Cleland and Ferry 1995; Dodoo and Ampofo 2001). It is no surprise, therefore, that national surveys typically show condom-use levels in single digits in most African countries. The decline in the proportion of people with multiple sexual partners (Konde-Lule, Tumwesigye, et al. 1997; Ntozi and Ahimbisibwe 1999; Malamba et al. 1994) and delay in the initiation of sex (Asiimwe-Okiror et al. 1997) have been highlighted as the key factors behind Uganda's unique success in containing the further spread of HIV/AIDS.

The emphasis on regional and national differentials in the prevalence of HIV often conceals substantial within-country variation in the burden of the epidemic. A wide range of surveillance data show that most urban areas have higher HIV prevalence rates than rural areas, despite the fact that urban residents tend to show greater awareness of AIDS and ways of avoiding it than rural residents. For example, in 2000 it was estimated that 13.5 percent of adults in Kenya were HIV positive. The HIV prevalence rate for urban areas was 17–18 percent while in rural areas it was 12–13 percent (Ministry of Health 2001). The higher prevalence of AIDS in urban areas has contributed to suspicion and complacency among some rural residents, who have tended to regard the disease as an urban phenomenon (Konde-Lule 1991; Caraël 1997). For instance, a study conducted in Kenya to ascertain people's perspectives about HIV/AIDS and identify ways that would enhance or impede changes in sexual behavior revealed that many rural residents regard their urban counterparts to be carriers of HIV and other sexually transmitted diseases (Bauni and Jarabi 2000). This suspicion is fueled by the apparent seasonal increase in the incidence of sexually transmitted infections around holiday times, when many Nairobi dwellers return to their rural homes. The fact that many of the earlier AIDS-related deaths occurred among urban dwellers, who were taken to rural areas to be buried, further enhanced rural people's perceptions of AIDS as an urban phenomenon. One explanation for the difference in the incidence of HIV infection between rural and urban areas is that urban residents' sexual encounters involve men and women from a broader spectrum (including commercial sex workers) than their rural counterparts, whose sexual networks mostly revolve around their extended kinship (Konde-Lule 1991; Geelhoed 1991).

Controlling the AIDS epidemic requires particular attention to the plight of the increasingly vulnerable and rapidly growing urban poor population. Over the past three decades, a continuous and substantial shift in population from rural to urban areas has occurred in sub-Saharan Africa. The projection that over half of all Africans will live in urban areas by 2025 (United Nations 1998) highlights the need to pay more attention to reproductive health needs and outcomes facing urban residents. Since 1960, Africa's urban population has grown, on average, by over 5 percent per year as compared to less than 2 percent in rural areas, and many cities have experienced growth rates exceeding 7 percent per annum (Todaro 1989a). For instance, while the Kenyan population grew at an annual rate of 2.8 percent per annum between the 1980s and 1990s, the city of Nairobi grew at an annual rate of 7.4 percent (and other urban areas grew by about 6.8 percent) during the same period (Obudho 1997). The city is projected to gain five million more people over the next 15 years. This growth will only aggravate the environmental, economic, and institutional constraints already facing the city and its residents. The lack of institutional capacity to provide services and jobs for the growing population will result in unprecedented growth of slums and shantytowns within the city. This problem already appears unbearable in Nairobi where over 60 percent of the city's population is estimated to reside in slums occupying 5 percent of the city's land area (Matrix Development Consultants 1993).

A clear consequence of rapid urbanization amid economic decline in Kenya is the disproportionate increase in urban poverty. The Welfare Monitoring Survey shows that while absolute poverty increased from 48 to 53 percent in rural areas of Kenya between 1992 and 1997, poverty in urban areas increased by a bigger margin, from about 29 percent in 1992 to about 50 percent in 1997. In Nairobi City, the percentage of people living in absolute poverty almost doubled from 27 to 50 percent over the same period (Central Bureau of Statistics 2000). The extreme poverty, high unemployment, and heavy disease burden that characterize slum settlements provide a conducive environment in which various social ills such as prostitution and teenage pregnancies among the unmarried widely occur. Across Africa, economic concerns incline women to risky sexual behavior, and many attempt to maximize their economic benefit by having multiple partners (Akuffo 1987; Schoepf et al. 1988a, 1988b; Schoepf 1988; Bassett and Mhloyi 1991; Gage and Bledsoe 1994; Meekers and Calvès 1997; Orubuloye et al. 1994). With continuing urbanization, the worsening socio-economic circumstances of urban areas promise to aggravate the living conditions of resident populations and, in turn, to worsen susceptibility to reproductive and health problems (Brockerhoff and Brennan 1998; Standing 1989; Timaeus and Lush 1995). The problems of slum dwellers are compounded by the fact that their settlements are deemed informal by the government, which, it claims, justifies its failure to provide appropriate sanitary, health, and other social services. This chapter examines how the living conditions of Nairobi's slums are related to harmful sexual outcomes.

Data

Qualitative data used in the study were collected by the African Population and Health Research Center in four of Nairobi's 19 slums in January 1999. The study, titled "Sexual Networking and Associated Reproductive and Social Health Concerns: An Exploratory Study of the Urban Informal Settlements in Nairobi, Kenya," had as its primary objective the understanding of the relationship between slum residents' living conditions and reproductive health outcomes, with a particular focus on sexual behavior in the context of the escalating HIV/AIDS epidemic. In addition to understanding sexual networking patterns among slum residents, the study covered other issues such as: general and reproductive health problems, coping strategies and support mechanisms, and other social problems such as prostitution, alcohol and drug abuse, street children, crime, and domestic violence. The four slums in which the study was conducted (Kibera, Majengo, Kahawa North, and Embakasi) were selected to reflect the major compositional differences in ethnicity, gender, age, marital status, and slum population size, while at the same time reflecting the geographical spread of the city's slum settlements. To ensure comprehensive coverage of these factors across gender and age, focus group discussions (FGDs) were conducted with men and women in four age groups (13–17, 18–24, 25–49, and 50+ years). Two additional FGDs were conducted in each of the four slums with community leaders and service providers, respectively. In total, therefore, ten FGDs were conducted in each of the four slums. One moderator and one note-taker, of the same sex as the participants in the age – gender groups, conducted the FGDs in an appropriate local language spoken by the participants.

All the FGDs were tape-recorded and detailed notes taken in English. The data were then transcribed verbatim, coded, and analyzed using NUDIST, a specialized software package for analyzing qualitative data. The data provide the social, economic, and environmental context of slum settlements, which is key to understanding the motivations underlying patterns of sexual networking in these contexts. The qualitative data are used to illustrate the major views that were expressed across various FGDs, and the quotes presented in the chapter are representative of the general views expressed in the study.[1]

Results

The extreme economic deprivation, with its attendant desperation, that characterizes slum life appears to be a core factor that provokes risky sexual behavior. People end up in slum settlements primarily because of the relatively low cost of housing compared to other city locations, and incomes that are inadequate to pay rent elsewhere in the city. Most slum dwellers without steady waged jobs generate money from sporadic petty trading and part-time work, both of which yield low and irregular incomes. As a result of their insecure financial status, slum residents generally struggle to make ends meet, to pay for basic needs such as rent, food, medical care, and children's schooling. The economic position of slum women is even more precarious than men's because the majority of the income-generating opportunities that slum residents depend on (such as working as commercial and residential security guards, manual workers in factories, etc.), mediocre as they are, are open only to men. The frustrations of unemployment and income insecurity promote high levels of alcohol and drug abuse among men, and consequently the responsibility of providing food and other basic necessities for children mostly falls on women's shoulders.

One key motivation for women in exchanging sex for money obtains when somewhat regular sources of money either do not pan out or are unavailable at times of need. The following excerpts demonstrate how economic deprivation fosters risky sexual behavior as a way for women to afford basic needs:

1: "People have different problems. Maybe this one wants to pay rent. Another wants to buy clothes; maybe another one just wants to buy milk. It happens, yes, that you might be having a [regular] source of getting money but at that time, you do not have a way of getting money. So, you just have to go [and have sex]; even if they tell you that they will give you 50 shillings [$0.71], you will go – depending on the problem you have." 2: "That time, you might not be thinking about the diseases because you have problems. That is the problem that women have. Now you see, I will not know if the man has a disease, because he has the money and I have a problem." (Embakasi, females aged 18–24)

1: "Now it is say 8:00 pm at night and you see that he has got money and you, you do not have flour, won't you just enter there?" 2: "Even there on the grass, even if it is on the grass we finish, and you are then given money to go and buy food for the children." 3: "You first run to buy food for the kids; after they have eaten and are satisfied, then you get one to sleep with or do it to get more money." (Embakasi, females 25–49)

These examples show that in the slums, sex is not a means for women to obtain luxury items as much as it is for basic survival. Sex becomes the last resort for ensuring that rent is paid and that children do not go to bed hungry. Lack of employment and lack of stable sources of income were highlighted by the respondents as critical factors that drive women to risky sexual behavior. The meager monetary returns that women get for providing sexual favors are no doubt determined by the poor economic conditions. In turn, however, they also make having multiple partners almost necessary in order to satisfy the most basic of needs. As the following excerpts show, the precarious employment conditions reinforce the thinking among women and men that the best strategy for women is to have a cadre of male partners so that, at any given time, some of them will be gainfully employed:

"Today she is with you. Tomorrow if you do not have money, you will find her with someone else. That is not love. This is selling the body. The problem is not selling the body. The problem is

lack of food. Can she sleep on a hungry stomach for two days when she knows that a certain man somewhere has money?" (Embakasi, male 50+)

"Girls may have many [men] friends because of this. If her problem is money and today she has been given 20 shillings, she goes with him. Tomorrow she won't come back to him. Maybe he is broke. She will get somebody else who has money and she will take from him. So that is not friendship, when it is being forced by circumstances." (Embakasi community leaders)

Men generally exploit slum women's economic vulnerability by paying them very little for their sexual services. Further, because sex is so cheap in the slums men can have a chain of women with whom they have sex, a phenomenon that increases impoverished women's vulnerability to STD/HIV infection.

1: "Now maybe this one is poor...me as a man, I am a man now, and I have seen this woman. I have gone to her place or I know her problems and because she has problems..., I will go to her and cheat her and give her this 10 shillings [roughly $0.14] and she will go and buy food and now a disease results from that." MODERATOR: "So they look at [for] the women who have problems?" SEVERAL: "Yes...they look at the women with problems." 3: "Yes, because they will be able to cheat them." (Kahawa North, female 50+)

1: "You can even give (pay) her 5 shillings [almost $0.07] so that she can buy *sukuma wiki* [a vegetable staple]." 2: "Or if you buy her meat from the butchery, even if it's a quarter kilo and it costs only 30 shillings [$0.42]." 3: "The rate is not fixed, it depends on how much you negotiate." (Embakasi, service providers)

"Others look for the stupid ones who accept chips or 20 shillings [$0.28] or a sausage. Others want only a soda!" "There are girls who live in California. They are called *Wabutoro*, meaning 'A packet of chips and soda is enough'." "Others can accept secondhand clothes from Gikomba [secondhand or used clothes sources] for twenty shillings only." (Majengo, female 18–24)

Because of the desperate economic circumstances in which many women live, men who have relatively decent incomes face an increased "risk" of having multiple sexual partners since they become obvious targets for women who are having a difficult time making ends meet:

"There are such cases because what people are after is money. Now she will move with that man, then she will leave him and start moving with this one, like that, like that. This is because this man has money. She can even see that they are dressing well. When one dresses well, that is an indication that you have money. Therefore, you could even get five or ten women. You see, women will be coming from you, and others coming to you, they are mostly attracted by money." (Kahawa North, female 25–49)

"Those men who are married do indulge in regular sexual activities because many of them are employed, working or are doing business and the way things stand now women like money. Those who are not married, most of them are not working and therefore lack money to give women, therefore these women do not like them, they prefer sugar daddies like this doctor whom they know, if they go to the clinic they are treated free of charge and besides they are assured of something small." (Kibera, male 25–49)

"Our children are jobless and there are these Njoroges and Kamaus [these are typical male names] who are employed. So the girls will go to them to be bought soda and so on in return for sex. What do they do? It is lack of jobs that drives them to practice these things, so everything has to do with money." (Embakasi, female 50+)

Men who live near, but not in, the slums also contribute to prostitution in the slums. These non-slum dwellers provide an important customer base for the proliferation of commercial sex work:

"Prostitution is there a lot because there are many companies here at the airport where people work as casuals. Others sell vegetables, but others do not work at all. Then there is that battalion of soldiers over here, the administration over there, and the police. I think that is why this village has become bad, because most of the promiscuity here, it is them who have brought it." (Embakasi, female 25–49)

Evidently, the demand created by available men soldiers, government workers, police, etc. plays a significant role in creating an unethical atmosphere in slums such as Embakasi, located near the Jomo Kenyatta International Airport.

Another salient feature of slum settlements is that they have a relatively large proportion of male migrants from rural areas who leave their spouses behind when they go to cities to look for work. The separation from spouses, as well as the relative oversupply of economically susceptible women, increases the risk of these men seeking other women for their sexual gratification (see also Caraël and Allen 1995; Anarfi 1992). Commercial sex workers in slums provide sexual havens for the many men, employed or otherwise, who idle around the slums and resort to alcohol and drug abuse.

Other studies have demonstrated how women's vulnerability to HIV infection is aggravated by economic hardship and inequality (Ulin 1992; Caraël and Allen 1995; Schoepf et al. 1988a, 1988b; Schoepf 1988). For example, studies in some urban centers in west Africa have linked women's involvement in petty trading to an increased risk of having multiple and extramarital sexual partners (Oppong 1995; Omorodion 1999). This is partly because women traders interact with more men, and many of their male trading suppliers or counterparts demand sexual services in lieu of financial payment in business transactions. The higher degree of social interaction between men and women and the relatively high incidence of commercial sexual activity in communities dominated by petty trading are some of the other factors contributing to the high levels of HIV infection in main-road trading centers, compared to both trading and non-trading villages (Konde-Lule, Tumwesigye, et al. 1997; Klitsch 1992; Serwadda et al. 1992).

Many women who live in the Nairobi slums encounter sexual harassment and exploitation by men who offer work and various favors to promote their businesses. Additionally, the interaction of female household headship and the high cost of living compels women to engage in risky sexual behaviors.

"If you go to a woman who is selling *chang'aa* [local gin] and buy a lot of it for yourself and friends, since you have promoted her [business], she can also offer to give you the other [sexual] service." (Embakasi, service providers)

"Especially in this village, there are very many women who stay on their own without husbands..." "This other one has a man and he is working and he has his wife. She will go to this one because of poverty...and you hear that she is married. Because you slept hungry and you have a husband who is not working, you will go to this one's husband because he is working so that you can get flour." "In fact that husband is ours both because..." (Laughter) "Yes, because he has money." (Kahawa North, female 50+)

"For instance if a woman stays [lives] alone, that is she is a single mother with children, and she wants to buy her children milk, the only solution would be to look for someone with money. She sells her body and gets the 20 shillings [$0.28] to buy milk." (Kibera, female 13–17)

Women who sell sexual services to supplement their income do not regard themselves as prostitutes since they have other mechanisms for generating income and they have relatively stable families (see also Schoepf 1988, 1992a; 1992b; Cleland and Way 1994). However, the rapid increase in the number of young female immigrants to cities and the paucity of income-generating opportunities for women have also led to an increase in the number of women working as commercial sex workers in slum settlements. In Majengo, which is considered the haven for prostitution throughout Nairobi, prostitutes are seen hanging around outside their houses waiting for men, even in broad daylight. The widespread practice of prostitution in the communities creates an environment whereby even children perceive it as an acceptable means of generating income.

1: "What is spoiling this place is that women sit in a line out there. They all do that kind of work [prostitution]. But they have to because they have no money." 2: "The *waziba* [foreign prostitutes] sit out there and wait for men. Our own girls also see that and go to the road. The children see them. Old men go with them and the youth also go with the same women." (Majengo, men 50+)

The idea of mixing generations seems to have caught these older men's attention. Many people deplore the exposure of children and youth to commercial sexual relations.

"Here it is about money. Because you can get a very young girl who already knows that sex is not for free; not like in the rural areas where love is born out of interest. Here it is a matter of give me and I give you." (Embakasi, male 25–49)

1: "There are those who sell sex. When a child sees a woman sitting outside her house and then a man goes in there, and the woman follows her and they lock the door..." 2: "Maybe I can control it in my house. Maybe, like me, I have my wife and two

children. My children are small. I could wait until they are asleep. You see something like that! I could use all my tricks. But from the fact that my neighbor is a sex dealer, will I have helped anything?" (Majengo, service providers)

Many study participants also expressed concern at the high level of sexual activity among teenage children. Young girls are typically exploited by elderly men because of their economic susceptibility, as the following example shows:

"I do not know if there is anything they [men] look at. Because if you walk around you find a small girl, may be it is when the breasts are coming out – a very young girl, and if you look at her, she is pregnant. Now tell me, this girl or this child cannot talk well with a man. You wonder, what did this man look at in this child? He left out those who are mature, someone like me or another one. He left them; he went for that kid. So what did he look at?" (Embakasi, women 18–24)

"Also this poverty here makes this girl to sin, maybe this child did not take supper and breakfast. She goes and meets with a person who maybe is an AIDS carrier. If he tells her I will give you a hundred shillings [approximately $1.44], she does not care whether he is very old or what. This makes this disease to spread." (Kahawa North, service providers)

An important side effect is that children are observing sex early and learning that it is a source of financial opportunity:

"Children do know what goes on but we just do it because you are his father. Even if they are 5, 6 years (old) they know because if you happen to see how they play you will just know they have a lot of knowledge on matters of sex [laughter]. You get one calling himself father and the other one mother." (Embakasi, male 25–49)

"You see, these houses of ours are small and children see a lot of wonders. That is why you see a child of 13 years is pregnant and it is because the parent did that and she saw and she went and tried it with another boy..." (Kibera, female service provider)

Often, the residential arrangements provoke haste among parents to complete the sexual act, and militate against protective behavior and caring sex. This contributes to the difficulty for parents of initiating discussions about sex and how to protect against contracting STDs, including HIV/AIDS. A corollary is that, because they share their small single rooms with their children and have sexual intercourse with the children sleeping in the same room, many parents feel they are deprived of the moral authority to counsel their children about sexual matters. Adolescent children often express discomfort about being in the same room with their parents when the latter have sex:

MODERATOR: "What do parents do when they want to have sex in these houses?" 1: "They switch off the lights." 2: "They wait for the children to sleep, and then they do their things." 3: "If you hear noise, you will just listen, you cannot wake up. You would not bother." 4: "If it is my age mate, I wouldn't be bothered. But parents – it is now a very bad story." (Kahawa North, male 13–17)

The relatively early initiation of sex is also aggravated by the high school dropout rates that characterize slum settlements. Children drop out early because of lack of money for fees and other school-related expenses, and they end up roaming the communities. Many others never start school at all. Consequently, boys typically start abusing drugs and alcohol at tender ages, and some become street beggars to generate income, much of which is contributed to family budgets. Because of the concern with sexual privacy, many teenage children move out of their parents' houses to share rooms with other youth. This undermines any control parents could have over their children, particularly, but not only, about sex. Adults speak of how they have to look away and pretend not to see anything when they come across their own sons or daughters having sex against the walls at night. The following excerpts show the extent of indiscriminate sex that takes place in these communities:

"Sometimes you may be asleep and hear someone knocking your iron sheet walls. You wonder what is it, only to find it is people trying to have their fun out there." (Embakasi, female 18–24).

"This village [slum] you know is not like Nairobi. Maybe here at night you would not like to pass here. Maybe your daughter is here, or it may be your friend's daughter. Just here outside; these people and cats are not different, you know, a cat does not do these things [sex] inside the house but it does it at night." (Kahawa North, community leaders)

"I used to work near those houses sometime back. I used to pass this road at around two o'clock at night. You would find them doing it on the roads, in the middle of the road. They only get up when you flash your lights. Sometimes they will simply sit when they are not able to get up fast." (Embakasi, men 50+)

Early initiation of sex among girls is also promoted by the need for children to contribute to the economic well-being of their families. While adolescent boys are sent to the streets of Nairobi on begging and scavenging missions, adolescent girls end up having to offer sexual services to men in exchange for money to augment the family income. The following excerpts show the dilemma that many parents face when poverty forces them to make ends meet by accepting financial contributions derived from their daughters' sexual services:

"Now you see, if you had three such rooms, which you are renting out and charge at least 500 shillings [$7.14] for each, even our daughters would stop this prostitution because we can feed them. They do this because of hunger. This is where and why they get cheated. Do you understand?" (Kibera, women 25–49)

"Sometimes it is we parents to blame. If I tell my daughter that I want a certain thing and she is a student and she does not have money; where will she get what I have asked for?" (Majengo, community leaders)

In some cases, parents actually send their children out with no option but to sell sex. When young girls with little or no schooling are sent out to bring home money, there is no mistaking what the instruction is, as they have little resource (other than their bodies) to exchange for money:

"Now if a girl is 13 years old or even 12 and she is told by the parent to go and search, and she goes and meets an old man like this one and she wants money and the old man wants the young girls. The old man will give money to the girl. And that child, her body is still tender and does not have energy, and this man has energy, so when they have intercourse this man will spoil the girl. The reproductive organs will be spoilt." (Majengo, service providers)

Conclusion

The rapid growth of African cities and the increasing proportion of impoverished people in cities underscore the relevance of the above findings for understanding both the HIV/AIDS epidemic and the means for controlling further spread of the disease. Because of the increasing urbanization and the size of the urban poor population, it is no longer sensible to ignore urban areas on the grounds that Africa is predominantly rural, and that rural areas are more disadvantaged than urban areas as far as health and social services go. Recent findings show that certain city dwellers are becoming increasingly disadvantaged compared to their rural counterparts in many measures of social development, including reproductive health (Brockerhoff and Brennan 1998).

The data presented in this chapter suggest that high-risk sexual behaviors in slum settlements are mostly influenced by the extreme economic deprivation and gender inequality that prevail in these settings. These behaviors are bound to raise susceptibility to HIV infection among slum dwellers. High unemployment and reliance on low-wage and unstable jobs push many women and their daughters into selling sex to supplement their incomes. The frustrations of unemployment and poverty promote drug and alcohol abuse, as well as domestic and other forms of violence against women. Slum parents' moral and social authority to control their children's sexuality is greatly undermined by the lack of privacy for sex that crowded living arrangements provoke. The result is a very early onset of sexual activity among children. Low levels of school attendance in slums also contribute to the relatively early initiation of sex in slums. The idleness associated with dropping out of school reinforces peer pressures that promote sexual activity among young people. Poverty, coupled with the deficiency and expense of reproductive health services in slum communities, limits people's adoption of preventive and curative measures against reproductive health problems, including sexually transmitted infections. These, in turn, increase risk of HIV transmission.

Considerable work remains to be done in this arena. For one, although we have pointed to slum residence as being a critical determinant of poor reproductive health outcomes, more direct evidence from surveys in urban slums should evince more support for these findings. The results presented in the chapter support findings of other studies that, in the absence of some improvement in impoverished people's economic circumstances, messages urging change in sexual behavior are unlikely to yield substantial success in the fight against HIV/AIDS in sub-Saharan Africa.

NOTE

1. Most of the quotes canvass statements made by several participants during the discussion, and we distinguish different speakers using numeric labels like 1, 2, etc. ALL or SEVERAL are used to indicate situations where all or several respondents made the statement or comment cited in the text.

Chapter 13

Mobile Populations and HIV/AIDS in East Africa

Maryinez Lyons

AIDS Knows No Boundaries

There has never been a time in modern history when human interdependency has been more critical to our survival. (Mhloyi 1995:23)

It has become clear that efforts to control the spread of HIV/AIDS and to cope with its impact will require cooperation across national borders. In early 1998, six east African countries, Uganda, Kenya, Tanzania, Rwanda, Burundi, and Democratic Republic of Congo (DRC), formed a new organization, the Great Lakes Initiative on AIDS (GLIA), and began discussing a regional plan to address the epidemic. The first priority selected was the two principal routes of the Great Lakes region, Mombasa to Goma and Dar es Salaam to Goma.

Uganda is a landlocked country bordering five countries – Sudan, Kenya, Tanzania, Rwanda, and Democratic Republic of Congo, each of which is severely affected by the epidemic. It is a public health nightmare, and especially so with a disease for which human beings are the vector. The region is volatile: there is war in Sudan and the DRC while in Uganda, insurgencies by the Lord's Resistance Army in the north and the Allied Democratic Front in the west seriously threaten the stability of the country. Displacement of population in the region has been of dramatic proportions (Famine Early Warning System 1996). Over the past few years, the waves of refugees across the borders of DRC, Rwanda, Burundi, Tanzania, and Uganda have created havoc in the region.

However, when one looks at Uganda carefully, the question: "Is Uganda an island of hope in east Africa's AIDS epidemic?" can be posed, and relates to the recent reports of a decline in HIV prevalence in Uganda. In the midst of the shrinking global community, with expanding communication and interaction of peoples, can any state in isolation stem the pandemic of HIV? Some observers question the reality of a decline in HIV prevalence in Uganda. They argue that the statistics of decrease are deceptive and reflect, not a true decline in prevalence, but more likely the impact of heavy mortality. Additionally, the detractors argue, antenatal surveillance is notoriously difficult to adjust for bias and the decline may be a result of the fact that fewer HIV-infected women are becoming pregnant. We have no idea of true incidence rates, which are extremely difficult to measure accurately.

Nevertheless, if indeed HIV prevalence has declined in Uganda, how can the country sustain the trend, surrounded as it is by neighbors with equally severe epidemics and destabilizing wars? According to the Uganda AIDS Commission, an "island of success in Uganda will be meaningless since the virus will ultimately cross borders if it is not checked diligently all over the world" (Nation 1999).

Social and Geographical Networks and Sexually Transmitted Diseases

There can be little doubt that the transmission of HIV in east Africa is related to the patterns of population movements and interpersonal relations in the region (Obbo 1993b). The long history of sexually transmitted diseases in east Africa demonstrates the complexity of the cultural, social, and economic context in which they occur and helps us to understand their resilience (Setel et al. 1999). Rapid transition from mainly rural, subsistence agricultural economies to capitalist forms has severely affected the social relations of many African societies. A recent volume on the history of STDs in sub-Saharan Africa reveals in study after study the enormous impact of rapid socio-economic change on the sexual health of Africans.

Epidemiologists have popularized several theories for the spread of HIV in Africa, including the "urban disease model" and the "truck driver model." The former focused initially not on the rural poor but instead pointed to privileged urban elites, while the latter theory marked truck drivers as the vectors of the virus. Many researchers believed that HIV was transmitted initially by the educated, professional middle classes from urban to rural regions. The emerging patterns of infection soon drew attention to the Trans-African Highway and the truck drivers who move between Mombasa, Kigali, and Kisangani (see Hunt 1989, 1996; Barongo et al. 1992). The two theories are based on the premise that the spread of STDs is enhanced by the *movement* of specific groups of people. Movement of people is one factor in the spread of the virus but equally important is the nature of sexual networking patterns within and between populations.

The transmission of HIV is linked to social and geographical networks in intricate and complex patterns. The first cases of AIDS were noticed in Uganda and Tanzania, not in urban centers but in remote and rural villages along the shores of Lake Victoria, and not among the educated, professional middle classes but among poor and disadvantaged rural traders and fishermen. A glance at the early pattern of the epidemic in the region reveals the flash points around the shores of Lake Victoria and along the major transport routes of the region. A number of careful studies have illustrated the differing rates of infection between populations located on or near major routes and towns and those located in the hinterland of villages and farms. I find useful the suggestion that we are confronted, not so much with a pandemic of HIV but more with a series of *microepidemics*, interlinking perhaps, but individual in character. Mobility of people is a major factor in the spread of HIV but the complexity of AIDS epidemiology defies easy explanations. "There is more to AIDS than 'truck drivers' and 'prostitutes'" (Bond et al. 1997:xi.). Before discussing other mobile populations, however, I would like to briefly sketch the epidemic in east Africa.

The East African Epidemic – a Brief Overview

AIDS was first noticed in rural east Africa between 1982 (Uganda) and 1984 (Kenya) and by 1987, Uganda, Tanzania, Kenya, and Rwanda had in place AIDS Control Programs. A major task for each country was to establish a surveillance system. In east Africa, surveillance is carried out by anonymous testing of blood drawn from first-time visits of women attending antenatal clinics, which is believed to indicate the prevalence, not incidence, of HIV in the general population. Extrapolating antenatal data to the general population has been criticized for not being representative, even after controlling for age, as antenatal HIV prevalence overestimates population-based prevalence in the younger clinic attendees, but underestimates in those aged roughly 23 and over. In addition, the somewhat ambiguous "sexually active population" aged

15–49 further weakens the extrapolation. Other statistics are derived from blood banks, while in recent years in Uganda the appearance of voluntary testing centers has provided additional prevalence statistics. We really have no idea of the true rate of HIV incidence, and prevalence rates are probably more impressionistic than accurate in gauging the epidemic. Incidence rates are expensive to collect and are only possible in carefully controlled, repeated studies of small populations. Thus, while prevalence rates are the best indication available at present, they should be approached with much caution.

It is surmised by some researchers that the infection rates in rural regions will gradually increase and perhaps reach the proportions now pertaining in high infection zones. It is further surmised that the major factor in the "leveling" of the epidemic will be sexual networking between urban elite and rural populations. There is a tendency to conceptualize the AIDS epidemic as a "wave-like" phenomenon, or perhaps more accurately, a series of waves, some flattening, others merging, but basically heading for a "leveling" of infection rates throughout the region. The waves are generated by movements of people. I now briefly examine each country in eastern Africa (for a map of eastern Africa, see Figure 13.1).

Kenya

There is no evidence that the epidemic curve in Kenya has reached its peak and, by the end of 1997, there were an estimated one and a half million HIV-infected people (National AIDS and STDs Control Program 1998:4). The overall urban prevalence in Kenya is between 12 and 13 percent while the rural prevalence hovers around 8 to 9 percent (Mulindi et al. 1998:22; Forsythe et al. 1996). As shown in Table 13.1, Nyanza Province, bordering Uganda and Tanzania, is one of the most seriously affected regions of the country (Republic of Kenya 1997:3). Even within Nyanza Province, rates vary considerably across geographic region and by age.

Kisumu town, a fast-growing urban center in Nyanza and hub of western Kenya, is the focus of migrants of both sexes in search of employment. Like migrant labor elsewhere in east Africa, Kenyans in Kisumu maintain close links with their rural homes so that there is movement back and forth. Siaya District, north of Kisumu, is one of the poorest and most important labor-exporting districts in the country; 30 percent of people born in the district have traveled beyond its borders.

Kisumu is located strategically on the major highway to Uganda, some 50 kilometers distant, and has a direct link with Tanzania to the south. For decades Kisumu has been a major trading link for Uganda and it is a major transit point for travelers through east Africa. A UNAIDS study of Kisumu town disclosed high rates of HIV infection, especially marked in younger women (see Figure 13.2 and UNAIDS 1997a).

Rwanda

Whether AIDS contributed to the tragic events in Rwanda in 1994 is a moot question. Some authors argue that indeed AIDS added to the political instability which led to the breakdown of Rwandan society and to ethnic violence. It is probable that AIDS contributed to a general atmosphere of tension in Rwanda, but, in comparison with other aspects of this question, which are economic, political, historical, and cultural in nature, AIDS in itself was a relatively minor factor. (Taylor 1995; see also Anonymous 1994:1; Anacleti 1996)

The 1986 national serological survey reported HIV prevalence slightly over 1 percent in rural areas and 18 percent in the general urban populations. Among urban adults between the ages of 26 and 40, levels reached 40 percent. HIV prevalence rates among antenatal women ranged from 22 to 30 percent between 1988 and 1991. Similarly, for female STD patients prevalence rates ranged from 70–76 percent and for male patients from 49–57 percent during the same period (Family Health International 1997a; Mayaud et al. 1997). The national AIDS program was established the following year. When antenatal surveillance is disaggregated by place of residence, we see the sharp differences pertaining between urban and rural communities. HIV prevalence among antenatal women by residence varied from 26.7 percent for urban residents to 8.5 percent for semi-rural residents and 2.2

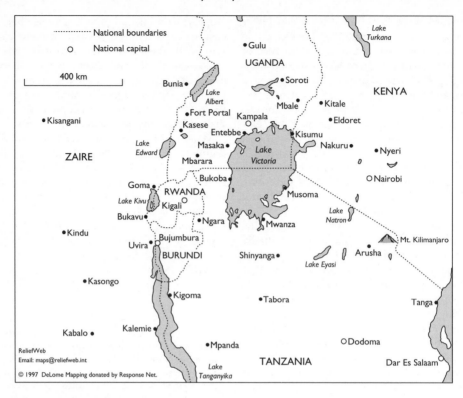

Figure 13.1 *Great lakes region*
Source: ReliefWeb <http://www.reliefweb.int/>.

percent for rural residents in 1997 (Ministry of Health 1997).

Tanzania

In Tanzania, AIDS was first seen in 1983 in the rural Kagera region, bordering Lake Victoria, Rakai District of Uganda, and Burundi. By 1991, the highest prevalence rates in the country were in Kagera (20 percent); the next most affected area was Mwanza (11 percent), also bordering Lake Victoria. By 1992, the World Bank considered the region around Kagera to "comprise the area of the world with the largest concentration of HIV infected individuals" (World Bank 1992b:16). By 1995, the Tanzanian AIDS Control Program estimated that 1.2 million people were infected with HIV in Tanzania (Family Health International 1997b).

As I mentioned earlier, HIV rates can vary greatly in relatively small regions, with higher rates along main roads and lowest rates in

rural villages. For example, in a study in the Mwanza region of Uganda by Barongo et al. (1992), it was found that rates of HIV infection ranged from 11.8 percent in town to 7.3 percent in roadside settlements and 2.5 percent in rural villages. Rates also vary greatly by age and gender. For example, among town residents aged 25 to 35, the rate of infection among women was twice that of men: 20 percent of women and 10.7 percent of men. Generalized statistics of HIV prevalence rates can be extremely misleading. Finer analysis can reveal important variations in rates of infection and show the danger of extrapolating from small data sets. For example, although Kagera was assumed in the 1980s to be the worst-affected region of the country, careful analysis shows important variation among socio-economic areas in Bukoba, the district headquarters. For example, Bukoba town had HIV rates of 16.1 percent for high socio-economic status wards and 42 percent for low socio-

Table 13.1   *Ante-natal surveillance for HIV seropositivity of pregnant women, Kenya 1990–7*

Province	1990	1993	1995	1997
Nairobi	12.1%	16.2	15.7%	15.9%
Central:				
Thika	2.5	9.6	19.6	23.1
Nyeri	2.9	5.4	9.6	10.1
Rift Valley:				
Nakuru	10.0	22.5	27.2	24.6
Mosoriot	–	2.0 (1994)	12.5	9.1
Eastern:				
Kitui	1.0	2.0	4.2	5.9
Karurumo	–	2.0 (1994)	10.3	26.6
North Eastern:				
Garisa	4.9	3.8	5.8	8.1
Coast:				
Mombasa	10.2	16.5	15.8	17.4
Tiwi	–	12.2 (1994)	24.1	–
NYANZA:				
Kisumu	19.2	19.6	25.3	34.9
Chulaimbo	–	49.2 (1994)	21.8	27.2 (1996)
Western:				
Busia	17.1	22.2	22.0	28.1 (1996)
Kakamega	5.3	8.6	11.7	10.0

Sources: National AIDS & STDs Control Programme and National Council for Population Development (1998) and Mulindi et al. (1998).

economic status wards. Bukoba rural and other rural districts had rates ranging from 4.5 to 10.0 percent in 1987 (Setel 1999:128). Setel (1999) notes that "the only clarity to emerge from the testing frenzy of the 1980s and 1990s was that the epidemic in Tanzania was anything but a 'monolithic blight.' Rather, an enormous degree of heterogeneity characterized the early manifestations of the epidemic across the country."

Uganda: An Island of Hope? – The Decline in HIV Prevalence

The Uganda AIDS Control Programme has reported that since 1982 about 2 million people had been infected with HIV of whom 1.5 million were still alive. This is not good news. The good news came near the end of 1995 when Ugandan researchers announced the first observable decline in HIV prevalence. The reduction in prevalence was limited to a specific group, young men. Most observers believe that changed behavior provides the explanation (STD/AIDS Control Programme 1996). This was very good news, not only for

Uganda, but for the entire region and those who had been working vigorously for years in the country's education and prevention programs.

The very high prevalence rates observed in urban areas indicate that at some stage in the past, HIV incidence rates must have been higher than those currently prevailing. There is general consensus that although HIV incidence levels must have declined, the main decline probably occurred before the studies of HIV incidence. No one knows what the incidence rate in Kampala, Rakai, or any other part of Uganda was in the period 1985–90. It is clear that the numbers of HIV-positive persons dying each year far exceed the new (incident) HIV infections during the same periods. The researchers from the Rakai [Columbia University study] cohort felt that excess mortality among HIV-positive persons could almost entirely explain the decline in HIV prevalence.

Indeed, the term "significance" has a specific definition in epidemiology, while "substantial" has crept into the literature with the implication that it is also a "scientific" term.

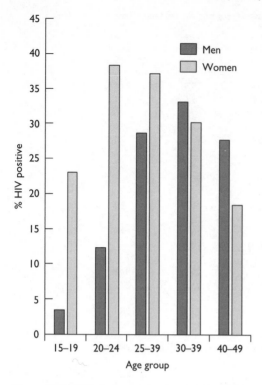

Figure 13.2 *HIV infection rates by age and gender, Kisumu Town, Kenya, 1997*
Source: Data from UNAIDS 1997a; *Multi-Center Study, Phase One: Qualitative Information* (A draft report of Kisumu study site). Kisumu, Kenya: Department of Community Health.

Statistical significance is derived through statistical methods which allow an estimate to be made of the probability of the observed or greater degree of association between independent and dependent variables under the null hypothesis (Last 1988:24). In 1997, the Masaka team was able to report the significant decline in the overall adult rate which moved from 8.1 percent in 1989 to 7.3 percent in 1997. In addition, the decreased prevalence rates among younger people continued. It can be argued that the Ugandan antenatal rates also declined and in some cases did so substantially between 1991 and 1995, as shown in Tables 13.2 and 13.3.

There is other data to substantiate the argument in favor of a decline. In Masaka the overall adult rates (those aged 13+ years) of 8 percent had remained stable for a decade but among young men aged 13–24 HIV prevalence

had declined *significantly* from 3.4 to 1 percent. In 1989, almost 12 percent of men aged 20–24 were infected; by 1995 it was almost 3 percent. However, young women had a much slighter decline in HIV prevalence. Women aged 13–24 had come down from 9.9 to 7.3 percent and women aged 20–24 who in 1989 were 21.3 percent positive had by 1995 come down to 19.4 percent (Mulder et al. 1995).

The international press carried the news, yet there were skeptics who argued that there has been no *true* decline in HIV in Uganda. They argue that the decline in *prevalence* is a result of the heavy mortality caused by AIDS and that *incidence* has remained more or less constant. [New infections are rapidly replacing the statistics of older, prevalent cases which are dying.] Those who agree that there has been a decline in HIV prevalence argue that it is most likely a result of observed behavior change. A series of studies of behavior change between 1989 and 1995 concluded that "This is the first report of a change over a period of 6 years in male and female sexual behavior, assessed at the population level, that may partly explain the observed decline in HIV seroprevalence in young pregnant women in urban Uganda. This result should encourage AIDS control programs to pursue their prevention activities" (Asiimwe-Okiror et al. 1997).

Risk and "High Risk Groups"

Let us agree for now that there has been a decline in the rate of HIV infection in Uganda. I would like to return to the question posed earlier in the title of the chapter: how can Uganda sustain the decline in HIV prevalence, surrounded as it is by countries at war and with high rates of infection? Here a few words on "risk" are relevant. The concepts of "risk," "high risk groups," and "risk behaviors" are much discussed in relation to HIV and AIDS. Is it feasible to think of a country "at risk"? Bond and Vincent (1997a) have proposed the concept of *multiple contingent risk* to encapsulate the multifaceted nature of the life situations of many individuals: unemployment, underemployment, poverty, forced separation from family and kin, lack of access to health services. I would add war and displacement to the list.

Table 13.2 *HIV Prevalence among antenatal women in Uganda, 1991–7*

Site	1991 %	1992 %	1993 %	1994 %	1995 %	1996 %	1997 %
Nsambya, Kampala	27.8	29.5	26.6	21.8	16.8	15.4	14.6
Rubaga, Kampala	27.4	29.4	24.4	16.5	20.2	–	–
Jinja	22.0	19.9	16.7	16.3	13.2	14.8	11.0
Tororo (Eastern)	12.8	13.2	11.3	10.2	12.4	8.2	9.5
Mbale (Eastern)	12.1	14.8	8.7	10.2	7.7	–	–
Mbarara (Western)	24.4	30.2	18.1	17.3	16.6	15.0	14.5

Source: STD/AIDS Control Programme (1996) and UNAIDS (1997).

Table 13.3 *Decline in HIV prevalence rates, Uganda*

	1989 %	1990 %	1992 %	1993 %	1994 %
Masaka study – overall	8.2	–	–	–	7.6
young men	3.4	–	–	–	1.0
young women	9.9	–	–	–	7.3
Rakai study					
adults 15–49	–	23.4	20.9	–	–
younger 13–24	–	17.3	12.6	–	–
Antenatal clinic surveillance – Kampala	28	–	–	16	–

Source: UNAIDS (various years) and World Bank (1999).

Other analysts suggest that AIDS can be best understood in the context of an *ecology of risk*. Obbo (1993b) has suggested that analysis of the *situations of risk* is more useful in understanding the epidemic than is the continuing emphasis on individual risk behaviors. Gilbert Herdt, stressing the cultural meaning of risk, suggests *risk milieu* (Herdt 1992).

The paradigm of risk behaviors has led to the categorization of certain *sub-populations* considered to be more at risk of infection. Conceptualized as free-willed individuals, capable of making choices, certain groups are considered *vectors* of HIV, *transmitters* of the virus. The burden of responsibility is on the individual, a very Western, European approach to public health. I would like to underline the importance of understanding the dynamics of social and geographical networking (sexual networking) in contrast to the facile labeling of certain groups of people as "core" transmitters of disease. All assumptions must be questioned. For example, a study of fishermen and bar workers, generally categorized as *high risk* groups, has shown that they "are less promiscuous than has been assumed, and there is a continuum of behavior both within

these groups and between them and the 'ordinary' citizen" (Pool et al. 1995).

Such studies illustrate the need to question a number of common assumptions: (1) HIV will spread quickly from high prevalence to low prevalence areas; and (2) sexual networking rates are higher in Africa than in other areas. The Masaka study concluded

> Given the high rate of partner change of a minority of men in both urban and rural areas HIV will continue to spread in both areas. But with the rarity of sexual contact between the high prevalence town (40%) and the low prevalence rural area (8%) it is unlikely that HIV prevalence in the rural area will "level up" to that of the town. (Pickering et al. 1996)

While there can be little doubt that highly mobile individuals can act as conduits for STDs, more attention needs to be drawn to the wider *milieu of risk*, for example, the socio-economic factors driving men and women away from the rural villages towards the roads and small towns and trading centers. It makes more sense to seek answers to the areas of high rates of HIV infection in east Africa in the socio-economic circumstances of their occasion. Research should focus more on the *ecology of risk* rather than the *risky behaviors* of individuals.

Other high risk groups frequently cited are long-distance truck drivers, migrant laborers, prostitutes, unemployed youth in urban centers, traders, and the military. Interestingly, refugees are not mentioned as often, in spite of their extraordinary mobility and extreme instability. I would like to discuss migrants and refugees in east Africa. I mentioned earlier the Great Lakes Initiative on AIDS in east Africa. The six countries have decided that the first focus for intervention in the epidemic should be the truck drivers and all other groups at risk of contracting HIV along the Trans-African Highway: bar owners, prostitutes, and transport company owners.

Trans-African Highway and the "Trucker" Paradigm for AIDS

The Trans-African Highway stretches between Mombasa and Kigali, passing through Uganda, Democratic Republic of Congo [DRC], Rwanda, and Burundi. It is considered to be a major route along which HIV has been spread. A number of busy small towns, or trading centers, have mushroomed along the highway. Ugandan examples are Lukaya in Masaka District, and Lyantonde, Kalisizo, Kyotera, and Mutukula in Rakai District. Studies have been made of the HIV prevalence rates and the sexual behaviors of groups considered to be at high risk of infection (see, for example, Muizarubi et al. 1991). These include truck drivers and their assistants, women who work in the hundreds of small bars and lodges along the route, and adolescents. A 1991 study in one of the busiest trading centers in Masaka District revealed an HIV rate in adults of 40 percent.

Another trading center on the Masaka highway was referred to in the 1980s as Uganda's AIDS capital. It then contained about twenty lodges and bars and on a busy night, thirty trucks and hundreds of women would be present. In the early 1990s, following frightening mortality from AIDS and with the civil war in Rwanda disrupting normal business, people fled the trading centers. But in recent years, trading centers have been returning to activity and "Business is once again booming, the

fastest selling commodity being sex. But things have changed. Today sex workers are more aware of the hazards of unprotected sex and so insist on condoms. So do their clients. The result is a high demand for condoms" (Sunday Vision 1997). The women claim that their clients are mainly Kenyan truck drivers and traders from the Democratic Republic of Congo (Sunday Vision 1997).

Female bar workers, who are often also prostitutes, have complex sexual networks. In the small back rooms of the many bars lining the highway, women sell cheap sex to men from the town or immediate rural area. Inside the bars, women sell beer and sex to passing truck drivers while more successful women own bars along the main roads. The back street bar workers are less able to negotiate safe sex and are at higher risk of contracting HIV and STDs (Bwayo et al. 1991; New Vision 1999; Talle 1995). In Kisumu, where a recent study enumerated 1,385 prostitutes, "bar owners admit commercial sex is part of the entire business and indeed it attracts more customers" (Kisumu Department of Community Health 1997).

In Kenya, near Mombasa adolescent girls are flocking to the truck stops along the highway. Young girls along the roads, as well as in home villages, are much desired by the older men who assume that they are free of HIV and therefore "safe" (Nzyuko et al. 1997:10). In a study of 200 adolescents, aged 15 to 19, 52 percent of the girls and 30 percent of the boys reported that they had had a sexually transmitted disease and 46 percent of the girls reported that they "usually had sex with truck drivers."

Borders and Trade

In the late 1980s and early 1990s when AIDS morbidity and mortality struck visibly in the trading centers along the Trans-African Highway in Masaka and Rakai, significant numbers of small-scale traders emigrated to the busy border towns near the Kenyan border: Tororo and Busia (Obbo 1993b:952; Witte et al. 1996). At the other end of the country, the conflict in Democratic Republic of Congo has created a bustling trade for Ugandans. In 1996, with "Banyamulenge" victories along the eastern side of DRC, traders were close behind. They rushed to the borders with Democratic Republic of Congo in the far northeast of the country in Nebbi and Arua Districts as well as the far southeast of the country at the Kisoro border. The border towns attract intermediary entrepreneurs of many types and of course, the women migrate to work in bars, lodges, and offer their sexual services.

In 1996, HIV prevalence along the Uganda–Kenya border ranged between 20 and 30 percent (Balthazar 1994; Balthazar and Okeyo 1996; Kenya National AIDS and STDS Control Programme 1996; Blair et al. 1997). Business women who frequent the border express fears that they are at high risk of AIDS. A recent HIV/AIDS project is aimed at sensitizing people about their *risk milieu*. Women were made aware of the potential risk of contracting HIV and advised how to conduct their border business more safely. They were discouraged from moving about in the border town at night. As a result, a number of women have rented small rooms to stay in at night and in that way have avoided the busy bars/lodges. Condoms have sold well and the women were encouraged to look at HIV-positive women more positively and to help each other. The women now prefer to do their business during the daylight hours. The women feel the risk has now decreased because border custom officials have been sensitized to assist them more quickly (Matu et al. 1996).

Migrants

Another highly mobile and most often disadvantaged population at high risk of contracting HIV and other STIs in east Africa is the many thousands of migrant laborers. A vast majority of these primarily younger people exist in a *milieu of risk*. In east Africa, most migrant labor is non-contractual: simply a matter of mobile individuals in search of employment in the rapidly growing towns and cities. Migrant labor is believed to contribute significantly to the spread of HIV in South Africa, Zimbabwe, Angola, and Uganda (Russell et al. 1990). In spite of this observation, the groups most studied in AIDS research have been truck drivers and prostitutes. Consequently, the role of migration in the spread

of HIV remains largely unknown and as a result, HIV/AIDS prevention and care programs are largely deficient in this area (Lamptey and Tarantola 1998; Anonymous 1997). Finally, migration status is traditionally not included in national-level surveillance systems for fear of stigmatization.

Migrant labor

Uganda was traditionally a *labor-importing* region. Hundreds of thousands of men came from Sudan, Rwanda, Burundi, and Congo, labor-exporting regions, seeking work in central Uganda. Most came without wives and families and most were employed without contract, not by the colonial state, but by Ugandan (Bagandan) farmers in the production of cash crops, mainly coffee. Many thousand others worked contractually on large sugar and tea plantations. Between 1920 and the late 1950s, migrant laborers were feared by the colonial administration to be carriers of disease (Lyons 1996).

After World War I, there were massive numbers of migrants arriving in Uganda: by 1948, immigrants comprised 34 percent of the total population in Buganda and by 1959, they outnumbered the indigenous population in several counties of Buganda. In Mbale town, not far from the Kenyan border, more than 50 percent of the population was immigrant (Dak 1968). At the last census in 1991, about 2.4 percent of the total population of some 18 million, or nearly 450,000 people, were immigrants in Uganda.

Uganda no longer imports migrant labor on a massive scale across borders; instead, most labor migrancy is internal. Nevertheless, there are still those who cross the borders seeking employment.

Migrancy and the "risk milieux"

The classic migrant laborer was male and often traveled far from his home area, leaving families behind for very long periods of time. Kakira and Lugazi are two large sugar plantations which still employ many thousands of men, many of whom are without their families. Long periods of separation cause great hardship for both men and women. Living conditions at the two sugar plantations are fair but most migrant laborers are outside the formal contractual system of the plantations and live in harsh conditions, in new disease environments without access to even a modicum of health care, and in such circumstances they often form temporary sexual liaisons. Women left behind in rural areas are confronted with increased work burdens, which often means decreased nutritional status for the family. For example, studies have shown that in many areas women cultivators, the sole providers of family food, have been forced by sheer workload or the declining fertility of the soil to switch from high protein crops like millet to less labor-intensive crops such as cassava or plaintains. The result was lower nutritional status of themselves and their families. The migrant labor pattern of east and southern Africa over the 20th century has led to the weakening, even breakdown, of stability in the family and formed an ideal milieu in which sexually transmitted diseases can spread.

In more recent times, women have begun to migrate about east Africa and beyond in search of economic opportunities ranging from trade to prostitution. It is widely assumed that the many women traders who travel to Dubai to purchase secondhand clothes for resale in Uganda top up their profits by prostitution while abroad. In Uganda from the mid-1970s many women joined men in a booming black market trade economy referred to as *magendo*. The smuggling of coffee from the Great Lakes region was highly lucrative and, together with the illicit trade in other commodities in exchange for consumer goods, has been implicated in the early days of the epidemic of HIV/AIDS, particularly among the many small, remote villages around the southern shores of Lake Victoria. On the Tanzanian side of the lake, the relatively prosperous young men who resulted from this trade were called *abekikomela*. Between 1980 and 1983, signs of AIDS were first noticed in these young men who were moving between Tanzania and the border of Uganda. The mortality rate among them was very high and at the time Tanzanians associated the disease with the Baganda traders and vice versa (Lwihula 1990; Obbo 1991).

Internal migration at present

In terms of the *ecology of risk* in present-day east Africa, it may be more important to focus on the many hundreds of thousands of younger people, mainly male, who leave the economically depressed rural sector to seek work in the relatively few urban centers. In Kenya in 1962, about 7.8 percent population was urban. By 1989, 27 percent of the population was urban, an increase of 19.2 percent. The annual urban increase in Uganda between 1980 and 1996 was 6 percent. But official figures do not capture the enormous flood of unemployed, disenchanted younger people in east Africa who come to the towns and cities for relatively short periods searching for economic opportunity. In Kampala there are whole slum areas inhabited by young people from traditional labor-exporting areas such as Kabale in the southwest, and Arua, Moyo, Gulu, and Kitgum in the north. They move back and forth between town and village, defying description as either. They constitute an ideal channel for the dissemination of sexually transmitted diseases.

For several years, I have resided near the central food market in mid-Kampala where I have witnessed a veritable explosion in the number of youthful, mainly male, population. As in all fast-growing urban centers in east Africa, there are many hundreds, thousands, of young men hanging about the streets in hope of a few hours' employment in a week. They tend to live in the surrounding slums, crowded together in small shared hovels without access to safe water and sanitation facilities. Most often unaccompanied by wives and families who remain in the rural sector, these concentrations of mostly underemployed/unemployed young men are at terrible risk of disease. They live in an extreme *ecology of risk*. Yet, these huge concentrations of rural migrants to African urban centers most often fall outside any official definitions of "migrant labor" and very little research has been carried out on their sociology. A group of women interviewed in Masaka explained

that men, especially under 35, spend time away from home conducting their business: marketing foodstuffs in local trading centers, or carrying produce such as bananas to Kampala for sale.

They said that when staying in trading centers and towns traders may feel lonely and thus engage in outside sex. Older women said that a man may take things from home to give to other partners in the trading center and the woman might resort to forming a liaison with another man in order to obtain the necessities she requires. (Nabaitu et al. 1994)

A long-term study of HIV / AIDS in rural Rakai District, carried out by Columbia University and Makerere University, reported *a strong association* between travel outside the district and HIV infection. Individuals who had migrated out of households in the study area were associated with high seropositivity (see Table 13.4; Musgrave et al. 1991; Kigongo et al. 1992; Hawkes 1992). In another analysis of the Rakai data, 28 percent of HIV-infected individuals had traveled outside Uganda and 24 percent had traveled outside the district. The HIV-positive people reported that 36 percent of their partners had traveled outside the country, 24 percent outside Rakai, while another 17 percent have traveled around inside the district. Only 9 percent of the HIV-positive individuals reported no travel at all (Kirunga and Ntozi 1997). People move about inside a country for a variety of reasons. Between 1988 and 1992 Ugandans moved for the motives highlighted in Table 13.5. The most predominant reason throughout the regions is work followed by war and then marriage.

Refugees in east Africa and HIV/AIDS

I would like to turn now to the topic of refugees in east Africa. It is well known that war is one of the worst *risk milieux* for STDs. Not so frequently mentioned, however, is one of its main consequences, refugee camps, and even less often mentioned are the increasing numbers of *internally displaced populations*. East Africa has an abundance of all three. The upheavals and displacements which force many hundreds of thousands of Africans to seek refuge away from their homes in east Africa is directly related to the incidence and prevalence of HIV and other STDs in the region. The risk to individuals is incalculable. In east Africa, the refugee crisis alters almost daily in the context of ongoing conflicts and wars. Uganda is surrounded on three sides by up-

heavals which seriously destabilize the region: the Sudanese war, depredations of the Lord's Resistance Army (LRA), and more recently the Allied Democratic Forces (ADF) in Uganda cause a shifting kaleidoscope of peoples around and over the borders. The ADF, based in the Ruwenzori mountains of western Uganda, is a combination of fundamentalist Tabliq Muslim rebels and remnants of another rebel group, the National Army for the Liberation of Uganda (NALU). It has claimed responsibility for a string of bomb blasts that have rocked the country, particularly Kampala. It also frequently links up with the ex-FAR/Interahamwe militias operating in the region and is particularly active in the Bundibugyo area of western Uganda. Lord's Resistance Army is more concerned with destabilizing northern Uganda from bases in Sudan, but has linked up with Interahamwe and anti-RCD rebels around the Bunia area. Likewise, the now largely defunct West Nile Bank Front (WNBF) also wreaked havoc. As of June 1999, UNHCR calculated half a million internally displaced persons (IDP) in Uganda.

In April 1994 the Interahamwe began the genocide which culminated a few months later when perhaps as many as 1.3 million Rwandese fled across borders. After four years of bitter war in Rwanda, the Rwandese Patriotic Front (RPF) drew near victory by taking Kigali. In the refugee camps of eastern DRC, huge numbers of people were herded together in circumstances ideal for the spread of HIV and other STDs. Most often, AIDS is overlooked in the immediate wake of a disaster, because there seem to be more important things to do. However, it is just at this time that AIDS threatens most. Women and children are vulnerable, especially those unaccompanied by a male relation. Where the military is involved, the risk for the weak is increased. For example, in the Tanzanian camps, rape was a major issue. Unaccompanied women and girls reported that at night men simply forced their way into the flimsy shelters and raped them.

The numbers of people involved in these movements are mind-numbing. We read of "hundreds of thousands," a statistic without reality. In September 1994, Benaco Camp in Tanzania contained more than 450,000 people (Taylor 1995:24). Kenya hosts large numbers of

Table 13.4 *HIV rates in Rakai study of those who travel and do not travel outside district*

	HIV+	HIV+	HIV–	HIV–	Total
Traveled	441	20.6%	1702	79.4%	2143
No travel	30	10.6%	252	89.4%	282

Source: Musgrave et al. (1991).

Table 13.5 *Motives for internal migration in Uganda*

Region	Work %	War %	Marriage %
Central	30	6	5
Eastern	28	15	9
Western	44	6	4
Northern	21	23	4

Source: Barton and Wamai (1994).

refugees, and their difficult circumstances and unstable economic, family, and community situations make them vulnerable to STDs and HIV infection (Brockerhoff et al. 1996:5). There are a number of "permanent" camps: three in the northeast contain about 120,000 mainly Somali refugees while Kakuma near Turkana houses about 51,000 Sudanese (Mulindi et al. 1998:32). In Uganda, the number of internally displaced people is rapidly increasing at present. In June 1999, the World Food Program was preparing relief for 146,000 displaced people in the district of Bundibugyo in western Uganda where the ADF is creating havoc (Xinhua News Agency 1999). Xinhua News Agency (1999) reported that the security situation in the Rwenzori Mountains of western Uganda had seriously deteriorated, noting further that:

> The IDP have been located in 46 camps all over Bundibugyo district ... The camps where they are living are overcrowded with wretched hygiene, sanitation, a lack of non-food items and inadequate medical monitoring. At present, the International Committee of the Red Cross [ICRC] closely monitors the health situation in the camps, where the main problems are malaria, respiratory infections and diarrhea ... A little to the north, in Kasese district, the fate of the civilian population also remains fragile, with the continued displacement of some 23,000 people.

HIV/AIDS and other sexually transmitted diseases are not mentioned in the reports. As I have said earlier, in the immediate crisis of refugee movement, there seem more important matters to attend.

War and displacement in Uganda

Northern Uganda today faces an acute humanitarian crisis which has a long history. The infrastructure in Gulu and Kitgum is in a state of collapse and the long civil war in Sudan has impacted seriously on Uganda in a number of important areas, including the epidemic of HIV. In the 1980s northern Uganda experienced dramatic flows of population as refugees streamed into Uganda and years later back to Sudan. In recent years, the activities of the Lord's Resistance Army of Joseph Kony have continued displacing many hundreds of thousands of people. The abduction by the LRA of thousands of children to use as slaves, soldiers, and concubines is a particularly horrible feature of the conflict (for a full detailed discussion see Ehrenreich 1997).

In terms of internally displaced persons, the Ugandan government has established a number of "protected camps" near Ugandan army installations, 19 in Gulu District and 9 in Kitgum District. By June 1997 there were 37 refugee settlements and transit camps scattered around Uganda. The intention is to decrease the vulnerability of civilians living in isolated rural areas of the north. The result may be quite different. Crowded conditions and lack of food, sanitation, and health facilities have rendered the population vulnerable to death from malnutrition and disease. Ten of the camps in Gulu district are situated in areas with no health care facilities at all. By 1998, 400,000 Ugandans were living in the camps where it was reported that monthly mortality was high (see Figures 13.3 and 13.4). In addition, 160,000 Sudanese were in Ugandan refugee camps (AVSI 1998). Finally, despite the nearby military presence, the camps remain targets for rebel attacks.

The rationale behind the protected camps is straightforward: by concentrating the civilian population in a few well-defined areas, the army hopes both to simplify the task of protecting people from rebel attacks and make it harder for the rebels to find food by raiding villages. There is no end in sight. The recent activities of the Lord's Resistance Army have turned Gulu and Kitgum into permanent battle zones, filled with burnt schools, ransacked homes, abandoned fields, and a

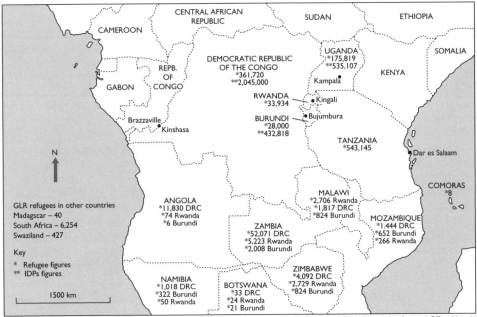

Prepared by OCHA Great Lakes Regional Office, Nairobi

Figure 13.3   *Great Lakes region: refugees and displaced persons as of September 2001*
Source: ReliefWeb <http://www.reliefweb.int/>.

huge population of internally displaced people.

Thousands of young people have been kidnapped and taken to Sudan as slaves, porters, and child soldiers while young schoolgirls have been taken for use by Sudanese military. In July 1999, a local representative announced that at least 11,000 children had been abducted from Kitgum District alone. For girls, life with the LRA is particularly onerous. In addition to military training, farming, and cooking, most adolescent girls are forced to provide sexual services.

World Vision, an NGO which manages a trauma center in Gulu, reported that 70–80 percent of the children newly arriving at the center test positive for at least one sexually transmitted disease (Human Rights Watch 1997a). Some of the girls are pregnant, while others, who tested negative for pregnancy, have stopped having their menstrual periods because of malnutrition and stress (Human Rights Watch 1997b). The trauma counseling centers do not test the children for HIV, reasoning that after their experiences in the

bush, the children are not yet psychologically ready to be told that they may have contracted a fatal illness. But with HIV infection rates of 25 percent in parts of Gulu and Kitgum, it is overwhelmingly likely that many of the children – especially the girls – have become infected.

Refugee camps

Refugee camps are a *milieu of risk* in which vulnerability to HIV is increased enormously. Refugees are not the only population at increased risk of contracting STDs. The surrounding communities are affected. The arrival of hundreds of thousands of refugees in predominantly rural and undeveloped regions creates instant economies. New businesses appear – bars and restaurants mushroomed along the major roads around the Tanzanian camps. Prostitution proliferates around camps as it is one way that women earn money to exchange for food. In most instances condoms will certainly be lacking (UNAIDS 1997b; Benjamin 1996). An interesting exception is this example

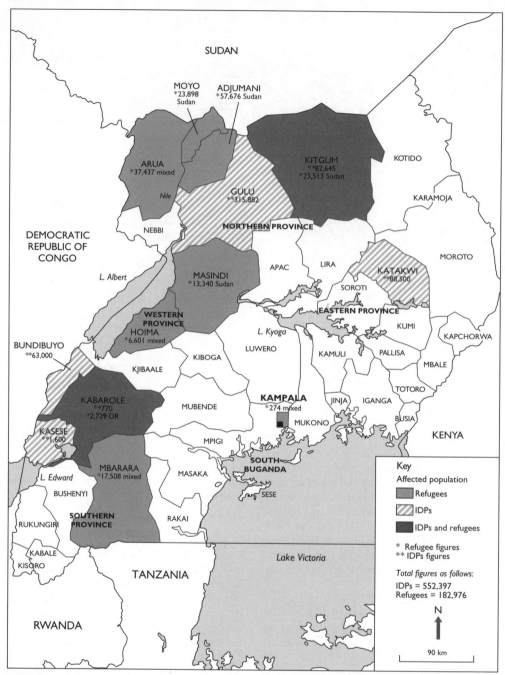

Figure 13.4 *Refugees and internally displaced persons in Uganda as of January 2002*
Source: ReliefWeb <http://www.reliefweb.int/>.
Note: In January 2002 there were a total of 552, 397 internally displaced persons and 182, 976 refugees in over thirty "protected camps" in Uganda, mostly concentrated in the northern part of Uganda.

of a UNHCR representative who visited Kigali during the Rwandan genocide in mid-1994 and reported that:

> Huge numbers of Rwandan refugees were continuing to pour into the camps in Zaire, specifically in Goma. It was a great surprise for me to see that one of the first things many refugees did was to ask for condoms – not food, not medicine, but condoms. Within two weeks we were able to get 2,000,000 condoms delivered. (Wernette 1994)

[Note: it is just possible that the requests were from the many thousands of Rwandese army and Interahamwe which used the huge mass of villagers as a "shield" to escape the RPF.]

A study of Benaco Camp revealed that many female refugees, with few or no relatives, used sexual relationships as survival strategy. Numbers of adolescent girls from local villages [were] hired to work as bar girls in Kasulo, the village bordering the largest camp, Benaco. The young rural girls provided a booming hospitality industry, some of whom were offering sexual favors after working hours. By September 1994 the village contained about one hundred commercial sex workers in little rooms behind the maze of small bars. They came from all over Tanzania "to take part in the economic boom that has accompanied the refugee influx. Their clients are mainly the businessmen and truck drivers who remain in town for a few days before returning home" (Wondergem and Brady 1994a:32). Sexual activity increased enormously in the camp, particularly with adolescents. Young men reported that "chasing girls has now become our main occupation" (Wondergem and Brady 1994b:28). In Benaco, 21 percent of people between the ages of 15 and 49 reported having had sex in the past year with someone who was not a regular partner and 36 percent of all sexually active men reported having had a new sex partner since arrival in the camp (Vogel and Wondergem 1995). UNHCR Guidelines prohibit HIV testing in refugee camps as it is thought that host countries might discriminate against seropositive refugees (AIDS Analysis Africa 1995:10).

In December 1996, the Tanzanian government, which had previously been one of the most welcoming to refugees in Africa, reversed its policy and ordered all refugees, over half a million, to leave by January 1. The result was a reversal of the flood of refugees, most of whom began walking back to Rwanda. Two hundred and thirty-five thousand headed for Uganda while others started towards Kenya, Zambia, and Malawi (New Vision 1996). On the same day, many more thousands of Rwandese who were trying to leave Rwanda were stopped and turned back at the Tanzanian border by Tanzanian police and troops. It was a scene of utter chaos. Frustrated by the seemingly endless spiral of disorder in the region, the UNHCR Commissioner complained that "refugees have become pawns in the hands of rogue political and military leaders in exile... The ordeal of exhausted Rwandans and Burundians in forests in the heart of Africa is one of the worst traumas of our times" (New Vision 1997c). But reflecting another widespread view among Africans, a Ugandan government minister was more blunt when she said that "Hundreds of thousands of people had become a 'lucrative business'... and a source of employment for the UNHCR and some NGOs with budgets that are mind-boggling" (New Vision 1998). In early July, Human Rights Watch [New York] noted that the 30th anniversary of the Organization of African Unity (OAU) Refugee Convention is marked by growing hostility and mistreatment of refugees in the Great Lakes region. The refugee crisis in east Africa is enormous and complex. It has created untold hardship for millions of terribly stressed people. This is a difficult time for east Africans.

Conclusion

In conclusion, it is perhaps no exaggeration to be reminded of the Four Horsemen of the Apocalypse: poverty, war, famine, and disease. Regardless of the explanation for the wars and conflicts which generate these massive movements of populations, the stark reality remains that even if peace and order were to come today, for many thousand tomorrows the millions of individuals already infected with HIV and their families and relations will continue to face the consequences of AIDS.

The HIV/AIDS pandemic in Africa can be conceptualized as a series of interlinking, yet separate, microepidemics. We can achieve a better understanding of the forces driving the epidemics through study of patterns of sexual networking and mobile populations which are major factors in the spread of HIV. Researchers and program designers need to broaden the scope of their enquiries and activities beyond prostitutes and truck drivers and the sexual behaviors of individuals. Equally important to the containment and prevention of HIV/AIDS are health programs designed to address the massive numbers of internally displaced people, refugees, and migrant laborers swirling about the landscape of east Africa.

At present, UN agencies are preparing a regional humanitarian contingency plan in anticipation of rising relief needs in the Great Lakes region in the near future because of the continued instability and the increasing vulnerability of populations. "We don't have an optimistic view of the situation," said a UN official (IRIN-CEA 1999). Yet, the newly formed Great Lakes Initiative on AIDS has chosen to focus on truck drivers, prostitutes, and the Trans-African Highway as its primary objective to combat AIDS in east Africa. I would like to suggest that, in light of the existing number of refugees, internally displaced persons, and internal labor migrants in the region and the fact that each of these categories of mobile population is likely to increase in the foreseeable future, the new east African regional AIDS program should refocus its attention.

Chapter 14

Understanding the African HIV Pandemic: An Appraisal of the Contexts and Lay Explanation of the HIV/AIDS Pandemic with Examples from Tanzania and Kenya

Gabriel Rugalema

Explaining HIV/AIDS: The Dominant Paradigm

In the late 1970s and early 1980s HIV/AIDS was concentrated among small pockets of urban population in many parts of the world. There was hope then that it might not spread systemically into the wider population (Turshen 1989). However, time and the relentless growth of the pandemic have invalidated such optimism. The pandemic was and is still mainly perceived as a medical problem and hence a domain of medical experts. The enduring hope has been that once the "causative agent" of the "disease" has been identified, a cure or a vaccine will soon be invented and the disease will be "controlled." Prevention efforts in Africa, where much of the HIV transmission is heterosexual, have focused on "risky sexual behavior."

The donor-driven National AIDS Control Programs (NACPs) found in almost every country of sub-Saharan Africa were initiated to spearhead the control of HIV. With few exceptions, the major preoccupation of most NACPs is to "control" HIV through provision of information, education, and communication (IEC) to the public at large and particularly those considered "at risk." Today the IEC model is the most dominant mode of intervention and control of HIV/AIDS in Africa.

IEC programs are premised on the Health Belief Model (HBM) (Rosenstock et al. 1988), which assumes that individuals will take responsibility or act rationally and desist from unsafe sexual behavior once they have been informed and educated about the dangers of contracting HIV and dying of AIDS. The IEC model is a standard one and is applied uniformly across countries and communities. To evaluate the "success" of IEC, researchers have resorted to attitudinal surveys widely known as knowledge, attitudes, and practices (KAP) surveys.

Results from various KAPs undertaken in sub-Saharan Africa indicate that almost everyone is aware of HIV/AIDS (Nyang' and Obudo 1996; Weinstein et al. 1995; Cleland and Ferry 1995). However, 20 years into the epidemic, there is no tangible evidence that HIV infection is going down. Even where some evidence suggests a falling HIV seropositivity trend, Uganda for example, credit is given to social cohesion and improvement in economic well-being rather than IEC per se (Barnett and Whiteside 1998).

The cornerstone of the paradigm of "risky sexual behavior" is the concept of risk. Beck (1992) has argued that increasingly we live in a "risk society." Other theorists are equally persuaded that "risk" is a central concept in social life, but prefer to take an institutional–functional approach rather than a social evolutionary perspective. In the well-known formulations of the neo-Durkheimian cultural theorists such as Douglas and Wildavsky (1982), Rayner (1992), cf. Johnson and Covello (1987), social context – specifically the limited number of ways in which institutions facilitate social accountability – determines risk selection. In this perspective, it is our institutionalization that tells us which risks to worry about and which to discount.

Life is a risky business, but risk has upsides and downsides. Classifying risky behaviors as "good" and "bad" has an important practical side. It is not hard to conclude that driving under the influence of alcohol is dangerous to others as well as the driver. But business ambition (supposedly) is good because it enriches us all.

As Douglas and Wildavsky (1982) and others point out, however, there is nothing clear-cut or self-evident about the moral "scoring" we apply to risky behaviors. They argue that the "badness" of nuclear energy is a moral badness. Rankings of risk on moral grounds reflect social organization and institutionalized values, and the moral hurt is at times a more powerful "pain" than anything else.

If risk assessments clash for moral reasons it is irrelevant to appeal to practical rationality as a way of lessening the danger or hurt. Sex is dangerous, but also fun, and a reproductive necessity. There is increasing evidence to suggest that "factual" appeal to "objective" hazard tends to have little impact on the at-risk group. Smokers continue to smoke, and young people continue to take drugs and engage in "high risk" sexual activity.

The reason "objective" evidence has so little impact – according to neo-Durkheimians – is that we all know, tacitly at least, that moral reasons and practical dangers are constantly mixed up. There is constant "leakage" between the two domains. Practical reasons are forever being cited to buttress moral arguments, and vice versa. Humans regularly discount between the two domains, and frequently suspect that evidence is being used for political purposes (as an attack on ways of life lived according to different institutional values).

Humans tend to believe what they need to believe to make social life work. Schemes for rendering social life workable do not come easily. Nor should we countenance discarding them until proven better alternatives are in place. So they tend to be protected tenaciously.

At present, medical professionals, the political elite, and other powerful groups have a more or less free hand to impose their own culturally constructed risk assessments on the general public (Rugalema 1997). HIV seropositives are thus "victims" of their own "risky" behavior. Working on the socio-economic effects of the HIV epidemic in various parts of east Africa, I argue (Rugalema 1999a, 1999b) that the pandemic is contextualized differently by different groups of people depending on location, occupation, gender, age, etc. HIV/AIDS in Africa is as much "socio-economic" as biological (a viral epidemic) and requires to be addressed through socio-economic negotiation and reform in which those "at risk" are thoroughly engaged.

Limitations of the Health Belief Model and policy action modeled on it have increasingly been acknowledged (Hubley 1988; Tawil et al. 1995). However, evidence to show that researchers have sought to analyze the views of those "at risk," that is, the views of those who are *living with the pandemic*, is still scanty. I argue that to understand the HIV pandemic in Africa is to understand how people who live with it explain it, or rather how they construct schemes of risk assessment in the face of it. It is by listening to the "stories" that we can understand the context in which the pandemic is constructed, including factors that may promote or constrain behavioral change. Such an understanding would be liberating to the participants in theoretical debates about the pandemic and public policy. In the next part of this chapter I present two case studies. One is from a rural setting, a village in Bukoba

District, Tanzania. Bukoba district, with an HIV prevalence rate of more that 25 percent in the adult population, is undoubtedly one of the areas of the world hardest hit by the HIV/AIDS pandemic. The second study is from five research sites in Kenya.

Explaining the HIV Pandemic: The Missing Voices

Throughout history, the perception of epidemics and pandemics has been a matter of power and authority (see, for example, Slack 1992). Lately, however, researchers have begun to analyze the perspectives of the people affected by AIDS[1] to try to understand the context in which the epidemic is constructed.

Why focus on lay discourse?

I contend that the way local people talk about the HIV epidemic reflects their perception and definition of the pandemic. It tells "us" not only the way "they" perceive the epidemic but more importantly the way "they live with it." The latter implies the way behaviors are negotiated, risks taken or avoided, corners cut, care given to the sick, funerals organized, and consequences mitigated or not. Analysis of the language of AIDS as coined and used by lay people is very relevant in the understanding, control, and mitigation of the epidemic. First, it helps in the understanding of the social construction of the epidemic. Social construction of disease is a product of institutionalization. Thus differences in perception of the epidemic by different social categories of people (based on gender, class, age, ethnicity, among others) should not be that surprising. As discussed shortly, the "scientific" discourse of HIV and AIDS is quite different from the lay discourse of the same epidemic. The second point is that perception predetermines response. The way people respond to a phenomenon is mostly foreclosed by what they make of it, how they perceive it. It follows that in the context of HIV, people of different cultural backgrounds have responded to the epidemic in the way that makes sense to them or in the way they define the epidemic.

Presently there is very little, if any, cross-fertilization between the "scientific" percep-

tion of the epidemic and the lay perception. If anything, the traffic is one way. "Scientific" evidence is constantly pushed to local people and so are the intervention programs informed by or modeled on that evidence. The reverse is not happening, mainly because policies and programs are made through an exclusionary process (Reid 1996a). Reid (1996a) points out that the words "we" and "they" have shaped the way "experts" exclude the perspectives of lay people in an entire spectrum of addressing the epidemic. In Reid's (1996a) own words, the attitude of the experts can be summarized thus:

They are at risk
They are affected
We need to design programs to educate them
We need to protect them (Reid 1996a:2. Italics are mine)

Inclusion instead of exclusion would seem to be the way forward for HIV policy. Lay discourse has to be researched, analyzed, and internalized into HIV control and mitigation programs, otherwise externally conceived programs are likely to record minimal achievements.

Language, like society, is organic and dynamic. Evidence analyzed in this chapter reveals that the lay language of AIDS has been changing over time to reflect either the lay internalization of scientific evidence or the changing boundaries of the lay-defined risk environment, or both. Thus the time dimension is an important aspect in the analysis of people's perspectives of the epidemic as old terminology becomes modified or discarded as a result of changing perceptions conditioned by changing times.

In the same vein, socio-economic factors are key determinants of differences in the perception of the epidemic within communities. Materials analyzed in this chapter clearly show that women and men, the young and old, have different perspectives of HIV. For example, age differences have a bearing on how individuals define risk environment and take risks. The same is true in respect to gender as men and women have different constructions of the epidemic mainly based on their gendered socialization, occupations, and access to social and economic resources, including information on HIV.

It would be counterproductive to propose that local people are always right in their perception of the epidemic and construction of the language around it. As the following discussion will show, local construction of the epidemic contains some myths, inaccuracies, and misinformation. This makes it all the more necessary to analyze lay discourse because while strong points have to be taken on board, inaccuracies and myths have to be corrected and demystified. This is not simply an academic issue, it is of critical importance in HIV policy development and implementation.

In the following case studies, perspectives of people living with AIDS in Kenya and Tanzania are described and analyzed. As each study progressed, it became apparent that there was a gap between the professional and lay explanations of the epidemic. It was therefore thought necessary to collect information pertaining to lay explanation of AIDS in different localities. The following discussion reveals that HIV/AIDS is viewed as a disorder of social (productive and reproductive) relations and that sexual behavior and risk taking cannot be divorced from such relations. To understand HIV/AIDS in Africa (and sexual behaviors that spread the virus) is to examine the political economy of production and reproduction whether the unit is a household, family, factory, or agro-estate.

Case Study 1: A Buhaya Village, Bukoba District, Tanzania

The study was conducted in Bukoba District, NW Tanzania between February and December 2002. A combination of research methods was used to collect data. The most important ones included a questionnaire survey of sample households, in-depth interviews among key informants from affected households, recording of daily time expenditure among adults in affected households, and focus group discussions.

Buhaya means "the land of the Bahaya people." Bahaya (part of the interlacustrine Bantu) are the largest single ethnic group that inhabits Bukoba district. The village where the study was conducted is situated some 14 kilometers west of Bukoba town (the district headquarters). The district lies on the eastern shores of Lake Victoria and is bordered by Uganda to the north.

What has made Buhaya susceptible to HIV/AIDS?

The risk environment and susceptibility to AIDS for this remote corner of Tanzania developed gradually throughout most of the 20th century and AIDS might be considered as a climax of the social and economic ills that have afflicted Buhaya. In short, one could describe the situation in terms of multiple risk factors and multiple contingency relationships (Bond and Vincent 1997a). Commercial sex work was already common in this part of Africa in the first decade of the 20th century. Bahaya women left Bukoba for commercial sex work in different parts of east Africa and were claimed to be aggressive and frugal businesswomen (White 1990). This does not imply, however, that Bahaya women are more sexually active than others or that they prefer commercial sex to marriage. To understand why Bahaya women went into commercial sex in greater numbers than any other ethnic group in Tanzania or east Africa, one has to examine the feudal, hierarchical, social, and political organization that characterized the district until the 1960s. Women's lack of access to land (except through marriage) meant that in the event of divorce a woman's livelihood would be threatened. In a place characterized by marital instability and a high rate of divorce (Sundkler 1980), commercial sex was and probably remains almost the only alternative for (divorced) often semi-literate women to support themselves and their dependents, especially children. As Kaijage (1993) observes, savings from commercial sex work were invested in buying land, educating children, and supporting elderly parents. In this way women earned their wealth and status (see also Weiss B. 1993; Swantz 1985). In both World Wars I and II Bahaya men were mobilized to fight in north Africa and Asia and this added to demographic flux in the area. However, it was not until after World War II that Bahaya men (especially educated ones) began leaving Bukoba to work in different sectors of the colonial economy. The same trend was maintained or even intensified after Tanzania's independence. Some have blamed the circular mobility in and out of Bukoba for the outbreak of venereal syphilis (and other STDs) that was so intense in the 1940s and 50s, to the extent that the Bahaya were classified as a "dying people" (Laurie 1958; Sundkler 1980). Generally, the constant and intense in- and outflow of Bahaya and others (e.g., Rwandese and Burundis) created a situation whereby social cohesion was gradually eroded and provided a good environment for the spread of diseases.

While the first sixty years of the 20th century were relatively economically secure, the last four decades have been an economic disaster for the district. This has been due to a combination of socio-economic, biological, and political factors. Poor agricultural policies adopted by Tanzania immediately after independence and the *Ujamaa* policy a few years later, coupled with falling world market prices for coffee, undermined the local agricultural economy (Hyden 1969; Tibaijuka 1984, 1997). The situation further deteriorated due to the 1978–9 Tanzania/Uganda war, which was not only fought in the district but the area remained "a front line" many years afterwards. The war paralyzed the infrastructure (much of it has never been repaired) and brought the economy of Bukoba to its knees. Moreover, heavy infestations of banana weevils and root-rot nematode disease have nearly devastated the banana crop, which for centuries provided a secure means of subsistence (Rugalema et al. 1994), and the near collapse of the Tanzanian economy in the late 1970s to mid-1980s has exacerbated the situation even further.

The declining economic fortunes gave rise to illicit trade, poor medical services and hence reliance on village injectionists (Garret 1994), sex liaisons for the sake of protection and economic provisioning, and high prevalence of STDs. It is against this background that HIV became a generalized epidemic in Bukoba district. The first Tanzanian cases of AIDS were diagnosed in Bukoba district in 1983 (Killewo et al. 1990; World Bank 1992b; Garret 1994) and since then the district has been characterized by high seroprevalence of HIV (de Zalduondo et al. 1989; Killewo 1994). De Zalduondo et al. (1989) cite a study that estimated an HIV seroprevalence rate of about 32.8 percent, while Killewo (1994) has estimated a maximum HIV seroprevalence of 24.5 percent. The 1988 population census shows that Bukoba district had a total of some 318,185 people. Only about 40 percent were adults of 15–64 years of age (Bureau of Statistics 1990). The actual number of AIDS cases is certainly not known (due to underreporting and misdiagnosis). A look at the number of AIDS orphans in the district provides a glimpse of the gravity of the situation. As depicted in Table 14.1, the number of AIDS orphans has been on the increase. More importantly, the rising number of orphans depicts the speed at which adults are succumbing to AIDS.

Villagers talking about AIDS

The term AIDS is widely known to people in the village and so is its Kiswahili equivalent, *ukimwi*. A variety of locally coined terms and euphemisms are also in use and these reflect changes in the perception of AIDS over time. At the very beginning, those who died of AIDS-related symptoms in the villages in Buhaya were mostly Tanzania/Uganda cross-border itinerant traders and their spouses or sexual partners. Cross-border trade, locally referred to as *magendo* (smuggling), reached its peak in the 1978/79–84 period when Tanzania experienced acute shortages of most kinds of goods (Maliyamkono and Bagachwa 1990; Kaijage 1993; Weiss B. 1993). The biggest market (source of goods) was and is still located on the Tanzania/Uganda border at Mutukula and is known as *kikomela*.[2] At that time, one very popular commodity was textiles, of which the most popular brand was *Juliana*.[3] Most *magendo* traders were young men and women from various parts of Bukoba district and beyond. They brought merchandise from Uganda for sale within the region and even across Lake Victoria into the rest of Tanzania. In Bukoba district most of the goods were sold locally in the villages and at weekly markets (locally known as *emijajalo*). Therefore, originally AIDS was known as *Juliana* because it was seen as a disease or affliction of *Juliana* or *magendo* traders. However, as victims of *Juliana* lost so much weight during their illness, the condition was dubbed *silimu* (a corruption of the English word "slim"). From the mid-1980s the term *silimu* became

Table 14.1   *Increase in child-orphaning due to AIDS in Kagera Region*

	Number of orphans			
District	May 1991	March 1992	March 1993	March 1994
Biharamulo	1344	2888	3034	5444
Bukoba(Rural)	**24812**	**26636**	**30262**	**31298**
Bukoba(Urban)	**2409**	**3059**	**3183**	**4714**
Karagwe	4297	4305	7411	9914
Muleba	12206	13447	18271	20306
Ngara	3056	3131	3781	6922
Total	**8121**	**53466**	**65842**	**78598**

Source: TAP (1994)

more dominant, not least because with trade liberalization in both countries, *Juliana* as an article of cross-border trade was no longer fashionable. But *Juliana* the textile brand also stood for the fluid situation in which, in the late 1970s to mid-1980s, wealth was acquired and spent. *Juliana* was a symbol of success, of modernity, and of fashion. *Juliana* traders had money in a district where poverty was already commonplace. Money enabled them to afford leisure, including alcohol and sex. This was not only a new experience, it was an exciting one. It wasn't difficult to get sex either. Most women, divorced or single, needed the money to survive. These were the years of centralized planning and commodity rationing throughout Tanzania. Cash was terribly scarce and probably sex was the only item women could use to buy *Juliana* and other necessities.

Since the late 1980s the preferred name for the disease has been *ekiuka* (a pest). The evolution of the term *ekiuka* is an analogy drawn between HIV infection of the human population on one hand and the infestation of the banana crop by weevils and nematodes on the other. The destructive combination of the weevil and nematodes leads to the falling over of immature banana plants (Walker et al. 1983). Much like AIDS, efforts to control the weevil and nematodes through chemical and other means have so far not borne fruit. As AIDS kills young adults, similarly banana weevil and nematodes kill young banana plants prematurely. As my informants explained, Buhaya is faced by two kinds of *ekiuka*: one pest is destroying the *kibanja* (banana/coffee farm) while the other is destroying human beings. The use of the term

ekiuka has wider implications than a mere comparison between the two afflictions. *Kibanja* is the archetype of Buhaya social stability, production, and reproduction. The demise of the *kibanja* farming system has destabilized the organization of livelihoods and forced people into various activities, including itinerant trade. It has also led to the commercialization of hitherto free goods and services such as the local brew, family and community labor, etc. Respondents claimed that as a result of the demise of *kibanja* and hence more dependence on cash for survival, there is nothing to be had for free. When everything has been commercialized, everyone needs cash to survive, and commercial sex is one part of the solution.

At present, the phrases *ekiuka* and *silimu* are used more or less interchangeably. However, there are other ways in which AIDS is perceived in the village. The increase in human mortality as a result of the disease has led to its being dubbed *lumara bantu* (the exterminator of human beings). Older informants (above the age of 50) perceived AIDS as *lwaka abazaile* (the disease that deprives parents of their children). Under normal circumstances elderly parents were/are cared for by their adult children. The epidemic is seen to reverse this normal course of events, exposing the elderly to insecurity in old age. An old woman crying over the death of her son said that his loss was like being "dumped in the middle of a desert without any kind of support" (*kunagwa omwirungu*). Asked why the old people can't counsel the young ones on issues of sexuality, I was informed that the young generation is unlikely to listen to the old one. Modern life has emasculated the old, yet they are expected to take care of their grandchildren when parents die of AIDS.

Young men (in the age group 17–30) have a different view of AIDS. Here, contracting AIDS is viewed as an "occupational hazard" (*enfuka kugwa omundimilo* or *ekihosho kugwa aki-konya* – the English equivalent of these two Luhaya phrases is "to break the hoe while farming"). Some young people told me quite seriously that they saw AIDS as an affliction of the age that will continue to kill many, but also many will survive, and with time the disease will go away. These views may seem fatalistic or irrational in that it is as if young people have already discounted themselves from the living, or that they are not aware of the dangers of contracting HIV and dying of AIDS. On the other hand, young people's views reflect their desire to go on with life in an environment in which social and economic circumstances are not favorable. They discount fear and anxiety in order to be able to carry on with what they do, even if that means taking some risks. Clearly, what the young people are doing is to assert life in the presence of death, a feature also noted by anthropologists working in war zones (Helander and Richards forthcoming). Young people in the village said that if they became afraid of AIDS they would probably not go out for work or for a drink. But more importantly, they emphasized the boredom that they have to live with. Comparing the 1960s to the 1990s, some middle-aged adults mentioned that people now drink and have sex more than in the 1960s because there is simply not much to do. The village football clubs, village music groups, etc. that were common in the 1960s have all but vanished. There is simply nowhere to spend free time after a day's work except in village pubs (*ebigata*). And when one is drunk the thin line between casual sex and HIV infection is no longer visible.

One of the fundamental impacts of AIDS is the decline in life expectancy. Young people in the village were quite aware that due to HIV few people are living beyond 60 years of age. In a discussion with a group of teenagers there was unanimity that people are dying younger than previously. They remarked that "the time is coming when a 40-year-old will be the oldest man in the village." Young people have

interpreted this trend in their own way. They want to reproduce early so as to leave their mark on the world. So when our discussion turned to the use of condoms for HIV prevention, the group was visibly not in favor of condoms.

On the other hand, (married) women view AIDS as a disease that they have no power either to control or to run away from. Blame was directed at husbands (or men in general) for bringing death "into the bedroom." But women were also quick to add that, being women, there is nothing they could do to stop that, since they are unable to control men. They implied that it was through the behavior of men that the disease is spread. Yet many widows were surreptitiously accused of bringing AIDS and hence death into families. Many of those who have died of AIDS have suffered in silence, without disclosing information on the possible source of their HIV infection and death from AIDS. This leaves ample room for accusation and victimization. The accusations, however, should be seen in the light of gender relations in Buhaya rather than a simple woman–man relationship. In a hierarchical, patrilocal Buhaya society where gender relations are skewed in favor of men, women have no power to question the sexuality of their husbands. Even if a wife knew that her husband was having a relationship outside, she would rather remain quiet than raise her voice. Neither do the prevalent gender relations and power structure allow women to protect themselves from unsafe sex. To have or not to have sex is a man's decision in which a woman has little, if anything, to say. And as I found out, for a woman to talk about condoms in marriage is like talking of abortion in the Vatican!

That Buhaya women are generally socially and economically vulnerable has been thoroughly discussed elsewhere (Swantz 1985). Marriage provides some social and economic security for women. The death of a husband makes the economic life of a widow and her children all the more difficult (see Table 14.2).

In my discussions with widows, most of them longed for remarriage or some kind of relationship that would help them to weather the difficulties imposed by widowhood. Indeed, a good number of widows maintained such relationships. This is a cycle in which HIV

Table 14.2 *Difficulties imposed by widowhood (n = 19)*

Perceived difficulty	Frequency of mention
Lack of cash income	19
Added responsibilities and shortage of labor	15
Neglect by in-laws	16
Worry of loneliness and thinking about deceased husband	19
Reduced consumption of some foodstuffs	14
Lack of enough land	8
Insecurity on land	5

Source: Author's fieldwork notes (discussion with AIDS widows)

infection in the village goes around. Villagers are well aware of it and more so the widows whose husbands have succumbed to AIDS. Yet they were quite clear that without some form of male "economic" protection, their lives would be terribly precarious. "If men don't come, we follow them, we entice them. Otherwise how can we survive without sugar, soap, paraffin, clothing, food, everything?" remarked one of the widows.

In local accounts, young adults have died and are dying of a condition known as AIDS, or *silimu* or *ekiuka*. In public, many villagers prefer to address AIDS as *endwala ya bil'ebi* (the modern-day disease).[4] *Silimu* and *ekiuka* are terms used widely in private, or when not talking about anybody in particular. When addressing the sick or caregivers, the term *ndwala ya bil'ebi* is more widely used. Indeed *silimu* and *ekiuka* are terms that still carry some stigma. Nevertheless, the young as well as the old in the village admit that many of their kinsmen, friends, neighbors, and fellow villagers have died of *silimu* or *ekiuka*. Villagers mentioned that those who get ill and die of AIDS suffer from a combination of symptoms, including chronic diarrhea (*okuharuka*), persistent fever (*okushagwa shwagwa*), vomiting (*okutanaka*), persistent dry cough (*olufuba*), oropharyngeal candidiasis (*ebilonda by'omukanwa*), herpes zooster (*ebilonda by'omubili*), swelling of pelvic lymph nodes (*okuzimba amahasha*), and genital warts (*endwala nkulu*), all of which culminate in a general wasting syndrome (*kuteba kuhwao* or *okusilimu*). The World Health Organization (WHO) diagnoses AIDS based on the combination of symptoms just mentioned (Ndiaye n.d.). I am not indicating any disagreement between science and local opinion on the symptoms of AIDS. What is distinctive

about the local views, however, is the integration of the disease with wider socio-economic problems, as opposed to the prevailing scientific approach in which HIV is seen to cause AIDS and consequently adult mortality. Villagers are not reductionists. Their view is that AIDS and its effects cannot be separated from the wider social and economic environment. So far, this discussion shows that behaviors that are labeled "risky" are shaped by the realities obtaining in the society and that the epidemic is spreading along the socio-economic fault-lines, some of which are as old as society itself. It is through these "lenses" that the HIV pandemic in Bukoba district can be understood and tackled. For more local terminology for the AIDS epidemic, see Box 14.1.

Case Study 2: Agro-Estates in Various Parts of Kenya

The study reported in this section was conducted in five agro-estates in three provinces of Kenya, namely, Nyanza (2), Rift Valley (2), and Eastern (1). I undertook this study between June and September 1998 as a consultancy assignment that was funded by UNDP (HIV and Development Program) and executed by FAO on behalf of the Government of Kenya.[5]

Risk environment and susceptibility to HIV in the agro-estates

Plantation agriculture in Kenya is a legacy of British colonialism. Plantations or agro-estates were owned by white settlers to produce cash/export crops on a much larger scale than was possible under traditional smallholder farming. The general aim was to sustain the colonial state through agricultural exports. The postcolonial government maintained the status quo and to date Kenyan agriculture is still characterized by two sub-sectors, namely, plantations and smallholder farming. Plantations are characterized by large-scale operations and employ a large number of un-skilled and semi-skilled laborers, most of whom live in congested housing estates pro-vided by agro-estate companies. The study found that the susceptibility of agro-estate workers to HIV is rooted in the political econ-omy of the agro-estates as economic units. The research team interviewed agro-estate employ-ees of all cadres and professions (managers to casual laborers) and the findings are discussed below.

It was found that all agro-estates are charac-terized by "high prevalence of commercial sex." Commercial sex in the agro-estates is driven by a number of social and economic forces. Spouse separation for a long period of time featured as one of the most important factors. When men migrate to work in agro-estates, mostly as unskilled workers, they leave their families in the rural areas. For those living hundreds of kilometers from their families, it is difficult, given the low income, to visit their families as frequently as desirable. The majority of (male) workers tend to depend on casual and commercial sex to satisfy their sexual desires.

Also important are the social and economic factors obtaining within and outside the agro-estates. One of these is *gender inequality* among agro-estate employees, particularly in terms of differential earning capacity for women and men. Throughout the entire spectrum of em-ployment, women earn far less than men. In some jobs we found that women's daily wages are just half of men's in a more or less compar-able job. And as women pointed out, most of them are job insecure. Job insecurity creates the need for women to sleep with their bosses in the quest to ensure their survival.[6] But the fact that women earn less (and a good number happen to be sole providers for their house-holds) means that they are driven by economic necessity to sell sex to make ends meet. Com-mercial sex is not limited to within the bound-aries of agro-estates. Much of it takes place just outside the fences of agro-estates, as well as farther away in urban centers.

All the agro-estates we visited are located next to small commercial settlements, also known as shopping centers, and these are the places where most agro-estate employees go to shop. They are also centers of commercial sex. Interviews with commercial sex workers in and around the commercial settlements revealed that HIV is spread by such factors as poverty, scarcity of employment for youth (particularly girls), and broken families. These were said to be the most important factors which have driven women (most of them were girls and women in their late teens and early twenties) to selling sex. In an interview with some com-mercial sex workers in Kisumu town we asked under what circumstances they would be pre-pared to leave the "business." They mentioned a need for a secure livelihood such as a job or small business. These are girls who had dropped out of school due to lack of school fees, lack of moral support from parents, or-phanhood, or a feeling that spending eight years in school is a waste of time if, in the end, there is no job to be had. With no educa-tion that can provide jobs, and no jobs that pay decent wages, they are indeed vulnerable. They told us that they rarely use condoms because they are entirely dependent on the decisions of their customers. Asked if they were not afraid of dying of AIDS, they empha-sized the lack of alternatives for survival. Some of them told us that they barter sex for food, just to survive from one day to the next.

Within the agro-estates there is an acute shortage of recreational facilities for junior staff. Most residential houses have no electri-city and this makes it impossible for workers to use electronic equipment such as music systems, TVs, or VCRs. The workers claimed that they go to commercial centers for recre-ation and to drink beer and that indulgence in commercial sex is a product of beer drinking rather than a conscious decision. All those inside the estates, including senior officers and medical officers, viewed commercial settlements as "risky places," particularly in terms of the high prevalence of STDs and HIV. Yet commercial settlements are an inte-gral part of social life around the agro-estates, and there is a lot of interaction between agro-estate workers and the settlements. For example, some of the workers not housed by companies live in them. Commercial settlements, with their many bars, guest houses, and bustling night life of beer drinking and loud music, provide fertile ground for the transmission of HIV and they invariably act as a bridge through which HIV crosses from the general population to the agro-estate population. The foregoing discussion shows how employees' welfare or rather lack of it, in this case lack of recreational facilities, might expose the workforce to a fatal disease. Provision of a variety of recreational facilities might be a cheaper, long-term HIV prevention strategy for agro-estate employees than any amount of IEC.

Commercial activities inside the agro-estates also promote commercial sex. Agro-estate employees are paid fortnightly. On each payday, traders and hawkers come into the agro-estates to sell a variety of items ranging from bread to clothing. According to farm laborers, some women who come as traders on paydays (selling clothes, for example) end up as commercial sex workers at night, spending a night with their sexual partners in the labor camps and leaving the next morning. Worse still, there is no guarantee that if a "business-woman" sleeps with a particular man on a particular payday she will be able to meet and sleep with him on the next payday. What is obvious, though, is that she will sleep with some man on the next payday.

The fact that sexual activities increase significantly on and immediately after each payday was confirmed by medical personnel who claimed that in the few days following a payday they attend more STD cases than in the days prior to paydays. We were also informed that over the years some AIDS widows (whose husbands had been employees of agro-estates) had settled in the commercial settlements to try to eke a living from petty trading and commercial sex. Asked whether such well-known widows could get sexual customers, the answer was affirmative. "A few months after losing a husband a widow regains her health and beauty," a respondent told us. Such an improvement in health convinces her customers that she is safe and that the husband might have died of illnesses other than HIV-related ones. If he died of HIV, they reason, the wife would also be showing symptoms of the disease. As discussed later on, we found that such discounting of risk is far more widespread than we had expected. We probed further into the factors that lead to widows settling in commercial settlements rather than their rural homes. It emerged that once a husband has died, the widow and her children become socially and economically vulnerable. This is more so if the widow has always lived with her husband at his place of work. Unable to provide for herself and her children and unable to marshal social and economic support from the extended family, a widow decides to migrate (with or without her children) to a commercial settlement or urban center. Her choice to settle in a commercial settlement near an agro-estate where she is well known is driven by the logic of "the devil you know..." A widow expects some form of support from her friends and the colleagues of her late husband if she lives nearby rather than far away. Widows are driven into commercial sex because of poverty and powerlessness.

Food insecurity among village communities in rural Kenya was said to be another reason why young people flock to commercial settlements near agro-estates. Ostensibly they come to these settlements to look for jobs and hence to earn some money to support themselves and, if possible, their needy relatives back home. Agro-estates are perceived as "islands of hope in a sea of want." Salaries might be too low for laborers but at least they are assured of a small income twice a month. Such security does not exist among many semi-subsistence smallholders. While some of the young people are able to get lowly paid jobs as casual workers or semi-permanent staff, many others do not. Those with lowly paid jobs (girls in particular) supplement their low income through casual sex while the unlucky ones survive entirely on commercial sex. It emerged from the interviews with youth that once they turn 18 or so, parents and relatives pressure them to leave home and seek jobs. Girls and boys seem to face the same kind of pressure to leave home but while boys might be able to find some form of employment (formal or informal), girls seem to be more disadvantaged.

In the Eastern province (which is dry and food insecure) we were informed that in years of low rains and hence lean food production, many more girls are driven to commercial sex along the Nairobi–Mombasa highway. Surprisingly, we found that surviving on commercial sex is also common among young men. For example, in the floriculture belt in the Rift Valley province we were informed that young men were in high demand to meet the sexual needs of many single women employed on the flower farms. These "flower moms" entice young men by providing food and accommodation in return for sex.

One of the significant findings is that sexually transmitted diseases (STDs) are common among adults in the agro-estate populations. Medical personnel attributed this state of affairs to a high degree of sharing sexual partners. Medical records revealed that STD-related complaints increase immediately after each payday. There are thus small epidemics of sexually transmitted diseases in the *middle and at the end of the month* which, as explained earlier, indicates that paydays are followed by intensive sex encounters. For example, a medical officer at one of the agro-estates said that he normally attends about 20 cases of STDs a week but this number jumps to 60 cases in the seven days or so after each payday. The most common STDs and reproductive tract infections are gonorrhea, syphilis, clamydia, genital warts, candidasis, and chancroid. Medical personnel insisted that in most cases these diseases manifest a syndromic clinical presentation (meaning that they occur in combination).

Data obtained from health centers around the agro-estates surveyed indicate that STDs are highly prevalent in the general population too. The data we obtained from these health centers clearly show that STDs are common even in young people between 11 and 19 years of age. This indicates sexual encounters at an early age, hardly surprising given the evidence presented in Table 14.3.

General health on the agro-estates

The prevalence of common infectious and contagious diseases in the agro-estates in Kenya is high. The outbreak of disease and the high mortality rates have been attributed to the appalling living conditions of workers and their families on agro-estates. Medical personnel on all the agro-estates surveyed confirmed that preventable diseases other than STDs were very common. Common diseases (from the medical perspective) were said to be malaria, gastrointestinal infections (diarrhea, vomiting, amoebic dysentery... all these were said to be associated with HIV infection), fungal infections (primarily skin diseases), typhoid, and amoebic dysentery. Others are TB (also associated with HIV infection and said to be on the increase), other respiratory tract infections, and cholera (sporadic but persistent epidemics over the years). Other respondents mentioned almost the same types of diseases but with varying emphasis. Women were more concerned with disease afflicting children, youth viewed STDs and AIDS as big problems, while men put emphasis on work-related injuries.

To explain the prevalence of common treatable diseases on agro-estates one has to look at congestion and poor sanitation[7] in the labor camps. Most housing estates are unkempt. Facilities, including toilets, bathroom, laundry, and water taps, are shared on a communal basis, and are insufficient to meet the needs of residents. Respondents claimed that their surroundings were infested with rats and cockroaches and that houses were infested with bed bugs.

In sum, it is worth emphasizing that because of the social and economic conditions obtaining in and around the agro-estates, the majority of the employees (and their dependents) are highly susceptible to HIV infection. The prevalence of STDs, common tropical diseases, casual sex, commercial sex, underemployed/unemployed youth, mixed perceptions on HIV and AIDS, lack of recreation facilities, overcrowding (and hence lack of privacy), high prevalence of other communicable disease, and alcohol (and drug) abuse render agro-estate communities susceptible to HIV.

In general, among agro-estate workers, knowledge about HIV and AIDS is widespread. Respondents were able to mention the modes of HIV transmission, common means of protection, the symptoms of an AIDS patient, and the impact of prolonged illness on AIDS sufferers and their families. In many instances low- and middle-cadre employees were more at

Table 14.3 *Age at first coitus of Kenyan adolescents*

Age at first coitus (years) n = 3,086	Percent
<10	6
10–14	30
15–18	61
19+	3

Source: Youri (ed.) 1993

ease discussing the disease than the managers. Most respondents were also curious to see or obtain information about the *female condom*. It would seem that if introduced, the female condom would be readily accepted. The majority of respondents acknowledged having seen one or more AIDS sufferers. The high level of awareness thus stems from both personal experience and information obtained through the media. Respondents mentioned that brochures, peer educators (where available), newspapers, radio, video/TV, places of worship, and political rallies (known as *baraza* in Kiswahili) were the main sources of information on HIV and AIDS.

Most respondents, regardless of age and gender, were aware of the disease and its implications. A recent study by Nyang' and Obudo (1996) found that 97 percent of the respondents were aware of AIDS. But such awareness is generally not being translated into action, as shown in Box 14.1. Respondents have a range of perceptions about the disease and its control and they legitimize their behavior based on their own perceptions rather than on the IEC messages or other medical information available to them.

Box 14.1 *Respondents' perceptions of HIV/AIDS*

"AIDS does not exist, if it does, it is everywhere and one can't escape it!"

"It is not AIDS, it is Chira/Jinni!"
Cultural perceptions vs. medical perceptions of the disease.

"So what? We will all die anyway!"
Women's fear of their husbands' reaction, if they (women) started talking about AIDS at home.

"Life is a chance, death is a destiny!"
A woman with small children, without any alternative but to eke out a living from commercial sex.

"It is just like stepping on a snake – you never know when or where you gonna meet it … it just happens, you step on it and it bites you."

"The bull dies with the grass in the mouth."
Better death than giving up having sex with a lover you so much desire. Risk taking as an expression of manhood.

"AIDS is just an accident at work."
A commercial sex worker who perceives AIDS as an "occupational hazard."

"Condoms promote extra-marital sex!"
Women's fear of husbands' having more casual sex if condom use is widely encouraged in the country.

"Condoms frequently burst!"
A rather common claim among our respondents.

"Condoms are infected with HIV!"
Common perception; in the Nyanza province this view was said to be publicly promoted by a politician.

"Nyama kwa nyama or Sox (implying condom) is for the feet not for the penis."
Claims that condoms prevent maximization of sexual pleasure were more frequent than we had imagined.

"It is El Niño."
AIDS perceived as a temporary rather than a permanent phenomenon.

Conclusion: HIV Epidemic in Africa, Which Way Forward?

Evidence discussed above shows that the HIV pandemic in Africa is a product of social factors upon which the virus has found fertile ground. However widespread the pandemic is, its "shape" varies from one society to the next largely because different societies are differentially susceptible to HIV transmission. The Buhaya village of Tanzania and the five agro-estates in Kenya might be experiencing the same HIV epidemic but the environment in which the virus spreads is significantly different.

The interrelationship between health, disease, and the social environment is a well-established one (Learmonth 1988) and the African HIV pandemic is a classical case of such interaction between biological and social factors. People living with the pandemic see and explain it in a wider perspective that reflects reality on the ground. They see it as a cross-sectoral issue rather than a narrow medical problem. Unless research and policy begin to address HIV in a context similar to that perceived by those who live with it, prevention efforts are likely to yield only partial success. The HIV pandemic, just like many other diseases before it, is a social event (Stark 1977). The pandemic has shown itself to be a more complex phenomenon than many had expected. To address it, there is a need to go beyond health and the Health Belief Model. HIV research and mitigation strategies have to be more sophisticated and must cut across the narrowly defined disciplinary boundaries. As we move forward, the need to consult widely and to enlist the support and understanding of those who live with the pandemic cannot be overemphasized. It is in this unified understanding of the pandemic that research can shed more light on the theoretical and policy challenges posed by HIV/AIDS.

NOTES

1. When I use the term "people affected by AIDS or people affected by the pandemic" I do not only mean those who have contracted HIV and/or are suffering from AIDS. I use the term in a broader sense to include people living in areas of high HIV prevalence where the risk of contracting the virus is very high but "life has to go on." This therefore includes the infected, the uninfected, and the affected (survivors of those who have died of AIDS).

2. I visited the *kikomela* during the fieldwork. I traveled with one of the orphans from the village who has taken up itinerant trading. Trade is still going on but it is now more liberalized and hence more open. It is therefore no longer called *magendo*.

3. *Juliana* was a polyester fabric from which dresses and even shirts were made. It was popular not because it was cheap but because it was almost the only good quality alternative in a country where shops were literally empty.

4. The way villagers use modernity to conceptualize HIV/AIDS reflects the changes that have happened in the area in the past 100 years or so. I was informed that AIDS is called a modern-day disease because it does not fit into the traditional frame of reference; it is not a disease which they consider to be an indigenous or Buhaya disease (i.e., it is not *kaitu kaila* = ours from time immemorial). AIDS is seen as a disease of modernity whose outbreak and spread hinge on the changing social, economic, and political realities of the 20th century and beyond.

5. The study was conducted by the author as head of mission in collaboration with Ms Silke Weigang (FAO Staff, Rome) and James Mbwika (National Consultant, Fibec, Nairobi). My use of the plural words "we" and "us" in this section refers to these individuals, including myself.

6. Similar experience has been reported in Zimbabwe commercial agriculture where Kay (1997) observes that "foremen tend to lure women in the workforce into sex, in return for favours."

7. We use the concept of sanitation in the broader sense to mean *environmental sanitation*, which refers to the environment not only outside the house but also inside the house. The fumigation of houses to kill cockroaches and bed bugs and the control of rats and other pests both inside and outside the houses should be complemented by cleanliness outside the houses.

Chapter 15

Socioeconomic Obstacles to HIV Prevention and Treatment in Developing Countries: The Roles of the International Monetary Fund and the World Bank

Peter Lurie, Percy Hintzen, and Robert A. Lowe

Introduction

By the year 2000, 90 percent of all HIV infections will have occurred in developing countries (World Health Organization 1992). Worldwide efforts to stem the HIV epidemic have to date emphasized inducing behavior change in individuals at high risk for HIV infection. In this review we argue that social and economic forces have also played a critical role in promoting the spread of HIV, and that these have been largely overlooked in favor of factors that operate at the individual level. The failure to consider all aspects of HIV transmission may be inhibiting our ability to reduce the spread of HIV infection. (Although our discussion focuses on socioeconomic conditions in developing countries, many of the same forces operate in the industrialized world.)

The epidemiology of HIV in developing countries reflects these powerful social and economic factors. HIV seroprevalence is generally highest in urban centers (Nzilambi et al. 1988), along trade routes (Carswell et al. 1989), among commercial sex workers (CSW) (Bonacci 1992), and among male migrant workers

(Parker 1991). These observations can best be understood by considering how social and economic forces predispose to certain risk behaviors, later manifested as HIV infection, rather than as some intrinsic property of the virus. In addition, recent evidence from Canada suggests that low socioeconomic status is an independent predictor of increased mortality from HIV disease, even after controlling for potential confounders such as age, disease stage, and access to health care (Hogg et al. 1994).

To understand these socioeconomic forces, one must consider two related economic concepts: macroeconomic measures and structural adjustment. Macroeconomic measures typically evaluate national economic performance using aggregate indicators such as per capita gross national product (GNP), employment rate in the formal economy, and inflation rate. Modern attempts to improve macroeconomic indices in developing countries fall under the rubric of structural adjustment, a complex of policies that aim to stimulate growth in the private sector and to bolster the export sector in countries suffering balance of payment deficits. In this review we argue that this approach, which took hold in the early 1980s and is spearheaded by the International Monetary Fund (IMF) and the World Bank, may have created conditions favoring the spread of HIV infection.

We are well aware of the hazards of describing the sorts of relationships described in this review as causal. Of necessity, this analysis depends in substantial part on ecological data, which by their nature require caution in interpretation. The legacies of colonialism, corruption, inefficiencies in production, global recession, and numerous other factors have no doubt also played a role in these phenomena. We do not, therefore, seek to posit structural adjustment programs as the sole cause of the relationships described here; in some cases they may have only exacerbated preexisting circumstances or simply failed to reverse adverse trends. Rather, we seek to extend the debate over the determinants of HIV infection in developing countries to include economic policies.

The Historical Origins of Structural Adjustment Programs

Between 1950 and 1973, growth in the economies of industrialized nations increased demand for the exports of developing countries, leading to a considerable expansion in exports from these countries (Murdoch 1980). Thus, many developing countries did not have substantial foreign exchange deficits and some even enjoyed foreign exchange surpluses (Harris 1986). The exports of many developing countries had guaranteed access to industrialized country markets, often at negotiated prices, and for predetermined quantities of goods (Hintzen 1995). Job opportunities for the growing middle class in developing countries expanded in both the public and private sectors. Benefiting from such prosperity, developing countries emulated the social policies of western Europe, providing government support for health, education, and welfare programs.

This relatively favorable economic environment suffered a devastating blow in the early 1970s. The Organization of Petroleum Exporting Countries oil embargo of 1973 quadrupled oil prices, producing a doubling of commodity prices in industrialized countries

and a 43 percent increase in the cost of exports (Girvan 1984). The resulting recession in the industrialized world led to significant decreases in demand for developing country products, and consequently to reductions in the prices and volumes of goods produced in these countries. Because of the inflationary conditions that accompanied the post-1973 recession, many developing countries found themselves with an excess of imports in the face of lagging exports, producing mounting debt (Todaro 1989b).

Initially, most developing countries responded to this loss of income by obtaining foreign credit to pay for vital services and the importing of such essential items as food, medicines, fuels, and raw materials. Because prevailing interest rates in the industrialized economies (particularly the United States) determine the interest rates on outstanding debts paid by developing countries, when inflation due to a second oil shock in 1979 drove interest rates upward (as high as 16 percent in the United States in 1981), developing country borrowing could no longer be sustained (Gillis et al. 1992). Debtor countries borrowing at flexible rates or seeking to refinance loans found themselves with enormous, unpredictable interest payments. An international recession in 1980 and 1981 further decreased demand for developing country export commodities (Gillis et al. 1992).

In 1982, private industrialized country lenders decided that further loans to developing countries were too risky and severely limited credit to many developing countries (Feinberg 1992; Frieden 1991). Rocked by economic crisis, developing countries were forced to turn to the IMF for loans to cover their foreign debts. This assistance came at the price of agreeing to "stabilization programs," an early form of structural adjustment. Under these programs, developing countries were forced to enter into agreements to meet specified macroeconomic targets – first with the IMF and later with the World Bank (Dell 1984). One critical element of both IMF and World Bank loans is that, unlike loans from private banks, these agencies cannot reschedule debt (i.e., allow a country more time to pay the principal and interest on its debt).

While IMF loans usually emphasize short-term stabilization, aiming to reduce inflation as well as budget and trade deficits, World Bank adjustment programs seek to remove economic distortions over the long term (Anonymous 1993a). Because the IMF offers both stabilization and adjustment programs, and because entering into an agreement with either the IMF or the World Bank is often a condition for lending from the other institution (Anonymous 1993a), we discuss both programs together under the term structural adjustment programs (SAP).

During the 1980s, the IMF, the World Bank, bilateral aid agencies, and private international banks increasingly cooperated to set similar preconditions for all forms of international credit. Developing countries, especially poorer ones, were often forced to enter into SAP in order to obtain IMF or World Bank loans and sometimes even as a precondition for borrowing on private financial markets (Harris 1988). Indeed, the incorporation of policies associated with SAP has become a leading criterion for assessing developing country creditworthiness. Consequently, many developing countries were compelled to institute their own "home-grown" economic recovery programs that included the structural adjustment elements advocated by the IMF and the World Bank (Loewenson 1993), amplifying these institutions' impact on the developing world economy and blurring distinctions between SAP and non-SAP countries.

In summary, worsening developing country debtor status over the last two decades created economic conditions that permitted industrialized countries to impose SAP. While some policy elements of SAP existed prior to the debt crisis, SAP for the first time consolidated and coordinated these macroeconomic policies, and then applied them in a manner that gave developing countries little choice other than to drastically restructure their economies along the lines mandated by the programs.

The Characteristics of SAP

SAP typically include eight components: (1) concessions to foreign investors, including tax incentives and tariff elimination; (2) economic and trade liberalization, often exposing developing country producers to competition from imported goods; (3) stimulation of economic activity directed toward export rather than toward domestic demand; (4) currency devaluation leading to higher prices for imported goods; (5) curbs on consumption in developing countries by making loans more expensive and less available; (6) increases in the prices of goods and services to bring them in line with world market prices; (7) personal income and consumption tax increases; and (8) reductions in government spending, including cut-backs in health and social services. In summary, these measures seek to stimulate the growth of the private and export sectors in developing countries (Stiglitz 1993), thus making their economies more competitive on the international market. From the industrialized country perspective, they enhance the security of loans, benefiting international lenders and others involved in trade with developing countries.

The expansion of SAP has been rapid. Whereas in 1980 only three sub-Saharan African countries were involved in World Bank SAP, in 1989 this had increased to 20 countries (Figure 15.1). Thirty-two of 44 sub-Saharan African countries entered into a World Bank SAP at some time between 1980 and 1990 (Elmendorf and Roseberry 1993). Worldwide, a total of 89 developing countries received 241 World Bank structural adjustment loans and 325 IMF stabilization or structural adjustment loans between 1980 and 1991 (Bello et al. 1994). At present, approximately one-quarter (about U.S. $5 billion) of annual World Bank lending is in the form of SAP (Elmendorf and Roseberry 1993).

An important consequence of these loan policies has been spiraling debt in the developing world, largely due to interest payments on loans. Total developing world debt rose from U.S. $562 billion in 1982 to 1020 billion in 1988 (Kanji et al. 1991); in sub-Saharan Africa debt now exceeds the region's annual GNP (Anonymous 1993a). Dependence on IMF and World Bank loans increased over the 1980s, until in 1988 40 percent of sub-Saharan Africa's U.S. $218 billion debt was owed to these two institutions (Kanji et al. 1991). While in 1979 there was a net flow of U.S. $40 billion from

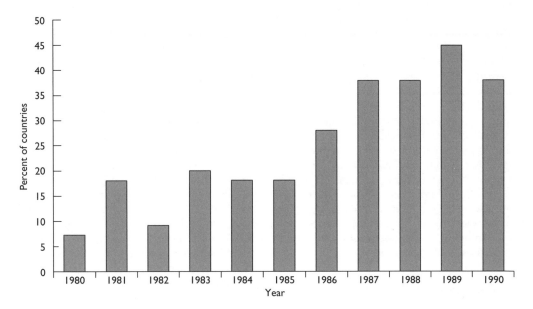

Figure 15.1 *Percentage of sub-Saharan African countries (n = 44) with World Bank structural adjustment programs 1980–90*
Source: Data adapted from Elmendorf and Roseberry 1993.

industrialized to developing countries, interest payments soon outstripped new loans, and by the end of the 1980s U.S. $60 billion was being transferred in the opposite direction annually (Kanji et al. 1991).

Ironically, even on the macroeconomic indices emphasized by the IMF and the World Bank, the performance of sub-Saharan African countries has been less than stellar. For example, per capita GNP in the 44 poorest countries had an average annual growth of 1.2 percent between 1965 and 1980; between 1980 and 1987 there was an average annual decrease of 1 percent in this index (United Nations Development Program 1990). The real value of exports from sub-Saharan Africa declined by 0.8 percent annually between 1982 and 1987 (Kanji et al. 1991).

Furthermore, a frequent result of the focus on national macroeconomic measures is to ignore other economic indices, such as poverty, unemployment, and income distribution. In the 1980s, per capita income in sub-Saharan Africa fell by over one-quarter and in most countries in the region unemployment increased (Kanji et al. 1991). In 1985, almost one-third of the population of developing countries, more than 1 billion people, were living below the World Bank-defined poverty level (World Bank 1990). If present trends continue, the share of income accruing to the poorest 40 percent of the population in developing countries will drop from 9.8 percent in 1975 to 6.5 percent by the year 2000 (Todaro 1989b).

These problems are particularly acute in sub-Saharan Africa. In Nigeria, a country that entered into seven IMF and World Bank SAP beginning in 1983 (Elmendorf and Roseberry 1993; Bello et al. 1994), oil exports were largely responsible for the 6.9 percent average annual growth in GNP between 1965 and 1980. However, by the mid-1980s living standards had fallen precipitously and were lower than they had been in the 1950s. GNP actually decreased at an average annual rate of 1.1 percent between 1980 and 1988. Similarly, while private consumption increased at an average annual rate of 5 percent between 1965 and 1980, it decreased at an average annual rate of 0.1 percent between 1980 and 1988. These latter trends, which were doubtless the result of many interacting social and economic factors including SAP, have intensified during the 1990s as the debt crisis worsens (World Bank 1990).

In recent years the World Bank has sought to limit the adverse social consequences of SAP by becoming more involved in health care issues. These areas include HIV prevention and treatment (U.S. $600 million in loans between 1986 and 1994) (Brown 1994), developing employment and training programs, and targeting health and educational programs toward disadvantaged groups. However, these efforts have been criticized as coming too late, being too limited in scope, too reliant upon the private sector, and consequently as reinforcing a two-tier health care system (Loewenson 1993; Bose 1994).

The Impact of SAP on the HIV Epidemic

The effects of these SAP have been documented by the United Nations Children's Fund (UNICEF) and others (Sanders and Sambo 1991; Anonymous 1990; Cornia et al. 1987). Four phenomena that may result from SAP have conspired to undermine the social fabric of many developing countries, potentially promoting behaviors that place their citizens at increased risk for HIV infection: (1) declining sustainability of the rural subsistence economy; (2) development of a transportation infrastructure; (3) migration and urbanization; and (4) reductions in spending on health and social services.

Declining sustainability of the rural subsistence economy

Currency devaluation, investment concessions, and other efforts to promote exports under SAP disrupt rural subsistence economies. Small farmers and craftspeople find themselves facing stiff and sophisticated foreign competition as declines in local income shrink the demand for their products. The shift to large-scale export agriculture, logging, and mining displaces rural subsistence producers. The rural population thus becomes a cheap labor pool for export manufacturing activities (which tend to be concentrated in large cities), export agriculture, and mining, and

people in rural areas are often forced to leave their families in search of work. Those who remain in the rural areas often depend on remittances from their migrant family members. Ultimately, these migration patterns may be linked to the spread of HIV, as we discuss below.

Even some agricultural exports undermine the rural economy. Small-scale subsistence farming is displaced to less fertile land (Hunt 1989) and the production of food for local consumption is replaced by the production of commodities suitable for export or for consumption by the growing urban population (Sadik 1992). Much of the wealth generated by agricultural exports does not devolve to the farmer; instead it is expropriated by urban international traders and later by industrialized country investors who benefit from the value added once these commodities arrive in the industrialized world. The need to purchase increasingly expensive agricultural materials further undermines the viability of the rural agrarian economy (Packard and Epstein 1991).

Between 1969 and 1985, per capita food production declined in 51 developing countries and increased in only 43. This decline led to deteriorations in food self-sufficiency, with cereal imports increasing substantially. Furthermore, food prices increased significantly, in part because of currency devaluation programs under structural adjustment (Sadik 1992). These factors may contribute to declines in nutritional status, potentially increasing the risk for HIV seroconversion (Moore et al. 1993).

Development of a transportation infrastructure

Transportation networks that developed in the 1980s (often as explicit components of SAP) tended to support the export-led economies promoted by SAP rather than the commercial or personal needs of subsistence farmers. Thus, networks connecting outlying areas to export centers (rather than to other outlying areas) developed, connecting rural areas to urban centers with high HIV seroprevalences. This facilitates permanent or seasonal migration to large cities by rural dwellers searching for wage employment.

Transportation routes may also facilitate the spread of HIV as truck drivers and other workers carry the virus from the cities to casual partners along the roadways (Carswell et al. 1989). At Kenyan truck stops, young girls often have intercourse with truck drivers and local boys have sex with the same CSW who serve the truck drivers (S. Nzyuko 1993, pers. comm.). In Tanzania, HIV infections cluster around truck stops, fishing camps, mining centers, and refugee camps (Okie 1992). High seroprevalences of HIV among truck drivers have also been reported in Kenya (Bwayo et al. 1991), the Sudan (Burans et al. 1990), and Nigeria (Gashau et al. 1992). Similarly, Abidjan, an international business hub and major port in Côte d'Ivoire, is a focal point of the HIV epidemic in west Africa (De Cock et al. 1989).

In India, 64–82 percent of truck drivers frequent CSW (Black et al. 1992; Ahmed 1992; Singh et al. 1992). Almost all the truck drivers on the Delhi–Bombay route have contracted sexually transmitted diseases (STD) at one time, and 6 percent of the truck drivers in one study were HIV positive, with projected increases to 30 percent within 5 years (Black et al. 1992).

Migration and urbanization

Structural adjustment and other development programs may also contribute to increasing HIV risk behavior by promoting urbanization, a phenomenon that preceded SAP but has been hastened by these programs' emphasis on export activity, which is usually concentrated in urban areas (Sanders and Sambo 1991; Hunt 1989). The annual urban population growth rate for sub-Saharan Africa between 1960 and 1990 was 5.2 percent, higher than in any region in the world (United Nations Development Program 1991). For developing countries as a whole, urban populations are increasing 3.6 percent per year – 4.5 times faster than urban populations in industrialized countries and 60 percent faster than rural populations in developing countries (Sadik 1992). While some of this increase was due to natural growth in developing country urban population size, 39 percent of the increase is estimated to result from migration (Harpham 1986).

These migration trends have profound implications for patterns of sexual relations. Male migrant workers may leave a single sexual partner in the countryside for multiple casual partners in the city. Indeed, in a study of male factory workers in Zimbabwe, HIV-positive men were more likely to live apart from their wives and to have multiple sexual partners than HIV-negative men (Bassett et al. 1990). Women in rural areas remain dependent on their male partners for financial support, decreasing the women's ability to negotiate for safe sex when the men return to the rural areas, and fostering the spread of HIV from cities to rural areas (Huband 1991). Women who remain in rural areas for protracted periods without their male partners may also take other partners, increasing their HIV risk (Packard and Epstein 1991).

Lack of adequate employment opportunity has forced workers from Botswana, Malawi, Swaziland, and Mozambique to seek work in South African mines; significant prevalences of HIV infection among blacks in South Africa were first detected among these migrant workers (Lone 1987). In Zambia, a country with nine IMF or World Bank structural adjustment loans between 1980 and 1991 (Bello et al. 1994), the Copper Belt contains 45 percent of reported AIDS cases, far greater than the percentage of the Zambian population that lives there (United Nations Development Program 1990; Black et al. 1992). Camps for predominantly male migrants working in the mining and forestry industries in Australia, Papua New Guinea, Malaysia, and Indonesia may also predispose to encounters with CSW (Moodie and Aboagye-Kwaneng 1993).

Events in Thailand, which had five IMF or World Bank structural adjustment loans between 1980 and 1991 (Bello et al. 1994), illustrate a possible cascading relationship between rural impoverishment, urbanization, and HIV infection. Road construction, reforestation projects, and logging encroach on the land of the rural population by turning vast areas of the countryside over to corporate interests. The rural population has become poorer, forcing them to migrate to urban centers such as Chiang Mai, where the HIV epidemic has been particularly severe (Nelson et al. 1993; Celentano et al. 1994). Faced with a declining rural economy and a paucity of jobs for women in urban centers (Hunt 1989), 1 million Thai women have gravitated to the sex industry, while men can earn money in the drug trade and may initiate drug use themselves (Kammeren and Symonds 1992). The HIV seroprevalence is 65 percent among some groups of CSW in Chiang Mai (Celentano et al. 1994) and 43 percent among injecting drug users in Bangkok (Choopanya et al. 1991). CSW who test HIV positive may be sent back to the rural areas where they originally lived, reducing their access to health care services and potentially introducing HIV into these regions (Sachs 1994).

Large-scale migration of CSW from poorer to richer countries is also common and may spread HIV infection. Approximately 10,000 Thai CSW work in Japan, while women from Laos, Myanmar (formerly Burma), and southern China engage in commercial sex work in Thailand (Moodie and Aboagye-Kwaneng 1993).

SAP also advocate increased investment in the tourist industry as a means for earning foreign exchange and meeting macroeconomic targets. Foreign tourists may have been instrumental in spreading HIV in some areas through sex with CSW (Smith 1990). In Thailand, sex tourism from Europe, North America, Australia, and Japan is common and, at least in the past, condoms were rarely used (Wilke and Kleiber 1991).

Brazil, which has one of the highest total foreign debts in the developing world and which received seven IMF or World Bank structural adjustment loans between 1980 and 1991 (Bello et al. 1994), also illustrates the role of commercial sex work as a link between poverty and HIV. There are now 8 million Brazilian children out of school, in part because the state decreased spending on education, and children were forced to enter the informal economy. With escalating poverty rates came an increase in child abandonment; many of these children were forced into commercial sex work to survive and may have initiated drug use. The prevalence of HIV infection among one sample of street children was 9 percent and is likely to increase (Perlman 1992). In many parts of the globe, demand for child prostitutes has increased as men seek partners less likely to be HIV-infected (Sachs 1994).

Reductions in spending on health and social services

While SAP create circumstances that could encourage high-risk behavior, they also decrease the resources available to reduce those behaviors and to treat HIV infection and its complications. Tax reductions and other concessions to foreign investors have decreased government revenues in many developing countries. Scarce government resources are frequently allocated to meet the infrastructural needs of foreign investors rather than the health and welfare needs of the local population, and consequently many services and facilities have been eliminated, particularly in poorer regions. Between 1980 and 1985 there was a 26 percent decline in spending on health, education, and welfare in sub-Saharan Africa (United Nations Development Program 1990). Spending on education for all low-income developing countries (excluding India and China) declined from 21 percent of national budgets in 1972 to 9 percent in 1988, and health spending dropped from 5.5 to 2.8 percent of national budgets over the same period (United Nations Development Program 1990). Because levels of per capita social spending were extremely low prior to the debt crisis, these figures are even more telling. The average annual per capita health-care expenditure by African governments at the beginning of the 1990s was U.S. $2 (Weeks 1992).

As a result, only 2.8 percent of global expenditures for HIV prevention go to sub-Saharan Africa, which contains 10 percent of the world's population and accounts for two-thirds of the world's HIV infections (Anonymous 1992, 1993b). The United States federal government spends U.S. $2.95 per capita annually for HIV prevention, a sum many would regard as insufficient, but still far greater than the U.S. $0.07 devoted to this task by governments in sub-Saharan Africa (Cameron and Shepard 1992). Under these circumstances, it is almost impossible to launch an effective campaign to reduce high-risk behavior or to provide resources such as condoms and sterile needles for preventing HIV transmission. High rates of illiteracy, in part the consequence of diminished educational expenditures, further reduce the effectiveness of HIV prevention programs that depend upon written materials (Chowdhury 1991).

While numerous economic studies have focused on the impact of HIV infection on developing country economies (Nabarro and McConnell 1989; Over 1992; Rowley et al. 1990), less attention has been paid to the huge potential savings that could be realized if HIV prevention activities were adequately funded. In 1993, the World Health Organization (WHO) estimated that a comprehensive HIV prevention program, which would include condom promotion and distribution, treatment of STD, education programs in the schools and media, screening of the blood supply, and needle exchange programs, could cut the cumulative number of HIV infections in the developing world in half (by 9.5 million infections) by the turn of the century. WHO estimated that a program of this sort would cost U.S. $2.5 billion per year but would save U.S. $90 billion in the direct and indirect costs of HIV infection by the year 2000 (Global AIDS News 1993).

Developing countries have been forced to charge fees for previously free medical treatment services (McAfee 1991), sometimes with devastating results. For example, when the World Bank mandated that Kenya impose charges of U.S. $2.15 for STD clinic services, attendance fell 35–60 percent, potentially increasing the burden of untreated STD and thereby increasing the risk of HIV transmission (Moses et al. 1992; Manji et al. 1992; Creenblatt et al. 1988). Similar decreases in clinic utilization following increases in user fees have been reported in Mozambique, Zaire, Ghana, and Zimbabwe (Kanji 1989; De Bethune et al. 1989; Waddington and Enyimayew 1989; Logie 1993). The Bamako Initiative, which advocates charging developing country residents for essential pharmaceuticals and using the proceeds to purchase more drugs, has been similarly criticized for potentially leading to the denial of critical health services (Kanji 1989; Anonymous 1988).

Decreased access to health services may have important implications for health status. In the northern Nigerian region of Zaria, the government reduced subsidies and introduced user fees. The 56 percent increase in the number of maternal deaths following these changes has been attributed to the Nigerian SAP (Ekwempu et al. 1990).

Treatment resources for the HIV-infected are also scarce. Whereas the United States spends U.S. $32,000 per year to treat each AIDS patient, sub-Saharan African countries average under U.S. $400 per patient per year (Cameron and Shepard 1992). Declining health expenditures, currency devaluation, and foreign exchange shortages have contributed to severe pharmaceutical shortages in many African countries, including Zambia, Uganda, and The Gambia (Sanders and Sambo 1991). In most developing countries, the cost of drugs to treat HIV and its complications is prohibitive and zidovudine or other antiretroviral drugs are essentially unavailable (De Cock et al. 1993). Resources for treating STD are similarly limited, although some recent World Bank loans have included funding for this purpose (Elmendorf and Roseberry 1993).

State cut-backs in health care spending can also lead to the emigration of professionals, technicians, and managers as their jobs are eliminated, their conditions of work deteriorate, and their costs of living escalate. Medical personnel, whose skills are in high demand on the international market, often leave their countries of origin at times when they are most needed. The number of foreign nurses admitted to the United States increased from 4,701 in 1982 to 16,237 in 1990, with most coming from developing, particularly Asian, countries (American Medical Association 1990). Fifty-six percent of migrating physicians in the world emigrate from developing countries and fewer than 11 percent of all migrating physicians have other developing countries as their destinations. In Jamaica, the efflux of nurses, many of whom had been trained using Jamaican government funds, was so substantial that nursing vacancy rates exceeded 50 percent, forcing the Ministry of Health to close wards and reduce services (World Bank 1993b).

The breakdown of health delivery systems that may accompany SAP also inhibits surveillance and testing for HIV. In many clinics in East and Central Africa, for example, patients are treated solely on the basis of their clinical findings, without even rudimentary laboratory support or HIV serotesting (Cameron and Shepard 1992). Even HIV screening of blood used for transfusion can be limited; in some countries only 50 percent of blood transfusions were screened (Cohen 1992). Funding shortages also encourage the reuse of disposable syringes, potentially contributing to HIV transmission (Mann et al. 1986).

Toward an Alternative Development Strategy

The preceding discussion highlights the need for social and economic interventions in stemming the spread of HIV and in treating those infected. While biomedical scientists worldwide have risen to meet the challenges offered by the HIV epidemic, the socioeconomic aspects of the epidemic have often been ignored. For HIV transmission in developing countries to be substantially reduced, economic policies that may have promoted disease spread must be modified.

What are the elements of an alternative development strategy? First, the satisfaction of basic human needs such as food, housing, and transport must become a primary goal; this can be accomplished in large part by reducing spending on military and luxury commodities (Stewart 1989). A relatively inexpensive example of this would be altering long-distance truck drivers' work schedules so that they spend less time away from home, potentially decreasing the frequency of sexual contact with casual partners. Second, to ensure regional self-sufficiency, emphasis should shift from the production of a small number of primary commodities for export to the diversification of agricultural production (Anonymous 1993a; Kanji et al. 1991; Logie and Woodroffe 1993). Third, marginal producers and subsistence farmers must be supported. Thus, large infrastructure projects that are often environmentally destructive and socially disruptive must be de-emphasized and more attention paid to smaller-scale projects using appropriate technology (Anonymous 1993a; French 1994). Fourth, because the economic value added in the production process results largely from the technological innovations that occur in industrialized countries, greater emphasis must be placed on human resource development in developing countries (Anonymous 1993a; Loewenson 1993). Fifth, the kind of paternalistic "top-down" approach favored by the IMF and the World Bank must make way for a truly cooperative development policy, in which the desires of developing country citizens can be heard (Kanji et al. 1991; Logie and Woodroffe 1993). Finally, the charters of the IMF and the World Bank must be altered to permit the cancellation or rescheduling of debt. In the meantime, those institutions should play a leading role in the restructuring of debt owed to private lenders (Logie and Woodroffe 1993).

HIV infection will be an unwelcome guest for the foreseeable future. In recognition of this, the IMF and the World Bank should require AIDS Impact Reports (analogous to the now common Environmental Impact Reports), which would require the parties to any loan agreement to explicitly stipulate the potential impact of the proposed loan on HIV transmission.

In closing, the advice of one commentator bears heeding: "[The] epidemic of HIV-1 seropositivity [in Africa] is a social event, not simply a biological occurrence. Although a biological understanding of HIV-1 is necessary, it is inadequate. The epidemic of HIV-1 seropositivity and AIDS in Africa must be understood socially, in its historically specific context, or not at all" (Hunt 1989).

ACKNOWLEDGMENT

The authors would like to thank Norman Hearst, Jeff Mandel, Mark Lurie, and the Institute for Health Policy Studies Writing Group for their thoughtful comments on earlier drafts of this manuscript. This paper first appeared in *AIDS* 9 1995, pp. 539–546 and is reproduced here by permission from the publishers of *AIDS*.

Part IV

Research Methods, Agendas, and Ethics

Introduction to Part IV

The predominance of top-down research in both biomedical and social scientific studies of AIDS is increasingly being recognized as having limited potential for shaping effective interventions because it overlooks the ways in which individuals themselves understand and subsequently negotiate HIV risk. There has consequently been a move away from the objectification of individuals and their sexual practices toward bottom-up research that incorporates individuals as agents who have much to say about AIDS and their location within the coordinates of risk. Kesby's chapter beautifully illustrates the insights proffered from a participatory observation approach when women diagram their own perspectives on risk, priorities for change, and possibilities for intervention. Kesby's documentation and analysis of these diagrams provide not only a wealth of information about women's own perceptions of risk and intervention, but also stand as an exemplar of how powerful participatory methods can be. As he suggests, it also counters critical assessments of participatory approaches that focus on their limitations rather than potential. Kesby's skillful use of participatory diagraming resonates with the growing call for "less study and more action" in the fight against AIDS by showing more clearly the possibilities for facilitating change.

Baylies in her chapter discusses the obstacles in doing community-based research that come primarily in the form of intractable funding requirements. By demanding study designs centered upon quantitative techniques and scientific "rigor," funding agencies overlook the promise of smaller-scale community studies utilizing interviews and ethnographic approaches. Yet Baylies also goes on to problematize community research itself, particularly in the context not just of high HIV/AIDS prevalence but of chronic poverty whereby "research," however bottom-up, is not always what is needed. Funding for a variety of social concerns is needed, and Baylies gives a poignant example of when researchers in a pilot study showed up at an appointed time only to find that participants assumed them to be beneficiaries rather than researchers with nothing but questions to offer. She also asks hard questions about how the benefits from research findings are to be made effectively available to the communities concerned. Baylies' chapter thus problematizes the sometimes overly romanticized notions of community research, while not vitiating the potential that reflexive, well-designed community research nevertheless retains.

Craddock's piece critiques the ethics of how medical knowledge about AIDS is sometimes produced. In part due to the greater regulation of human subjects' research in the U.S., clinical trials are frequently conducted with U.S. funding and principal investigators, but with subjects recruited within poor countries. Though there are sometimes good reasons for this,[1] the primary rationale for this division of labor parallels other sectors of the global economy where cheap "labor," lax regulations, and reduced costs reign supreme over concern for individual welfare. In the case of the AZT trials investigated by Craddock, designs that would not have been approved within the U.S. but were implemented in several African countries raise questions concerning what a global ethics of medical research should look like. More visible in the global spotlight is the related issue of drug pricing. Because the high prices of life-prolonging antiretroviral drugs (ARVs) have made them available to less than 5 percent of individuals with AIDS in poor countries (World Health Organization 2002), intense controversy has been generated over the legitimacy of patent regulations when so many lives are at stake. The World Health Organization has recently placed many ARVs on their list of essential medicines, which will aid somewhat in making these drugs available to those who need them. It will not, however, solve the problem of access. What these two cases of clinical trials and drug pricing point toward is the fact that AIDS is not just an epidemic but an industry. With researchers increasingly contracting with biotech and pharmaceutical firms and resources going into products that sell rather than save lives, trenchant questions are being raised about the implications of corporatizing medicine for AIDS and other global diseases with little profit potential.

NOTE

1. Since different subtypes of HIV pertain in different regions, for example, some trials specifically investigating a particular subtype would need to be located in the relevant region.

Chapter 16

Participatory Diagraming and the Ethical and Practical Challenges of Helping Africans *Themselves* to Move HIV Work "Beyond Epidemiology"

Mike Kesby

Introduction: The Social Embeddedness of HIV in Sub-Saharan Africa

Mobilized through various processes of body fluid exchange, the HIV virus can infect the human body regardless of its age, race, class, gender, or sexuality and is doing so on a global scale. Why then are 70 percent of the cases of both HIV and AIDS concentrated in sub-Saharan Africa? (UNAIDS 2001b). We can begin to answer this question using a biomedical lens at the scale of individual bodies. HIV is primarily transmitted through sexual intercourse but not every coupling between an infected and uninfected body is equally at risk of transmitting the virus. Rates of transmission in a population will increase in line with the frequency of *unprotected* couplings and the complexity of sexual networks. Bodies that are ruptured in the genital area due to untreated STDs are much more likely to transmit or receive HIV. Once an infected body's immune system becomes impaired, it will succumb more rapidly to opportunistic infection if that body is malnourished, frequently exposed to virulent disease, or fails to ingest

compounds that suppress related infections or the virus itself. On this biotic account then, bodies located on the African continent are disproportionately at risk from HIV/AIDS.[1] In Zimbabwe, for example, while overall contraceptive use is relatively high, most is non-barrier and regular use of the male condom is very low. STDs are pervasive and the accompanying sores and ulcers facilitate transmission of HIV. Multiple partnering and payment for casual sex is common among men of all ages, marital status, and social class. Poverty is growing and health funding declining as structural adjustment policies bite and political and economic crises loom (see Adamchak et al. 1990; Ankrah 1996; Boohene et al. 1991; Civic and Wilson 1996; Gregson et al. 1997a; Latif et al. 1989; Mbizvo and Adamchak 1992; Moyo et al. 1993; Runganga et al. 1992; Wilson et al. 1990). Thus scaling HIV only at the corporeal level ignores the broader political, economic, social, and cultural phenomena that unequally position human bodies in relation to the risk and consequences from HIV infection. Therefore, while analysis might begin by focusing through a biomedical lens, a complementary social scientific lens is necessary if a three-dimensional understanding of the global pandemic's concentration in Africa is to emerge.

What contribution then might social scientific research make? All too many possible lines of enquiry exist. The one pursued here is an investigation of the role that regionally specific gender relations play in the transmission of HIV. In this task extreme caution is required, however, especially from a white, European, middle-class intellectual. Sex must always be analyzed in context, not judged against idealized models. In the African context (while generalization are always dangerous, and this chapter is based on the Zimbabwean case), we can say that culturally, sex is seen in terms of reciprocity (men promise material support but not fidelity to their partners), has never been confined to marriage (nor marriage to monogamy), and has always been intimately associated with reproduction. Indeed, fertility is so central to heterosexual identity that even serodiscordant married couples feel obliged to have unprotected sex in order to conceive. Historically, the geographical division and social dislocation associated with colonial migrant labor systems instigated now-persistent patterns of multiple partnering and payment for sex by men. Economically, many African women's continued dependence on resources controlled by men means that they habitually demand material recompense for their sexual services. Sex becomes yet more commodified for women, whose survival strategies include seeking multiple boyfriends, pursuing serial monogamy with informal husbands, or entering fully commercialized sex work. Analysis must be cognizant of these contextually specific experiences and meanings if it is to be accurate and have practical utility (see Ankrah 1991; Bassett and Mhloyi 1991; Caldwell et al. 1989; Gage and Meekers 1994; Jochelson et al. 1991; Meursing 1997; Meursing and Sibindi 1995; Schoepf 1993).

The Ethics of Social Scientific Research on HIV

Nevertheless, while absolutely vital, such cultural sensitivity can seem simultaneously to negate the very possibility of research in this field. In the swirling wake of the self-reflexive turn, social scientific research on HIV in rural southern Africa might seem hopelessly compromised by ethical and epistemological dangers. The unequal power-relations inherent in academic enquiry, the unbridgeable positional differences between researcher and researched, and the impossibility of transparent representation all threaten to stultify investigation (e.g., see Callaway 1992; Clifford 1986; Stacey 1991; Staeheli and Lawson 1994). These perils notwithstanding, from the perspective of researched subjects themselves, engagement in research on HIV in rural Africa might seem a lot less dangerous than actually engaging in unprotected sex in the same context. Similarly, while unequal, the power-relations endemic to a social science research project are unlikely to be the most oppressive that respondents will have encountered, nor indeed the most hazardous. In Zimbabwe, for example, gender fundamentally and unequally structures lives and constructs rural women as deferent and dependent "outsiders" in households owned by men (see Kesby 1999). In this power-filled context, steadily improving knowledge of HIV has failed to facilitate behavioral change. Only commercial sex workers have thus far developed the leverage to ensure that their (paying) partners use condoms. Most African women have great difficulty communicating about safe sex with their partners and a veil of silence surrounds HIV and AIDS at the domestic and local scales. While men are no less the victims of HIV, their existing understandings of masculinity, dominance of heterosexual relations, failure to take the safe-sex initiative, and frequent use of sexual coercion mean that they bear unequal responsibility for transmitting the virus. Thus, while cultural sensitivity and reflexivity in research are critical, they cannot be allowed to stultify research. Existing behaviors cannot go unchallenged nor can historically produced and relatively unstable contemporary gender relations be allowed to blind people to the possibility of future change (see Adamchak et al. 1990; Ankrah 1991; Bassett and Mhloyi 1991; Baylies and Bujra 1997; Kesby 2000a; McFadden 1992; Meursing 1997; Meursing et al. 1995; Ngugi et al. 1996; Reid 1996b; Schoepf 1993; Ulin 1992; Vos 1994; Wilson et al. 1990).

It is therefore not that self-reflexivity is unimportant, but rather that our concern with it has become disproportionate to the impact it actually has on the lives of the researched themselves. The obsession with what we can *know* through our research has left enquiry into what we can *do* through it neglected. Those privileged enough to spend time contemplating lives more dangerous than our own miss a fundamental dimension of self-reflexivity if we neglect to inspect our own potential capacity to facilitate change in those lives, not merely represent them. Ironically then, despite our myriad other differences, a little discussed *academic* positionality unites all who reflect on reflexivity. Too often we end up locating *ourselves* and our *texts* at the center of the research process (conceived as being between researcher and researched) even as we attempt to make room for the other (see Nast 1994). What remains at the margin of autocentric critiques of research are the relationships between researched people themselves and efforts to make these a central feature of what the research process might be about. What is missed in the struggle to open spaces for the contestation of meaning in text is the realization that researchers can also work to open up material and discursive arenas for such contestation in the field. My point is not that we abandon the insights offered by poststructural textual critique, but that we restructure its geography and struggle to negotiate its implication in action-oriented fieldwork praxis. When the issues under investigation is as appalling as HIV in Africa, the ethics of post-structural methodology need to extend beyond simply recording the nuances of multiple voices in texts. A major goal for future research should be the development of approaches that facilitate African people's *own* critical reflection on, and communication about, sexual behavior, even as we study it.

In the case of Zimbabwe, several exciting action-oriented projects have already been undertaken, using focus groups and one-to-one counseling (see Civic and Wilson 1996; Meursing 1997; Meursing et al. 1995; Ray et al. 1996; Wilson et al. 1990). Further work is necessary, however, since the benefits of initiatives with special groups (e.g., commercial sex workers, factory workers, and people testing

positive at urban hospitals) are not "trickling down" to the community generally because of the continued veil of silence surrounding HIV. More work is also necessary in rural communities where the majority live and where sexual networks are no less complex and indeed include those of urban/special groups (Bassett and Mhloyi 1991; Laver et al. 1997; Meursing 1997; Munguti et al. 1997; van der Straten et al. 1995). This chapter draws on a small pilot project conducted in Zimbabwe in January 1998. The visual diagraming techniques it used and the participatory epistemology it attempted point to ways in which the task of addressing some of the many issues raised above can begin. Many ethical and practical problems arose from this exercise and remain to be addressed by future papers and projects. I hope my exposition of the advantages and practicalities of the approach will inspire others to carry it further forward than I was able to do at that time.

The Epistemology of Participatory Research

Although originally developed in the area of agricultural systems research, participatory diagraming techniques have increasingly been applied to sexual health (Butcher and Kievelitz 1997; IIED 1995; IDS 1996, 1997a, 1997b; Kaleeba et al. 1997). The research techniques that have so far emerged are very exciting, but it is the question of how these methods are deployed that is perhaps primary. The most "radical" of techniques can sustain the most conservative research traditions if they are employed in projects that simply extract data from the field and confine research design, analysis, and knowledge dissemination to distant academic institutions (see Edwards 1989; Goss and Leinback 1996; Hagey 1997; Katz 1994; Patai 1991). Those who have developed the techniques emphasize, however, that participatory diagraming *can* be deployed through epistemologies that enable the power-relations of "research as usual" to be disrupted, open up spaces for the renegotiation of meaning and behavior in the field, and facilitate ordinary people's self-empowerment.

In such a deployment the meaning of the term "participant" (rather than "informant" or "respondent") has pivotal significance.

Participants are not simply providers of information but enter into reciprocal relations with researchers and become increasingly active in the whole research process. They set and develop the research agenda by using diagraming techniques to physically generate visual data on issues they define as relevant. The results of these intellectual labors are immediately available to participants who can begin to analyze them there and then in their own communities. Through their active engagement in the research process participants learn about their own problems *and strengths*. Simultaneously, they develop communication skills and organizational capacities that empower them to *act* on the results generated even as the process of investigation evolves. External researchers facilitate participants' communication and negotiation across axes of difference (enabling them to safely transgress discursive and behavioral norms) and to create a physical and social environment in which this process can begin to take place. Thus research will already have had beneficial impacts in the researched communities before researchers undertake their more familiar roles as advocates and academic commentators (see Chambers 1994a, 1994b, 1997; Cornwall and Jewkes 1995; Hagey 1997; IDS 1996, 1997a, 1997b; Lather 1991; Leurs 1996; Maguire 1987). Given that poor communication about HIV is facilitating its continued spread in southern Africa, the deployment of diagraming techniques through this kind of epistemology would seem to be particularly relevant in this context.

The Methodology of Participatory Diagraming

Participatory diagraming has similarities with focus group interviewing except that participants produce visual data in addition to discursive information and work with people they already know, in order that post-exercise action among group members may be facilitated. Participants initially work in peer groups (widows, older married men, young unmarried women, etc.). These *exclusive* groupings enable participants to share experiences and develop ideas independently of those with different and/or competing positionalities. In their groups, participants, facilitated by researchers, set, tackle, and analyze research questions by generating models and diagrams. To facilitate the contribution of non-literate people, these can be created entirely without written scripts as long as participants agree on the meanings of the symbols used. In the developing world, diagrams are usually constructed on the ground from locally available materials (seeds, bottle tops, pebbles, sticks, straw, household objects or representations drawn in the soil, etc.). In the developed world stationery (card, marker pens, etc.) is more commonly used. Loose materials have the advantage that participants have fewer inhibitions about changing and adapting diagrams as they work through their ideas. The visual and tactile nature of diagraming can facilitate the contribution of less dominant personalities, allowing them to express their "voice" without necessarily requiring them to "speak." Because the data generated are immediately available (rather than simply removed for analysis in distant research institutes), diagrams act both as a stimulus for further detailed questioning by the researcher and as a focus for participants' own analysis and discussion.

There are many different diagraming techniques but they all employ a similar methodology: (1) a specific research question is generated (by the researchers in "shallow" participatory research, or reciprocally with participants in "deeper" programs); (2) a diagrammatic tool is nominated and explained to (or invented and developed by) participants; (3) the "focus group" discusses possible responses to the question posed; (4) they cooperate to produce a large diagram that visually represents their response to that question; (5) while participants are engaged in this activity the researchers observe and record group dynamics and facilitate the process if difficulties arise; (6) once "completed" the diagram is photographed and sketched; (7) the researchers then "interview the diagram," soliciting detailed explanations about its elements, interrogating its coherence, comparing it to other diagrams or other sources of data, and pursuing the conflicts and consensus that arose during its creation; (8) participants should be encouraged to respond to the facilitator's questions by analyzing their own responses and fine-tuning their diagram; (9) the participants record their final interpretation by transferring their data to a large poster which is their own copy and a resource for use in future group or inter-group sessions; (10) finally, participants and researchers decide what to do with the data generated (e.g., hold further diagraming sessions to explore particular points, elect delegates to present the data to other groups or influential decision makers, and/or act on the data locally).

The bold posters produced in peer group sessions provide participants (particularly those from marginalized social groups) with a powerful mechanism through which to voice their (often previously muted) experience and perceptions. Armed with these visual aids, peer groups can gather for *inclusive* plenary sessions where all participants can be exposed to the diagrams, and thence perspectives of others. Plenary meetings can then become arenas in which the social renegotiation of the phenomena under discussion can begin to take place. This final point highlights the fact that the whole process of a participatory action research project is important, not just the results it generates. It is through the process of participation that people can empower themselves by developing the skills, knowledge, and capacities that enable them to begin to locate and solve problems around issues like HIV/AIDS.

In the section below, a practical attempt to use "participatory diagraming" in sexual health research is explored. Readers should note that at this pilot stage of the program, my deployment of the techniques was *not* exemplary of the epistemology and methodology discussed above. Rather it was a somewhat more "shallow" venture into participatory research (see Cornwall and Jewkes 1995). The project followed a conventional "extractive" format; the researcher's agenda dominated proceedings; its pattern was short-lived, one-off encounters rather than an extended program of meetings; detailed analysis was segregated in space and time from the field; and the outputs were primarily academic rather than action oriented. Nevertheless, the approaches described certainly have the potential to shift the balance of the research process towards action in the field. The challenge for the future work of the author, as much as any reader, is to develop that potential.

Piloting Participatory Diagraming in Gender-Sensitive HIV Research

In a short pilot survey conducted in January 1998, I attempted to explore the possibility of using "participatory" diagraming as a means to facilitate communication about sexual health in two rural areas of Zimbabwe. Given the need to win researchers over to the idea of pursuing action-research, my first aim was to establish whether diagraming techniques would generate the kind of data that social scientists would valorize. Secondly, I aimed to discover whether rural people would be comfortable using the techniques as a means to describe and discuss their sex lives. Time constraints resulted in the study being confined to work only with women, the assumption being that it was their voices that most needed to be facilitated and heard.

Methodology and techniques

Two groups of ten women were recruited in two locations by "snowballing" from a key informant. They were rather undifferentiated and included women of different ages (late twenties to mid-fifties), marital status (single mothers, married, divorced, widowed), and wealth (principally a function of access to their own or a partner's off-farm income). One group consisted of members of an HIV peer education project connected to the non-governmental organization (NGO) with whom I was collaborating, the other (in a community in which I had previously worked) comprised "ordinary villagers" linked by bonds of kinship, friendship, and mutual help. Expected differences between the groups in levels of knowledge about HIV promised to make for interesting post-fieldwork comparisons. The first group met at two one-day workshops in a hospital clinic; the second met on three consecutive evenings in the house of the key informant. Meetings were intensive but participants' efforts were rewarded with refreshments and, in this primarily academically driven project, payment appropriate to the hours worked.

The groups were asked a number of open-ended questions addressing three basic themes. The first theme was *level of understanding about HIV and AIDS*. Participants were asked to address three questions separately and sequentially: (a) "what are the most serious health risks faced by people in this area?" (b) "where do you get your information on HIV and AIDS?" and (c) "what factors put local women at risk of catching HIV and AIDS?" The second theme was *the context of sexual decision making*. In this section participants were asked (a) "how and where does sex take place?" (b) "who makes the key decisions about your sexual health and who is responsible for seeing that they are carried out?" and (c) "what strategies, if any, have you used to influence your husband's sexual behavior?" The final theme was *identification of future goals for sexual health*. In this section participants were asked (a) "what future changes in sexual health do you desire?" and (b) "what forces would help or hinder the achievement of your goals?"

In response to each of these questions, participants collaborated to produce a number of large ordinal and relational diagrams that visually represented their responses. They chose to write in English rather than to use pictures, symbols, or the local language and made their diagrams on the ground using card, string, stones, and bottle tops. Using the basic methodology described above, two types of diagrammatic technique were utilized. The first was *matrix ranking and scoring*. Here, participants generated a list of elements they felt were relevant to the topic under discussion, wrote them on cards, and arranged them vertically in rank order of importance. This was followed by a process of "free scoring," in which participants attributed various numerical values to these elements, indicating their relative importance. Next, a further list of variables by which the first set could be judged was generated. These were arranged horizontally. The scores (stones/bottle tops) attributed to each element in the initial ranked list were then distributed in turn along rows under the columns formed by the second set of variables, forming a matrix. The second technique involved the production of *flow diagrams*. Here, the central issue under discussion was written

on a card and placed on the ground. Through discussion with each other, participants generated a number of factors that they felt were relevant to this question, wrote them on cards, and arranged them around the central issue. Factors that the women felt were connected were linked with arrows made of string. Following the researcher's suggestions, some diagrams were "free flow," allowing arrangement and connection of factors in any order, while others were "tree diagrams" that divided strategies (roots) to solve a problem (trunk) from their effects (branches). Still others were "force field diagrams" that showed factors for and against future change (pushing up or down an inclined slope connecting the "present" and "future"). In some instances the factors were scored to indicate their importance and/or frequency. Participants chose either to "free score" the factors or to use a closed percentage scale. All scores indicated the *relative* importance of factors compared to others within the same diagram (i.e., they were not absolute, quantifiable values). The diagrams then provide an agenda for discussion that took place in a mixture of English and Shona translated by field assistants (for more details about techniques, see Kesby 2000b).

Results: the gendered context of sexual decision making

It soon became clear to me that there were strong similarities between the two groups, indicating that women face many common problems in the area of sexual health. Furthermore, early work on the first theme revealed that even the "ordinary women" possessed a fairly good understanding of HIV and its transmission (gleaned from mass-media education campaigns and NGO outreach work). Given this, the crucial question then became: Are these women able to act on the knowledge they possess? Thus, for the purposes of this chapter I will concentrate mainly on the material that was generated around the second major theme: *the context of sexual decision making* (for full results see Kesby 2000a). The data generated in this section of the research highlighted the central importance of the gendered social barriers that continue to stand in the way of the development of safe sexual practices *despite* growing knowledge about HIV.

Both sets of women generated "free flow" diagrams to illustrate the conditions under which they believed sexual activity takes place. They were very similar. For their part, the HIV peer educator group visualized three distinct contexts (Figure 16.1 shows my formalized reproduction). To each they attributed a closed percentage score to illustrate the relative frequency at which sex occurred within each context. Forced sexual activity with drunken husbands was judged to be the most common experience. After discussion, both groups separated "forced sex" (within marriage) from "rape" (outside marriage). While no absolute measurement of the prevalence of rape was possible, it was mentioned repeatedly throughout the research. These depressing data are compatible with other, more conventional surveys of the abuse of women (and children) in southern African (see McFadden 1992; Meursing 1997; Mhloyi 1990; Njovana and Watts 1996; Ray et al. 1996; van der Straten et al. 1995; Vos 1994; Wood et al. 1998). Discussing the diagram, women indicated that they knew that forced sex put them at risk of HIV infection because many suspected their husbands of having multiple partners. Thus while they possessed *knowledge* (especially the peer educators), in the common context of coercive sex, safe practices, and even the discussion of risk, become impossible.

Aggression, violence, and a desire to dominate women were thought natural and inherent male characteristics (see also Meursing et al. 1995). Nevertheless, with further debate, both sets of women began to identify social structures that legitimate and facilitate men's sexual domination of women (although in this predominately academic exercise their discussion was curtailed). Women move from father's to husband's household at marriage, while bridewealth travels in the opposite direction. Husbands are said to refer to this payment when they demand unrestricted access to their wives' bodies regardless of the woman's own feeling or desires. Similarly, they use their ownership of the family home, land, and assets, and associated threats to divorce/evict wives, as a means to subdue wives who resisted their sexual advances. Thus significant social and material geographies underpin gender relations in this context (see Kesby 1999) and position women in ways that make it difficult for them to encourage men to address sexual health issues.

Mutually negotiated, pleasurable, and loving sexual intercourse between married partners emerged in discussion as the relationships that both groups of women desired the most. Yet this was judged to occur in only a minority of sexual encounters. Significantly, even the HIV peer educators suggested that a culture of poor communication between couples on sexual issues made articulation of these desires extremely difficult in their own private lives. Wives who attempted to *initiate* pleasurable lovemaking were likely to be rejected, even assaulted, by husbands who assumed that only infidelity could be the source of such assertiveness. As a result, wives tended to reject husbands' attempts at sexual innovation and experimentation, only to have this cited by men as justification for their seeking "more loving" partners outside marriage. Both groups believed that married women are also increasingly seeking lovers to satisfy their sexual and emotional needs and to provide material tokens of appreciation. In addition to their frequency, the reported context of these illicit liaisons is not conducive to safe sex and seems likely to increase the risk of HIV transmission (see Figure 16.1).

The group of "ordinary women" undertook an additional matrix-scoring exercise focusing on the gendered division of sexual decision making under conditions of *freely negotiated sex* between married couples. The women's sense was that in this context they shared power with men. However, their responses indicated a clear gender division of responsibilities (see also Mbizvo and Adamchak 1991). Although respondents judged that a balance existed between their own responsibility for non-barrier contraception, contribution to pleasure, and mutual genital hygiene, and men's responsibility for initiating sex, condom use, conception, and treatment of STDs, men's dominance over the key decisions pertinent to HIV transmission was obvious to the outsider. Thus, the prevalence of coercion notwithstanding, cultural norms seem to ensure that even in conditions of mutually negotiated sex between

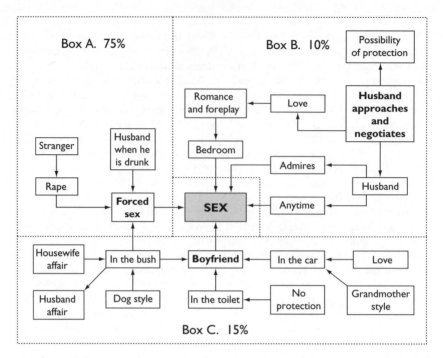

Figure 16.1 *The peer educator's free-flow diagram of the conditions under which sexual activity takes place*
Source: Kesby 2000a, reproduced with kind permission, © Elsevier Science Ltd.

stable partners, rural women are not well placed to use their basic knowledge to protect themselves or their partners.

The final question in the section of the research discussed here invited the two groups to produce structured "tree diagrams" as a means to express the strategies they employed to influence their husbands' sexual behavior. Significantly, despite their greater technical knowledge of HIV, the peer educators' strategies were similar to those of the "ordinary village women" and were largely limited to traditional mechanisms (Figure 16.2). The diagram produced by the "ordinary women" suggested the additional strategies of (i) mobilizing traditional intermediaries (such as aunts and elders) to persuade violent husbands to reform, and (ii) seeking STD clinic consultations, which often led to husbands being called for treatment and prescribed condoms (men's use usually declined as symptoms receded, however). While traditional strategies were said by both

groups to be effective in securing marriage, they subsequently had very mixed rates of success. In fact the group of "ordinary women" suggested that *not* trying to influence husbands' behavior, for fear of "driving him away to a girlfriend or prostitute," was one of the best strategies to ensure a "good relationship." The peer educators constructed their diagram around the statement *"what makes your husband love you"* rather than around the question I had asked: *"what strategies do you use to influence your husbands' sexual behavior?"* This suggested that, in the context of poor communication and frequent male violence, even these well-informed women primarily deployed existing strategies to elicit affection and mutual pleasure, *not* safe sex. This interpretation was confirmed through discussion of the diagram. Depressingly, even the peer educators suggested that actually discussing HIV with their own partners was rarely attempted (Figure 16.2).

Branches (Effects)

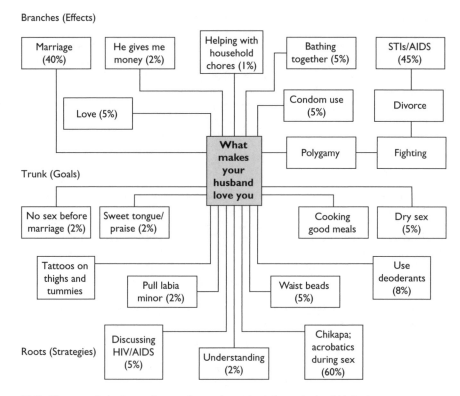

Figure 16.2 *The peer educator's tree diagram of strategies used to influence husbands' behavior.*
Source: Kesby 2000a, reproduced with kind permission, © Elsevier Science Ltd.

The success of diagraming as a technique

While sessions were long and exhausting and required considerable prior preparation, diagraming proved an extremely successful technique for data gathering. In addition to producing data comparable to that generated using more conventional methods, this short pilot study yielded rich material on topics that other methods either could not access or would take much longer to approach. Rural women were both willing and able to use the techniques to describe and discuss their private sex lives and to breach the silences surrounding HIV. They did this despite the gravity of the topics under discussion and notwithstanding my positionality as interviewer/facilitator. The tactile and physically engaging nature of diagramming, together with the back-seat position I took after introducing each research question and technique, was key to this success. Moreover, once diagrams

were complete and sensitive issues were already (visibly) out in the open, it became much easier for me to pursue them and for participants to discuss them. With the data laid out before them, considerable debate was generated *between participants themselves*. Moreover, as I "interviewed the diagram" the women had the opportunity to confirm or challenge my interpretations of the data generated and to participate in the production of the analytical categories, which I would later use in my textual representations of their lives.

Results from the research certainly seemed to suggest that biomedical research on the HIV pandemic must be complemented by social scientific work on phenomena that unequally position African bodies in relation to this virus. In Zimbabwe, unequal gender relations, poor communication between couples, men's disproportionate control over crucial aspects of sexual decision making, and the prevalence of coercive sex all make the discussing of HIV

and the negotiating of risk avoidance extremely difficult. In such a context, efforts
simply to improve the public's knowledge of
HIV will not necessarily lead to the development of safer sexual practices (see also Ankrah
1991; Vos 1994; Campbell 1995a; Meursing et al.
1995; van der Straten et al. 1995; Reid 1996b;
Meursing 1997).

Remaining Practical and Ethical Challenges

The greatest and most immediate challenge
(for this author as much as anyone) is of course
to develop the potential of these techniques
beyond mere data collection. Notwithstanding
the valuable insights that the research may
have brought to outsiders, my shallow and
extractive pilot did little to facilitate the long-
term analysis, communication, or action of Africans themselves. My failure to engage men in
the project (not unlike other HIV/AIDS projects that target women by design or default)
also did nothing to achieve this goal, as my
participants pointed out. If these techniques
are really to facilitate dialogue between ordinary Africans and provide an arena and mechanisms through which they can empower
themselves to become active agents in mapping and reshaping their own sexual health,
then the techniques must be deployed through
a more fully participatory and action-research-
oriented epistemology. This said, even where
research achieves these goals many ethical
challenges and practical problems remain. I
would like to use the last lines of this chapter
to flag a few of these issues.

The limits of "community"

The concept of "community" is often central to
projects that attempt a participatory approach
but requires careful consideration. First, the
tendency to assume that "communities" are
small, bounded, and distinct *spaces* (Cornwall
and Jewkes 1995; Madan 1987) commits the
fallacy of uncritically imposing a scale on
"the field" of investigation without first contemplating at what scale a social process actually operates (Duncan and Savage 1989; Nast
1994). It also emphasizes territory over social
networks. In Africa, the phenomenon of HIV,
with its complex socio-sexual networks that

link town to country, presents HIV prevention
projects that attempt to be "community based"
with many difficult challenges.

Second, there is a tension at the heart of
many participatory projects. On the one hand
lies a notion of "a community" as a socially
coherent group whose shared values and
knowledge researchers wish to valorize, and
whose wishes they wish to facilitate. On the
other sits a recognition of social difference,
diverse knowledge repertoires, and inter-
community conflict that makes researchers
skeptical about finding "community consensus" and inclined to concentrate on the voices
of the marginalized (see Cornwall and Jewkes
1995; Long 1992; Mayoux 1995). The myriad
divisions between "insiders" are often
obscured by the kind of "insider/outsider"
dichotomy famously used by Chambers
(1994a, 1997) to galvanize "outsider" researchers to consider participatory approaches. Managing these divisions can be central to the
practical success or failure of participatory research, however. Thus if researchers set out to
find and promote "the community's view,"
dominant groups may utilize participatory
programs to "officialize" their own interests
as those of the community as a whole
(Maguire 1987; Mosse 1994). Alternatively,
faced with unsolicited external enquiry into
sensitive topics, communities can conjure an
image of social coherence as a defensive mechanism. Worse still, where researchers are successful in promoting the voices of the
marginalized, they can provoke a backlash
from dominant groups resulting in project collapse (Cornwall and Jewkes 1995).

Practitioners have offered two practical solutions to the problem of difference. The first
(as previously described) involves facilitators
dividing "communities" into peer groups
based on wealth, age, gender, etc. Within
these, marginalized people can develop their
ideas without interference from dominant
social groups and then report them with new-
found confidence to community-wide plenary
sessions that confront issues of difference (IDS
1997b; Jonfar et al. 1991; Kinnaird and Hyma
1993; Welbourn 1991, 1992). Researchers
should, however, avoid simply imposing
homogenous meta-categories like "women"
(i) without considering intra-category subdiv-

isions, (ii) seeking participants' opinions on appropriate categories, or (iii) exploring the relational nature of positionality and the effect that group membership and context have on the way certain people will act in each other's presence. Moreover, simply airing differing perspectives is no guarantee that they will be resolved. No single set of predefined "ground rules" can hope to dissolve *all* the unequal relations of power between participants (Ellsworth 1989). A second approach avoids the problem of difference by defining the community to be researched on the basis of shared interest, experience, or risk (BenMayor 1991; Maguire 1987). Such an approach can prove very therapeutic for participants but can also leave them depressed, frustrated, and unable to act if the phenomenon under investigation operates at a different social scale to that of the "interest community" identified (for example, an HIV project that works only with abused wives without also working to change the behavior of abusive husbands).

The conclusion that participation "works best in less stratified communities" (Woelk 1992; Ugalde 1985) is depressing news for those sensitive to the myriad axes of difference in any "community." The challenge for participatory HIV projects in rural Africa is precisely to find ways to facilitate negotiation across such differences so that participants can build affinities that will protect their mutual health (Baylies and Bujra 1995). This will be difficult in practice.

Problematizing "participation"

"Participation" is an increasingly popular discourse; however, its meaning can range from people being contracted into pre-designed projects, or consulted before interventions are made, to more collaborative endeavors in which participants contribute actively to all aspects of research design and implementation (Cornwall and Jewkes 1995; Seeley et al. 1992; Smith and Blanc 1997; Woelk 1992). Few programs reach the higher levels. Most remain to a greater or lesser extent projects conceived, imposed, funded, and controlled from outside (Cornwall and Jewkes 1995; Hagey 1997; Lather 1991; Maguire 1987; Mayoux 1995; Oliver 1997). Even where this is not the case,

equitable relations within a single project do not fundamentally change the broader political economy (see Madge 1997; Oliver 1997, 1999). For example, while HIV is never the only problem Africans have to worry about (Wallman 1997, 1998), outsiders may be forced to retain power over the macro agenda (analysis of HIV/AIDS), despite locally identified priorities (TB, malaria), in order to satisfy their sponsors (see Kesby 1999). Disparities in command over resources can limit reciprocity in other ways; for example, researchers have time to "participate" while participants may not (Kitchen 1999). In these ways and others, participatory programs can end up being rather similar to more conventional "top down" projects (Long and van der Ploeg 1989). Advocates of participation should also be aware of their position within a wider context in which international financial organizations simultaneously encourage governments to cut public spending at the same time as encouraging programs that facilitate "local knowledge and local solutions." Community-based, participatory HIV programs could be seen as capitulating with this strategy, risking that participants will be left to shoulder the blame for any project failures while the broader macroeconomic policies that handed them the burden to succeed will escape unscathed (Long and van der Ploeg 1989; Madan 1987; Schoepf 1998; Villarreal 1992).

Other difficult questions about the power-relations of research arise from the tension between the desire to facilitate the voices and priorities of "the community" and the desire to facilitate the empowerment of the marginalized *within* the community. At what point does the outsider's political commitment to, say, women's equality become an imposition that annuls the participation of some or all insiders? Conversely, when does cultural sensitivity become collusion with a system of domination? (McFadden 1992). Opinion is mixed. Some encourage researchers to assert their politics (Batliwala 1994; Mayoux 1995; Patel 1996), others condemn this (Patai 1991; Gilbert 1994). Certainly, while indigenous knowledges and practices must be valorized, they are not beyond criticism and often transmit oppression even when recounted by the marginalized (Cornwall and Jewkes 1995;

Kesby 1999; Lather 1991). Nor should researchers consider themselves to be the only ones who can benefit from cultural critique. The case of HIV powerfully illustrates the need for researchers to facilitate participants' own reflection on the limits of their existing social knowledge and practice (Schoepf 1993). Balancing these conflicting imperatives in practice will be very challenging.

Conclusion

Clearly then, participatory approaches do not dissolve the power-relations endemic to research, nor do they enable researchers to avoid the difficult ethical questions raised in recent post-structuralist textual debates. Indeed advocates must identify and explore these continuing challenges themselves; if not, others will make the criticism that because "participation" is no panacea it can be dismissed. The point is that, while not perfect, participatory approaches can at least develop tangible mechanisms through which researchers *and participants* can produce partial, practical resolutions to ethical questions in the arena of the fieldwork praxis itself, rather than simply leaving academics to rehearse their absolute intractability in texts (see Gormley and Bondi 1999; Herman and Mattingly 1999; Rundstrom and Deur 1999). Notwithstanding the need for researcher self-reflexivity, then, the greatest challenge for social scientific investigation into HIV in Africa really is to find ways to help Africans *themselves* move HIV work "beyond epidemiology."

ACKNOWLEDGMENTS

This chapter is based on papers originally presented at the Association of American Geographers 96th Annual meeting, April 4–8, 2000, Pittsburgh, Pennsylvania. I am indebted to all the women who agreed to participate in this study, everyone at the Women and AIDS Support Network and the Zimbabwe PRA Network, and to Mary Sandasi and Ivy Tendere for their translation and assistance in the field. Many thanks to Graeme Sandeman for his excellent cartography and to Elsevier Science Ltd for allowing its reproduction here. This research was made possible by a research grant from The Carnegie Trust for the Universities of Scotland.

NOTE

1. In Britain, there are no significant differences in the time that migrant Africans survive with full-blown AIDS, compared to other UK population groups (DelAmo et al. 1998).

Chapter 17

Community-Based Research on AIDS in the Context of Global Inequalities – Making a Virtue of Necessity?

Carolyn Baylies

Introduction

Questions of ethics are close to the surface of all research around AIDS, not just because of the stigma a diagnosis of HIV confers, but by virtue of the global inequalities which set the context for differential rates of infection and uneven capacities to combat the epidemic. With reference to research on community-based initiatives, this chapter explores a range of questions relating to potential harm and benefit. It deals with ethical issues which emerge in the research process itself, but also, more widely, which relate to how research agendas are set. A specific concern is with the way researchers intent on examining and facilitating community-based action around AIDS can sometimes be drawn toward making a virtue of necessity. They may find themselves focusing attention on coping strategies or prevention initiatives at the community level precisely because funds which might otherwise serve to arrest the epidemic and assist those affected are not forthcoming, whether from poor governments or from those richer nations where AIDS, while still a problem of significance, has been largely contained.

In a perverse manner, social science research assumes greater importance in the context of AIDS in Africa, not less, as medical advances in treatment possibilities emerge (Becker et al. 1999). New therapies bring with them the increasing potential for the emergence of two AIDS syndromes (Farmer 1999b) – one in the north where medical treatment regimes become increasingly a preoccupation and AIDS becomes increasingly routinized as it is progressively medicalized, and one in the south where poverty at both national and individual levels limits access to new treatment regimes and heightens vulnerability to infection. Where medical interventions are limited or accessibility to them is restricted, an appreciation of the social dynamics of transmission is essential if inroads in prevention are to be made. An understanding of the way community resources may be mobilized to assist with the care of those who are ill is all the more necessary where state resources are minimal and public welfare provision skeletal.

Because so many other avenues remain closed or obstructed, communities are frequently compelled and encouraged to fall back on their own resources, and researchers may be drawn in to assess and facilitate this process. Treichler's reference to the human sciences often assuming the role of handmaid to the biological sciences in respect of AIDS, doing "their best to ease suffering and combat ignorance until the laboratory can find the 'ultimate solution'" (1992b:66), may apply here as more broadly. Yet in practice, the social sciences have much more to offer by virtue of their capacity not just to illuminate the dynamics of social behavior, but also to critically appraise the inequalities which systematically construct vulnerabilities to HIV and differential access to care, with market relations and positioning of national economies affecting the life chances of individuals on the ground. This critical stance needs to be directed not only toward the international inequalities which configure the AIDS epidemic, however, but also toward the practice of AIDS research, the way it is funded, its agendas formulated and its outcomes utilized.

While examples will be drawn more widely in discussing the ethical questions which can emerge around research on community-based AIDS initiatives, particular reference will be made to a research project with which the author was involved. This study (hereafter referred to as the Gender and AIDS Project) sought to investigate how existing organizational capabilities of women (and men) might be harnessed for work around AIDS. Conducted primarily in 1995 and 1996 but with follow-up continuing through 1999, it involved teams of researchers in Tanzania and Zambia, working in six different locations.[1] The research design incorporated an initial survey and focus group discussions, followed by an evaluation, and at some sites, facilitation, of community-based initiatives in care or prevention. While successful in many respects, there was occasional slippage in this project, as in many others, between principled intentions and actual practice, with the emergence of unforeseen problems and missed opportunities. Reflection on these may inform broader consideration of the conduct and impact of research in this area.

From the Quest for Knowledge to Support for Interventions

Posing the question "what is this social science knowledge good for?," Herdt has declared, "it is not enough … that we conduct an AIDS study. We must also provide the means to translate the knowledge into education and prevention measures" (1992:7). AIDS has generated the conviction among many researchers that an activist stance is essential to ensure that knowledge gained is utilized for the specific advantage of groups whose marginalization puts them at risk of HIV infection (Lindenbaum 1992). This was expressed with considerable passion by an AIDS activist in Zambia when the Gender and AIDS Project was being formulated, who asserted that it was past time when research could be conducted for the sake of it. It must be linked to interventions, facilitating protection and care. Similarly emphasizing the need to build strong linkages between research and action in work on livelihood mobility and AIDS prevention, Painter (1999) has urged researchers to identify existing community-based organizations geared toward mutual assistance and to assess their potential or enlist their involvement in AIDS prevention programs.

This emphasis on linking research to community-based organizations parallels a call for AIDS interventions themselves to be community based. Bond and Vincent regard as a "critical moment" the realization by professionals that "community response and organization promises to be more effective than campaigns launched by national and cosmopolitan centers" in AIDS prevention (1997b:111). In the same vein, Parker refers to intervention being increasingly "reconceived as a collective dialectic process, driven as much from the bottom up as from the top down" (1996:S29–S30), with community mobilization seen as potentially more effective in combating the epidemic than earlier models. In recent years, donors and non-governmental organizations (NGOs) have actively promoted this concern, with many programs at local level being initiated and supported. But many initiatives have emerged "on their own," given recognition of pressing need by those "on the ground" to offer comfort and support to their neighbors and the absence of external support. Numerous presentations and posters in the stream on "community responses" at the X1th International Conference on AIDS and STDs in Africa (ICASA 1999), as in other similar meetings, bear witness to the extensiveness of such activities, detailing the successes they have realized and the problems they have encountered. Research is not always an integral aspect of such interventions, but recognition of the need for community-based and -led initiatives and, moreover, of the necessity for attention to underlying structural inequalities, if such interventions are to be successful, lays down a firm imperative for social science input. Research may be critical prior to an intervention in providing an understanding of existing beliefs, capacities, and social structure, in facilitating an intervention through investigating organizational dynamics and resource allocation, or as an adjunct to monitoring and evaluation.

This tying of research to interventions around AIDS at community level has resonance with broader tendencies in the development field, where participatory methodologies of development practice, often employed at community level, increasingly intersect with participatory research methodologies (Seeley et al. 1992; Nelson and Wright 1995; Robb 1999). Especially if linked to collective reflection on pervasive inequalities and if stimulating collective action, participation is believed to serve as an antidote to the subordination which has prevailed in the past. Applying these ideas to the research process implies the assumption that individuals become agents of their destiny by virtue of their collective involvement in analyzing their situation and pressing for justice and equality (Fernandes and Tandon 1981). These are noble ends and not always (or perhaps often) achievable via the research process. But they may be as important in some aspects of research on AIDS as in other research geared to achieving development objectives.

Increasingly, then, the community has become an important context for the linking of research with interventions, and knowledge with means of AIDS prevention (Campbell and Williams 1999). At the same time, research skills have been increasingly deployed to progress the work of community-based initiatives (Leonard and Muia 1998). In both cases, principles of participation, democracy, and inclusiveness are often aspired to as part of a process which utilizes local knowledge, develops local expertise, and expands capacity for action. These principles in turn call for critical analysis of the concept of community itself and a recognition of the heterogeneity of interests which communities invariably incorporate. In the context of AIDS, awareness of such internal inequalities is crucial to an understanding of patterns of vulnerability and identification of targets for intervention.

Adherence to the Principle of No Harm

Of the range of ethical issues which can emerge in research aimed at facilitating community-based AIDS interventions, many are common to research around AIDS more generally. Some of these can be highlighted with reference to the Dakar Declaration of the African Network on Ethics, Law and HIV, issued in 1994, and with ongoing salience for work around AIDS. The Declaration affirms the principles of partnership and empowerment, including the right to knowledge and freedom of choice, all of which have implications for research. But it also comments explicitly on research ethics, affirming as fundamental that:

> the interest of the research subjects or communities should be paramount. Research should be based on free and informed consent, be non-intrusive, and the results should be made available to the community for timely and appropriate action. (African Networks on Ethics, Law and HIV 1994)

The framing of this principle suggests its immediate – though certainly not exclusive – application to a model of research involving passive subjects, whose rights must be respected. Much research continues to accord with this model and the ethical issues attending it must, of course, be carefully considered. But taking account of principles of partnership and empowerment – as also incorporated in the Dakar Declaration – we will argue that a stronger and wider ethical stance may be postulated, especially in reference to research aimed at facilitating community-based initiatives.

But we begin with reference to a more narrow consideration of ethical issues which arise in the research process itself. One of the most basic components of an ethical stance is that research should not harm those who are its subjects or who are touched by the research process. Questions of consent and confidentiality bear strongly here. The stigma which continues to be attached to a diagnosis of HIV [COMMENT1]and the extent to which such a diagnosis may have repercussions not just for a single individual, but for sexual partners, children, and those yet to be born, means that AIDS is a subject around which deep sensitivity must be observed. The pursuit of knowledge about AIDS must always be balanced by the harm to individuals which may accompany that pursuit, all the more so if such knowledge does not immediately or automatically feed back into practice or policy in such a way as to assist those who have comprised samples or otherwise participated in the research. As Lindenbaum notes (1992), ethical concerns also imply responsibility to research subjects who have yielded sensitive information, to guard against use of findings in ways that further stigmatize.

The need for such sensitivity as well as for confidentiality is broadly acknowledged (Schoepf 1991a). As the Dakar Declaration (African Networks on Ethics, Law and HIV 1994) affirms, "every person directly affected by the epidemic has a right to confidentiality and privacy." But research often delves into the private domain and can sometimes inadvertently breach confidentiality or cause discomfort. In some cases stigma may be conferred by the mere association with AIDS research, which guarantees of confidentiality may be insufficient to staunch. Ensuring informed consent is less common in research involving community-based samples than those situated within the medical arena, and arguably less necessary if ascertaining HIV status is not at issue. Yet even then, and indeed even when the protocol and objectives of a research project are communicated, and consent formally or informally requested, inclusion in a sample in connection with AIDS research can cause worry, raising questions at the back of the mind – and sometimes articulated: "Why are you visiting us or interviewing me? Is it because I have AIDS or we have AIDS in this household?" ("Is it because you know something which I do not?")

Certain methodologies, such as the focus group discussion, increasingly used in community-based research precisely because of the candor which it can encourage and the richness of data it can generate (Irwin et al. 1991; Kitzinger 1994; Morgan 1997), can pose particular problems relating to confidentiality. Asking women in this context, for example, who is to blame for HIV transmission can result in instructive tales about wandering husbands and precautions taken. However, it can also expose to public view errors of judgment and self-deception, bringing to light dangerous miscalculations about safety. If significant as a learning experience and potentially a means of building solidarity through sharing, such sessions also have the capacity to breach confidentiality and contribute to personal discomfort.

This can be illustrated through reference to a focus group discussion of women during the Gender and AIDS Project.[2] One participant explained how she had discovered that her husband had been visiting a sex worker, his indiscretion coming to light after he left his jacket at the sex worker's home. He expressed great remorse and she forgave him and welcomed him back to her bed. But not long after this episode he died. She attributed his death to a stroke, yet it was clear as the discussion progressed that she was troubled with worry that it might have been from AIDS. She tested her reasoning with the group. Surely the fact that she was still alive and her child was thriving meant that she was not infected? She was disconcerted to learn in the course of the discussion that matters are not so straightforward and that the state of her child's health could not be taken as a reliable measure of her own HIV status. Having so freely shared her experience, she realized that she had inadvertently revealed, in light of this new information, the fact that she might in fact be HIV positive.

Another of the women then told her own story. Her husband had gone off for some time, during which he had a number of sexual encounters. When he returned, she, too, welcomed him back without conditions. As she explained, "at that time all that was in my mind was love and seeing him back." Now, she said, she was pregnant. "If I am infected I will just have to die. There was nothing I could do."

The aftermath of these revelations was shrouded with unease, not least because of the critical comments made by other women in the group. As one said in respect of the second woman's story, "you should think more of your own life." Another chided her for not insisting that her husband take an HIV test. Those involved in community-based research may be attuned to the enormous anxiety which AIDS continues to generate and may indeed aspire to defuse it. But the greater transparency and opportunity for public scrutiny sometimes built into research intended to feed into local interventions can sometimes entail unwitting disclosures and unintended distress. Sensitivity on the part of the researcher is not always enough to guarantee lack of harm in so deeply stressful a situation and one where stigma continues to operate to damage an individual's sense of worth.

That harm may in some cases be an unintended and unanticipated outcome of research is partly a consequence of the way different layers of harm potentially apply in contradictory ways, with benefits to one group within a community implying harm to others, or protection from harm on one dimension creating danger along another. Drawing on an episode from her own work, Bond (1997) demonstrates the myriad ethical pitfalls which can attend the research process. Ironically in this case (and probably not uniquely), the situation was exacerbated by a commitment to link research to intervention and benefit. She describes how her concern to limit the danger from AIDS to young, underage girls working on a commercial farm in Zambia's Southern Province contributed inadvertently to their being dismissed from work, when knowledge of this legal transgression reached the ears of the farm manager. In the event the girls were potentially thrust into a situation of even greater risk, insofar as they sought to compensate for lost income through exchange of sex for material gain. As Lindenbaum affirms (1992), the misuse or unintended use of information acquired in the context of research is an all-too-recognizable dilemma.

Questions of Who Benefits, How and for How Long

The Dakar Declaration sets out the principle that "results should be made available to the community for timely and appropriate action" (African Networks on Ethics, Law and HIV 1994), emphasizing the importance of benefits from research feeding back into practice and highlighting the responsibility of researchers to research subjects in this regard. In the case of research facilitating community-based action around AIDS, the principle may be even more strongly articulated and extended to incorporate a more direct engagement with questions of who benefits from research, what the benefit consists of, and what its duration may be. But there are prior and broader questions which must also be taken into account. Benefits follow from the nature of the research and the way research agendas are set, and the issue of who exerts control or claims ownership at these levels is crucial.

Given limited resources in many African settings, the necessity to deal with external funders means that initiative, agenda setting, and full participation seldom rest with those at community level. What funders will countenance always places parameters on questions addressed and methodologies utilized (Farmer 1992a); the amounts which are on offer in turn set parameters on the scope of research designs; eligibility requirements place limitations on access to funds. Applicants must display their credibility, their institutional ties, their track record, and sometimes their creditworthiness. While donors and other funding bodies may increasingly direct their resources toward NGOs, particularly as regards interventions, research monies are more typically oriented toward those in the academy or private research institutions. Thus funds are often skewed toward northern researchers or those with affiliations with northern academic and research institutes. In turn, agendas may be influenced more by principles of cost effectiveness or ongoing theoretical debates than by need.

Obbo (1999) notes how ownership may apply on a number of levels, between researchers from the north and the south; between researchers and their "assistants"; and between researchers and the subjects of research. Power-relations infuse the research process across these various levels. Yet these reside in turn within a larger context. For in practice funding bodies often have a considerable role in setting agendas for researchers of all complexions and positions and sometimes exercise this overarching control in ways that undermine collaborative intentions or aspirations to ensure greater participation. The points highlighted by Obbo were an issue of discussion and some contention with the Gender and AIDS Project from its beginning. Funds made available early on (by an agency which in the event was not the ultimate source of project money) permitted preliminary consultations regarding agenda and research design among at least some of those who eventually made up the research teams, although not with the ultimate subjects/participants. And though efforts were made to build in equity among the research teams, the requirements of the granting body and of northern universities which formally hosted the project and oversaw the budget sometimes militated against this. In this as in other areas, inequalities based around resources can intrude, even where unintended and undesired.

All of this of course begs the question of who *should* carry out research. Perhaps this is better – or more comfortably – phrased as who is best positioned in terms of their attributes, be they skills, expertise and experience, knowledge of context, or linguistic facility. Collaborative approaches may be particularly valuable to the degree that they combine different skills and knowledge most effectively. Yet it is sometimes more a matter of status and control of resources that determines division of labor and ownership than questions of what is most effective and more likely to generate good and useful knowledge and to bring the greatest benefit. What is important, as Obbo (1999) stresses, whether researchers are local or "from the north," is that they listen carefully, that is, that "experts" do not rest on their reputations and their preconceptions but do research "away from our offices and desks."

But what of the benefit to research subjects? How are such subjects transformed into beneficiaries? At the least, it is important that findings be communicated to, and disseminated among, those who have contributed to them through participation in group discussions or as interviewees or members of a survey population. But as has been noted, the Dakar Declaration goes beyond this to affirm that findings should be made available to communities for "timely and appropriate action." Yet the question still remains of who should initiate, fund, and monitor that action. At best, it would be hoped that findings feed into better practice, greater protection, and more informed policy through a process of full consultation with beneficiaries and, moreover, that community members be enabled to determine what constitutes appropriate action and to direct its implementation. But while perhaps most fundamental, however, these are not the only benefits accruing from the research process.

"We are not a donor agency" – the boundaries in practice between research and interventions

Conducting research in conditions not just of high prevalence of HIV/AIDS, but also of persistent poverty, raises questions about immediate material benefit (and costs) as well as long-term, vaguely promised health improvements. The point was cogently made in the context of an interview with an elderly man in Zambia who said with great simplicity but considerable eloquence that he was unable to participate in an interview because he had not eaten that day. Recognition of immediate and pressing needs and questions of compensation are matters of importance but also of much debate, applying not just to research participants but also to those who are encouraged to become involved in community-based initiatives. And the matter is not just whether there should be compensation, but how much.

The issue was raised in the workshop that inaugurated the Gender and AIDS Project in Lusaka by a local academic who was involved in both research and the facilitation of peer education projects around AIDS. While those with whom she worked received some compensation in the form of allowances, it was minimal, because she was concerned that their involvement be, if not voluntary, then as much for personal and community benefit in respect of AIDS prevention as possible, rather than for monetary gain. She was disturbed by plans of an international NGO to mount a peer education project in the city where allowances would be considerably greater. While accepting the need for some compensation, she worried that this could well escalate expectations and convert community service into employment opportunities.

If applying to community initiatives, then perhaps the principles at issue also apply to participants or subjects in research projects. Here too it may be more than a matter of courtesy to provide some compensation, even if minimal, for the time that individuals give. This issue of participation and the benefit attached to it can be slippery and problematic, however, as noted by Seeley et al. (1992) in respect to AIDS research in Uganda, where groups and individuals competed for the immediate benefits the project offered, not least in the form of employment as interviewers, mobilizers, census takers, home visitors, or counselors. Resentment of the unequal distribution of these benefits was evident from the grumbling complaint that some were "growing fat" at the expense of the community.

On a much smaller scale, similar issues arose in that part of the Gender and AIDS Project carried out in Zambia's Luapula Province. Differential payment of individuals within the team sometimes led to resentment and grumbling, with competing claims about who was doing the "real" work. It was evident, moreover, that many within the community wished to participate, and a number readily volunteered to do so, with a view to becoming paid research assistants. In a context where few apart from the government, donors, and international NGOs appeared to be offering funds and even temporary and partial employment, individuals could hardly be faulted for trying to gain access to what might be put to personal advantage from a research project in their midst.

But this particular study also threw up other issues relating to compensation. Because it was geared to exploring how women's (and men's) organizational capacities might be harnessed around campaigns of protection against AIDS, it necessarily encountered some of the same dilemmas about the degree to which community work should (or can) be voluntary

or entail compensation that emerged in connection with peer education projects in Lusaka, referred to above. An example may be given of an initiative which emerged quite spontaneously from a focus group discussion held in Mansa (Bujra and Baylies 1999; Baylies forthcoming).

The group consisted of a number of market women, recruited from their stalls one afternoon and invited to participate in a discussion the following day to consider issues of who was at risk from HIV, who was to blame, and what collective action might be taken around prevention and protection. They continued to discuss these issues among themselves in the days following the focus group and decided to form themselves into a drama group and perform plays which demonstrated the dangers of AIDS. The success of this group can be measured by its longevity. Three years after its formation, it was still going strong, having survived some rough patches and membership circulation. Throughout, however, questions of material benefit, or at the least of compensation for its community outreach activities, preoccupied its members. Although they did not articulate it so directly, their position could easily have been described through a rejoinder to members of the research team that "we are doing all the work but you are getting paid (and you are probably getting paid far more than we could ever imagine)."

Another example from the same research site, based on a degree of miscommunication, illustrates the extent to which presumptions about benefit may vary as between researchers and "subjects." We met with the officers of a village women's club which was in the process of re-formation after an initial false start and asked if they might be willing to participate in the project, with their members constituting a focus group. When we arrived at the appointed time, there were many more people than we had anticipated, but it also soon became clear that they understood us not to be researchers interested in logging their opinions, but as potential benefactors or sponsors of their club.[3] In the end, they graciously agreed to a group interview and we made a modest donation to the club's funds. The collective experience seemed to strengthen them in their resolve both to progress their own initial agenda and to take up some work around AIDS, but it was evident that their immediate priority was material assistance.

It was in Mansa, as well, that one of our key informants, who had been involved in pre-test counseling since shortly after the epidemic came to local medical attention, asked for the donation of a video recorder which he said would be immensely important to the carrying out of health education initiatives. He was right. It was impossible to deny it. But this would run counter to the budget as set out. In this and other cases, it seemed necessary to explain that, although the difference might be hard to discern from the outside, we were involved in a research project and were not a donor agency, nor even connected with one.

But in the course of this research it became increasingly clear that the sort of project we had embarked on, which aspired to prompt members of the community to reflect upon and build on their commitment and their skills in collective endeavors, precisely needed to include in its budget the provision of seed money for community initiatives. In a very small way, we endeavored to provide such seed money,[4] but it was evident that this could be no more than a gesture of support and a far from reliable form of assistance, and we included a recommendation in our final report to the funders about the need in future to incorporate more extensive seed money in similar projects. The distinction that donors or funding bodies often draw between interventions and research, however, may make for particular difficulty in fashioning projects that try to bring these two together. An increasing emphasis on dissemination does not satisfy the obligation to "give something back" to research subjects. It is facilitation of community initiatives and implementation of findings that are of foremost importance, and, even more fundamentally, mobilization of the resources needed to support them.

The issue of material as well as moral support for community-based AIDS work is a persistent and serious one and among the outcomes of the Gender and AIDS Project was recognition of the extent to which this must be reckoned with. Our discussions with the market women's drama group touched on questions of benefit, along a range of dimensions. How far could benefit be seen in respect of their personal empowerment, through the augmentation of their ability to ensure protection of themselves and their children? How far did their drama assist the wider community through increasing awareness of the dangers of AIDS and of preventive means? How far might it serve to stimulate discussion about the way in which gender relations contributed to the vulnerability of women (and men) to the HIV virus and through collective reflection contribute to a transformation in the content of these relations? But while these wider goals and their partial achievement were sometimes acknowledged, questions about meeting immediate material needs remained high on the personal agendas of individual participants, underlining relations of economic inequality which accompany patterns of vulnerability, not just on a local, but, more importantly, on a global scale.

The wider ethics of promoting self-help and of facilitating communities to "help themselves"

These issues about economic inequality which emerged in the context of our research raise larger questions about research agendas which focus on facilitating local action. When the women's drama group requested allowances, members of the research team asked them to reflect on why they were doing the AIDS work. Were they doing it *for* the research project or for themselves and their community? If the latter, what was the rationale for the research project "paying" them? If having some logic, this may have been in some sense a fatuous response, given the wider relations of inequality with which the project itself was bound up. It was in order for the research team to further reflect on its own practice and on the consistency (or lack of it) between the funding assumptions on which it rested and the altruistic behavior it was hoping to assess and ultimately to encourage.

Any such altruistic (but ultimately self and community preserving) collective activity should be valued wherever it appears. On occasion we begrudged the fact that so little spirit of volunteerism seemed to be in evidence. Many more had been trained in community AIDS work, counseling, or peer education in this area than were involved in this work on the ground at the time of the research. Indeed there appeared to have been a series of initiatives begun over the years, often by donors, which had flourished for a short while, only to drift into decline. Although there was still strong evidence of concern and commitment, individuals frequently felt unable to continue without compensation. It sometimes seemed that only under the auspices of the church, backed up by notions of Christian charity and compassion, were some people willing to give their time truly voluntarily (perhaps seeking less tangible or at least less worldly rewards). Yet the apparent resistance to altruism was not irrational, given the context of immediate needs and competing demands which many experienced. And if reasonable on an individual basis, it may be similarly so on a broader scale.

Discussion of participants in a focus group held in conjunction with the Gender and AIDS Project, in Kanyama, on the outskirts of Zambia's capital, Lusaka,[5] further illustrates both the inclination toward altruism and its limits in respect of AIDS work. The focus group involved members of a Resident Development Committee (RDC) who had been elected by people in the community, demarcated into zones, under the auspices of an international NGO in an attempt to foster grassroots participation and community responsibility for local development initiatives. The RDC had identified several development objectives, including the improvement of the local water supply and drainage around water taps, and work toward this end had been initiated. The member of the research team acting as facilitator of the group discussion tried to tease out the link between their personal involvement with the RDC, which was formally on a voluntary basis, and community benefits which might accrue from its work:

Participant 1: We are expecting some achievement. For example, working on water, we shall get the reward by sacrificing ourselves.
Facilitator: Aha, nobody is paying you?
Participant 1: No.
Facilitator: You started working because you had identified that there

was a problem? But the benefit would be water?
All: Yes.

The question was then put to the group – might this principle be applied in work around AIDS? The responses of some group members revealed their skepticism about activities which might not bear immediate fruit and concern about the balance between volunteerism and personal benefit. In contrast to water, AIDS seemed a problem whose solution was much less concrete and indeed for one man – revealing his own prejudices or perhaps his inability to see how his own behavior might change – elusive.

Participant 2: We are only seven, sharing our ideas. How can we prevent HIV/AIDS? You are saying water was a problem. Yes, we worked on it and gained clean water. The answer to the AIDS problem is, unless you remove the ladies from the earth, we cannot be cured. Otherwise, no cure can be found.

Others were more forthcoming about the need to do something and of the value of collective work in this area: "we agree we need to help prevent HIV/AIDS from spreading." But they also acknowledged that they needed assistance in the form of training and funds:

Participant 3: We need you to teach us ways in which we can work properly...So whenever you call us again we are willing to meet. Money alone cannot help [is not enough], but this could be a supplementary to the work we are doing.

The economic burden of AIDS lies heavy on many communities, flowing from the loss or displacement of productive labor through illness, death and the care of those afflicted, loss of income, and additional expenses associated with care and funerals. As a review of Zambia's AIDS program has indicated, given the lack of funds from external sources, "communities are responding simply because they have to" (Republic of Zambia 1997:13). But they do so at enormous financial and psychological cost.

A crucial question to be posed, therefore, is why those who are most needy in terms of the AIDS epidemic should be required to "help themselves"? In the north the history of AIDS has also been characterized by very significant voluntary sector activity. Indeed this can be credited as a significant contribution, with new models of support being devised. In that context community mobilization was initially a product of relative neglect by authorities in some countries, particularly when AIDS seemed to be confined to the gay community. Yet northern voluntary sector AIDS organizations have to a large extent been quite generously supported by public money. In the UK, where community-based support fit well with the then government's ideological stance on devolving care to the community, largesse during the late 1980s (albeit subsequently substantially reduced) can be credited with the veritable burgeoning of locally based AIDS support groups.

The pattern is very different in much of Africa. Here the promotion of NGO and community-based work around AIDS follows in large part not so much from a reluctance to lend support as from the dearth of government resources. As other solutions appear impractical and improbable, communities are exhorted to help themselves. This is surely important, but also exposes the inequalities that pervade the story of AIDS. The introduction to an *HIV/AIDS Bibliography* (NASTLP and UNICEF 1996) on research on HIV/AIDS in Zambia makes the important and valid point that "as we understand more of the way the virus moves, interacts with other diseases, manifests itself, how people learn to live with HIV/AIDS and how households and communities respond, then these feelings of hopelessness are converted into optimism, empowerment and ultimately positive action" (1996:1). This is crucial. Yet empowerment and positive community responses, while important, are not sufficient to meet current and future need and to break the destructive power of the epidemic. They cannot of themselves make good the costs involved.

Increasingly, the depth of inequality on a global basis is starkly revealed, whereby UNAIDS estimates suggest that 70 percent of the global total of those living with HIV/AIDS live in Africa (UNAIDS 1998a, 1999d), but few have access to new modes of therapy which can prolong their lives. When a human rights discourse is comprehensively applied to AIDS, the injustice of this situation is evident. Increasingly, this is recognized as a question of ethics transcending national boundaries.[6] Increasingly, pressure is put on multinational pharmaceutical companies to incorporate ethical criteria into the mechanics of pricing and calculations of profitability,[7] to make therapies more widely available where need is greatest, and to reduce the penalty placed on people living with HIV and AIDS by virtue of the level of development of the country in which they happen to reside and the social location they occupy within it.

The Africa Partnership against HIV/AIDS launched in April 1999 (UNAIDS 1999a) reflects recognition of the depth of the present emergency and the level of need, even if still placing a substantial and perhaps disproportionate burden on those states and the communities within them which are most affected (Baylies 1999). But as the Partnership's statement of intent suggests, an enormously increased level of resources must be directed at the epidemic in Africa if the prevailing injustice is to be redressed. In this context, Matchaba's (1999) suggestion in a letter to the *British Medical Journal*, April 1999, of a novel form of conditionality warrants serious consideration. As he said, "perhaps it is time to write off old debts and earmark any future aid for the sole purpose of reducing the perinatal transmission of HIV, treating TB and financing public health programs." The suggestion has subsequently gained credence, as indicated by its promotion at the ICASA meeting in Lusaka in September 1999. But the claim can be extended further. What is needed is not just additional funds devoted to medical interventions, but a multi-pronged approach targeting gender-sensitive poverty alleviation, alongside effectively supported programs of prevention and support.

Conclusion

Social science research on AIDS at community level has made many and varied contributions. In general, work in this area is informed by a strong sense of purpose and urgency, and in many instances a strong commitment to action. Researchers generally are attuned to the sensitive nature of their work and to the ethical dilemmas which often attend it. In ensuring that the principles of the Dakar Declaration are upheld and that interests of subjects and communities remain paramount, however, greater inclusiveness may be increasingly required, with communities and groups within them being brought into the process more directly to set agendas and determine what appropriate action should follow from research findings.

Ethical questions attending the harm or benefit of AIDS research are not, however, confined to the nexus of researcher, community, findings, and appropriate action. They extend to the broader, global context in which vulnerabilities to AIDS and differential access to means of protection, care, and treatment are constructed. Indeed the way in which citizenship both enables and constrains claims on health and health care is increasingly revealed as the foremost ethical issue associated with the AIDS epidemic. Research on AIDS is not disconnected from this context, nor immune from its repercussions. It is important, therefore, for social science research to keep critique of the factors underlying and perpetuating global inequalities and injustice in respect of AIDS to the fore. Researchers need to reflect on the way in which their agendas in some cases make a virtue of necessity. Investigations of potential survival strategies and creative accommodation to the impact of AIDS need not always bow to the global inequalities which entail a process almost of "going it alone." Community-based strategies of support and protection are crucially important, but alongside their advocacy, there is need to contest the nature of such global inequalities and to call for justice in distribution of resources and assistance. Moreover, there is need for advocacy of greater global responsibility in assisting communities to cope with AIDS in ways which help them to set their own agendas, define their needs, and secure appropriate support.

ACKNOWLEDGMENTS

While I bear full responsibility for the ideas and arguments presented here, due recognition and an expression of gratitude must be given to all who were involved in the research project from which examples have been drawn, as well as, of course, to the participants in the research. Janet Bujra was co-grantholder with me of the ESRC grant (R00235221) which funded the project and a member of the research team working in Tanzania. Members of the Zambian team, with whom I worked, included Beatrice Liatto-Katundu, who was local coordinator, and Tashisho Chabala, Arnold Kunda, Lillian Mushota, Olive Munjanja, Faustina Mkandawire, Caroline Shonga, and Anne Sikwibele.

NOTES

1. See Baylies and Bujra (forthcoming) for a detailed account of this research and its findings.
2. Focus group discussion, April 9, 1996; facilitator T. Chabala. The group was composed of five married women and one widow, among them a retired teacher and three community workers.
3. Lukakula Village, April 16, 1996; facilitator T. Chabala.
4. Attempts were also made to liaise with and encourage connections between groups and potential funders within the NGO/donor/government nexus.
5. Focus group, Kanyama, RDC, September 18, 1996; facilitator F. Mkandawire.
6. This emerged as a dominant theme in contributions to an Ethical Issues in International Health Research Discussion List, sponsored by the Harvard School of Public Health (bioethics@hsphsun2.harvard.edu; May 8, 2000).
7. While an ongoing process, some progress has been registered through agreements by pharmaceutical companies to reduce costs of drugs for treating HIV ("Health-L [Zambia]," health-l@hivnet.ch, [543] Cost of AIDS Drugs for Africa).

Chapter 18

AIDS and Ethics: Clinical Trials, Pharmaceuticals, and Global Scientific Practice

Susan Craddock

Whereas much has been done to address the HIV/AIDS pandemic in a multidisciplinary way, very little has been done regarding legal and ethical issues.
Nsubuga K. Yusuf, Uganda Network on Law, Ethics, and HIV/AIDS

Introduction

It is difficult to contemplate AIDS in the world today without contemplating human rights and social justice. As other chapters in this book attest, the huge death toll from AIDS in Africa is a painful testament to inequitable location in global economies, inadequate health-care budgets, and national and international neglect of human lives and the complex antecedents of a devastating syndrome. Yet AIDS recently has made other facets of human rights and ethics more visible. The conduct of several clinical trials of antiretroviral drugs in African and other nonindustrial countries in the past several years has generated intense debate within the scientific community over trial designs that would not have met standards of ethical scientific prac-

tice in the U.S. Nine of sixteen of these studies were funded by the U.S. government through the Centers for Disease Control or the National Institutes of Health; the rest were funded by other governments and by the UN AIDS program.[1] All nine U.S.-funded studies and six other studies used a placebo-arm in investigating interventions into mother–infant (vertical) HIV transmission even though the antiretroviral drug AZT is known to effectively intervene in vertical transmission. Two similar studies being undertaken in the U.S. ensured that all women received AZT for the duration of the study. According to several physicians and lawyers contesting the design of the sixteen studies in poorer countries, the result of using placebos on HIV-infected pregnant women is that approximately 1,502 infants may be expected to die unnecessarily (Lurie et al. 1997).

That these studies would not have been allowed to take place in the U.S., that they were conducted instead in impoverished African countries, on pregnant women and their infants, has raised a multitude of questions over what is ethical in the production of scientific knowledge involving human subjects. As scientific practice becomes increasingly global and commercialized, these trials highlight unprecedented tensions being played out among individual rights, disease prevention, and corporate profit. They also point painfully clearly to what has become expedient in the short term for thousands of women with no other means of access to life-saving drugs. In part these issues revolve around interpretations of ethical recommendations guiding scientific practice since Nuremberg. But they also suggest larger questions, namely concerning ideologies of nation, race, and class buttressing apparent differential valuations of human life inherent in transglobal scientific practice and the institutions that support it; pharmaceutical power and privileging of profits involved in medical research on AIDS and other diseases; and the degree to which medical research is both contributing to and exploiting a globalization characterized by untenable aid packages and inequitable flows of capital and commodities. In the rest of this chapter, after a more thorough description of the trials, I will address some of these issues with the intention of raising more questions than I answer concerning scientific practice and its implications for Africans living with the AIDS epidemic. My main argument, however, is that bioethics and medical communities must attend to the larger social and economic contexts which have enabled these trials to take place, and which indeed have made them desirable for those communities cited for the trials. Getting beyond the impasse of ethical debates requires this recognition that medical practices and the contexts they currently exploit constitute larger questions of social justice and human rights that cannot be addressed simply by rewriting ethical guidelines for medical practice. They must be addressed rather through more comprehensive changes in the status quo of global economic and political practice.

The Trials

In 1994 a team of medical researchers published the result of a study that has come to be known as AIDS Clinical Trials Group (ACTG) Protocol 076. The purpose of the study was to test the efficacy of zidovudine, or AZT, in preventing transmission of HIV from pregnant women to their infants during pregnancy and delivery. Between 1991 and 1993, 477 pregnant women around the U.S. were enrolled in a randomized, double blind, placebo-controlled trial. Approximately half of the women who enrolled were randomly selected to receive AZT while the other half received a placebo; neither the women who participated in the study, nor the researchers conducting it, knew who was in the placebo or the AZT groups. At the time the study took place, AZT's effectiveness in diminishing viral load in most seropositive individuals was established. What was not known, however, was whether AZT could be similarly effective in preventing transmission between mothers and children. As the authors of the study note, maternal–infant transmission "is the primary means by which young children become infected with HIV type 1 ... [with] fifteen to forty percent of infants born to infected mothers becom[ing] infected in utero, during labor and delivery, or by breastfeeding" (Connor et al. 1994:1173). In the U.S. or elsewhere, HIV infection in infants almost always proves fatal.

Women in the study received AZT (or a placebo) beginning in the second trimester of pregnancy or later, and during delivery of their infants; infants in turn received treatment for six weeks after birth. The results of the study showed that AZT was indeed highly effective in preventing vertical transmission. The proportion of infants infected at 18 months of age in the zidovudine group was 8.3 percent on average, versus an average of 25.5 percent in the placebo group (Connor et al. 1994:1176). In other words, infection was reduced by 67.5 percent, or two-thirds, in the AZT group (1994). AZT was so effective in reducing mother-to-infant transmission that the study was halted early; in the opinion of the researchers, it would have been unethical to continue to withhold treatment from the women in the placebo group (Lurie et al. 1997:2).

It is necessary to know the findings of the Protocol 076 study in order to understand the ethical questions raised by subsequent studies performed in Africa and elsewhere on interventions into vertical HIV transmission. The primary motivation for the studies was commendable: the duration of AZT treatment as indicated by the Protocol 076 study was an average of 11 weeks during pregnancy, during labor and delivery, and for six weeks to the infant after birth. The cost of this standard course of AZT is approximately $1,000 per patient. With average per capita annual incomes in much of sub-Saharan Africa less than half of this amount, and average per capita government health-care expenditures a small fraction of this (Bayer 1998:568), virtually no one in African countries could afford to take advantage of the treatment despite the fact that vertical transmission is a far greater problem in much of Africa than in industrial countries. The exciting findings of the ACTG 076 study were significantly diminished, then, by the fact that those countries in greatest need of the regimen were those that could not afford to access it. Addressing this discrepancy, the World Health Organization in June of 1994 called for studies to be launched testing the efficacy of a shorter course of AZT that might be affordable to a much larger number of women in poorer countries (Bayer 1998:568).

It is the design of the trials that has subsequently come under scrutiny. Medical research today is guided by a number of documents outlining what is ethical in research and what basic principles medical investigators should follow in designing and implementing their clinical trials. As aptly stated by Troyen Brennan of Harvard Medical school, "the heterogeneous foundations of research ethics are the result of revulsion" (Brennan 1999:527), that is, revulsion generated by abusive experiments performed without consent on human subjects in Tuskegee, Alabama, and during the Nazi regime. The Nuremberg Code of 1947 was a response to Nazi experiments, and its numerous principles of scientific research are clearly aimed at safeguarding individuals from potential abuse in the pursuit of medical knowledge. Its most notable guidelines state that research participants "should be so situated as to be able to exercise free power of choice," or the principle of informed consent (quoted in Loff and Black 2000:292); that experiments should not be random but instead should "yield fruitful results for the good of society, unprocurable by other means" (Loff and Black 2000:292); and that experiments should be designed and conducted in such a way as to avoid any possibility of harm to the research participants (Lurie et al. 1997:6).

The World Health Organization issued its own response to Nazi science in 1964 with the Declaration of Helsinki, a document that adds to the principles of the Nuremberg Code. Specifically, two statements contained in the Declaration of Helsinki bear repeating here: that "the interest of science and society should never take precedence over considerations related to the well-being of the subject," and that "In any medical study, every patient – including those of a control group, if any – should be assured of the best proven diagnostic and therapeutic method" (1989, quoted in Angell 1997:847).

By incorporating groups of women who do not receive the best proven therapeutic treatment, the designs of the post-Protocol 076 trials appear to be in direct violation of the unambiguous principles contained in the Declaration. Reaction accordingly has been vehement. In a now famous commentary published in the prestigious *New England Journal of Medicine*, Marcia Angell, the then Executive Editor of the journal, likened the design of the HIV intervention trials being conducted mainly in southern Africa to the Tuskegee medical experiments conducted in the U.S. under the U.S. Public Health Service (1997). In that study, 204 poor southern African-American men with syphilis were followed but not treated from 1932 to 1972 to trace the "natural history" of the disease. Within a few years of the study's inception penicillin came out as an effective treatment for syphilis, yet the study continued without providing participants access to the drug. Nor were the participants ever asked for their consent to participate in the study – indeed researchers deliberately deceived the men as to the purposes of the research. As Angell points out, the arguments in favor of the study suggested that these men would not have had access to treatment anyway given their poverty and rural isolation, so researchers were just observing what would have happened even if the study were not done. As one physician purportedly commented, the study was a "never-to-be-repeated opportunity" given the imminent widespread availability of penicillin (quoted in Angell 1997:847).

Outrage was quick over this comparison of HIV intervention trials to the most notorious chapter in U.S. medical history,[2] but Angell's analogy was not chosen arbitrarily. One of the primary arguments of proponents of the AZT intervention trials centers around "standard of care." The simplest version of the standard of care argument is that it is ethical to conduct a placebo-controlled trial in a country where trial participants would not receive therapeutic treatment anyway because of widespread poverty and the expense of therapy. To the question of why an African woman with AIDS would knowingly take a placebo in a trial when American women with AIDS would not, a writer for *The Economist* responds that the answer is cruel but simple: because an effective alternative is not available to the African woman (1997:19). In an African setting, then, the question is whether a less expensive treatment is better than none at all, and that is what the interventions were designed to answer. Likewise, David Ho of the Aaron Diamon AIDS Research Center in New York responds that the intervention studies were designed "to be responsive to local needs." Invoking the support of local researchers to buttress his point, he adds that "African scientists have argued that it is not in their best interest to include a complicated and costly AZT regimen for the sake of comparison when such a regimen is not only unaffordable but logistically infeasible" (Ho 1997:83; cf. Mbidde 1998). Though not exactly responding to the principle of the Declaration of Helsinki, the point proponents make is that there is not one standard of care that can be, or even should be, incorporated into the design of clinical trials. On the contrary, standards of care vary significantly across the globe, and trial designs need to reflect such variations in local conditions if they are going to be helpful to the communities in question (Karim 1998).

An extension of the standard of care argument emphasizes the dubious applicability of Protocol 076 results to non-Western countries. This argument responds more specifically to the charge made by critics that after the establishment of Protocol 076, only equivalency rather than placebo-controlled studies can be considered ethical. Equivalency studies would compare short-course regimens of AZT in one group against the longer Protocol 076 regimen in a control group. The efficacy of the short versus the longer course of AZT would then be determined. But proponents of placebo-armed trials contend that equivalency trials would not work. The trials for 076 were conducted in the U.S. under conditions of relative prosperity, good nutrition, and adequate health care. Conditions in poorer countries are not necessarily similar, and where undernutrition is more common, health more compromised by infectious and respiratory diseases, and medical care inadequate if not nonexistent, the generalizability of 076 results (i.e., of a two-thirds reduction of HIV vertical transmission) is claimed by proponents of placebo trials as negligible (Karim 1998; Varmus and Satcher 1997).

In fact, according to Salim Karim, a South African researcher, even the rates of vertical HIV transmission within South Africa cannot be generalized because they are changing over time: one study conducted in 1990–1 found a 27 percent vertical transmission rate, while a 1993–4 study found one of 38 percent (Moodley 1994, cited in Karim 1998:565). If a baseline vertical transmission rate is not known, and if it is uncertain whether the standard Protocol 076 therapy would result in 66 percent reduction of vertical transmission rates for South Africa, then it is impossible to determine without a placebo whether a short-course therapy is as effective as Protocol 076 in different settings, or indeed whether a short-course AZT regimen is effective at all. A placebo-controlled study then becomes more ethical, according to proponents, because only with this design can a clear understanding be gained of the efficacy and applicability of a short-course AZT regimen for particular regions (Karim 1998; Varmus and Satcher 1997).

These arguments of regional context are compelling, yet the larger background of international research and institutional practice of which these trial debates are a part is more complicated. When the WHO called for post-Protocol 076 trials to be conducted, it specified that these trials should use randomized placebo-control designs (Bayer 1998). The impetus for this bias toward use of placebo-arms in trial protocols comes largely from agencies such as the National Institutes of Health (NIH) and the Food and Drug Administration (FDA) who determined that randomized clinical trials incorporating placebo-arms constitute the best method for obtaining rigorous scientific results. Without even addressing the disciplinary history explaining why this determination was made, the more important point is that it has had widespread material repercussions. The FDA in particular has significant influence over international research practices because it prefers "the gold standard" of placebo-controlled medical research for approving new drugs no matter where the drugs are tested, or whether they constitute a new class of drugs or an alternative to existing treatments (Lurie and Wolfe 1998; Temple 1982 1996; Jost 2000). Yet the NIH is also influential because of its control over research funding. In the case of a Harvard University-based trial in Thailand testing effectiveness of AZT interventions into HIV vertical transmission, the NIH insisted upon a placebo-arm trial design as a contingency for funding. Despite this mandate, the Harvard School of Public Health's ethics review board refused to include a placebo-arm in the trial design, insisting that such a design would be unethical. Harvard finally won, but it has been the sole exception in NIH-funded international AZT trials (Wolfe and Lurie 1997).

The applicability of placebo-armed trials in cases of no known effective treatment is apparent, yet the insistence on this particular design across all therapeutic circumstances and regional contexts exemplifies Haraway's comment that "the power to define what counts as technical or as political is very much at the heart of technoscience" (Haraway 1996:89). I would turn that statement around, however, to say that the power to define what counts as technical in technoscience is very much political. Many European countries, Japan, and New Zealand consciously avoid reliance upon randomized placebo-controlled trials, allowing them only in cases where no known treatment is available, or where minor ailments such as headaches or insomnia are involved (Jost 2000:182). The reasons given by medical researchers in these countries for shunning placebo-arms pivot around medical ethics and the rights of individuals involved in research. The point is also made that other study designs provide equally legitimate results (Jost 2000:182). In light of such extensive opposition, the U.S. reliance upon placebo-arms in medical research illustrates the politics involved in determining what counts as (technical) knowledge, and in arguably determining the prioritization of "science" over human rights. The FDA's and NIH's normalization of placebo-arm trials also condones, however indirectly, the practice of this protocol design by pharmaceutical and medical device companies eager to demonstrate as quickly as possible for marketing purposes that their products work, rather than to test whether they work more or less effectively against other products (Jost 2000:176).

A separate issue involved in the trial design debate revolves around an apparent lack of communication among researchers concerning what was known or not known about the effectiveness of short-course AZT regimens. As Wolfe and Lurie note (1997), the Protocol 076 trial itself contained data relevant to those researching the effectiveness of a shorter course of AZT. Protocol 076 enrolled women at different stages of their pregnancies, and the results were classified according to how many weeks women had received AZT. Those women receiving an average of seven weeks of AZT showed an HIV transmission rate of only 7.7 percent versus 22.9 percent in the placebo-arm, a clear indication that a shorter course of AZT was as effective as the longer course (66.4 percent versus 65.1 percent reduction, respectively), and certainly more effective than a placebo. Though this breakdown of data according to duration of AZT was not included in the primary Protocol 076 publication, it was presented to the NIH Data Safety Monitoring Board in February of 1994 (Lurie and Wolfe 1997:2). Data from other studies testing the efficacy of shorter-course AZT in vertical HIV transmission have also been published subsequent to Protocol 076. A study done in the Bahamas showed transmission rates of 12.5 percent versus 11.5 percent among women receiving AZT for less than two months and more than two months of pregnancy, respectively (Gomez et al. 1997, cited in Wolfe and Lurie 1997). And perhaps more importantly, a Thai study published in 1998 showed a 51 percent reduction of HIV transmission among women taking a short course of AZT, results that prompted the CDC to end placebo-arms in that study as well as one in the Côte d'Ivoire (Studdert and Brennan 1998). Why these study results were not taken into consideration by those researchers designing the post-Protocol 076 trials, nor the Institutional Review Boards (IRBs) approving the studies, remains unclear.

Drug Availability

The question of whether and how post-Protocol 076 trials should have been conducted is itself a subsidiary of broader ethical debates largely kindled by the AIDS epidemic and increasingly gaining the attention of the medical community. One of these issues is whether a drug found to be effective is made available to the communities that participated in testing it. Though the post-Protocol 076 trials are ostensibly about finding a less expensive regimen of AZT to ensure greater access among women in poorer countries, it is far from clear that even a shorter course of AZT will be affordable to the vast majority of women in most African countries. One editorial focusing on South Africa's HIV-positive pregnant women, for example, accuses Glaxo of "allowing thousands of avoidable infant HIV infections to take place" because the company's pricing policies make AZT unaffordable to most South Africans, even in short courses (Ekambaram 2000:23). South Africa's case is made somewhat more complicated by the vacillations of its Health Minister, Manto Tshabalala Msimang, over whether the South African government would buy AZT and make it available to pregnant women, or whether limited resources were better spent on education and prevention (Baleta 1999). Yet even with reluctant state support of AZT, problems have ensued in acquiring the drug from Glaxo at prices that the government can afford, and in amounts that will be anywhere near proportional to demand (Baleta 1999). Short course or not, AZT's price keeps it beyond the purchasing capacity of most African governments, not to mention their more impoverished constituencies. Until

recently (see below), the pharmaceuticals' response to their high-priced drugs was exemplified by Peter Moore, Glaxo's medical director for sub-Saharan Africa, commenting that "I'm not really sure it's our responsibility to be involved in the ethical issues..." (Finkel 2000:A09).

The concern over making drugs available after a trial's completion does not end with AZT trials, but extends to drug trials in general and most recently, to AIDS vaccine trials (Rothman 2000). Drug availability also raises related ethical questions concerning whether trials should be conducted in countries where participants and their communities are unlikely to benefit from research findings, or whether individuals in poor countries are being exploited in research geared toward patients in richer countries where subject recruitment would be more difficult (Wilmhurst 1997:840; McLean 1997; King 1997). More will be said about vaccine trials below, but the primary concern here is that individuals from poor countries might play the part of guinea pigs in order to determine the safety and efficacy of drugs or vaccines whose primary markets, if effective, will be industrial countries like the U.S. As summarized by Wilmhurst, pharmaceuticals conduct research in African and other poor countries because of "lower costs, lower risk of litigation, less stringent ethical review, the availability of populations prepared to give unquestioning consent, anticipated underreporting of side effects because of lower consumer awareness, the desire for personal advancement by participants, and the desire to create new markets for drugs" (1997:841).

It has become increasingly obvious that those markets are not located in Africa or in most other poorer countries where testing takes place. Pharmaceutical companies have come under increasing fire recently for their drug pricing policies, placing antiretrovirals out of reach of almost everyone outside of industrial countries. Out of over a million people estimated to be infected with HIV in Malawi, for example, only about thirty people are on drug cocktails; yet even for these individuals access is tenuous, dependent on the ability of employers or the Malawian government to continue purchasing them (Finkel

2000). Answering increasing international criticism of their pricing policies, several pharmaceutical companies (including Glaxo, Bristol-Myers Squibb, Merck, and Boehringer Ingelheim) agreed to offer their AIDS drugs to targeted countries at significantly reduced prices. Though a step in the right direction, there are two problems with this move. The first is the sluggish pace at which deals are being negotiated with individual countries. After several months of negotiations, only a few countries have signed contracts and begun receiving drugs at reduced cost. One example is Senegal, which brokered a deal with Bristol-Myer, Glaxo, and Merck to begin supplying several antiretroviral drugs at prices up to 90 percent below market cost (Schoofs and Waldholz 2000). But the second problem is that even with prices significantly reduced, drugs are beyond the capacity of most individuals or governments to purchase. The combined cost of the reduced drugs supplied to Senegal, for example, is well over $1,000 per person, beyond the reach of all but the wealthiest few (Schoofs and Waldholz 2000). This concern is above and beyond the logistical problems of getting drugs to individuals in remote areas and ensuring long-term adherence.

A serious contestation of drug pricing policies recently came into play, however, when two Indian drug companies, Cipla and Hetero, announced a proposal to begin producing and selling AIDS drugs at even greater price reductions than those being brokered by the major pharmaceuticals. The drugs would be distributed to agencies such as Doctors Without Borders, and at prices of $350 to $600 would seriously undercut the major pharmaceutical price reductions (Zimmerman et al. 2001). The action had drawbacks, such as covering only a few patented AIDS drugs (Zimmerman 2001),[3] but the reaction of pharmaceuticals was nonetheless immediate. While accusing Cipla and Hetero of tenuous legal grounds in their intended actions, Merck, Bristol-Myers Squibb, GlaxoSmithKline, and others simultaneously began announcing greater price reductions of their drugs to match those announced by Cipla and Hetero. Merck also reversed its policy of country-by-country negotiations, instead setting a standard price for each drug for purchase by any country or organization (Schoofs and Waldholz 2001). The reversal was generated by the threefold need to save face, to regain a hold on the market, and to combat the potential for governments and international organizations to rescind patent rights (Schoofs and Waldholz 2001).

Pharmaceutical face-saving was relatively short lived, however. Two other potential means of acquiring cheaper drugs involve either manufacturing or importing generic versions of patented antiretrovirals, practices called compulsory licensing and parallel importing, respectively. Both practices are legal under a loophole of the World Trade Organization's regulations concerning drug patenting and intellectual property. That loophole states that in countries hard hit by a disabling or fatal disease, national governments may permit companies to manufacture essential drugs without the authorization of the patent holders but with compensation of 1–10 percent of sales of the drug to the patent holder (Singh 2000). The drugs are produced far more cheaply and sold at a fraction of the price demanded by the patenting pharmaceutical, thus allowing governments to purchase higher quantities for their populations in need.

The initial problem with these alternatives is that despite their legality under World Trade Organization regulations, pharmaceuticals and even the U.S. government threw impediments in the way of countries' attempts at parallel import and compulsory licensing. The most visible example of this has been the case of South Africa. Backed by powerful pharmaceutical lobbies, the U.S. until recently threatened trade sanctions against South Africa after its 1997 Medicines and Related Substances Control Act cleared the way for compulsory licensing of AIDS drugs (Ireland 1999). As one report stated it, "pressure has been put on the government ... of South Africa to safeguard profits of U.S. pharmaceutical interests against the needs of the people" (Singh 2000:30). Subsequent international criticism toward the U.S. during a presidential election year caused a reversal in that policy that so far has held: the U.S. now no longer stands in the way of countries attempting to manufacture or import cheaper AIDS drugs. Despite this reversal, GlaxoSmithKline and the South African Pharmaceutical Manufacturers Association recently sued the South African government for abrogation of intellectual property rights in passing the 1997 Medicines Act and in allowing South African drug companies to manufacture cheaper versions of major AIDS drugs. The suit went to court, with South Africa's Treatment Action Campaign (TAC), a local AIDS lobbying group, joining the defense and claiming that patients' rights should be placed above pharmaceutical profit in the fight against AIDS (Block 2001). International criticism of pharmaceuticals escalated during this highly publicized case, with pharmaceuticals increasingly seen as placing "patents over patients" in a nation contending with an estimated 4.7 million HIV-positive people and virtually no access to life-prolonging therapies. The result of this criticism and its attendant public relations nightmare was that by mid-April 2001, the 39 pharmaceuticals unconditionally dropped their case against the South African government (British Broadcasting Corporation 2001).

Ethics and AIDS Vaccines

Though the virtual impunity with which pharmaceuticals have been pricing their drugs is seemingly over, the ethical questions arising from AIDS and its prevention continue. Vaccine research is gaining visibility as another arena for concern about enabling scientific progress through neocolonial relations and the differential valuation of individuals' lives in poor countries. According to a recent World Bank report, most of the money for AIDS vaccine research is allocated for HIV subtypes more common in North America and western Europe (World Bank 2000/2001, cited in Sharma 2000). Yet people in poorer countries make better participants in trials testing the efficacy of those vaccines both because they are "treatment naïve," meaning they have not been exposed to drug regimens, and because, apparently, it is acceptable for them to be exposed to HIV during the course of a vaccine trial.

Testing the efficacy of AIDS vaccines, for example, is trickier in countries where individuals have broad access to antiretroviral drugs and where medical standards encourage drug treatment early in the event of HIV seroconversion. Antiretrovirals make it difficult to determine whether a vaccine might be effective in blocking the impact of HIV on the body, since they also work in varying ways to block HIV's ability to damage the immune system. Institutional review boards in the U.S. and other industrial countries also require researchers to counsel trial participants on avoiding risky behaviors and on where to obtain access to condoms, clean needles, and medical assistance. The unfortunate irony, however, is that it is impossible to know the efficacy of an AIDS vaccine if trial participants have not been exposed to HIV. Vaccine trials are thus better conducted in countries with higher prevalence of HIV, less stringent requirements on counseling, less effective educational outreach programs, and few regulations on partner notification; where participants are more likely, in other words, to be exposed to HIV (Rothman 2000). Finding a vaccine with the potential to save thousands of lives, then, apparently requires the sacrifice of hundreds. As Barry Bloom, the chair of the UNAIDS Vaccine Advisory Committee, stated, "Determination of the protective efficacy of HIV vaccine candidates may only be possible in trials in developing countries where the resources are not available to provide antiretroviral drugs" (1998, quoted in Rothman 2000:63). And where the seroconversion and potential death from AIDS of participants, it would seem, is less of a concern. Indeed, it is a bonus. Treatment does not have to be given in trials in most poor countries in the event of HIV seroconversion. If and when subjects contract AIDS during the course of a trial and are not given AIDS drugs such as AZT, then, "researchers would learn more about other properties of the vaccine, including whether it reduced the severity of the disease or the infectiousness of the virus" (Rothman 2000:63). Hints of Tuskegee all over again.

Ethical concerns of vaccine trials become even more trenchant in light of two recent developments. The first involves proposed changes to the Helsinki Declaration, and the second involves changes in the structure of international medical research. The Helsinki Declaration is only a set of guidelines for medical research, and as such they are not enforceable; the trials described in this chapter have clearly abrogated those guidelines. Yet the Declaration nonetheless serves an important function in setting standards by which research should be conducted and by signaling a consensus among the medical community on issues of ethics and patients' rights in the pursuit of scientific knowledge. Yet some in the research community contend that rather than seeing recent trial protocols as abrogations of the Declaration, they should signal the need to rethink the Helsinki guidelines in light of the recent shift toward globalized medical research. Accordingly, recent revisions to the Declaration have been suggested which would dilute those clauses ensuring patient rights and informed consent. A summary of those changes follows (taken from Loff and Black 2000:295):

II.3. *Current*: "In every medical study, every patient, including those of a control group, if any, should be assured of the best proven diagnostic and therapeutic method. *Proposed*: "In any biomedical research protocol every patient-subject, including those of a control group, if any, should be assured that he or she will not be denied access to the best proven diagnostic, prophylactic or therapeutic method *that would otherwise be available to him or her*" (italics added).

II.3. *Current*: "This does not exclude the use of inert placebo in studies where no proven diagnostic or therapeutic method exists." *Proposed*: "This principle does not exclude the use of placebo or no-treatment control groups if such are justified by a scientifically and ethically sound research protocol. When outcome measures are neither death nor disability, placebo or other no-treatment controls may be justified on the basis of their efficiency."

II.5. *Current*: "If the physician considers it essential not to obtain informed consent, the specific reasons for this proposal should be stated in the experimental protocol for transmission to the independent committee." *Proposed*: "When permitted by applicable law, the requirement for informed consent may be waived by the independent research ethics committee."

These proposed revisions have not been passed so far, and in recent international meetings of the medical community discussion of them has either been inconclusive, or significant opposition has been voiced about the implications of the proposed changes to patients'

rights (Stockhausen 2000; Lurie and Wolfe 1999a, 1999b). In particular, there is a fear "that these revisions may inappropriately cause a shift to an efficiency-based standard for research involving human subjects and weaken the principles of the investigator's moral commitment to the research subject and the just allocation of the benefits and burdens of research" (Brennan 1999:527). Indeed, it is clear that the proposed revisions to the Helsinki Declaration are designed to better enable medical researchers to perform research cheaply and with fewer impediments. The first proposed revision listed above reverts to the standard of care argument, meaning that if no drugs or prophylactics are available in a poor country, none need be provided by researchers to trial participants. In the second proposed revision, use of placebos if justified by "scientifically and ethically sound research protocol" leaves wide open the interpretation of what constitutes a sound research protocol, and whether there are any conditions in which placebos should not be used. The first two revisions not only potentially reduce costs to researchers, but also enable implementation of trial designs that would be unethical in industrialized countries.

Proposing to conduct research without informed consent, however, is perhaps the most explicit testament to the diminished value being placed by some medical researchers on the lives and well-being of individuals in poor countries. Informed consent is already a contentious practice in any context (Rothman 2000; Jost 2000), but especially when language and social understandings are profoundly disparate between researcher and researched or when contexts of poverty render questionable the very notion of "consent." As stated by a Zimbabwean virologist, "In an environment where the majority can neither read nor write and is wallowing in poverty and sickness, hunger and homelessness, and where the educated, the powerful, the rich or the expatriate is a semi-God, how can you talk of informed consent?" (cited in Lurie and Wolfe 1999a:3). Nonetheless, eliminating even the most flawed attempts at gaining the understanding of potential participants about the process and agendas of a trial, and ascertaining their willingness to participate in that process, is an ominous prospect. It indicates either that the lessons learned from Nazi medicine have been forgotten, or that those lessons only need apply to white bodies in rich Western countries.

The second trend involves a shift away from university-based research and toward research performed by for-profit organizations (Rothman 2000; Brennan 1999). Pharmaceuticals in particular are moving toward contract research organizations (CROs) as a way to speed up the process and reduce costs of getting drugs tested and out onto the market. The speed-up occurs in part because using CROs bypasses the institutional review boards (IRBs) and human subjects committees connected to university-based research. Bypassing IRBs, in turn, means a greater likelihood that CRO research protocols will have fewer oversights ensuring ethical design and conduct – stipulations that tend also to increase costs and add time to design and implementation phases of research. The trend toward CROs has not surprisingly been rapid. In 1991, academic medical centers were recipients of 80 percent of pharmaceutical funding for clinical trials; by 1998, this proportion had dropped to 50 percent (Bodenheimer 2000:1540, cited in Rothman 2000:63). The implications of moving toward for-profit research organizations and away from the oversight of institutional review boards, however flawed, are disturbing. It indicates an increased emphasis on efficiency and cost of research, and a heightened trend toward using individuals in poor countries to test drugs ultimately slated for western markets. As stated by Brennan, "the marketplace [does not] tolerate well the principle of commitment to an individual patient or research subject" (Brennan 1999:528).

More specifically, "the marketplace" is driven by individuals from pharmaceutical executives to drug representatives to medical researchers in for-profit organizations who have no qualms about acknowledging the neocolonial conditions necessary to the new structures of global research making their lives more profitable. At a meeting in London sponsored by pharmaceuticals and attended by CRO representatives, the theme was "Unleashing the Untapped Potential of Clinical Trials in Southeast Asia" (Rothman 2000:63). Conference programs were explicit in outlining the benefits of doing biomedical research in China, Malaysia, and South Korea: per patient trial costs are up to 25 percent lower than in the U.S. or Europe, many Asians are "treatment naïve" and thus will not sully research data, and the "changing disease profile" of many Asians means more research is possible on cardiovascular disorders, one of the most profitable markets for pharmaceuticals in Western countries. As summarized by David Rothman, "In this way, global economics goes hand in hand with global medicine" (Rothman 2000:63).

Conclusion

The question that arises from a discussion of globalized biomedicine is whether equitable research is possible between countries and institutions that are often vastly inequitable in resources, and with individuals who potentially have no other means of access to health care and drug therapies (Loff and Black 2000). Attempts to answer this question have generated numerous suggestions from the medical community. One answer is simply to ensure that the same basic standards of ethics pertain for all clinical research, no matter where it is conducted. If placebo-arms would not be used in the U.S. in post-Protocol 076 trials of AZT in pregnant women, for example, then they should not be used in Africa (Lurie and Wolfe 1998; Rothman 2000). This is not to suggest that all research should be conducted in exactly the same way, without regard to differences in cultural understandings of medicine and the body, or without sensitivity to differences in how decisions get made within communities vis-à-vis trial participation or informed consent (cf. Christakis and Fox 1992; Ijsselmuiden and Faden 1992). It does suggest that all trial participants everywhere in the world should have equal access to the same (best) treatments and medical care during clinical trials, and continued access to effective drugs after trial completion. More detailed responses of how equity should be met and maintained in clinical research focus on the importance of guidelines such as the Helsinki Declaration that have not been diluted in their commitment to patients' rights, and that have in fact been revised to better ensure patients' rights within changing norms of internationalized medical research (Stockhausen 2000; Report 1999; Brennan 1999). Others propose new protocols for designing and implementing clinical trials that incorporate greater community involvement, stricter justifications for conducting research among disenfranchised populations, greater oversight of potential exploitation in clinical research, and greater scrutiny of possible short- and long-term repercussions of a trial (Loff and Black 2000; UNAIDS 2000; Proceedings 1999).

These suggestions are all commendable to the extent that they demand a recommitment to patients' rights and an enhanced understanding of, and commitment to, globalized equity in clinical research. They also implicitly redress the racialized ideologies of difference informing those trial protocols incorporating ethical standards at variance with international medical guidelines. It is no coincidence that the emphasis on efficiency and cost in clinical trials comes at the expense of lives already devalued by extreme poverty, neocolonial global relations, and narratives of "overpopulation" in currency since the 1970s. Acknowledging these broader contexts enabling differential valuation of African (or Thai or Chinese) bodies is critical to reversing ominous trends in global biomedical research and ensuring safeguards on the lives of disenfranchised individuals.

But there is a sense in which these recommendations remain embedded within a discourse of medical experimentation that itself deserves scrutiny. Ensuring that individuals do not get hurt in the course of a clinical trial is a minimal safeguard, but is it adequate? As Solomon Benatar and Peter Singer suggest (2000), current recommendations to address perceived breaches of ethics in globalized clinical trials maintain a reactive posture signaling ontological roots in the post-Nazi era of medical research. The kind of equity proposed in most recommendations from the medical community, in other words, is largely limited to the design and implementation of clinical trials themselves. Left relatively unexamined are larger contexts of inequitable global relations, market forces, and funding structures that de-

termine not just how research is conducted, but what kinds of research are conducted. Also left unscrutinized in the recommendations for individual equity in research is the role medicine itself has played historically, and continues to play, in generating racialized narratives of global citizenship. Researching cardiovascular disease rather than malaria in Malaysia, no matter how well trial participants are treated, signals the unworthiness of addressing a disease that affects only individuals in poor countries, even if those affected individuals number in the millions. Ensuring better treatment of trial participants in Uganda will also not guarantee that the AIDS vaccines tested there will be designed for those subtypes of HIV most common in Uganda rather than the U.S., nor guarantee their affordability to the majority of those desperately needing it. Guaranteeing equitable treatment of trial participants, in other words, does not address the fact that currently 90 percent of annual funds spent worldwide on health research goes toward those diseases affecting 10 percent of the world's people (Sharma 2000:787). It also does not address those factors such as poverty, lack of sanitation, and access to health care that severely impinge on the quality of life of most individuals in poor countries. Leaving trial participants unharmed means implicitly condoning the status quo of resource inequity and overlooking medicine's potential for ameliorating it.

A more profoundly restructured research ethics, then, might be one grounded in the context of global health and systemic poverty (Benatar and Singer 2000). More precisely, a new "proactive" research ethics "must more forthrightly address the social, political, and economic forces that widen global inequities in health, and ... must ultimately be concerned with reducing inequities in global health and achieving justice in health research and health care" (Benatar and Singer 2000:826). Possibilities for what this restructured ethics might look like include performing research only on those diseases commonly afflicting the study community, undertaking research that benefits the study community, translating research findings into components of accessible care in the study community, and ensuring that research builds capacity of local health-care professionals and does not inadvertently drain resources away from other health care needs (Benatar and Singer 2000:825–826). This is of course only a partial list, but it nevertheless suggests a reconstitution of what is viable and ethical not just for the design of clinical trials, but more broadly for the focus of medical funding and research. When as much emphasis and money is placed on researching malaria as on marketing profitable drugs, and when poverty and social deprivation are considered issues to ameliorate rather than capitalize on in medical research, then a new era of global medical ethics will truly be launched.

ACKNOWLEDGMENTS

I would like to thank Ida Susser, Jane Huber, and Brooke Schoepf for reading earlier versions of this chapter and for their insightful comments. The views and arguments contained within the final version remain solely my own.

NOTES

1. The other governments were France with two studies, Belgium, Denmark, and South Africa (Lurie et al. 1997:1). The countries in question are the Côte d'Ivoire, Uganda, Tanzania, Malawi, Ethiopia, Burkina Faso, Zimbabwe, Kenya, Thailand, Dominican Republic, and South Africa (Bayer 1998:568).
2. Two members of the editorial board of *The New England Journal of Medicine* resigned over the comparison, and at least one of them, David Ho, made a rebuttal (1997); a rebuttal was also made by Harold Varmus and David Satcher, directors of the NIH and CDC, respectively (1997).
3. Only three of ten AIDS drugs were on offer from Cipla, namely Zerit from Bristol-Myers, 3TC from GlaxoSmithKline, and Viramune from Boehringer Ingelheim (Zimmerman et al. 2001:B13).

Part V

Understanding the Repercussions/ Impacts

Introduction to Part V

It is difficult to summarize all of the impacts AIDS has had on African economies and communities. One of the elements not easily encapsulated within any analysis of AIDS is the degree of emotional suffering by those either afflicted by AIDS or watching a loved one die. It is virtually impossible to portray what it must feel like to live in a hard-hit community in Africa today; the funerals, the classrooms with no teachers, the children struggling to run households with no parents, the hopelessness and despair as the epidemic progresses with few means of treating the ill or tangible means of intervention.

Kaleeba's chapter depicts the unimaginable personal tragedies caused by AIDS for many in sub-Saharan Africa. Yet through her portrayal of the formation of TASO, an organization in Uganda to help those affected by AIDS, there is evidence of strength, compassion, and hope emerging from such profound loss.

Eaton's chapter provides some insightful portrayals of two musicians as they negotiated AIDS. Eaton's point of entry is to suggest the complex "social pragmatics" that sometimes preclude openly articulating visible instances of AIDS when disease is integrally connected to sorcery. Eaton weaves a highly personal and insightful portrayal of religious beliefs, social practice, and medical approaches surrounding AIDS in its earlier days, and the ways in which these are all inter-related. Eaton tells a story of what it is like to come to terms with a disease about which so much is not known except the seeming inevitability of its progress.

It might seem comparatively easier to calculate the toll on regional economies, and this is what Brown has tackled in her chapter on the impacts of HIV/AIDS on economic growth. What she insightfully points out, however, is that the usual indicator of economic growth or decline, the GDP or Gross Domestic Product, ends up being an inaccurate index for calculating the impact of AIDS because it pivots upon corresponding population growth figures. The significant losses of life have outstripped economic decline, thus ironically in some cases driving the GDP up rather than down. So, Brown concludes, a better indicator of impact is the

UNDP Human Development Index, which among other variables takes into account life expectancy. The HDI for hard-hit countries consequently has declined dramatically. Brown's extremely thorough and thoughtful analysis is a testament to the difficulties of measuring human devastation. Her last point is perhaps surprising given the emphasis on poverty's role in driving HIV/AIDS. Brown provides statistics showing accelerating rates of HIV/AIDS concomitant with regional economic growth spurts and raises the question of whether economic growth can actually bring with it the potential for increased AIDS. Clearly, alleviating poverty through economic growth is not a simple redress for AIDS; *how* poverty is addressed matters.

The fourth and fifth chapters in this section cover in very different ways the subject of AIDS orphans. Ghosh and Kalipeni provide an overview of numbers of orphans, potential impacts on child development and survival, and the difficulties of caring for them in such significant numbers. Many countries in Africa have tried various means of addressing this pressing issue, including state-run orphanages or subsidizations for extended-family care, but so far no solutions have proven adequate. Orphans are still very much at risk in most communities, where a paucity of funds and people to care for them means a greater likelihood that they will be malnourished, not go to school, and end up on the streets and in sex work. As Schoepf points out in her chapter in Part III, the growing emphasis by African states on community care of orphans is a travesty given the severe strain on community resources that AIDS has created and the rising numbers of orphans to care for. Guest's chapter provides a complement to Ghosh and Kalipeni's chapter with an insider's view of what life as an orphan is like. Tracing the lives of several South African orphans and their struggles for survival, Guest's portrayal is at once poignant, heartrending, and hopeful in the knowledge that individuals and communities find ways to mitigate loss.

One obvious element missing from this part is an inside view of the multiple and varied organizations that have developed at the community level to address aspects of AIDS. Africans, in other words, are not simply "victims" of an epidemic. From well-funded NGOs to small-scale movements, the proliferation of these organizations gives testament to the ability of communities to rally in varied and innovative ways. Whether they provide small loans to financially struggling households, help find treatment for the ill, care for orphans, or provide educational outreach, these organizations constitute a hopeful counterpoint to the inadequacies of higher-level interventions. Indeed since individuals understand best their communities' social practices and interpretations of risk, it is more likely that grassroots intervention strategies with adequate funding could better succeed in mitigating the progress and impacts of AIDS.

A final chapter might also have ended on a hopeful note with discussion of an imminent AIDS vaccine. The social, economic, and political forces driving HIV/AIDS are so profound and seemingly ineluctable that many argue AIDS will not see a decline in Africa until the advent of an effective vaccine. Unfortunately, one is not forthcoming in the near future. Pharmaceuticals have funneled disproportionately few resources into vaccine research relative to drug development because drugs have the better profit potential. With increasing global pressure and the financial help of nonprofit organizations like the International AIDS Vaccine

Initiative (IAVI), there are now a number of vaccines being tested, including in Uganda and Kenya. Yet the majority of these are only in Phase I trials which test for the safety, not the efficacy, of the vaccine. Only one type of vaccine so far is in Phase III testing for efficacy, and these trials are in the U.S. and Thailand. The African AIDS Vaccine Program recently met in Cape Town in an attempt to lure more international partnerships and funding for vaccine research to Africa, and to coordinate research across the continent. Initiatives such as IAVI and AAVP will undoubtedly speed up development and help with delivery of a vaccine for African countries. A vaccine is still many years away, however, and questions remain about the financing and logistics of distribution. Controversies abound as well around conduct of vaccine trials that depend upon HIV exposure to test efficacy (Craddock this volume; Schoepf 1991a; Rothman 2000). The consequent implications for individual welfare, ongoing regional intervention programs, and global medical ethics are profound, yet the resolution of these holds much promise for future interventions. Vaccines thus stand as further testament to the paradoxes of despair and optimism characterizing the fight against AIDS.

Chapter 19

Excerpt from *We Miss you All:* AIDS in the Family

Noerine Kaleeba

Part I: AIDS in the Family

The fateful telex

AIDS came to my house on the afternoon of June 6, 1986, when the British Council sent me a telex to tell me that my husband Chris was seriously ill in a hospital in England. He had gone to Hull University to do his postgraduate training the previous year.

I often wonder what my life would have been like today if that telex hadn't come. I know that Chris was already ill and dying, long before the telex was sent, but I always connect my misery and subsequent suffering to that telex.

During our last telephone conversation in May, Chris had told me that he was not coming home, as we had been anxiously expecting. His request to register for a Ph.D. had been accepted by the British Council, and so he would be away for another year. The political atmosphere in Uganda was also getting better, so the prospect of another year without him was not as desperate as it would have been a year earlier.

It never crossed my mind that Chris might be ill. So when I went into the British Council the next morning, and was given the telex, I was shocked. My husband was critically ill in a British hospital. He had been unconscious for three days. He seemed to have meningitis. He was not in pain, but his condition was critical. Everything was being done for him. The British Council staff were very solicitous, offering tea, and comforting me. They suggested I return the next day for more news.

The following day I went back with my friends Mary and Margaret to the same news. His condition was still critical; everything that could be done was being done. He needed me. But the Council people had to ask London first.

I went to a friend in the microbiology laboratory to ask him what he knew about meningitis. He suggested that I find out what type Chris had. I went back to the British Council with the question. The following day the answer came, cryptococcal meningitis. My microbiology friend reacted in a funny way and asked if I was sure it was cryptococcal.

I went back to the British Council and asked [them] to write it down for me. My friend in the laboratory then asked me to find out if they had done an HIV test. I vaguely wondered what the HIV test had to do with it, but I went back the next day and asked the question. Everybody looked at each other.

They said they would relay the question, and asked me to come back the next day to talk to the doctor on the phone. I can't quite recall quite how I got through those days, but I remember that the days merged into nights and I was crying a lot. The girls were devastated by my tears, and I couldn't even support them. All I knew was that Chris was dying. When I went back the next day, Dr. Symonds told me on the phone that the HIV test results were positive.

The news did not register right away. I was already saturated with misery. I did not believe it. There was no reason whatsoever to associate my husband with a white homosexual disease, which was what we knew about it in Uganda at that time. I did not believe it, and I did not know the magnitude of the stigma associated with AIDS, so I told my friends at work and the neighbors. I told my in-laws, and my parents. I told anyone who came to sympathize with me.

Meanwhile arrangements were being made for me to go to Chris.

My first encounter with AIDS

In 1983 some doctors in Uganda had started reporting cases of a disease that seemed similar to one being reported in the USA. The reaction of the Ministry of Health was that we already had enough problems with the war and the poor state of the economy, without trying to deal with AIDS as well. The attitude was: forget about AIDS: deal with the issues that you can do something about. After all, if people in the USA cannot cure AIDS, then what would be the point of saying that we have AIDS too?

At the same time it was a sensitive issue. People were asking, where did AIDS come from? Was it from America? Was it Tanzania? The instruction from the Ministry of Health was not to talk about AIDS, to avoid creating a scare that couldn't be dealt with then.

As a physiotherapist, at Mulago Hospital, I had heard intermittent reports of this mysterious and deadly illness, caused by a virus that did not respond to treatment. The early reports connected the illness with white homosexual men in San Francisco. Like many people, my reaction was to dismiss the illness as having nothing to do with us in Uganda. But then in 1983 we began to hear reports about a similar illness that was affecting people in the Kesensero area on the southwest border with Tanzania. There was also a strong rumor that the disease was contagious, and highly infectious sexually. I still dismissed the problem since there was nobody I knew in that area, nearly 200 kilometers from where I lived.

Meeting Chris

I was born at Seta Nazigo, a small village 35 kilometers southeast of Kampala, the third of ten children. I was educated at a missionary boarding school. After my O levels I was accepted for training at the Mulago Hospital School of Physiotherapy.

I was in my third year at the school when I met Christopher. He was handsome and smart, about 25 years old, from the same tribe as I. He said that he loved me. I had had other boyfriends before, but there had been no one I wanted to marry. I found myself head over heels in love with him. Life with Christopher was different. Exciting. My first exposure to love. Chris and I lived together for a year and a half, and had our first baby, Elizabeth, before we had saved enough money for the wedding. We had a modest Christmas wedding on December 27, 1975. Our second daughter, Phiona, was born in April 1976.

Phiona was a lovely child, but Chris was disappointed not to have a son. It was even more of a disappointment for Chris because he had wanted to have only two children, while I had wanted six. Now that there were two girls, he would have to have a third child, a boy. This was a hard time in our relationship. We were struggling to make ends meet, and we had two very young children.

We quarreled a bit over the first baby, over the second, maybe even a little over the third. One of our problems was dealing with family planning. We tried various family planning methods, including condoms. I did not fare well with the pill, and was scared to use an intrauterine device. So we used condoms, despite the fact that Chris did not like them much. He would use them, but became sulky afterwards and behaved as if he was unsatisfied.

Around this time Chris began a relationship with another woman, in search of a boy child. Although I suffered the stress of deprivation during this time, I did not feel betrayed, deserted, or angry at the other woman, because polygamy was something we had all grown up with. Another reason we didn't argue about the other woman was simply because our battles during that time were over the struggle to make ends meet. Our battles were not due to sexual jealousy, but over shortages in the house or the children going without something basic. Throughout this time Chris, because he loved me, did not behave in any way that showed that the other woman's presence divided his love.

The result of Chris's boy-seeking ventures was another bonny little girl, Julliet.

In the meantime, Chris had been studying privately for his A levels, and was accepted for a first degree at Makerere University. We were once again living happily as a family, and by the time Marion, our third child, was born in April 1980, we were a happy hardworking couple. I was working as a physiotherapy teacher, and Chris was studying sociology and social administration at Makerere. We suffered the life of married undergraduate students, but we were in love. Chris didn't seem to mind this time that Marion was a girl. Perhaps the shock of having tried for a boy elsewhere and getting a girl instead had taught him a lesson. We were maturing, and began to talk in a more constructive manner and plan our future.

In December 1980, I was awarded a British Council scholarship to study orthopedic physiotherapy in the UK. I was away for ten months, from January 1981.

When I returned to Uganda, I was appointed Principal of the School of Physiotherapy.

Chris was making plans to go to England for further education. When the news came of his acceptance at Hull University on a British Council scholarship we were all overjoyed. He was very happy because he was finally going to realize his life's ambition to become a university professor. If Chris returned with a Ph.D., it would mean a better job and a better way of life.

Chris left for Hull in July 1985, and registered for a Master's of Education in sociology and social administration. His families were all there to see him off, together with the girls and me. We were full of hope for the future.

We were not to know on that day at the airport that it would be the last time we would see him looking so tall, smart, and handsome.

The War

After Chris left for England the girls and I settled down to the life of a family separated by distance but bound closely by the love they shared in letters and a telephone call once a month.

By about October 1985 Chris's letters began to contain complaints of stomach discomforts and the total lack of any foodstuff that was appealing. I put this down to his inability to cook. In all the time I knew him he never cooked anything other than coffee or tea. I teased him about living in England and wanting to eat in Uganda.

By December 1985 the war that eventually brought the National Resistance Movement (NRM) led by Yoweri Museveni to power had reached a climax. Kampala was surrounded and mail was not moving. The second week of January 1986, which saw Kampala fall to the NRM, was a nasty experience. I had to hide with the four girls in the basement of our flat, where we stayed with no food and little water for three days. The departing soldiers were molesting, stealing, and raping women as they went, and it was God's great mercy that by the time they came to our house we had already gone into hiding.

> Five years ago in Uganda one man with a gun could walk through the door and take everything you had – just one man with one gun will make you lie down under the table and cover your face, while he takes everything. After you go through an experience like war, you come out a different person. Either you go down with the experience, or you rise, you are enhanced by the experience. So one of the things that the war experience has done for Ugandans is to produce a feeling of getting involved, a feeling of not wanting to suffer under the table. (Women and AIDS Support Network Conference Report, 1990:19)

I missed Chris terribly through this experience. I know now that during this time Chris was ill on and off with fever, loss of appetite, loss of weight, and mouth sores. He was working hard to complete his Master's degree and register for a Ph.D. His professor told me afterwards that he did not look after himself well enough. Chris's explanation to himself for his ill health was that he was missing the staple Ugandan food (matooke), was working too hard, and was lonely and missing his family. On June 2, 1986, he was referred by the University Health Centre to Hull Royal Infirmary where he collapsed and was diagnosed as having cryptococcal meningitis (an infection of the brain linked to AIDS). He was transferred to the care of Dr. Nanda at Castle Hill Hospital. It was there that the diagnosis of AIDS was made when he was found to be HIV positive. In view of the grave diagnosis, and the fact that he was critically ill, the hospital asked the British Council to contact me in Uganda.

My journey to Chris in England

I was finally able to leave Uganda to see Chris on June 12, 1986. I hardly remember the journey, which I seemed to make mechanically. I was met at Heathrow by a British Council guide, escorted on a three-hour train journey to Hull, and on the afternoon of June 13 I entered Ward 4 of Castle Hill Hospital. Dr. Symonds, the house officer, came in to explain once more that Chris was gravely ill, that I would probably not recognize him, and that I needed to be very strong when I went into his room.

I heard all this and nodded as he explained, but my only thought was to go to Chris. I still held on to a tiny possibility that this was all wrong, that I would get there and find that it had all been a mistake, a dream, a scare. Anything but not real. Finally he asked whether I wanted to see Chris and I said yes. I had to wear a sterile gown, footwear, gloves, and a mask, as they feared I would infect him because of the state of his health. As I entered Room 10, and was met with what was left of what had been my handsome young husband, two things struck me quite vividly. First, that I did not have a husband any more: he was dying, virtually dead. Second, I would have to be very strong for myself, for what was left for

Chris, and for the girls. I didn't cry then. I moved towards his bed like a zombie. He was awake and recognized me instantly. He lifted his frail arm, the one which was not strapped with tape and monitor leads, and attempted a smile.

"What took you so long?" he asked.

In hospital in England

As I write this I am having to fight hard to keep the tears back. I cannot understand how it was that I did not cry in front of Chris, then or ever. It was not that I did not have any tears, for afterwards in my room I cried for a long time, until I fell into an exhausted sleep.

The nurses were very afraid for me. I was impressed from the start by the attitude of the staff toward us. It was not long before I established that we were the only black couple on the ward, and their first heterosexual patients living with AIDS. Despite having two ingredients for stigma, we were treated with such care and compassion that it left an everlasting mark on me. It was then that I resolved that if God would allow me time and life I would like to return this kind of care to patients. They all went out of their way to be nice to us. Apart from the sympathetic way they nursed Chris, bathed him, combed his hair, dressed his wounds, they each did small things for him, like bringing him a flower from home, sending him a postcard when they were off duty for a few days, sharing their family photographs, and so on. I remember on his birthday, August 23, Sister Ann made a big cake with Happy Birthday Christopher on it. Everybody brought a card, and the staff came singing *Happy Birthday*. Although Chris wasn't happy at all, he managed a smile. This, his 36th birthday, was to be his last.

It was during the second week that Dr. Nanda, the consultant, asked me if I would consider taking an HIV test. It was the first time that I realized that Chris's being HIV positive had direct implications for me. Up to that time all that I had focused on was that he was dying. I sat down with Dr. Nanda and Dr. Symonds, and they explained that AIDS is a sexually transmitted disease and what the implications of this were for me. They asked me many questions, including whether I knew where Chris could have got the infection. I didn't. I couldn't think at the time. Then they asked me if Chris had ever had a blood transfusion. Yes. He had had a blood transfusion. Chris had been given eight units of blood when he was involved in an accident. He may have got the virus from that blood transfusion, which meant that he could have been infected in Uganda.

The accident

I was at work on July 7, 1983, when I was informed that Chris had been brought into casualty, bleeding profusely, having been run over by a bus. I rushed to casualty to find him on a trolley, his left leg twisted at a funny angle, and the doctor shouting for blood. In Uganda, like in many developing countries, blood for transfusions has to be found from relatives or volunteers, since there is never enough blood in the blood bank. I rushed around looking for blood donors. I was four months' pregnant and unable to give blood myself. I rang all of Chris's family around Kampala and informed them of the accident and of our desperate need for blood. Godfrey, his younger brother, was teaching at a nearby secondary school and rushed in to donate a unit of blood. As he was the same blood group as Chris, his unit was transfused straight away. Chris had to be given eight units altogether. He was hospitalized for two months and then discharged with a slight limp.

Later that year, our fourth child, Christine, was born. I was working hard, and had an additional part-time job. Things between Chris and me had seemed much better since Marion was born, but by the end of 1984 we were having problems again. Looking back now, I know why he was feeling weak, but at the time I couldn't understand it. Chris seemed to have lost interest in work, and was frustrated by his lack of success in registering for a Master's degree. He had been making plans, before the accident, to go to England for further education. Often I would return home after my two jobs to find him in bed complaining that he was tired or not feeling well.

In November 1984 he developed a skin rash and sores in his throat. The sores cleared up, but the rash persisted for three months.

This is when we started having major domestic problems again. In the time before he secured the scholarship to go to the UK our marriage was in trouble. Essentially I thought he had another woman, and so we were quarrelling most of the time. This didn't help our relationship. I was working at two places, and would only get home about six in the evening. Chris would already be in bed. When he was asked why, he wouldn't be able to explain it. He would say "I'm not strong enough. I am not feeling well. I'm not sick, but I'm not strong."

When the news came that he had been accepted at Hull University, we were all overjoyed. While he prepared for his departure we had a glimpse of the good old days. He was a happy, loving husband, and all the tiredness, which had characterized the previous few months, seemed to have evaporated. We had a lot of friends, and we began to plan to build a house.

The news of the scholarship came at a time when Chris particularly needed it. His younger brother, Godfrey, had just died, in April 1985. Godfrey had been ill for about a year, with a skin rash, fever, loss of appetite, steady weight loss, and finally death from meningitis. Chris and Godfrey had been very good friends, so his death affected Chris greatly. We did not suspect, at that time, that Godfrey had probably died of AIDS.

My HIV test

When I was asked by Dr. Symonds whether I had had sex with Chris after the accident and blood transfusion, I couldn't tell him everything about the quarrels and irregular sex. There are some things you can't even tell a doctor. I told him that we had had a time of normal sexual relations after the accident, and he said that meant that I was at risk of being infected [and] insisted that it was very important for me to know whether I was infected or not.

The next day a social worker was sent to talk to me. I don't know if she had been through a counseling course or not, but she rushed me through the whole counseling process – up to "What would you like to happen to your children if your test is positive?"

I wasn't just thinking about Chris, I thought about the children a lot. I was thinking about him dying, and how I was going to cope with the children on my own. But after the blood was drawn I also had to think about myself. Six days later they came and told me, "I'm glad to say the results of your test are negative." But they were very strict, very intent on not giving me false hope. From what I had told them they felt that the chances were high that I was positive, but that it didn't show up yet. They stressed that the results were preliminary, and another test would be needed six weeks later to confirm that I was in fact negative. I felt relief, but I did not feel happy about the result. In fact, the day I received the negative result it didn't mean that much to me. It really didn't. I knew it was a good thing. I knew that from the nurses, everybody was so excited for me.

I didn't tell Chris about the result that day, and when I did tell him, it was in rather an offhand manner. His first reaction was relief that I would be there for the children, although throughout his illness he was worried that I would marry again, or feared that I would become infected and die and leave the children with no one. He repeated this over and over. But from the day I told him the test result he started to plan for the future. The instructions were numerous. You have to do this. You have to take charge. You have to tell my mother this. You have to remember to tell my father that he should finish the house. You have to remember to do this and that.

Dr. Symonds had explained to me the implications of Chris's having AIDS. I tried to find out everything I could about the illness. I spoke on the telephone to people in the Terrence Higgins Trust in London, and was put in contact with two people, Mark and Johnny, who were starting a "buddy service" in Hull. This was a kind of volunteer support system for people living with AIDS. They came to see us and were very supportive and sympathetic listeners, although the issues that Chris and I were having to deal with were a little different from theirs as homosexuals. They spoke about stigma associated with AIDS, but not having been exposed to it we did not understand what they were trying to tell us.

Chris's major problem was still diarrhea and an inability to eat anything. He was being fed intravenously. After intensive therapy with amphotericin B, the cryptococcus was finally cleared from his cerebral fluid, and with intensive intravenous feeding with a specially formulated fluid he was able to restore some weight and enough strength to get out of bed to be taken to the toilet.

Going home

We were at the hospital in Hull for a long time, an agonizing experience. Chris would get better, then he would be bleeding through the nose, the next day the diarrhea would be less, the next week he would have a cough and fever. Through the ups and downs we received a lot of support from many different people.

The time came when we started talking more seriously about the future. At first, I had understood that Chris was going to die. Then it seemed that although his condition was too far gone for him to live totally normally, he would steadily recover and would be able to go back to university to finish his work. He knew that his only chance to complete his studies was to remain in England where he had access to medical care. What we totally underestimated was his need for support other than medical care. I mean the support that comes from family and friends.

We made the decision that I would go back home to the children. My sister was looking after them and although we were communicating with them regularly, their letters indicated that they were suffering from our absence, because they missed us and because of the uncertainty.

I had taken photographs during our stay in hospital, pictures of Chris at different stages. I put them in an album to send home so that the family could see what good progress he was making. What I didn't realize was that I had become used to his appearance. When the album reached home, and people compared how he looked in the pictures to the way he looked before he left for England, it only depressed them even further. By the time I got back everyone had lost hope and was convinced that he was dying.

When I returned home I found that things were not really the same. During the months I had been in England with Chris the AIDS issue had exploded in Uganda. Many cases were diagnosed but they were clothed in secrecy so that gossip about them flourished. People talked about them in moralistic and judgmental terms. Because HIV is transmitted through sex, it was a popular belief that those infected must have been immoral and promiscuous. This was the time I was first exposed to the stigma associated with HIV and AIDS.

The children started by telling me how they had been stigmatized at school, how people were asking questions about whether Chris or I had died of AIDS yet. I also began to notice that a few, not all, of my neighbors were very anxious to move on whenever we met them. Some of them stopped coming to the house. One or two neighbors tried hard to cover their anxiety and supported me in their own way.

I was beginning to feel the stigma myself. Whenever others did small or big things I felt they were being done deliberately. I expect everybody is exposed to stigma if they are in a situation like the one I was in. Some people don't understand, and you have to find explanations for the things that happen. So much of stigma comes from inside. People become so sensitive about everything that is said that even those who are being kind are misinterpreted.

I went straight back to work and began to notice that some of my colleagues, too, were finding it hard to deal with me. I learned that AIDS was being recognized in the hospital and was being talked about. The Ministry of Health had plans to institute an AIDS Control program, treating it as an infectious disease. I had been prepared for some of the stigma by Mark and Johnny, my buddies from Hull, who told me the problems faced by gays with AIDS in the world outside Castle Hill Hospital. But I was not prepared for these reactions from my own people. I would walk into the staff room and everyone would suddenly stop chatting. Suddenly it was time for everyone to go back to their work on the wards. I knew I was not included in conversations, or people would talk to me in excessively kind tones. I was surprised by this kind of behavior from fellow health professionals who had access to know-ledge and information, and who were trained to behave in a sympathetic manner. If they were unable to deal with me as an ordinary human being, how were they relating to their AIDS patients on the wards? I had to think back to my own training to examine the attitudes I myself had had.

My work as a physiotherapist

In my own career as a physiotherapist, in my work and interaction with my patients, one thing I am sure of is that I was a competent professional. I was given very comprehensive training by my beloved teachers, and my basic upbringing did not allow for a lack of discipline. What I do question now is my treatment of patients as people, as human beings with souls and emotions.

I remember working on the trauma and orthopedic ward during one of the troubled times in Uganda. The whole ward was filled with young men in their twenties who had been shot and were in wheelchairs for life. Young men whose lives had just begun found themselves stopped by a bullet. Suddenly they had no plans, no future.

I remember, vividly, that sometimes I would come to the ward with the best intentions, to teach someone to get out of bed into a wheelchair, to exercise his arms, expand the muscles of his trunk, so that he could cope with the chair. I would find him in a bad mood. No amount of coaxing or cracking jokes would get him out of bed that day. I would get very angry with this man who did not know what was good for him. I had a job to do. If he preferred to stay in bed for the rest of his life, he could suit himself. The following day, if he was in a better mood, I would tease him about the tantrums. I had no perception of his feelings. I couldn't even begin to appreciate the various emotions he was going through.

At other times I would be part of a major ward round. Like teaching hospitals all over the world, these rounds included the consultant, registrars, house officers, interns, a fleet of nursing staff, medical students, nursing students, physiotherapists, occupational therapists, and so on. They would congregate around one case and the discussions would go something like this:

The consultant asks the registrar, "How is this man getting on?" The registrar looks at the notes made by the intern and house officer. He reports back. "Is he taking his drugs, Sister?" Sister consults the drug chart and reports back. "Is he in pain?" All these questions are asked and answered within the group. Explanations are shared by the group in medical jargon and no effort is made to include the subject of the discussion. Decisions are taken, and orders barked to the juniors: Every time someone says something, the subject turns in that direction in the hope that he will be asked or given an explanation. In vain. Soon the whole group moves on to the next patient, and as it does so the subject may grab one of the friendly-looking physiotherapy students in search of an explanation. All he may receive is a sympathetic smile, a shrug of shoulders, a promise to return later to answer questions. A promise which doesn't materialize.

This kind of scenario was often described by Chris as the most inhuman part of interacting with people who were supposed to restore patients to full health.

Fighting in the open

I felt betrayed by the negative attitudes of those health care workers. It took me time to understand that the emergence of this new disease for which there was scanty information was causing panic. This panic, combined with the fact that the disease was associated with the two taboo subjects of sex and death, was the source of this deep stigma. There was an urgent need for clear information about HIV, but also for the fear to be confronted. It became increasingly evident to me that if I was going to fight this disease in any way, I would have to fight it in the open.

I did not really have a timeframe or a definite plan, or know what strategies I was going to adopt, but the one thing that I was sure of was the decision to remain open. In any case I didn't really have a choice, because I had already told everyone, when I first received the telex, that Chris had AIDS. I suppose I could have retracted the information if I had really wanted to. I could have said that it was all a mistake, that Chris had cancer or tuberculosis. But I decided, quite instinctively, that I wanted

to stick to the truth. It helped me that Chris and I discussed it before I left Hull. I explained to him that I had already told people his diagnosis, and he felt it was the right thing to do. The crucial part was that he didn't feel that having AIDS was something to be ashamed of.

I didn't really know what to do, but hoped for the best. Chris was making steady but slow progress. Just before the end of October 1986 I had another message from Hull, this time that Chris was coming home. Either he had been thrown out of England, which I didn't think was possible, or he had reached a state where he would not benefit from further treatment, which meant that he was coming home to die.

I was able to speak to Chris on the phone, and he told me that it was his decision to come home. I was surprised to hear that he was able to eat, and the people at Castle Hill were going to give him the medication he needed to come home with. He wanted to be home with the family, because he felt that without us life was just bare existence. In these circumstances I couldn't argue with him about the need to be near excellent medical care. We also badly wanted him to be home with us. I was very excited at the prospect of his coming home, but was also very apprehensive about how he would cope with the stigma I had already experienced. I was counting on his family. When I told them he was coming home, they agreed it was for the best.

Why I Came Out in the Open

For several years I was different from almost everyone else in Uganda, willing to share the experience of AIDS in my family. This was for a number of reasons. In the beginning I had already declared Chris's illness, and couldn't retract that. I suppose I could have opted not to tell the world, just suffered in the family. But I was increasingly convinced that AIDS was a disease that thrives in secrecy. It was prospering because people were choosing not to talk about it.

I reasoned that if people could see how it affected us, an ordinary average family, not a poor one, not a rich one, they would understand the importance of coming out. If it could happen to us, it could happen to anybody. The support that I received after Chris died was in response in my coming out. If I'd covered my head, been miserable and cried, I don't think I'd be where I am today.

Chris's return home

The day came when Chris returned home, we returned to his parents' house where a big meal had been organized. A big crowd turned up. The majority had come to sympathize, but there were some who had come to see what a person with AIDS actually looked like.

Chris handled the situation brilliantly. He was very excited, and he ate well. There is a photograph of him eating this whole mountain of food and he told me that the food had revived him. After this beginning he was able to eat small amounts of food, although he did vomit intermittently. That day the experience of seeing the children and his family gave him new life.

Before Chris came home I had held many discussions with God. I constantly asked for a miracle. Christopher's coming home was like rising from the dead. From the hospital bed in Castle Hill to being able to come home was the first miracle that I can recall in the whole terrible experience. I was later to think that there was another miracle, my good health. But the first miracle was when Chris came home, and was able to live with us again, in our home. It was nearly two months before he became ill again.

We had arranged that Chris would go straight to the hospital on his return. We expected him to be tired, and to need time to recover his strength under medical supervision before he returned to the house. He was in hospital for only two days, but in that time we were exposed to what it was like to be known to have AIDS in a hospital in Uganda. Despite a private room with the best facilities Mulago Hospital had to offer, I was made aware from the outset of the extreme stigma that existed. Even the nurses were unwilling to come anywhere near him.

The doctor Chris had been referred to never came to see him. To the doctor there was no point in wasting time over someone who was dying anyway. I resolved then that, if he fell ill again, I would do everything possible to nurse him at home, rather than take him back to the hospital.

After two days he came home, and we were able to live a very close life as a family. It was as if we all knew that the time we had together was very short, so we shared our loads. Chris was physically very ill and a sexual relationship was completely out of the question. During this time I really loved Chris, but it was like a maternal love, a deep caring for him. As a family we were very close and loving. The girls enjoyed his company. Christine, the baby, always jumped into his bed and wanted to sleep with her daddy. Chris fixed things around the house. The whole month was as fruitful as could be.

The search for a cure

On our return home from the hospital the struggle to keep Chris alive started. The whole family joined in, including Chris's family, my family, and friends. A prominent feature of this time was the search for a local cure. Everyone started looking for herbal preparations that they had heard were effective. The biggest problems then were Chris's lack of appetite, vomiting when he ate solids, and intermittent diarrhea. He was very thin and had a very itchy skin rash. However, the meningitis had cleared, and he wasn't really in pain, which was a blessing. Chris was a very good patient and laughed and joked a lot with the children.

Running from one place to the next in search of a cure, the one thing I never succumbed to was witchcraft. This was suggested many times. A traditional healer would be able to tell us precisely why Christopher had got this disease and what to do about it. The only reason I didn't go was because I was a Christian and was therefore opposed to witchcraft. Otherwise, I can assure you, when you are dealing with AIDS you get to the point of desperation, in which even the most deeply felt principles are put to the test. If I had had any doubts, or if I had not been given the information and counseling I needed in England, I might have consulted a traditional healer. I knew Chris had an illness that could be explained scientifically, and it had already done enough damage. I agreed to use the herbal medicines in the hope that they might help his symptoms.

It was during this time that we began to think about what we could do about AIDS generally. I started to seek out other people on the wards at Mulago Hospital who had been diagnosed with AIDS. When I met David he was actually nursing his wife, who died a few months later. I encouraged them to come to the house, just to talk or to share meals. I was away at work a lot and they became regular visitors for Chris. These were the meetings that eventually gave birth to TASO.

Chris's final illness

Every day, before going to work, I would make preparations for Chris, so that everything he required was within easy reach. He was a good patient, but at times he would get very bad spells of depression, and then it was difficult for us. He wouldn't talk for a whole day. Even though I had been prepared for the different moods that are likely to occur when someone is dealing with problems of this magnitude, it was a very difficult time.

I tried to deal with the problems as they came up. Sometimes Chris would react to his dependence on me by being irritable. Many women who are nursing their husbands experience this resentment, a natural and understandable emotion. Chris would sometimes get possessive, not wanting me to go to work, but to remain with him to talk and to be a wife in the house. I recall this vividly because of the day he fell really ill again. I got up in the morning and, as usual, prepared all the things he would need in his room for the day.

He asked how he could get better if he didn't have somebody constantly to look after him. I replied that we wouldn't have any money if I didn't go to work. It was a small domestic quarrel, but it showed the kind of communication failure that can happen when you are caught up in something. After I had arranged everything I went to work. Perhaps I didn't react with compassion that day. If I had stopped to ask him why he was feeling like that he may have told me that he had had a bad night and that he had a fever. I may have realized how insecure he was feeling.

When I came back at lunchtime he was very ill. He was feverish, with a temperature of about 40 degrees, and had collapsed in the bathroom where he had gone to get a wet towel.

I helped him out of the bathroom, took him back to bed, and realized that he was very ill. I gave him some medication and went for a doctor, who said that he had pneumonia and started him on a course of antibiotics. The fever persisted for the next few days. I sent a message to his mother, who came immediately, with his sisters. He started vomiting and complaining of a headache. This was a persistent headache that didn't respond to painkillers. When he also started having diarrhea we set up an intravenous drip. I was quite determined to nurse him at home, as far as possible. As a result of our earlier hospital experience I wasn't happy about the idea of taking him to a hospital. I nursed him for ten days, but he didn't get any better, and eventually he started to cough up blood. We realized that he needed a blood transfusion, and there was increasing pressure from the family to take him to the hospital.

On the tenth day, we went to the hospital and he was admitted and transfused with two units of blood, which seemed to revitalize him. His temperature subsided, but the cough and diarrhea didn't improve. He grew weaker and weaker. He was in hospital from that time until January 1987, getting worse and worse. On January 23 he died. He died in great pain.

I can't even begin to describe the kind of pain he was in. He had this terrible headache, which lasted for five days. He never lost consciousness. He suffered all that pain, and we felt the pain with him. The children would come into the room and he would ask for a wet towel to be put around his head. Even today my baby Christine, who was barely three at this time, remembers daddy's headache, and if any one says that they have a headache Christine becomes very anxious.

Our experience with the hospital staff was an uncomfortable and distressing one. They did not know how to help us in a compassionate way, and their personal fears and prejudices were very evident. The nurses would arrive as a team, on their routine ward rounds, and stand at the door to our room to greet us with their hands held behind their backs, not daring to cross the threshold. I became defensive and reluctant to ask them for anything, because of their manner.

Everything, all the nursing, cleaning, feeding, and caring, was done by my mother-in-law, Chris's sister, my friend Mary, the girls, and me. Even when the intravenous fluids needed replacing, or if the cannulas needed repositioning, it was up to me to find a doctor to attend to it. Often I would try to do it myself. Soon all the veins were too damaged to take the intravenous cannulas. I persuaded the junior doctor to attempt a cut-down. This is a minor surgical procedure where the skin in the leg is cut and the vein exposed for direct introduction of the cannula. The doctor was not experienced in this rare procedure, but Chris was very dehydrated and desperate for fluids. I scurried around to find the cut-down set in the hospital stores. The nurses who should have been assisting were standing at the door watching curiously. One of them made a comment I have never forgotten: "Imagine such a fuss being made about someone who is already nearly dead, a skeleton with AIDS." All this time Chris was awake and in agony, begging us not to hurt him any more, promising he would do his best to drink and not vomit. The doctor and I did the cut-down. I was reading from a textbook and the doctor was following instructions. This provided Chris with fluids for 48 hours, which was when he died.

He died in a lot of pain, and this is something that I cannot take. Even today. I can't understand why. He had withstood so much, and he could have died peacefully, but he didn't. It was too much pain, and afterwards I couldn't take it any more. I couldn't take it. I was surrounded by family and had a lot of support, but after the funeral I went away. I was completely devastated. I had known all along that Chris was going to die, but I wasn't prepared for the way that he died. Such undignified pain and suffering. So I went away, to my mother-in-law, away from the house. I wanted to be near the place where Chris was buried. I was away from home for three weeks.

> Sometimes, when I'm talking about these things, like the headache the week Chris died, I relive the moment, and the pain is deep in my bones. I have a feeling that my daughter Elizabeth also responds like this. She would just sit and look at her father, especially when he was in agony, when he was vomiting, when he was so ill.
>
> There is a special thing that happens when vomiting with AIDS. You begin to vomit, and just vomit and vomit forever, even if all the food is finished, you just keep retching. I would hold Chris and hold him, he would go on and on, and then start sweating, until he lay down exhausted. When I think about this, it still brings goose pimples to my skin.

Part II.   Tackling AIDS with TASO

> **There is a saying in Uganda:**
> If a snake comes into your house, do not waste time asking where the snake came from, but kill it first and ask questions later.

After Chris's death, I had to pick up the pieces and start over again. I soon discovered that I couldn't function the same way as before. I couldn't carry on working as if nothing had happened. I was going through a profound change in my thinking about HIV and AIDS. I decided I had to concentrate on supporting people living with AIDS who were going through the experience I had gone through. I began to plan for the future. Despite having taken a test, and receiving a negative result, I did not believe that I was free of infection. I first asked God to give me a little more time. I specifically asked God to give me one more year, to see whether I could use that year to do something useful for people living with AIDS.

By this time some of the original people I had contacted had already died of AIDS. I managed to trace some of the people who had originally met with Chris, and made contact with others who were living with AIDS. We started meeting again, and talking more constructively about starting a support group. Initially the group was big, but it fluctuated, becoming bigger and then smaller, bigger and smaller, as members of the group died and new members joined it. Within the first group I was the healthiest. I decided it would not be useful to share the information about my test in England and the negative result with the others. Whenever I was asked, I said that I hadn't taken the test. This way the group could relate to me better than if they knew that I had had a negative result.

Why I Chose to Live Positively

Through all of the years I worked with TASO, I chose to conduct myself as if I were HIV positive. My reasoning was like this: whether the results of an HIV test are positive or negative, we need to behave in a way that neither exposes others to infection nor exposes ourselves to infection from others. It is not the test results that are important. It's what we do with the results, how we conduct ourselves – to avoid infection or to spread infection.

Often it crossed my mind that I should take another HIV test. If it came out negative it would reassure my children, but otherwise what difference would it make? Although I'd had the negative blood test in Hull, the fact that I had been exposed to infection made me unwilling to take a second test.

After Chris died there was a lot of talk of my having AIDS. Would I die soon or not? More information was becoming available on HIV. People were learning more about it. Everyone knew that if a man died of AIDS then his wife would die soon after him. It was not a question of whether I would die, but when, as though everyone was waiting for me to die. I hadn't told people that I had had a test in Hull. I didn't think it would be useful, and I didn't think people would believe me. In any case, I had been told that I should have a repeat test to confirm the first one.

In fact the test, even though it was negative, didn't mean much to me. I didn't believe the result. Initially I simply didn't understand what it meant, but later, having learned a lot about HIV and AIDS, I couldn't believe that I was genuinely negative.

As I'll describe later on, the matter eventually came to a head, not for medical reasons, but for political ones.

At first we met informally, sharing whatever information we had. Then we began to get information from organizations like the Terrence Higgins Trust in the United Kingdom. This went on until we began thinking seriously about starting an organization of our own. We didn't know what we would do for money. We were not aware of the possibilities. However, as we reached out to other people who were infected, we found that a lot of the time they didn't have food, or medicines, or

transport to the hospital. Helping to meet these needs began to stand out as an important aspect of starting an organization.

We realized that we would have to obtain government clearance to start an AIDS organization. In October 1987 I went to the Director of the AIDS Control Programme (ACP) in the Ministry of Health. I told him about my husband's having died of AIDS, and of our intentions. He was skeptical about whether I really had the courage to carry the idea through, and discussed the implications of starting an organization, and the difficulties of getting adequate funding. I said that as an NGO we would look for donations, but we already had a group of committed people. Much to my surprise, he told me to go ahead. He asked us only to put our proposal in writing, and he would give us the support we needed. This was a tremendous boost to us because it gave us confidence in what we were doing.

Around that time I heard that President Yoweri Museveni was going to set up a national committee on AIDS. I went to him and asked to be included on the committee. He asked why, and I told him about our organization and the fact that my husband had died of AIDS. He said, "Oh my God, what about you?" I told him I wasn't sure if I was infected or not, but at this moment it was not a big concern to me. He said, "Put this woman on the committee," and that was that. At the time, I was the only person on it who had direct contact with AIDS, in the sense of having "AIDS in the family."

We were fortunate at this time to meet the Director of ActionAid in Uganda, Colin Williams. I had kept my friends in England informed about my plans for a support group, and our need for funds to begin work. They introduced me to Colin, who came to one of our meetings, just to listen. Actually, I had approached a few agencies prior to approaching ActionAid. The reaction from these agencies had been very cautious. They were honest with me. They said that what I was proposing had not been done before, so they didn't have a model for comparison. Funding and support were therefore a risk that they were not prepared to take at that time.

I think that Colin, by coming to a meeting, was able to feel the heartfelt enthusiasm of the group, despite the fact that we were people living with AIDS who didn't have a guaranteed future. He asked us to prepare a budget proposal and gave us some support to begin with, promising further resources if we could demonstrate what we could do. With this assurance we started getting very involved. Much the same happened with other early supporters, World in Need and USAID. They came to our assistance as a result of one person from each organization sitting down and listening to what we were saying.

We formally founded The AIDS Support Organization (TASO) in 1987 with 16 people, including 12 with AIDS. We wanted the word AIDS in the name, to break the silence and stigma of this disease. At that time people with AIDS were being managed without being told their diagnosis. In some cases the family would be told the diagnosis but without counseling or support. The results were that such families would abandon their loved ones for fear of catching the disease.

One of the disturbing features of our start was that within one year all 12 of the founders who had AIDS had died. But in the same year we registered 850 other people who used our services. We accepted people who had been exposed to HIV through their relationships but did not know their HIV status. Some of these people turned out to be HIV negative in the long run, but their survival over the years gave us a continuity that would not have been possible if only people with AIDS had been involved. Many of our members who had not been tested were living positively as I was, but could not face the reality of a test.

This was the beginning of TASO. When we began we were just a group of "lunatic" people. We met to talk, to cry, to pray, to share, to let off steam, to give each other courage and hope. Although many of our founding members were practicing Christians, we made it a point to concentrate on practical issues in people's lives regardless of whether they had faith or not. By working together in TASO, we managed to prove to the world that it was possible to involve people living with AIDS, people like me who have lost family to AIDS, and other people who have been personally touched, in campaigns against the disease.

Living positively with AIDS

We adopted as our slogan "Living positively with AIDS" to emphasize that there is life beyond a positive diagnosis for two main reasons.

First, at that time the public health messages were saying "Beware of AIDS, AIDS kills." In other words, "You catch it and you are as good as dead." There were no messages for those people who were already infected. What was implied was that people who were already infected should die and get it over with. People living with HIV and AIDS were seen as dying. We adopted the slogan "Living positively with AIDS" in direct defiance of that perception. We emphasized living rather than dying with AIDS.

Second, we emphasized that, for us, it was the quality rather than the quantity of life that was important. Once infected with a deadly virus like HIV, people needed to take definite steps to enhance the quality of whatever life they had left. They needed to develop a positive attitude to life.

As we developed this concept, we defined having a positive attitude as:

- Knowing and accepting that they are infected;
- Knowing and understanding the facts about AIDS;
- Taking steps to protect others from their infection;
- Taking care not to expose themselves to further HIV infection or other infections;
- Taking special care of their physical health, and treating symptoms of ill health as soon as possible;
- Having access to emotional support;
- Continued participation in social life; and
- Eating well and avoiding or learning to cope with stressful situations.

Nowadays this philosophy seems more obvious. But when we started we had to show that this way of life was attainable. Achieving positive living is a process, with ups and downs, in which we all need support. It is part of working through the various feelings that having HIV may bring: shock, denial, anger, bargaining, acceptance, and hope. Counselors, carers, and friends need to recognize this instability, and not be frustrated when progression through the stages seems erratic, and people regress to former emotional reactions. We need to be accompanied through these stages by sensitive, understanding friends who pledge to be there for us.

> The TASO slogan, "Living Positively with HIV and AIDS," addresses everyone in society, infected or non-infected. It calls on HIV-positive people to live responsibly with the HIV infection, and not spread it around, by making the effort not to infect others. It also calls upon people who are infected to look after themselves better, and preserve themselves until a cure comes. It calls to people who are infected to remain actively involved in society, and in social activities within society.
>
> It also calls upon the rest of society to support people living with HIV infection so that they can fulfill their obligations. It calls on those who are not infected, or don't know whether they are infected, to accept people living with HIV and AIDS, to recognize that they cannot catch HIV through casual contact. Acceptance of people living with HIV or AIDS within our community is an important starting point for dealing with the problem.
>
> HIV affects ordinary people. It does not only affect "the poor." It does not only affect "the affluent." It affects a cross-section of people. HIV and AIDS affect you and me.

The starting point for living positively with HIV within our own bodies or within the family is to know that we have HIV. This information must be given accurately, consistently, and sensitively. I believe that people must be told about their HIV status. But a negative test is not the end of the matter. Whether the blood test is negative or positive, people must understand that they have been exposed. After they have been exposed to the virus, and whether infected or not, what is important is that they aren't exposed again, and that they don't expose others.

Next, living positively with AIDS means people not just knowing but *accepting* that they are HIV positive. They must then learn about AIDS, and expose themselves to information about the disease. Some people say, "I don't want to hear anything about AIDS. I'm infected and that's enough."

We cannot live positively with AIDS if we don't have good information about it. There is a lot of stupid talk about AIDS, which may be worrying for those who are positive but don't know enough about the infection. Stupid things, like the idea you can catch AIDS by sharing a drinking glass or sitting next to someone who is infected. If people living with HIV don't have reliable information to defuse these myths, it is difficult to live positively.

> After Chris died I started to eat obsessively. I was reacting to stress, the stress of the stigma, the stress of having to live life without Chris. I was also pushed by the need to show people that I was not sick. I think I was deliberately eating to become fat. To be fat is to be fit and healthy, and I remember constantly, without having to think about it, needing to show that I wasn't fitting into my clothes any more, that I had to buy new clothes.

People have to know the facts about transmission. Is it safe to hug their children? It is very painful for mothers who know they are HIV-infected.

Living positively with HIV requires learning about HIV and coping with stress. This is one side of living positively. It is also very important to take definite steps not to infect others, and ensure that they are not exposed to further infection themselves. This needs to be explained quickly and clearly to people with the infection. Many people think that once a person is infected with HIV they can't catch other infections.

> **Personal Victory over the Virus**
> It is important to impress upon people that if they don't pass the HIV infection on to anyone else, this will be their personal victory over the virus itself. The virus that they have in their blood cannot outlive them in any other way than to go into another person's blood. If they allow the virus to move out, they allow it to survive and prosper, even long after they die.
> This is the only way the virus lives on. The virus doesn't want to kill you, because the day it kills you it also dies. It only intends to multiply, but in doing so it kills you. It is only while you remain alive that it can spread. The day you die the virus that is in you is buried with you and is finished.
> We had interesting sessions in TASO's day centers putting this kind of scenario into plays. We found that once people understood the

> virus in this way by using role-plays, they could see that the virus could also be defeated. At that moment they knew that they couldn't kill the virus, but they could defeat it.

Although primary prevention of HIV is rightly the focus of many programs, it cannot be separated from care and support for people living with HIV. Communities cannot take on the reality of HIV in their midst if there is nothing to offer for those who are sick. You have to provide for their immediate needs.

An essential aspect of positive living is social life. It's very important to avoid isolating people with HIV. For instance, during most of my time with TASO, during which I was assumed to be HIV positive, I was almost never invited to a wedding. If a person is going to continue participating in social activities, society must accept them. If someone arrives at a wedding and everybody turns their heads to look at them, it is very uncomfortable. In TASO, we started having our own weddings. In the day centers, weddings were arranged for people who had been living together and wanted to get married. People were also re-baptized by a priest who came especially to baptize them. These were big functions. They allowed people to have some social interaction and to mark important life events. Fortunately, TASO doesn't have to do this any more, as Ugandan society has become more accepting and tolerant. Another important celebration, held every year, was the birthday of TASO, which also celebrates all those who were still alive at each birthday. But even if there isn't a specific occasion to mark, part of positive living is simply to celebrate each day of life as a precious gift, the gifts of health and continued healing, as well as the memories of loved ones no longer with us.

As more and more people are living with AIDS, the old-fashioned attitude that if you have AIDS you are dead or dying is being thrown out. Given improved care, and a better understanding of the disease, people are living longer and better quality lives.

Coming out and denial

We try to protect our privacy by not coming out, and by not declaring our HIV status. This is one way. Our status is not written on our foreheads, although, as I mentioned earlier, full-blown AIDS is hard to hide. However, there is a need to balance the advantage of privacy against the disadvantage of the anxiety about others finding out. Some high-ranking people have even succumbed to blackmail from people who know their HIV status. Yet they are dealing with an infection that can't be kept quiet forever. When it flares up, there will be nothing that they can do to stop it.

The mind plays a very big part in how we deal with an infection like HIV. Until I had my confirming test in 1995, I lived in perpetual fear that I might become ill with AIDS. What I feared most were the early manifestations of HIV infection, particularly acute herpes zoster and meningitis, because they are such painful conditions. I lived in fear of that terrible pain that Chris had. Wherever I went, I traveled with a course of acyclovir, an antiviral drug used for herpes infections, especially if I was going away from home for a bit. I feared the infection and pain. I carried the drug with me so the moment that I saw a rash I could use it straight away. We kept a stock of it in TASO all the time. People used it as soon as they got a rash. If you start immediately it dries up within two days, and it stops the rash from getting infected. However, we never had enough because it used to be expensive. In fact, it took up so much of our budget that we didn't use it for anything but genital herpes.

Even though we feared AIDS like this, I always thought we needed to come out in the open with it.

Love carefully

As we began our work at TASO, AIDS was becoming recognized as a danger throughout the world. People were beginning to react, to begin initiatives to respond to the epidemic. A lot of these initiatives were geared to prevention. This was a good thing because, in the absence of a cure, prevention is the best way to fight this illness.

The public health messages that were being used then had a serious shortcoming. They all said "Don't catch AIDS, if you do you'll die," or "Beware. Don't catch AIDS. AIDS KILLS."

One popular slogan used in AIDS control in Uganda was "Love carefully." The church's slogan was "Love faithfully." The campaign based on this slogan contributed to the stigma associated with AIDS by relating it to low morals and death. But the very phrase "Love carefully" implies that the person with HIV has loved carelessly.

These slogans were coming at people in Uganda left, right, and center, as part of a massive campaign begun in 1986. The messages were all the same. There was nothing for the person who was already positive and diagnosed with HIV infection. As a result of these early messages, many people living with HIV and AIDS reacted adversely. We at TASO had to really struggle to keep going, not only with the physical illness in our family but also with the mental torture and torment of these people.

It has been argued that it was necessary to use messages that would shock people into realizing the seriousness of the AIDS problem. But the "Love carefully" campaign stigmatized people with AIDS. It said look, these are the people who have loved carelessly. This may be particularly stigmatizing in a society like Uganda, which is almost 90 percent Christian. The Christian stress on moral values, even speaking against polygamy, can contribute to stigma in this situation. TASO began as an organization which would provide counseling and support facilities for people living with HIV, and preventive counseling for families and communities. It aimed at impressing upon people in the community, especially at the grassroots, that the person living with HIV or AIDS was not dangerous. They need our compassion, our concerted effort to be supportive. We need to be in a joint fight against the disease. The emphasis is on positive living.

Traditional versus modern: polygamy as I grew up with it

To understand the complexity of the HIV situation in an African country like Uganda, you have to understand the way relationships between men and women work there. I am not an expert in how things work in other parts of the world, but I know that African women and men are in the middle of huge social changes, and it is not easy to resolve the traditional past with the rapidly changing present.

There are many traditional practices that are in direct confrontation with the HIV messages that we are giving. Culture and traditional practices are things that have been passed on from generation to generation, and we can't confront them directly by going to the people and saying "Stop, or you must perish." A better strategy is to educate them to realize that what they lose by no longer following a traditional practice is much less than the risk they run of contracting HIV infection. This is a gradual process. A particular example in Uganda is male polygamy.

My father had eight wives at different times, and my mother married him, as a fourth wife, at the age of 14. She was so young that one of the other wives came to the main house to help her. She often says that she was actually brought up by her co-wife. My parents were married in the Catholic Church, although my father had kept all other wives as traditional wives in separate compounds. My father was a chief, and an affluent man, who always went to church. It was considered proper for him to have a church-wedded wife, but my mother was the only one he married in a church.

I grew up, therefore, knowing and accepting the idea of male polygamy. Chris's father too had four wives. The idea of polygamy was not foreign to us, and Chris and I discussed it from time to time.

We had a very nice childhood by our standards. We each knew who our own mothers were, but we could go and sleep at each other's houses whenever we wanted to. I remember that we ate at each other's houses after school, and our mothers never had to worry that we had not eaten.

There were a total of 28 children in the family, including my father's adopted children. In my tribe there is a ritual where two men, if they loved each other, would cut their arms and then hold the cuts against each other to make them blood brothers. After this, if either of them died, the other would adopt his wife and all his children. If in the ritual they said that all that is mine is yours, this agreement, for inheritance purposes, would supersede even the claims of blood relatives. This was how some of my father's wives were inherited. When we grew up we were very careful never to discriminate between blood relatives and adopted relatives.

Loving faithfully: where does it start?

With the spread of Christianity, and the education of women, some women now have more say in the house. They are not as accepting as they had to be in the past. In this changed situation one of the first things the woman says is, "If I ever catch you with another woman, I'll kill you." The man really loves his wife, and he doesn't want to offend her. He knows that she is serious. At the same time, polygamy hasn't left him. It has only been suppressed by the circumstances. It will only remain so as long as they are happy.

Let me describe one possible scenario in this kind of relationship. Something happens at home, the husband and wife have a quarrel in the night, and he wakes up and goes to the office in a bad mood. There, he finds someone who is nice and kind and is looking for a man. He sees this seemingly happier person. A relationship begins to develop, but one of the first things he says to the girl is, "Look, I have a wife, and I don't want her to know about this relationship," and she accepts it.

Inevitably the girl is of a lower social class, and values this access to the boss, so the relationship builds. He doesn't go to her often, he goes there when there is a quarrel in the house. The girl knows he has a wife, and agrees to remain in the secondary role, not make any noise, but she's not really happy, she also wants a man of her own.

So another relationship starts for her. She meets a man who sympathizes with her because her boss treats her badly and only visits her when he feels like it. The new man says he would be available whenever she wants him. So he comes into the relationship, understanding that her boss visits her every Saturday. Every Saturday he makes himself scarce. Then, perhaps, the new man has another contact somewhere, and so it goes on. This happens in the majority of marriages that I know. I know many "big men" in this situation, with not one but two or three other women.

This man we are talking about is a busy man. Not only does he have a family and children to take care of, but he has a job, which sometimes takes him to Vienna or the US, or wherever. I was talking to a man in this kind of situation, with four women (his wife and three others). He was scared about AIDS. What could he do now? All these women have his children. He said to me, "But my situation is not so bad because I don't go to these women often." He was willing me to endorse his feeling that he was not at high risk because he didn't visit them often, only once a month. Most of the time he spent with his wife. But these were his children. So he said, "When you say 'love faithfully,' where do I start?"

If we tell people who already have a number of stable partners to love faithfully, what will happen to the other women? What are we giving the others who are not the ones to be loved faithfully? What are we putting in place of the man they have been depending on? We tell him, stick to one partner, but which partner? The one he married in church? What are the criteria? Why should he choose this one? What are the factors that took him away from the first wife in the first place? We don't know. If we are saying stick to this one, are we saying that the attraction for the others is completely severed, and that he won't be attracted to another person?

To make the situation more complicated, traditional practice has become very confused because of Christianity, affluence, education, and so on. Wives used to respect each other and actually formed a very tight group. Today a woman, because of affluence, Christianity, or education, tells her husband when they marry that she will not allow another woman in his life. When he finds one, the lies begin. This is the kind of situation that is bringing problems. Women say they are happy to remain behind doors, but they are not happy. So they look for somebody else who will not keep them behind doors, who will promise to be theirs alone, and the chain continues.

Talking about sex

Most women find it difficult to begin a discussion on AIDS in the home even now, but back then it was just about impossible.

Quite a few things not usually discussed could be raised, depending on how they were brought up. I remember going back to the School of Physiotherapy to talk about HIV. I asked the women how many of them had ever discussed HIV with their husbands. Almost none had done so, and those who had tried to discuss it had done so in a negative way. They accused, "You, John, you really are moving around too much. You are going to bring AIDS into this house."

For some women, even though they are married, there's no joking about sex. In a situation like that you can't just raise the subject.

There are exceptional families where safer sex can be discussed and remain between the two of them, but generally, if the man has not agreed to use condoms, they can't discuss the matter further. But with HIV we have to, especially when we live in cultures where men control sex.

Particular groups of women may have a particularly difficult task introducing condoms. Second and third wives, for instance. How can you present a condom in this situation, when he's visiting once a month? If the woman believes that this situation is right, she will not change no matter how long you talk with her. She will not speak up to a man, belittle him. She may believe that he should make the decisions.

Teenage sexuality

Before I met Chris, when I was about twenty years old, I had an affair with a man in his forties who was a friend of my older brother and my father. Right from the outset he told me he would marry me, and would therefore protect me from pregnancy until I finished at the School. I soon realized that my brother and father approved of this arrangement. Although I knew that he was already married, and in fact had two wives, the prospect did not alarm me. Being taken as a third wife, however, was not what I wanted out of life. So while I enjoyed his attentions and gifts, I was always looking for a younger man whom I could love and marry in church.

Even so, I was infatuated by this man. I had just started my first year at the School of Physiotherapy and I was very flattered by his attentions.

At boarding school, when we were about 18, the nuns taught us that sex led to pregnancy,

and that there were several different methods of contraception that could be used, including condoms. So when my friend suggested sex to me, I told him I was afraid of getting pregnant. He told me he would look after me and wanted me to finish at the School. I knew he wouldn't let me get pregnant because of his friendship with my brother and father. He had gone home to tell my father that he wanted to marry me. My father had agreed but said that I needed to finish my education first.

So many young girls fall into the trap of going out with older men who "look after them," as I did. They end up either pregnant or with HIV, and thrown out of their homes. If any one of my daughters had told me that she was having an affair like mine while she was still young, I would have found the man and killed him! I once asked my friend how he would react. He said he would kill the man who did with his daughter what he did with me! The situation is, of course, much worse now with AIDS. Girls can end up both pregnant and HIV positive when they first start having sex, and it is an added tragedy to have unintended pregnancies with HIV. The main way to prevent children being born HIV positive is first to prevent HIV in young women, but also to prevent unintended pregnancy.

My early experience is probably why I feel that we need to give our children information. I think we need to explain to our children that sex is healthy, that the feelings they have about sex are normal, natural, and can be expressed without putting themselves at risk. They have to know exactly what the risks are.

When I talk to young people, I try to simply give the facts about sex and contraception, what protects against pregnancy, and what protects against AIDS. I don't give advice, partly because of the counselor instinct in me, but also because teenagers don't take advice easily. They listen and pick out what they need. What is important is that they receive straightforward, not distorted, information.

I have long been convinced that in order for young people to be able to protect themselves from HIV, other sexually transmitted diseases, and unwanted pregnancies, they need four things:

- access to accurate information on sexual issues;
- skills to negotiate situations;
- practical and realistic options to chose from; and
- support and encouragement to maintain the course of action they choose.

Teenagers get a lot of their information from each other. Sometimes you go to tell them something, or to explain something, and you find they have already discussed it between themselves and know all about it. This is another reason why they need access to accurate information to pass around, through what programs call peer counseling or peer facilitation.

Talking to my own children about sex

Although I have often boasted (oh, the sin of pride!) about the open, honest relationship that exists between the girls and me, the issue of sex education has not been easy.

My early, timid efforts were not a shining success. As a frontline AIDS activist, I assumed that I should be able to manage it. But as an African woman, with all the baggage of taboos regarding talking about sex, it proved the hardest of tasks. Actually, in talking with women from other cultures, from the most industrialized countries to the poorest ones, I have found this to be true for almost all mothers.

In the hustle and bustle of getting TASO off the ground, it dawned on me that both Elizabeth and Phiona were now attractive, popular teenagers and that they might soon become sexually active. My first strategy was to expose them to TASO's work and all the basic information that was being generated about AIDS. I hoped this exposure would help them to fear the virus while learning to love and care for people living with it. To a great extent, that was what happened. But it still didn't address *my* problem of talking to them directly.

One day, I brought a box of condoms and left it in the girls' bedroom, hoping that they would use them if they needed to, but at the same time praying that they would not. I was tempted several times to check the box to see if its contents were decreasing but never had the courage to look (oh, sin of cowardice!).

It was not until Elizabeth actually broke the ice by asking who had placed the box in their room that I owned up. We finally had a discussion, which I survived by clicking into counselor mode – almost as if this was a client rather than my daughter. In any case, Elizabeth assured me that she had already learned something about condom use in school and from talking with friends, and if she needed them she would know where to find them.

This experience showed me that even when we are involved in this work we need help with our own families when it comes to discussing these sensitive issues. Every parent will choose to believe that their child is not yet sexually active and would want to wait for that time before providing the support the child needs for protection. This, despite the fact that we all know that we did not tell our parents the first time we became sexually active!

And what about the grandparents?

Children belong to the husband's clan in our tradition, so if one of my sisters-in-law died her husband's children would have to go to my mother-in-law, who lives in a village about 20 miles from Kampala.

In the past, this system worked quite well because the system of extended families and village life was "elastic" – it could always stretch to find a little more food and somewhere to sleep and so on for a few children. But AIDS has stretched traditional social safety nets to the breaking point, reducing the number of adults in their prime and piling fresh responsibilities on elderly people. My mother-in-law has already raised ten children of her own, and she's old and heartbroken. She is a very hardworking woman, and grew her own food well into her sixties, but more responsibilities would be beyond her, not just physically but emotionally. Today, at the age of 75 she has lost six children, four of them to AIDS. She doesn't like to talk about it. Her grandchildren remind her of the children she has lost, and my girls sense that when their granny looks at them she remembers their father. It is difficult for her when she visits us because we talk about Christopher a lot. She either keeps quiet or changes the subject.

We went to visit daddy at his resting place today for the first time in two years, the silent grave that I have stood over from the age of three. I think about things to say to him when I go and wonder if maybe he'll say something back. It's not really talking, it's just in my head. It's amazing how such a beautiful, peaceful place is unable to suppress the sadness. The neat row of relatives, many of which I've never known. And my grandmother, who each day from her veranda has to watch her children and grandchildren sleep without a stir. (Christine Kaleeba, January 2002)

AIDS continues to ravage my family

You have only to look at the statistics and reports that UNAIDS publishes every year to know that the AIDS pandemic is still growing in much of the world. On a global level, our best estimate for the year 2002 was that 42 million people were living with HIV/AIDS, of whom 3.2 million were children under the age of 15. About 29.4 million of those infected live in sub-Saharan Africa. The disease is killing a lot of people, about 3.1 million in 2002 alone. But it is stalking and catching people even faster: in the same year, five million people were infected with HIV.

Uganda is one of the few "success stories" in this tragic situation, having reduced the rate at which the epidemic was growing in its population. I am proud of my country, and pay full tribute to the efforts of our government, and also the many international agencies, NGOs, church groups, and community organizations that have helped achieve this. At the same time, I have to put quotation marks around the word "success" every time I use it, because although the statistics are impressive, it certainly doesn't *feel* like a success to me or to anyone I know. Too many are still dying and suffering.

Since the first edition of this book in 1991, AIDS has been back again and again to steal more of my family members. First to be snatched was my sister Rose, who died in 1992. Her spouse had died soon after Christopher. Then in 1994 my sister Harriet and her spouse were diagnosed. Mercifully, Harriet struggles on but her spouse died seven years ago. My brother Andrew, and his spouse, and my niece Veronica were diagnosed the same year. Veronica died in 1995.

Since then I have lost 12 close family members. All of them have left children who now constitute the 14 children for whom I am the sole breadwinner.

In countries where there are increasing numbers of people falling ill with AIDS, it poses a big challenge to all of us who are talking about AIDS in whatever capacity. There are a lot of scientists working on research in AIDS and producing epidemiological data. There is a lot of talk about HIV and AIDS. People stand up at conferences and say what should be done, but a lot of this has not been translated into action. One very real way in which we can show action in AIDS is by caring and offering support to people who are diagnosed positive, whether they are friends, people living with AIDS, people living with HIV infection, or their families. I have sat time and time again with elderly mothers and grandmothers whose talk of their dying loved ones has left an indelible mark upon my heart.

TASO Today

TASO has become a key player in the Ugandan response to AIDS and has made a significant contribution to Uganda's success in curbing the spread of HIV. It also continues to have a high international profile, and to serve as a model of "best practice" in its various activities. Some of the countries that have received training from TASO include Botswana, Kenya, Malawi, Rwanda, Tanzania, Zambia, and Zimbabwe.

TASO is a fully registered NGO, offering counseling services, outpatient clinical care, and community care for people living with AIDS and HIV infection. With seven centers across Uganda, the organization also offers awareness and sensitization programs for a cross-section of the community, from medical personnel and political leaders to village community workers.

TASO still has a special mission among the poorest sections of society, the people that are infected or affected with HIV/AIDS and unable to afford the expensive services in the market place. Two-thirds of the clients served are female. In the year 2000 alone, over 21,000 individual clients were served. As well as those provided directly with services ranging from counseling to medical care, TASO provides HIV/AIDS education to over 100,000 people annually.

(For more about TASO visit its website at www.taso.co.ug)

Chapter 20

Understanding AIDS in Public Lives

David Eaton

This chapter presents case studies of the problems posed by AIDS in the lives of two eminent Congolese men: Luambo Makiadi, a musician and composer, and Sony Labou Tansi, a novelist and playwright. Recognized as among the great creative artists of their time, these men influenced and defined sensibility in their respective domains in the adjoining cities of Kinshasa and Brazzaville, which together form a great urban center of francophone equatorial Bantu-speaking civilization.[1] Moreover, as exemplary embodiments of collective experience, and as original voices of social critique, they are important figures to comprehend in thinking across communities in this region of Africa. Their legacies are complex sites in which we participate in the construction of the person and can consider issues of cultural production and imagination within the history of these modern communities.

To the best of my knowledge, neither of these men publicly confirmed a diagnosis of AIDS. Their public lives, however, included their public deaths, almost certainly from AIDS, and each one's relation to his illness was shaped by his involvement in cultural and political struggles. The ways that each

man engaged his own experience – and more broadly, the social dimensions of the epidemic – illuminate arenas of discourse through which these dangers were managed in their societies. I hope the interpretive accounts which follow honor their memory, and help us better grasp the simultaneously personal and public stakes of AIDS within specific histories of language, power, and responsibility.

I look first at Luambo Makiadi's life, focusing on several songs and an interview in which he spoke out about AIDS. Then I turn to Sony Labou Tansi, considering responses to his death in Congo, and examining his political commitments and his enigmatic final novel for insight into how AIDS has been represented and interpreted. These accounts yield evidence of plural languages and idioms of affliction; of the complex terrain of secrecy and charged speech in which ill fortune is encountered and expressed; and of the possibilities for activism amidst the dangers of rumors, accusation, jealousy, and occult powers. They show also how social histories of ethnic and generational conflict within the politics of each nation fundamentally shape the ways in which AIDS has been experienced and understood.

Luambo Makiadi

Luambo Makiadi, also known as "Franco," was the most influential artist of his generation in Congolese urban music, with its center of production in Kinshasa and Brazzaville. Though a Zairian citizen who spent most of his life in Kinshasa, Luambo – as he was widely known – was a towering figure in popular consciousness across the river in the Republic of Congo as well.

Leader of the ensemble OK Jazz from 1957 to 1989, Luambo's hundreds of songs about love, politics, and daily life helped define an emerging sense of nationally shared life in the decades following independence. Luambo himself had risen from a humble family to exemplify masculine well-being, social consciousness, and generativity in national and transnational idioms.[2] He was called *"le grand maître"* and "the sorcerer of the guitar," and has been described as "the Balzac of equatorial Africa." "He educates, he inspires," said one young man I spoke with in a Brazzaville market, attesting to the respect held for Luambo by so many. "If you listen carefully to all of his songs, you will be honest on this earth." The sophisticated and vibrant popular music of his OK Jazz and other Congolese ensembles, with their assimilation of Cuban *rumba* and other Latin influences into distinctly African forms, spilled across national borders throughout Africa beginning in the 1960s (see, for example, Bemba 1984; Mukuna 1992; Mukuna 1999; Stewart 2000; White 2002).

Luambo's cross-cutting dimensions as a national figure were evidenced in his range of public identities: as a "missionary" eulogized in the Catholic church despite his conversion to Islam for a period beginning in 1978; as a dissident who spent time in then-President Mobutu's jails but who was one of the ruling party's most important supporters at times; and as a voice of the people who was also a successful businessman, always attentive to his own finances, who was reported to observe that money "rules the world" (Stewart 2000:364). The scope of his influence expressed the close relations between patriarchy, voice, and state authority in Zaire at the time, as well as his success in the regimes of capital accumulation and the fields of charisma and magical power which were so central in national affairs.

Attention na SIDA

In 1987, Luambo released a song entitled *Attention na SIDA* [roughly, "Beware of AIDS"] warning of the dangers of HIV and AIDS. The 16-minute piece became arguably the single greatest public contribution to AIDS awareness – as defined in secular Western and biomedically informed terms – in francophone central Africa in the decade. The song's lyrics broke public silences and spoke powerfully to the emerging crisis. Declaimed in French and Lingala,[3] they were heard throughout francophone Africa in the years that followed.

In French, the urgent appeal to listeners was clear:

> Teach those close to you
> Time presses
> With each day
> Die the victims of AIDS…

Calling to researchers, Luambo invoked the spirits of Pasteur and Fleming, singing:

> We await vaccines
> We await medicines
> Seven, eight, ten years
> *Share* your knowledge
> Don't work in closed circles! …
> It is now your turn –
> Conquer this evil which terrorizes humanity
> …

(Makiadi 1987)

A fuller selection reveals more of the politics present in the shifting languages of the song. The explicit and didactic exhortations of Luambo's voice in French – an authoritative transnational collective subject citing Pasteur and Curie in its appeal for reasoned action and education – are juxtaposed with plaintive and personal verses in his voice in Lingala, which convey the suffering and abandonment of ill persons. The unified chorus of soaring voices, also in Lingala, returns again and again between these twin solo discourses to call for solidarity among the "brothers and sisters," who are all those who are listening.

Thus these three components of the song present contrasting aspects of the crisis, separating by language and performance those vulnerable and afflicted from those with authority, resources, and understanding. In Lingala, Luambo sings plaintively in the first person for those stricken by AIDS:[4]

Sida ekaboli bikolo
Sida ebomeli ngai libala
Sida epanzeli ngai famille
Baliaka na ngai bamelaka na ngai
Bakomi nde kokimi ngai
Balobi mpo ngai nazwi maladie ya sida
Baninga nyonso bakimi ngai
Naleli epai ya nani?

AIDS divides nations
AIDS destroyed my marriage
AIDS scattered my family
They ate with me and drank with me
But now they shun me
They say it's because I have AIDS
All my friends abandon me
Who can I cry to?

The refrain of the chorus, a soaring phrase shared by several men's voices, appeals to listeners as members of a human family all endangered by AIDS. It is in Lingala as well:

Benda nzoto ngai nabendi nzoto mama
Benda ya yo ngai nabendi na ngai
SIDA eponi ekolo te mama
SIDA eponi loposo te mama
SIDA eponi age te mama
Bamama tokeba
Batata tokeba

Protect yourself as I protect myself
Save yourself as I save myself
AIDS strikes all nations
AIDS strikes all races
AIDS strikes all ages
Mothers [/women] let's beware
Fathers [/men] let's beware

It is in French that Luambo's voice again assumes individual authority, giving specific information on means of protection, speaking to specific social groups and institutions, and exhorting listeners to take all means to educate others and contribute to the struggle.

Youth
Attention
AIDS attacks you
Especially you
Force of life in society

If you want to protect yourself ...
Avoid dangerous sex ...
Avoid many partners ...

Governments of the rich countries
Help the poor countries
Offer them means to fight AIDS
Not weapons
Which incite them to killing
The real struggle
Is the fight against AIDS
Brothers and sisters ...

(Makiadi 1987)

Although *Attention na SIDA* constructs AIDS as it is understood in the secular West, in other materials from Luambo's life we see this illness understood in other ways which also play important roles in collective understanding of the epidemic in this region. Indeed, the complexity of the overlapping discourses through which threats of AIDS have been negotiated belie the dichotomous form of Luambo's *Attention na SIDA*, with its voices dividing the world into linguistically marked domains of cosmopolitan reason (French) and African vulnerability and solidarity (Lingala).

If God exists

After *Attention na SIDA* was released in 1987, stories began circulating about Luambo's health, even saying that he was dead. Luambo, for many years an enormous man, began losing weight at about this time. In a television interview in 1989, recounted in Gary Stewart's *Rumba on the River* (2000), he expressed the uncertainty and the search for meaning that so many have experienced in relation to HIV. Speaking of the rumors that he was suffering from AIDS, Luambo gave one complex account of how his own malady might be understood:

"I can't defend myself in any way, but people won't believe I don't have AIDS ... If I have this illness, I'm going to die, and they'll do an autopsy to find out. If God exists and I don't have this illness and I feel better, I'm going to ask those people who are gossiping, one by one, 'You said I had AIDS, why am I still alive?'

Now that I have been praying to God, I don't find the protections [that I used to carry, against witchcraft] necessary ... But now that

I've thrown them away I have a big problem.''
(Stewart 2000:363)

In the interview, Luambo also questioned the ubiquitous jealousy which threatened him as a successful man, saying he had started with nothing and worked hard to get where he was. He concluded by imploring his family to ignore the rumors. ''I know you are suffering because of me. People are laughing at you because of me. Be patient. That's the way the world is ... Leave everything to God'' (Stewart 2000:363).

Luambo's comments construct a number of issues as unresolved: whether he in fact has AIDS; whether God exists; whether protections against witchcraft are really necessary. The indeterminate and ambiguous quality of these constructions is familiar to those who have studied discourses of witchcraft and sorcery (the two are often not clearly distinguished in contemporary central Africa), which have proven extraordinarily flexible in adapting both to the presence of Christianity and to the socio-economic and political changes of the years after independence.[5] These understandings may offer simultaneous support to a broad array of interpretations of suffering and ill fortune, as Peter Geschiere has pointed out, ''making any attempt ... toward 'unification of meaning' and 'the imposition of interpretative control' ... extremely difficult'' (1998:159). Further, such interpretations can accommodate and complement other explanations. As Gruénais notes (1993:218), this is particularly true with AIDS, where remissions may give the impression of efficacious care, only to be followed by apparently renewed attack.

Luambo's remarks suggest that faith in God can protect both against AIDS and against witchcraft, and can neutralize the gossip and malicious laughter of others. More generally, his comments furnish a charged picture of the human condition. On the one side life and health are associated with God, protections against witchcraft, hard work, the respect and goodwill of others, and prosperity. Against these are arrayed forces of destruction which threaten Luambo and his family: AIDS, illness, rumors attributing illness, witchcraft, derision, and jealousy. The broad and deep

relations between these latter terms are almost palpable.

Les rumeurs

In October 1988 in Brussels, Luambo had recorded several songs explicitly addressing rumors about him and alluding to his impending death. The songs – Les rumeurs (Baiser ya Juda) [The rumors (Kiss of Judas)], Batela makila na ngai [Protect my blood/family], and Laissez-nous tranquilles [Leave us in peace] were all released only posthumously in 1994. Whereas in Attention na SIDA Luambo had taken on the voice of a person abandoned due to perceived AIDS, in these songs he laments the malice and hypocrisy which he sees in those around him.

In Les rumeurs, the chorus sings in Lingala:

Balobi bakoti lopitalo
Balobi bamoni ye na Ngaliema
Balobi akendi Bruxelles ...
[na Anvers, Paris, Genève, America]
Parti-état efuteli ye tike o

They say he's been hospitalized
They say they saw him at Ngaliema [hospital]
They say he went to Brussels ...
[and Antwerp, Paris, Geneva, America]
The [ruling MPR] party bought his ticket

Luambo himself sings in Lingala:

Ebele ya bato oyo balingi ngai te
Lelo namoni na miso ...
Bamosusu bakoseka
Bamosusu bakofinga ngai
Mpo nazwi mpasi na mokil''

So many of these people don't care for me
Today I've seen it with my eyes ...
Some just laugh
Others insult me
Because I'm suffering in this world

Then, in French, Luambo characterized his betrayal by others as a ''kiss of Judas,'' saying:

All my enemies whisper among themselves against me ...
He's dangerously ill
Look at him lying there
He won't get up again
Even those with whom I was at peace
Who had my trust
And who ate my bread

Turn against me
Psalm 41, verses 6 to 10[6]

As the song continues, Luambo returns to Lingala to ask:

Nini boye mpona nini boye?
Moto akokufa bango
bakoseka ye ...
Epaye bakoleli ebembe epaye ya kobina musique
Epaye bakoleli ebembe bakoloba maloba mabe ...
Mpona nini Nzambe asala bato?
Bato atinda na Zaire mosala koseka bato
Bato atinda na Zaire mosala koseka bato ya malade ...
O baninga
Famille nini ezwaka mpasi te na mokili? ...
Nayebi eloko nini bolingi nzoto na ngai te
Nazali nde moto lokola bino
Nani azwaka mpasi te na mokili?

Why? Why are things this way?
A person is dying and they laugh at him ...
At the wake they dance to [modern] music
At the wake they exchange evil gossip ...
Why has God made [such] people?
Those he sent to Zaire simply mock others
Those he sent to Zaire mock others who are ill ...
My friends
What family doesn't suffer in this world? ...
I don't know what you have against me
I am a person like you
Who doesn't suffer in this world?

(Makiadi 1994)

Luambo's lament about lack of respect or compassion for the dying was not unprecedented in Zaire. Indeed, Ndombe Opetun of OK Jazz had commented at length on these problems in 1984 in *Nayebi ndenge bakolela ngai* [I know how they will mourn me], singing in the voice of the deceased who witnesses the disgraceful actions of the living at his wake (Ngimbi 1997:13–14). In Kinshasa, lack of respect for the dead would become increasingly evident in changing funerals, especially of younger people, marked by conspicuous consumption, aggression, accusations of sorcery, drug use, sexual encounters, and obscene language.[7] Luambo's indictments of the bad faith he saw around him reflected a broader decline in Zaire, as conditions in the country continued to deteriorate toward the economic abyss and civil war of the 1990s. Many dominant gerontocratic institutions in Kinshasa and elsewhere were being eroded as generational

tensions opposed often-unemployed youth to their elders in family, church, and state.[8]

"For Ever"

By 1989, it was evident to all who witnessed Luambo's sporadic performances that he was severely afflicted. In February he completed a four-song album with Sam Mangwana entitled "For Ever." The release featured a cover photo of Mangwana alongside a startlingly gaunt Luambo, who seems abstracted, staring into distance. I had been surprised to see this photo on the cassette cover in a Kinshasa music shop. When I asked the proprietor what was wrong with Luambo, she looked at me carefully, and said in a measured voice *"il est malade"* ["he is ill"].

Perhaps this is the most respectful diagnosis one could offer in this situation. In this region of Africa, however, it is congruent with a widespread reluctance to refer specifically to AIDS or to identify individuals as suffering from its effects. Urban healers at this time, for example, often advertised treatments for wasting, prolonged diarrhea, *herpes zoster* – without a mention of HIV or AIDS. Such practices reveal, of course, not simply absence or denial, but rather both biomedically informed diagnoses and the delicacy of the social pragmatics of discussion of the disease.[9] They also reflect the fact that in equatorial African societies, in which the origins of illness are so often located in social relations and personal malevolence, bringing AIDS into speech is burdened with particular dangers and problems of personal and public responsibility.

Luambo died at Namur University Hospital outside of Brussels on October 12, 1989. A number of other Zairian musicians also passed away in the next year, several after a progression of AIDS-like symptoms (including Empopo Loway, who had taken over as *chef d'orchestre* of OK Jazz). None of these musicians spoke of having AIDS (Stewart 2000:370–371). It was common to attribute these deaths not only to battles of sorcery among musicians, but also to the fact that some of them, like Luambo, had sung about AIDS.[10]

A consideration of the aftermath of Luambo's death indicates the dimensions of this public figure who, more than any other performer, had embodied Zairian cultural expression in the years since independence. On the news of his passing in October 1989, Mobutu declared a period of national mourning. In Kinshasa, hundreds of thousands lined the route from Ndjili airport into the city to catch a glimpse of the coffin, "surrounded by flowers with a large portrait of [Luambo] at its head," carried on top of a station wagon in a cortège that stretched for more than a mile. The body was transported to the Palais du Peuple to lie in state. The next morning, a state ceremony was held promoting Luambo to the rank of commander in the National Order of the Leopard. "Then, his coffin draped with the flag of Zaire, he was taken to Notre Dame Cathedral for a solemn funeral mass" (Stewart 2000:365–366). The eulogy described Luambo as "an upsetting force ... because his message, frank and direct, called his listeners to consciousness. He was a missionary who understood his mission well. And he himself said that his mission was to provoke, to denounce, to say the truth ... He remained faithful to his mission until the end" (Stewart 2000:366–367).

Sony Labou Tansi

Across the Congo river from Kinshasa in Brazzaville, capital of the Republic of Congo, Sony Labou Tansi, the country's renowned novelist and playwright, suffered two years of debilitating illness beginning in 1993. After being treated in Paris, Sony (as he was known) had reportedly abandoned medicines prescribed by European physicians in favor of consultations with Congolese healers. He passed away June 14, 1995, fifteen days after his wife Pierrette, both from conditions reported in the international press to be AIDS. As with Luambo, the ways in which his illness and death were represented reveal important aspects of the politics of representation of AIDS in equatorial Africa.

Sony's novels and plays convey a surreally intense and fantasmatic inhabitation of the conditions of daily life in Brazzaville and Congo in these decades, in which economic underdevelopment and political oppression exist together with an extraordinary depth and plurality of cultural traditions and expressive genres. But Sony was not only an electrifying creative artist. As an increasingly militant deputy in Congo's National Assembly, he had become a crucial figure in the ethnic polarization of Congolese society which accompanied the contested multi-party elections of the early 1990s and which eventually led to the country's disastrous 1997 civil war. His passing was a profound loss to the Kongo-Lari community in the Pool area surrounding Brazzaville, from which he came and whom he represented.[11]

In considering aspects of Sony's life and work for the purposes of this chapter, I begin by quoting selections from a memorial to Sony published after his death in a Lari journal in Brazzaville. The absence of any mention of AIDS in the journal, and the invocation of occult malevolence as the cause of Sony's death, together raise issues of hidden knowledge and double consciousness in Congolese social life. I discuss how these issues were expressed in Sony's own political activism. I then look at Sony's last novel, completed as he was suffering from AIDS and as Congo was convulsed by factional warfare. Working closely with these disparate but interrelated materials yields insight into how problems of HIV and AIDS in Congo, as elsewhere, are embedded in imaginations of history and the politics of knowledge.

God has cheated

La Rue meurt, a partisan weekly journal of Lari news and opinion, dedicated much of one issue to Sony soon after his death. A drawing and a text in verse appear in large format on the front page, together articulating a composite – in some senses "double" – memorial vision of his life and death. The drawing portrays Sony as a thoroughly modern individual in Western formal dress, seated alone atop outsized copies of seven of his published works in French. The verse accuses a God of the Kongo people of killing Sony in an archetypal act of occult consumption. Entitled *Bon Dieu a triché* [roughly, "Good God has cheated"], it reads:

Nzambi a Mpungu, God of Kongo,[12]
What have you done? ...
Do you understand that you have betrayed the
contract?

Cannibal that you are,
irremediably,
the thirst for human flesh
burns your throat
without end

You had the right ...
according to the lineage contract
to take your game
among our people of the Pool[13]
Because you are related to me
truly through the maternal side

But the clause, the last clause stated,
you remember, that you could
take anything, anything except your geniuses/
spirits ...
Why have you betrayed the contract? ...
Why have you cheated by mowing down Sony?

You have chosen the best of all
The sacrilege is irreparable

... And what recourse
do you leave me when you yourself,
in shame, disappear
by the back door,
weeping for Sony?

(David 1995:1)

In these verses we see a reading of affliction
very different from that presented, for
example, in Luambo's *Attention na SIDA*, or
in biomedical diagnoses. Sony's death is attributed to the malevolent power of a God who
belongs to the matrilineal clan. Such appetite
for the vital energies of others, called *kindoki* in
Kikongo, is understood as an inevitable component of social life. Although it may be used
for evil, it is also necessary for protection of
the family and matriline.[14] Simon Bockie, a
member of the Bamanianga group like Sony,
describes *kindoki* as a component of a "complex system of social checks and balances that
works for the health and wholeness, the pre-
servation and continuance, of the community
... a subtle cultural science that serves a vital
function" (Bockie 1993:82).

Across Congolese communities, it is understood that AIDS or its symptoms, as with those
of many other illnesses, can be the result of
kindoki and other occult powers and entities.[15]

A diagnosis of HIV infection will therefore be
considered within the context of family history
and tensions. Indeed, the actions of the very
human god accused of killing Sony in the
verse above are those of a powerful elder
who has abused such powers. Further, what
the author of the verse objects to is the choice
of prey, not the murderous act itself. A family
head who chooses victims among his own maternal kin to protect its members is considered
quite differently from a witch who devours
others simply for personal gain.[16] The shame
comes from the "irreparable sacrilege" of
choosing Sony, "the best of all."

Secrecy and double consciousness

Beyond this front page with its drawing and
verse, several other pages of this memorial
issue of *La Rue meurt* were filled with homage
from Sony's peers across the country and in
France. At no point in the entire newspaper,
however, was there any other mention of the
causes of Sony's death, or of AIDS itself. This
public silence – similar to that of the urban
healers noted above, who advertised treatment
symptoms of AIDS without mentioning the
syndrome itself – hints at the secret, private,
and taboo qualities of AIDS as an element of
thought and discourse. And indeed, in both
countries at this time HIV tests were seldom
spontaneously sought out and rarely disclosed, and very few individuals had come
forward publicly with a seropositive diagnosis.[17]

The secrecy so often shrouding diagnoses
of HIV and AIDS in this region of Africa, as
elsewhere, stems partly from the pragmatic
need to protect vulnerable individuals from
the potential stigma, discrimination, and abandonment which can arise from a seropositive
diagnosis.[18] But this silence about AIDS is also
part of much broader economies of hidden
knowledge which situate individuals within
social groups and pervade understandings of
political life. Indeed, Jean-Michel Devésa, in
the introduction to his book on Sony's life
and work, calls Congo, in all its regional components, "a society of the unsaid ... dominated by the secret and its inverse, the rumor"
(1996:10).

Concealment and secrecy can be seen as inherent properties of systems of wealth-in-people (such as those common in Congo), given the asymmetries of knowledge in relationships of dependency and subordination, as Rosalind Shaw has suggested.[19] Writing of Temne-speakers along the upper Guinea coast, she describes practices of secrecy as "forms of self-defense" and as "established techniques for defining and promoting the membership of a group" (Shaw 2000:37–38, 42). Such economies of hidden knowledge and secret practice shape representation and practice in relation to AIDS in equatorial Africa, as has been noted above. More generally, they are present throughout social life, in which uncertainty is often managed – and modern life negotiated – through occult techniques anchored within family and clan.[20] Sony's roles within ethnic and national politics give evidence of such economies as they have been shaped by Congolese history in the 20th century.

What one may see in Sony's political life – as was also evident in the memorial drawing and verse cited above – is a modern public individual existing within a matrix of hidden clan-based powers. On the one hand, Sony took outspokenly liberal positions in international venues, especially in France, calling for democracy, pluralism, and political dialogue (Clark 2000:51). He was famous for the scathing and unrelentingly original denunciations of dictatorship in his work, beginning in 1979 with La vie et demie. In the years that followed, his international reputation as a human rights advocate was reinforced by his public critiques of Congo's Marxist one-party system in the 1980s.

However, Sony's humanist and democratic image was undermined by his involvement in ethnically based and sometimes clandestine projects in Congo, as Phyllis Clark has described in a recent article. Indeed, after the 1991 Congolese National Conference which brought a transition to troubled multi-party elections, Sony was reported to have been involved in secret nocturnal attempts to manipulate the political system on behalf of Kongo-Lari organizations. These contravened the principles of transparency and interethnic association which had been agreed upon in the Conference. Many of his peers were surprised

to learn after his death of these alleged involvements, including initiation into a secret society (Clark 2000:51–53, 58–59).[21]

Such a "double discourse" emerges from the recent history of a society split in two by colonialism, as Clark suggests, drawing on the work of Wyatt MacGaffey and others. The double order of the colonial period operated by two sets of rules: mu kindombe (African) and mu kimundele (European). Each domain included its own etiquette, modes of communication, language, and techniques of the body (MacGaffey W., 1986:16; see also MacGaffey 1994). The two sectors of colonial society – on the one hand, bureaucratic (encompassing Christianity, education, taxation, wage labor; in French) and, on the other, customary (including marriage and interpersonal relationships; in Kikongo) – created a pervasive syncretism and "double-consciousness" among BaKongo in daily practice and perception. These two sets of social rules – one official and public; one ethnicized and semi-secret – had continued into the postcolonial period, accentuated by the exclusion of BaKongo, including Lari, from the highest levels of national government since the late 1960s (Clark 2000:49).

Thus while Sony called for openness and pluralism in international forums, in publications and manuscripts in Brazzaville he advocated a sacred nationalism based on Kongo identity.[22] In these latter documents, he portrayed Kongo-Lari as not only rightful leaders of the transition to democracy, but also as a chosen people persecuted and martyred by evil enemies identified as ethnic and political rivals.[23] In one unpublished manuscript, Sony linked the BaKongo to the Jewish people and their sufferings, describing his ancestors as "the first in history to invent monotheism with the cult of Nzambi a Mpungu." "The God of Jacob is with us," he wrote. "We must organize ourselves to prevent the genocide of the Kongo" (Tansi [n.d.], cited in Clark [2000:57].

Le Commencement des douleurs

A fusion of these terrible forebodings with a sense of sexual sin and consequent suffering can be seen in Sony's last published work, Le Commencement des douleurs [The beginning of sufferings]. The book was completed while he was suffering from AIDS and the Republic of Congo was reeling from the armed conflict of 1993–4. It describes the apocalyptic afflictions and rebirth of a civilization, brought about by a casual but too-tender embrace of a young girl by an older man. This one gesture causes endless social dislocation and eventually draws all nature into cataclysm. To Clark, these narrative strands suggest "that Sony recognized that his illness had contributed to the manifestation of his extremism" (Clark 2000:61).

In the novel, the protagonist delays the socially expected marriage and consummation of this relationship for one reason after another, waiting, among other things, for a specially forged chastity belt to be completed. Eventually, despite his son's discovery of a "generalized immunity" for all human beings – vigorously resisted by medical professionals who stand to lose their livelihoods – the culmination of disaster is the approach of a vast "black hole" in the sky which threatens to destroy the community. Some readers have seen this as an obvious potential symbol of the female genitals.[24]

Although in one sense these narrative elements may index the dangers of sex in a time of AIDS, they more fundamentally invoke larger resonances of belonging, engulfment, and vulnerability in the context of BaKongo matrilineal society.[25] Consummating one's involvement in society through marriage and procreation is the ultimate commitment to the social order, yielding life which is always vulnerable to illness and death through the actions of one's kin and even oneself. As we have seen above in the memorial verse discussed at the beginning of this section, it is Sony's existence within these generational continuities of the Kongo social body that permits his annihilation by *Nzambi ya Mpungu*.

It may also be worth noting that themes we have noted in *Le Commencement des douleurs* bear similarities to narratives of collective misfortune long established among Congolese peoples. Another Kongo author, Kusikila-kwa-Kilombo, for example, writing in 1966, had explored related ideas in his account of the history of illness among BaKongo. Kusikila wrote then that the arrival of whites had brought great sickness to a healthy people, and a "foreign" death contrary to the will of God. The cause was carnal debauchery, due to the reduced effectiveness of sanctions against adultery. The resulting host of foreign diseases, he said, had murdered thousands of unborn through infertility, terminating whole races in the unfulfilled descendance of barren women (Janzen and MacGaffey 1974:49).

Sony's narrative in *Le Commencement des douleurs* yields no simple reading of this kind, of course. Devésa refers to the deep influence of Sony's mastery of Kikongo, with its symbolic and cryptic usages and its metaphorical and oracular turns "completely unavailable to a speaker using the language as a simple tool of communication" (Devésa 1996:61). He quotes Sony as saying "in the language of my mother there is a sub-language beneath the language, a subtext beneath the text, like the sugar in the starch – one must chew hard to taste it properly" (Devésa 1996:61). Other important influences in Sony's creative work included Tchicaya U Tam'si, Shakespeare, Soyinka, Borges, Garcia-Marquez, and the Bible – especially the Book of Job and the Revelation of St. John.[26]

From these reflections, we may gain some insight into the ways Sony's literary imagination, his political activism, and his understanding of affliction were shaped by composite cultural histories particular to his people and to this region of Africa, as well as by his experience with AIDS. The boundaries between individual and collective dimensions of these aspects of his life are difficult if not impossible to draw. Like Luambo, as a creative figure of great power and influence, Sony tapped into deep currents of life around him, and in their homage after his death, his peers wrote of his extraordinary presence and gifts. "*C'est un monde qui s'écroule quand on a été très proche de l'homme*" ["The world collapsed on itself when one was very close to this man"], said one. Another wrote: "*Sony a été plus humain que tout ce qu'on peut imaginer*" ["Sony was more human than anything one could imagine"].[27]

Conclusion

What can we learn from considering these elements presented from our consideration of the lives and works of these two men, Sony and Luambo? What do they tell us about the complex relations of AIDS and activism in public lives?

Luambo's *Attention na SIDA* galvanized public consciousness about AIDS perhaps more than any other single event of its decade in equatorial Africa. As we have seen, this 1987 song broke through public silences to reach millions of people, giving voice to the suffering of individual Africans while invoking histories of biomedical reason and exhorting its listeners to social responsibility. Its clarity and simplicity of message stood in contrast to Luambo's more complex and contradictory representation of his own illness in other venues. The enormous power of his engagement in this song stemmed from a number of circumstances related both to its composition and to his position at the center of power in national and international circuits of mass media. In contrast, although humanitarian organizations in Africa have often sponsored musicians in the creation of works which address AIDS, few such pieces that I am familiar with have received more than minor and local attention.

In *Attention na SIDA*, Luambo proposed one highly schematized interpretation of the interrelation between cosmopolitan and local worlds, compartmentalizing and juxtaposing languages and experiences of AIDS widely disparate in their tone, content, and social location. In contrast, a more embedded and contradictory plurality was evident in his personal therapeutic choices, and in his statements about his condition and its relation to the jealousy of others around him. As we have seen, in other songs he wrote during this period, he lamented the malevolence of rumors about his condition, and the lack of sympathy and respect which he (and others) saw as characterizing many people in Kinshasa.

But it was *Attention na SIDA* – the most enduring and influential legacy in his creative work in relation to HIV and AIDS – which achieved a kind of public diagnosis of the epidemic which could move millions toward safer lives and to greater compassion and solidarity in the face of social catastrophe. Despite its inadequacy as an accurate representation of the pressures and contradictions of his own engagement with AIDS, the song accomplished this by separating African and European languages and performative genres, by instituting a "talkability"[28] about some issues of the epidemic while leaving others in silence, and by providing points of reference to which the individuals of his audience could return for inspiration and education at moments which were appropriate to the circumstances of their lives. The outpourings of grief and mourning which followed his death reflected not only Luambo's centrality in primary institutions of Zairian popular consciousness, and the knowledge that what had felled him was reaping the lives of many among his audience. It revealed also the deep respect felt by so many for Luambo's willingness and ability to forge cultural works which conveyed shared experience in esthetically refined, pleasurable, socially insightful, and courageous ways.

Sony Labou Tansi also, like Luambo, died from what was almost certainly AIDS. Like Luambo, he can also be understood in some ways as a broker of disparate worlds, whose creative work and social commentary consistently defined public sensibility among varied audiences both within and beyond Congo. As with Luambo, his engagements with AIDS were complex, layered, and only partially discernible to any analysis. These can be understood only by situating them within larger problems and concerns of person, history, and the imagination of affliction and social responsibility.

Sony infused into his final novel his projection of civilizational apocalypse as the consequence of the most minimal gesture of erotic excess. In doing so, he drew not only on Biblical and Western literary traditions but also on Kongo storytelling and on the diagnoses of earlier Kongo intellectuals of community afflication. Further, Sony's suffering from AIDS at the end of his life conjoined with the increasingly violent breakdown of national order in Congo at this time. Indeed, Sony's final novel was suffused, Clark observes, with a sense of "irredeemable offense" (Clark 2000:61), cast in the novel as the consequence of sexual excess, mirroring the political ruptures which characterized his social world and the nation as a whole. Similarly, perhaps, the "irreparable sacrilege" of his death, invoked by the author of the memorial verse discussed at the opening of this section, must be understood – at least in part – through cultural sciences which situate his suffering in the histories and imaginations of this region of Africa.

Sony's imagination and personal destiny were unique. Like Luambo, however, his life was only one among those of millions of individuals in Congo and in equatorial Africa who have faced these difficult conjunctures of civil conflict and the challenges of HIV and AIDS. I hope this glimpse into the complexity of their experiences and choices lends irreducible depth and life to the exercise of interpretation on which our understanding of these problems is necessarily founded.

ACKNOWLEDGMENTS

I am grateful for support provided for research in Zaire and the Republic of Congo by the Social Science Research Council, the Wenner-Gren Foundation for Anthropological Research, and the Rocca Memorial Scholarship program at the University of California at Berkeley.

NOTES

1.   Kinshasa is the capital of the Democratic Republic of Congo (formerly Zaire), and Brazzaville is the capital of the Republic of Congo. The two are separated physically only by the Congo River.

2.   For biographical studies, see, for example, Ewens 1994 and Stewart 2000.

3.   Lingala is a vehicular language widely spoken upriver from Brazzaville and Kinshasa, classified in Guthrie group C among Bantu languages.

4.   Excerpts given in the original Lingala are followed immediately by the English translation.

5.   See Geschiere (1997) on this issue with specific reference to Cameroon.

6.   "And if he come to see me, he speaketh vanity: his heart gathereth iniquity to itself; when he goeth abroad, he telleth it. All that hate me whisper together against me: against me do they devise my hurt. An evil disease, say they, cleaveth fast unto him: and now that he lieth he shall rise up no more. Yea, mine own familiar friend, in whom I

trusted, which did eat of my bread, hath lifted up his heel against me. But thou, O Lord, be merciful unto me, and raise me up, that I may requite them" (Holy Bible, King James version).

7.   Ngimbi (1997); see also the selections in Grootaers (1998).

8.   See, for example, De Boeck (n.d.). But see also Devisch (1996) on alternative social ethics and renewed cultural tradition in healing churches and prayer groups, among diviners and healers, and in family councils and grassroots women's associations.

9.   See Whyte (1997:217) on this question.

10.   See Nlandu-Tsasa (1997:130). He names 22 famous Zairian musicians as having died, presumably from AIDS, by the early 1990s.

11.   Sony was a member of the BaManianga group of BaKongo. Born in what is now D. R. Congo, his family had fled across the border to the Republic of Congo in 1964. See Devésa (1996) for a critical consideration of his life and work.

12.   Janzen and MacGaffey (1974:14) discuss the traditional KiKongo expression *Nzambi a Mpungu Tulendo*, saying that it may mean something like "God Almighty," but that it has also associations with *min'kisi* (charms and medicines). They write that "the parallel between the biblical 'God' and the African *Nzambi* is sufficiently close that protracted scholarly debate has failed to discover how much the modern concept of *Nzambi* owes to missionary teaching, and the equivalence of the two terms has been universally accepted in Kongo for many generations." See also MacGaffey (1986:6, 120) re the hierarchy of various *nzambi*.

13.   The Pool is a southeastern region of the Republic of Congo, home to Sony's Kongo-Lari group. It is named after the Malebo Pool of the Congo river, which fills a large basin just above Brazzaville and Kinshasa.

14.   See, for example, Bockie (1993:46, 56); also MacGaffey (1986:6–7; 160–161).

15.   As Hagenbucher-Sacripanti (1994) has described in his study of Vili and Yombe healers of the Pointe-Noire region.

16.   As Hersak (2001:628) has noted for other Kongo groups (Vili and Yombe) of the coastal Kwilu region.

17.   See, for example, Gruénais (1993) on the reluctance of physicians to disclose seropositive diagnoses in Brazzaville at this time. Fassin (1994) discusses at length the practice of "not telling" and the reasons to keep quiet. In an earlier co-authored article, he made the case that acknowledging AIDS could be seen as threatening the legitimacy of the state itself in Congo and elsewhere in Africa (Dozon and Fassin 1989). The Congolese government nonetheless showed great openness as the first African country to publish open AIDS statistics in 1986, and in its extensive radio and television campaigns and government

programs, especially those led by President Lissouba in the early 1990s. Further, clinically based studies in the capital cities of Zaire, Uganda, and Kenya in the early 1990s had already shown that the use and effect of HIV antibody testing could be quite different. In these interventions, relatively high standards of medical care, counseling, and confidentiality were provided together with testing. All reported constructive outcomes and effective reduction in risk behavior among clients provided with such testing and counseling services (Kamenga et al. 1991; Moses et al. 1991; Muller et al. 1992). More recently, effective combination therapies for HIV infection have transformed the stakes of testing and disclosure wherever these have been become available (see Nguyen 2002 for a discussion of these changes).

18. Although both Gruénais (1993:218) and Bockie (1993:38) argue that there is solidarity within the family for the ill person, Gruénais notes that some families would not spend scarce resources on care for a person believed to have AIDS.

19. See also Guyer and Belinga (1995) on wealth in people and in knowledge in equatorial Africa.

20. See, for example, Desjeux (1987) for a fine explication of how kinship and occult power among rural Sundi-speakers (like Lari, also Kikongo-speakers of Congo's Pool region) structure interpretation of modern social relations.

21. See Devésa (1996) for Sony's interest in Lemba, a secret society and cult of affliction in the lower Congo since precolonial times (for the social history of Lemba, see Janzen 1982).

22. See Bernault (1996:72 ff.) for a description of the origins of Kongo-Lari militancy in the amicalist movement of André Matsoua, founded in 1926, and his subsequent martyrdom at the hands of French authorities in 1942.

23. Further evidence of these themes in Sony's private devotions is provided by Clark through an iconography of the ancestral and Christian shrine in his home in Makelekele in Brazzaville (Clark 2000:44–45, 51).

24. Sony had spoken publicly in criticism of prevalent sexual mores in Brazzaville. See also Martin-Granel (2000) for a further exploration of sexuality in Sony's fiction. He refers to "a relationship with Sodom that was an obsession of Sony's during the 1970s" (Martin-Granel 2000:98).

25. These themes may perhaps be informed by aspects of Sony's childhood experience. Although he is quoted as saying that a Kongo boy is expected to leave his mother to join his father once he is seven years old, his experience was quite different (Devésa 1996:64). He instead left his father's village in Kimwanza, in the then-Belgian Congo, for the extended family of his mother in Boko, in the then-Moyen (French) Congo, where he also began his schooling in the French language. As the eldest son of a second wife, his concern with the human condition of shame – of "being a refugee under one's own skin," in his own words – seemed to stem partly from his own "accident of birth" and from the sense of simultaneous estrangement and belonging which this move between families entailed.

Apparently, because of conflict between his parents, his mother did all she could to keep him from seeing his father, and Sony is quoted as saying he only came to respect him later in life. He spoke rather of his mother and maternal grandmother as great sources of his love of Kongo language and of literature, referring to the stories "without end [and] without beginning" he learned while living with them (see Devésa 1996:57–65; also Krzywicki 1997).

26. Kyrzywicki 1997, drawing on Devésa 1996 and Layraud 1988.

27. Quotations from homages by Nicolas Martin-Granel and Nicolas Bissi (David 1995:12).

28. Christine Obbo's phrase (Obbo 1993a).

Chapter 21

Economic Growth Rates in Africa: The Potential Impact of HIV/AIDS

Lynn R. Brown

Since the HIV/AIDS epidemic started around twenty years ago, more than 60 million have been infected, five million people in 2001 alone, with 3.4 million of these in sub-Saharan Africa. In 2001, 14,000 people per day were infected with the HIV virus, 95 percent of these in the developing world. In the past two decades some 14 million adults have died of AIDS, 82 percent in sub-Saharan Africa. In 2001, three million people, adults and children, died of AIDS, 2.3 million of them in sub-Saharan Africa.

In the early days of what has become a pandemic, HIV/AIDS was seen only as a health problem but is now increasingly recognized as a development problem reversing many of the hard-won development gains of the past decades. Unlike the developing world, the size of the epidemics in developed countries, combined with the immense resources available for prevention and treatment activities, has contained the epidemic with no perceivable economic impacts.

Today, more than 95 percent of all HIV-infected people live in the developing world, where, in 1998, more than 23 percent of the population lived on less than U.S. $1 a day and 800 million people were food insecure. In sub-Saharan Africa more than 48 percent of the population lives on less than U.S. $1 a day. Development, by whatever definition one chooses, is still a goal limited by tightly binding resource constraints. Recognition that the HIV/AIDS pandemic was more than a severe health issue and would drive overburdened development budgets near bankruptcy was slow in coming. But, in the past decade, the perceived impact of HIV/AIDS has shifted from one of a disease affecting individuals to a disease which potentially affects the development of nations (Forsythe and Rau 1998).

"Development" was measured in the past by economic growth in terms of gross domestic product, measured in per capita terms, and a money metric of poverty. More recently there has been a recognition of the importance of the human and social dimensions of the development paradigm. Some would undoubtedly argue it has been a long time coming and that the paradigm has still not shifted far enough. Examination of the impacts of HIV/AIDS from an economist's perspective has in some sense followed the same paradigm shift. Initial work tended to focus on direct cost estimates of treatment and prevention, and then moved toward indirect costs, essentially counting human life in terms of value to society in lost productivity terms, and macroeconomic models of HIV/AIDS impact. Most recently there has been a shift to looking at a broader concept of the impact of HIV/AIDS on human development or social welfare.

This chapter will begin by looking at some of the pathways through which HIV/AIDS impacts on economic growth. It will then follow the lines of the paradigm shift, looking at the direct cost, indirect cost, macroeconomic models, and finally the human development/social welfare approach to examining the economic growth impact of HIV/AIDS.

HIV/AIDS Pathways of Impact on Economic Growth

The impact of HIV/AIDS on economic growth is highly complex but originates in its impact on the labor force, in terms of both growth and productivity. The impact on the former is more intuitively obvious through AIDS-related mortality. HIV/AIDS will impact on productivity growth through several channels. Increased morbidity of HIV-infected individuals will reduce productivity. If sick people, who are not HIV-infected, are unable to obtain health care from a health system overburdened due to HIV/AIDS, the burden of disease in countries will increase and impair productivity.

Through its direct and indirect impact on health status, and indirect impact on human capital formation, it also impacts on the relative returns to capital and thus capital formation. The increased demand for health care services, both preventive, such as blood screening, and treatment, may crowd out other government investment in health and other sectors. The savings rate in the economy may fall both relatively and absolutely. HIV-infected people will face lower incomes and rising health expenditures, increasing consumption expenditures, and reducing savings. As the epidemic spreads, if people adopt more fatalistic attitudes and perceive shorter life-spans then they may choose to save less for the future. Lower savings result in lower resources for investment. Lowered rates of productive investment result in slower economic growth in the future.

A critical factor in the development process and in generating future economic growth is investment in human capital by government. Investment in health and education, particularly at the primary level, is generally subsidized by government because of the social benefits to society. It is a good investment, promoting the demographic transition[1] and improved child health, among other things. Rapidly growing populations require increased levels of investment in human capital just to maintain existing average per capita human capital stock. A shift in the demographic structure of the population due to AIDS – a movement toward younger rather than older populations – will result in shifts in relative social service expenditures. If health care expenditures are higher for the young than for the old, then higher health-care expenditures will be required regardless of the additional direct health costs of preventing and treating HIV/AIDS. Similarly, although the absolute numbers of the younger population may be falling as a result of AIDS, the relative proportion will grow, resulting in higher demand for education expenditures. This produces a shift in the dependency on social sector spending and the tax resources to finance it.

The argument is similar to the current debate in many developed countries as the post-World War II baby boom generation comes up to retirement. There have been numerous debates in the U.S.A. with regard to the funding of social security. Social security for the elderly today is largely funded from current taxation revenues. As the "baby boomers" retire, and spend longer in retirement than their predecessors due to earlier retirement and lengthening life-spans, a smaller tax-paying population base has to support a relatively large aged population. In the future, current taxation revenues may well be insufficient to support social security and welfare systems, thus raising present-day questions about the viability of the system in the future.

The situation in heavily AIDS-affected developing countries will be similar except that the dependent population will be the young. Despite the relative increase in demand for government health and education spending by the young, AIDS will lower the social returns to public investment in both health and education by shortening life expectancies and thus the time over which society recoups its initial investment. On a more positive note, providing investment in the young can be at least maintained once the AIDS epidemic is curtailed, and the fertility transition is completed, there will be the equivalent of a "baby boom" population when the number of workers relative to dependents will be high. This could potentially result in rapid economic growth.

Similar to its impacts on the social returns to human capital investment, AIDS will affect the private rates of return to human capital investment in health and education, particularly with the introduction of health and education user fees as a result of structural adjustment programs. If parents believe their children are unlikely to survive long enough to support them in old age, then they may reduce their investment in preventive health care, such as immunizations, for their children. Parents also face a dilemma regarding educational investment: if AIDS strikes at the more educated, productive worker, a skill shortage may be created, increasing the wages of skilled workers and therefore the private rate of return to education. But households facing labor shortages due to HIV/AIDS infection of members may have to choose current child labor over future gains from education, offsetting these long-run benefits.

One consequence of AIDS is an increasing number of orphaned children – 13.2 million have been orphaned since the onset of the epidemic – cared for by extended family members or by the state. Before the onset of the AIDS epidemic, around 2 percent of all children in developing countries were orphans. By 1999, 10 percent or more were orphans in some sub-Saharan African countries. An assessment of demographic and health survey data from eight countries[2] revealed that only one, Zimbabwe, had school enrollment rates higher for orphans than non-orphans and then only orphans who had lost both parents (World Bank 1997a). Figure 21.1 shows that in a study on the Kagera region of Tanzania, enrollment in school is low for all children aged 7–10 years but particularly for orphans in poor households.

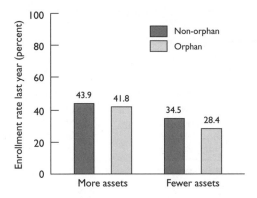

Figure 21.1 *Enrollment rates (age 7–10), by orphanhood and household assets, Kagera, Tanzania*
Source: Based on information in figure 14.4 World Bank 1997a.

Thus, HIV/AIDS puts pressure on both governments and households in terms of investing in human capital. Reduced levels of human capital investment will have negative consequences for future economic growth by virtue of a less educated workforce in poorer overall health.

AIDS will, however, have a more immediate and direct impact on the costs of maintaining human capital and thus current economic growth. AIDS-related morbidity will increase demand for curative health care. The increased demand for health care services, particularly in urban areas, where AIDS is currently concentrated, is crowding out other health care demands.

Table 21.1 shows that in all hospitals except Kenyatta National Hospital, over 50 percent of hospital beds were occupied by AIDS patients. It is highly unlikely that these beds were empty pre-AIDS epidemic, which suggests that some non-AIDS patients can no longer gain admittance. The Mama Yeo Hospital in Zaire had always operated at full capacity; however, in 1988, 50 percent of beds were occupied by AIDS patients, indicating that non-AIDS patients must have been turned away (Hassig et al. 1990).

In Kenyatta National Hospital, Nairobi, the average number of HIV-infected patients admitted per day doubled between 1988 and 1992 but the number of HIV-negative patients fell by 18 percent (Figure 21.2). In the same

Table 21.1 *Percentage of beds occupied by HIV-positive patients, Kenyatta National Hospital, Nairobi*

City	Hospital	Percentage of beds occupied by HIV-positive patients
Chiang Mai, Thailand	Provincial	50
Kinshasa, Congo DR[a]	Mama Yemo	50
Kigali, Rwanda	Central	60
Bujumbura, Burundi	Prince Regent	70
Nairobi, Kenya	Kenyatta National Hospital	39
Kampala, Uganda	Rubaga Hospital	56

[a] Formerly Zaire.
Source: World Bank 1997.

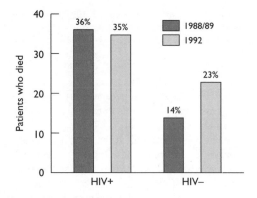

Figure 21.2 *Impact of AIDS on mortality at Kenyatta National Hospital, Nairobi*
Source: Based on figure 4.2 World Bank 1997a.

period the mortality rate for HIV-negative patients increased from 14 to 23 percent, suggesting that HIV-negative patients were more seriously ill on admittance than in the past, probably a function of rationing of scarce hospital beds (World Bank 1997a).

Shifts in the allocation of government health expenditures in favor of tertiary health care facilities, hospitals, and specialized services may shift the current donor-led emphasis of health care expenditures away from primary, particularly rural, health care. Health ministers face difficult choices: emphasize treatment or prevention expenditures with regards to HIV/AIDS; emphasize AIDS or non-AIDS patients with respect to hospital treatment. Governments face the additional decision of what priority to give the health ministry budget in the light of AIDS versus other activities such as education, social welfare programs, etc. Increasingly, resources will be allocated to health

sector expenditures and health care, in some sense maintenance expenditures, rather than to productive investment. Governments will be less able to secure overall health and education improvements for their citizens, resulting in stagnant rather than increasing productivity. The long-run results will be lower domestic capital formation, diminishing the capacity for future economic growth.

The next section will briefly assess the impact of HIV/AIDS on population growth and thus on the denominator of GDP per capita as a measure of development.

Population Impacts on Economic Growth

Economists' traditional yardstick of economic growth has been gross domestic product per capita. This metric is dependent on both aggregate economic product in a country and overall population levels. Thus one, and perhaps the least complicated, pathway through which HIV/AIDS will have an impact is through its effect on population size, the denominator in this metric.

Brown (1996) examined population forecasts for 15 sub-Saharan African countries to 2020 from the World Bank, United Nations, and The U.S. Bureau of the Census. The published forecasts of all agencies assumed a cessation in HIV infections at some point between 2005 and 2010. None of these forecasts predicted population growth rates below 1.2 percent in 2020 – the World Bank forecast for Zimbabwe. A commissioned set of U.S. Bureau of Census forecasts for Brown (1996), which relaxed the assumption of no new adult HIV infections post-2010, forecast the 2020 population growth rate for Zimbabwe to be 0.44 percent. Recent forecasts by the U.S. Bureau of Census now predict population growth will be negative 0.5 percent by 2010 for Zimbabwe. Life expectancy without AIDS in Zimbabwe in 2010 would be 70 years but the latest forecast now suggests it will be just 35 years. A similar halving of life expectancy over a no-AIDS scenario is true for other countries, including Botswana and Zambia.

Paradoxically, using GDP per capita as the indicator of development could translate the human tragedy of the HIV/AIDS pandemic into a "development gain," providing stark evidence of the inadequacy of GDP per capita as a development indicator. Improvements in welfare or "development," measured by gross domestic product (GDP) per capita, can be achieved only if GDP growth increases faster than population growth. Average annual GDP growth rates in sub-Saharan Africa were just 1.6 percent from 1980–90 and increased marginally to 2.5 percent from 1990–2000. The World Bank estimates it would take sustained GDP growth rates of around 5 percent to reduce the numbers living below U.S. $1 per day by 50 percent in sub-Saharan Africa by 2015, the Development Assistance Committee's Goal (DAC) of OECD[3] (Demery and Walton 1998). Very few sub-Saharan African countries have sustainably achieved close to that during the 1990s and many experienced negative growth in the 1980s. Therefore, some have argued that, although AIDS is a tragedy, it is also a Malthusian-type phenomenon. Its negative impact on population size will reduce pressure on available resources, improving the ability of the world to sustain and feed itself.

The IFPRI impact model appears to support this view, using global food security as a measure of welfare.[4] A simulation using the UN low-variant population forecasts indicates that global per capita food availability in 2020 would be 5 percent higher than in the baseline scenario founded upon the UN medium-variant population forecasts. This would translate into a reduction of 33.5 million in the forecast number of malnourished children in the developing world in 2020. About 31 percent of this reduction would be in sub-Saharan Africa. At the same time, net imports of cereals to the region would be 2.5 million metric tons less than in the baseline scenario in 2020.

The major caveat to these results in terms of drawing parallels to the impact of the HIV/AIDS pandemic, however, is that the low-population-variant scenario assumes that the productive capacity and economic structure of the economy will not change from the baseline scenario. If HIV infection and AIDS are not randomly distributed across a population, but concentrated spatially and/or in particular population subgroups that have higher than average economic productivity, then the effect of AIDS on domestic capital formation will be magnified. Those with higher wages are likely also to have higher levels of saving, both relatively and absolutely. Under this scenario, if the negative effect of HIV/AIDS on the productive capacity of the economy is greater than the effect on population growth, then the per capita availability of food in 2020 may be less than that of the baseline scenario. We will see a higher incidence of hunger and malnutrition.

The modes of transmission and its age-group selectivity, striking people in their most productive years, make AIDS a "clustering" disease and thus it is highly unlikely that HIV/AIDS will have uniform impacts on all sectors of an economy. Cohen (1998b) indicates that the HIV epidemic has a bi-modal distribution with peaks among both the poorest segment of the population and the richest and most educated. In a 1997 speech at the World Economic Forum, Peter Piot, the Executive Director of UNAIDS, reported on some of the impacts of HIV/AIDS. Barclay's Bank in Zambia lost most of its senior managers to AIDS; in Uganda more than 40 percent of the military are infected; and up to 30 percent of schoolteachers are infected in Côte d'Ivoire, with one teacher dying per day. A 1999 report in The Economist highlighted power shortages in Zambia as a result of the number of engineers who had died of AIDS. In Kenya, Forsythe et al. (1993) estimated that the average annual income of a worker with AIDS was 31 percent higher than the average national income. A 1995 sentinel survey report for Malawi indicated that the HIV infection rate among farmers was 11.5 percent, rising to 34.5 percent for professionals (Vella 1998, cited in Over 1998). The evidence indicates strongly that HIV/AIDS is neither evenly nor randomly distributed throughout the economy. Thus, the argument that the decrease in population growth could be "good" for development, in any sense, however perverse, as measured by GDP per capita, is fatally flawed, and starkly reveals the inadequacies of such an indicator as an isolated measurement of development.

Researchers have attempted to assess the economic effect of HIV/AIDS, or gross domestic product effects, in a disaggregated sense by estimating the direct and indirect costs, and at an aggregate level using computable general equilibrium (CGE) and Solow-type growth macroeconomic models.

Direct Cost Estimates of the Impact of AIDS

Direct costs of AIDS are defined as the costs of treating HIV-and AIDS-infected individuals.

Estimates of the direct costs vary tremendously, not only across countries but within countries, depending on the socio-economic characteristics of those infected and the quality of services to which they have access. Table 21.2 shows the diversity of estimates.

What is clear from Table 21.2 is that in all but the lowest of country-specific estimates, the direct costs of AIDS per case exceed per capita gross national product (GNP). They also exceed average per capita public expenditures of $5 on health care in most sub-Saharan African countries. Ainsworth and Over (1994:225) estimated the total costs, public and private, of treating the estimated number of AIDS cases in Zimbabwe, Kenya, Malawi, Tanzania, and Rwanda. These costs ranged from 23 percent of 1990 public health spending

Table 21.2 *Estimates of the direct cost of AIDS, per case, selected countries*

	Direct costs				GNP per capita
	Low[a]	Mean[a]	High[a]		
Country		(U.S. $)		Ratio of costs to GNP/capita	(1992 U.S. $)
Zaire (1987–88)[b]	132	n.a	1,585		110
Tanzania (1987–88)[b]	104	n.a	631	1/5.7	110
Tanzania (1990)	n.a	290	n.a	2.9	110
Tanzania (1996)[g]		414		0.7	591
South Africa (1991)[c]	2,857	n.a	7,143	1/2.7	2,670
Malawi (1989)[d]	n.a	210	n.a	1	210
Kenya (1992)[d]	n.a	938	n.a	3	310
Jamaica (1987)[d]	n.a	1,807	n.a	1.4	1,340
Zimbabwe (1991)	64	614	2,574	0.1/1.1/4.5	570
Thailand (1993)[e]	987	n.a	1,524	0.5/0.82	1,840
Thailand (1996)[g]	n.a	2,516	n.a	0.4	6290
Korea (1993)	n.a	2,010	n.a	0.3	6,790
Malaysia (1993)[f]	n.a	3,000	n.a	1.1	2,790
Rwanda (1989–90)	n.a	358	n.a	1.4	250
Cote d'Ivoire (1996)	n.a	2,335	n.a	1.7	1,373
Mexico (1996)[g]	n.a	13,868	n.a	2.0	6,934
Brazil (1996)[g,h]	n.a	27,639	n.a	3.0	9,213

[a] Rate of estimates is based on type and quality of treatment sought. If only one figure is cited, it is shown as the mean.
[b] 1985 U.S. $.
[c] Based on an official exchange rate of R2.8 to U.S. $1.
[d] 1991 dollars.
[e] Based on 18-month life span with AIDS.
[f] Based on 12-month life span with AIDS.
[g] International dollars for all figures.
[h] São Paulo state only.
Sources: Table 4 Brown 1996; Thailand, Tanzania, Côte D'Ivoire, Mexico, Brazil, 1996 in Shepard 1997.

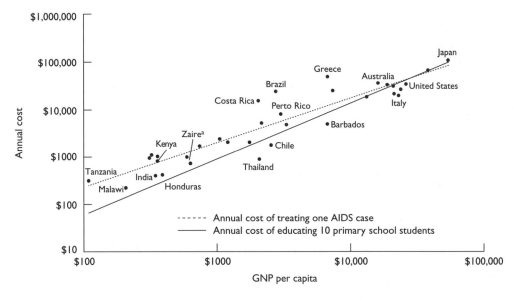

Figure 21.3 *Annual treatment cost for an AIDS patient correlated with GNP per capita*
Source: World Bank 1997a, figure 1.8.

in Kenya to more than 65 percent in Rwanda. Not surprisingly, the estimated total treatment costs per year per AIDS patient, including public and private costs, are correlated with GNP per capita, as shown in Figure 21.3.

On average, for the countries shown, the total annual treatment cost per AIDS patient is 2.7 times per capita GNP. An illustration of the trade-off facing governments, particularly in poor countries, when considering financing these treatment costs is that for an equivalent expenditure they could fund an additional ten primary school education places (World Bank 1997a). This trade-off is significant given the percentage of adults illiterate in some of the worst-affected sub-Saharan African countries – Botswana 26 percent, Burundi 50 percent, Kenya 31 percent, Uganda 52 percent, and Rwanda 50 percent.

Indirect Costs of the Impact of HIV/AIDS[5]

The indirect costs of HIV/AIDS are defined as the discounted healthy years[6] of life lost per individual to society as a result of AIDS-related mortality or, when valued in economic terms, the value of production forgone as a result of AIDS-related morbidity and mortality. This approach underestimates the contri-

bution of the under- and unemployed, assuming they do not spend all their productive years in this state, and overestimates the loss of those whose salary is made up in part of economic rents rather than productive activity.

Examples of the approach are provided by Over et al. (1988) for Zaire and Tanzania, and Forsythe et al. (1993:16) for Kenya. In Zaire and Tanzania, preventing one case of HIV infection saves 8.8 discounted healthy life years,[7] a number that ranks fifth after sickle-cell anemia, neonatal tetanus, birth injury, and severe malnutrition in the number of healthy life years saved.[8] It is notable that the first four diseases are largely diseases one is born with or that are acquired in early childhood. AIDS counts for greater savings in discounted healthy life years than many other endemic adult diseases such as TB and malaria. In Kenya, Forsythe et al. (1993:16) calculated that ten years of discounted productive life years were lost with each new case of AIDS, or more than three-fifths of an individual's undiscounted productive years. In Zaire and Tanzania, Over et al. (1988) used three categories of labor to arrive at an economic valuation of healthy life years lost: rural adult, urban adult with primary education, and urban

Table 21.3 *Estimates of the indirect costs per case of HIV infection in Zaire and Tanzania (1985 US$)*

	Zaire		Tanzania	
Labor category	Average annual income	Cost of HIV infection	Average annual income	Cost of HIV infection
Rural	144	890	391	2,425
Urban				
Primary	287	1,780	626	3,880
Secondary	431	2,669	821	5,093

Source: Table 3 Brown (1996), compiled from information in tables 3 and 4 in Over et al. (1988)

adult with secondary schooling or more. The results are shown in Table 21.3.

Forsythe et al. (1993:15) valued the discounted life years on the basis of age, income, and industry distribution of new AIDS cases and calculated that the average annual income of a person with AIDS was U.S. $650. Assuming a loss of ten discounted productive life years per AIDS case, the indirect costs per case would be U.S. $6,713. Therefore, for these three countries the indirect costs of each AIDS case far outweigh both the direct costs and, therefore, gross domestic product (GDP) per capita (the indirect costs per new adult AIDS case in Kenya were 23 times per capita GDP). The HIV seroprevalence rate in Kenya in 1991 was estimated at between 3.4 and 5.1 percent of the total adult population. This represents a considerable potential indirect cost of AIDS to the Kenyan economy in the period from 1991 to 2001, dependent on the conversion rate of HIV into AIDS. By the year 2000, Forsythe et al. (1993:17, 24) estimate that the direct cost of AIDS (that is, the cost of treating AIDS patients) in Kenya could be as high as 4.7 billion 1991 Kenyan shillings.[9] The indirect costs, however, could be as high as 40 billion Kenyan shillings (in 1991 shillings).

One flaw in using the discounted life years approach in combination with a valuation of human capital is that it ignores lost savings. When a worker becomes too sick to work, not only is a productive lifetime of earnings lost but also the proportion of earnings that would have been saved. These savings contribute through investment to capital formation in

the economy. Similarly, the human capital approach assumes a constant income loss per worker lost. The standard economic production function approach generally assumes diminishing marginal productivity[10] of each additional worker. Thus, as the epidemic begins to bite, each worker lost is more valuable than the one before. To overcome some of these difficulties in the human capital approach, various attempts have been made to use CGE and Solow-type growth models[11] to forecast the effects of AIDS on various aggregates in the macroeconomy.

Potential Macroeconomic Impact of HIV/AIDS

An example of the CGE approach, applied to Cameroon, is provided by Kambou, Devarajan, and Over (1992). In a dynamic model they portray AIDS as a shock to the labor market, resulting in the loss of 10,000 workers from each of the three labor categories (rural, urban unskilled, and urban skilled) in each year of the simulation between 1987 and 1991. A savings closure rule is used (that is, foreign savings are determined outside the model, exogenously, rather than by the model endogenously) such that investment varies directly with the level of domestic savings. The reduction in workers causes the economy to contract sharply, with GDP growth falling from 4.3 percent in a no-AIDS economy to 2.4 percent in the AIDS simulation. The decline in growth is triggered by falling investment (a result of stagnating private savings) and falling government savings (a result of declining trade revenues when exports decline).

To further investigate the selective impact of AIDS on more productive categories of labor, Kambou, Devarajan, and Over reran the simulations by reducing 10,000 workers from one labor skill category at a time. The removal of 10,000 rural sector workers each year seems to have little effect on the economy. The prime reason for this is that 10,000 workers represent just 0.4 and 0.3 percent of the rural and entire labor force, respectively. Because rural labor supply grows 2 percent per year in the model, labor force growth in the rural sector is still positive, despite the impact of AIDS.

The result is similar when the reduction is 10,000 urban unskilled workers in each year. The most striking result occurs with the removal of 10,000 urban skilled workers in each year of the simulation. Government savings plummet by 20.6 percent per year on average, resulting in a fall in fixed investment growth from 5.1 percent in the base year to 1.7 percent per year in the simulation. The assumption of this model – a constant yearly fixed loss of labor – may not be realistic. What is clear, however, is that an unequal loss of labor concentrated among the skilled workforce has devastating effects, reducing long-run economic growth from 4.3 to 2.6 percent per year. In Cameroon, where the average annual population growth from 1986 to 1995 was 3 percent, the difference between these two economic growth rates is the difference between increasing per capita GDP and declining per capita GDP.

Cuddington (1993a) has used a Solow-type growth model to explore the macroeconomic impact of AIDS in Tanzania. He first used a simple neoclassical model in which the economy adjusts to maintain production with efficient allocation of all resources, including labor – assumptions that are unrepresentative of Tanzania, or indeed many African economies. The model considers only one type of labor and focuses on the direct effect of increased health-care costs on savings. The model uses the population and AIDS-prevalence forecasts of Bulatao for Tanzania, in which AIDS prevalence rises from nine in one thousand adults in 1985 to 315 in one thousand adults in 2010.

Simulations were performed using alternative values for the annual labor productivity lost per AIDS-infected worker (from zero effect to 2),[12] and the proportion of AIDS-related medical expenses financed by reduced savings (also from zero to 2).[13] The simulations show that, depending on the assumptions made, the Tanzanian GDP in 2010 may be reduced by 15 to 25 percent from a no-AIDS scenario. This translates into a per capita income reduction of zero to 10 percent, depending on assumptions relating to labor productivity and health care financing.[14] Cuddington and Hancock (1994) applied a similar model to the Malawian economy. The simulations were limited to a maximum 100 percent reduction in labor productivity of the infected individual only, and a maximum of 100 percent of health care costs met from savings (that is, zero to 1 in both cases). The simulations showed that in 2010, under a medium forecast for the prevalence of AIDS, average real GDP growth would be 0.2 to 0.3 percentage points lower, and per capita GDP growth 0 to 11 percent lower, than in a no-AIDS scenario.[15]

One potential criticism of these models is that the underlying classical economic assumptions are invalid. Assumptions about the homogeneity of labor productivity and education in the face of an epidemic (which has initially hit the most productive workers disproportionately) and fully flexible labor markets are likely to result in an understatement of the true effects of the AIDS epidemic. Cuddington (1993b) subsequently modified this approach for Tanzania by relaxing the full-employment assumption and considering a dual-economy labor surplus situation, a more valid assumption for both the Tanzanian and other sub-Saharan African economies. This is achieved by introducing a formal sector, with sticky wages, and an informal sector, with wages equal to the average product of labor rather than the marginal product, to the model.[16] Results from the simulations, using the same alternative parameter values for declining labor productivity and reductions in savings, are similar to the results using the one-sector model. In a scenario in which wages adjust slowly, the impact of AIDS is a reduction in GDP of between 11 and 28 percent, depending on the assumptions made about the decline in labor productivity and savings behavior. Similarly, the effect on per capita GDP ranges from a 3.6 percent increase in a no-AIDS scenario to a decline of 16.1 percent in the scenario where AIDS reduces the productivity of a worker and a caregiver by 100 percent, and the decline in savings parameter is set to 2.

Over (1992) takes the modeling one stage further by incorporating a high-productivity urban sector and low-productivity rural sector as well as three types of workers: uneducated, those with primary education, and those with more than a primary education. Although the model makes no allowance for reductions in labor productivity as a result of AIDS, it does allow for assumptions to be made in relation to risk of infection for different skill categories of workers. These range from an assumption that the epidemic disproportionately affects the least-skilled worker to one in which the worker with more than a primary education is 16 times more likely to be infected. Like the models described in the previous paragraphs, health care costs can be financed to varying degrees from savings.

The Over model is applied both to an aggregate of 30 sub-Saharan African countries and to a subgroup of the 10 countries most affected by AIDS. Results indicate that, as the likelihood of more-educated workers being infected increases and the percentage of health care costs financed from savings increases, the negative impact on annual GDP per capita growth for both the 30-and 10-country aggregate increases. In a situation where the epidemic affects those with no education most, and none of the health care costs are financed from savings, annual growth rates of GDP per capita are reduced by 0.56 percentage points. Where those with more than primary education are 16 times more likely to be infected and all health care costs are financed from savings, the negative impact on annual GDP growth per capita is 1.08 percent. For the 10 worst-affected countries, the impact on GDP growth per capita ranges from a decline of 0.73 to 1.47 percent. Neither of these extreme scenarios is likely, but they reveal an inevitable conclusion – per capita GDP growth rates are likely to be decreased by at least 0.6 percent and possibly

as much as 1.4 percent. This is a substantial reduction in relative terms for many sub-Saharan African economies, given that the sub-Saharan African average annual GDP per capita growth rate was –0.8 percent from 1980 to 1992, 1.7 percent from 1980 to 1990, and 2.1 percent from 1990 to 1997.

Like the direct and indirect cost approaches, these models are not without their problems. Unlike costing models, they do include cross-sector links but they cannot include feedback loops based on changes in behavior. The models assume that agents always base behavior on the information available at the initial date and consequently there is no account made of changes in behavior that might alter the path of the epidemic. Bloom and Mahal (1997) argue that for this reason and the fact that AIDS is now emerging as a disease of poverty, these models overestimate the economic impacts of the epidemic.

In an effort to address these issues Bloom and Mahal use well-established empirical growth equations with cross-country data on AIDS to estimate the impact of AIDS on income growth per capita between 1980 and 1992. This approach explains the past as opposed to predicting the future, and looks for an impact of AIDS on economic growth. Initial estimates did show significant impacts of AIDS on economic growth, but when other factors that impact on economic growth were introduced, these effects disappeared. They conclude that "there is more flash than substance to the claim that AIDS impedes national economic growth." The problem with this approach is that by using per capita income growth as the outcome of interest, the impact of HIV/AIDS on population growth is masked. Also, non-epidemic countries are acting as the controls, or counterfactual cases, for countries with HIV/AIDS epidemics.

In the preceding sections evidence has been presented indicating that the direct and indirect costs of HIV/AIDS are substantial but these costs cannot be translated into accurate estimates of the impact on economic growth due to the lack of cross-sectoral linkages. Most of the macroeconomic models permit the inclusion of cross-sectoral linkages but at a relatively primitive level, and are unable to incorporate behavior and structural change when predicting the impacts on economic growth. The estimates of economic growth impact range from positive to negative 28 percent depending on the macro-model of choice. Ultimately no macro-model can truly capture the impact of HIV/AIDS on economic growth for a country in a "with and without AIDS scenario" as, by definition, one state does not exist.[17] Equally, alongside this range of empirical evidence, raw observation of the growth performance of some of the worst-affected sub-Saharan African countries shows GDP growth ranging from negative 6.3 percent in Rwanda to positive 7.2 percent in Uganda.

This could be a disheartening result, but perhaps more to the point is whether we are asking the right question. Ultimately economic growth is used as a proxy indicator for development because it signifies an increasing resource base in the belief that this translates into reductions in poverty and improvements in welfare. As Over (1998) points out, "the deficiencies of per capita income as a measure of social welfare are well known, but the example of the AIDS epidemic throws them into stark relief." As we saw earlier in this chapter, the negative impact of HIV/AIDS on population growth rates can paradoxically turn a human tragedy into a development gain, when gross domestic product per capita is used as the lone indicator of development as was the norm for many years.

The most recent studies on estimating the macro-level impacts of HIV/AIDS have moved beyond the impact on economic growth and focused on the impacts on the UNDP Human Development Index (HDI). This index, introduced by UNDP in their Human Development Report in 1996, is a weighted aggregate of life expectancy, adjusted income per capita, measure of schooling enrollment, and the adult literacy rate. Based on a sample of 56 countries, Bloom et al. (1996 cited in Cohen 1998b) concluded that between 1980 and 1992, countries on average lost 1.3 years of human development progress. For the most severely impacted countries these losses were much higher – more than ten years for Zambia, eight years for Tanzania, seven years for Rwanda, and six years for the Central African Republic. When considering human development as proxied by the HDI, a 1 percent in-

crease in HIV prevalence rates leads to a 2.2 year loss of human development on average (Godwin 1995). While HIV/AIDS has an impact on all components of the index, the biggest determinant of the loss in human development is the impact of AIDS on life expectancy, which carries a weight of about one-third in the HDI. As Cohen (1998b) points out, this impact is over a period when the HIV/AIDS was in its early stages and the HIV seroprevalence rate was far lower than it is today. Thus it is reasonable to expect that these impacts will be far greater in the future. Cohen (1998b), using projections of movements in the HDI between 1996 and 2010 for Botswana, showed that, instead of enjoying an increase in its HDI index, Botswana would see a fall in its HDI index in 2010 to a level lower than in both the with and without AIDS scenario of 1996. Human development is being lost, not gained, and the story is similar for other severely effected countries in southern Africa.

Over (1998) uses a social welfare function approach, which essentially parameterizes the arguments of the HDI index – life expectancy, school enrollment, income per capita, and adult literacy rates. Using a reasonable, although arbitrary, parameterization of a Cobb Douglas social welfare function, Over estimates that ten years of a sustained HIV seroprevalence of 13 percent in Malawi will rob it of welfare worth 13 percent of its per capita GDP.

Conclusions

The jury would still appear to be out in terms of the impact of HIV/AIDS on economic growth. Even if it has a measurable impact on GDP growth, that impact has to be greater than its impact on population growth for the traditional indicator of economic development to worsen. However, the HIV/AIDS pandemic really highlights the inadequacy of this measurement of development. The focus of our interest should be on sustainable human development, not the performance of an imperfect proxy indicator. As such, the recent work examining the impacts of HIV/AIDS on the HDI seems to indicate unambiguously negative impacts. Some may argue that most of these impacts are driven by changes in life expectancy, but surely that is a critical component of sustainable human development.

This chapter has, however, not looked at the other, and potentially more important "side of the coin," from a proactive viewpoint. What is the impact of rapid economic growth on the spread of HIV/AIDS? A vibrant, growing economy is generally associated with rapidly growing centers of economic activity and with integration and mobility of both capital and people. These centers become the focus of migrant labor, leading to increased population density even though the population may be very transient. Over time, market infrastructure, such as roads, and communications networks are set up. This essentially creates an environment conducive to the spread of HIV/AIDS. Average annual GDP growth in Botswana, home to one of the worst HIV/AIDS epidemics in sub-Saharan Africa, from 1975 to the early 1990s exceeded 10 percent, the highest in the world. In the past few years South Africa has been home to one of the fastest-growing HIV/AIDS epidemics in the world. Is it a coincidence that in much the same time period South Africa has been striving to integrate its peoples and economy internally and has reintegrated in the global marketplace with the demise of apartheid? We have known for some time of a locus of HIV infections along truck and trade routes and we need to scale that knowledge up when we think of economic growth and development.

In the future, development activities, designed to lead to economic growth, must recognize the potential for those same activities to exacerbate the spread of HIV/AIDS and take steps to mitigate it. The World Bank requires environmental assessments (EA) for all projects requiring financing. These assessments take into account the natural environment (air, water, and land); human health and safety; and sociocultural, transboundary, and global environmental aspects. It is encouraging that the EA for a large pipeline construction project between Cameroon and Chad included assessment on the potential spread of HIV/AIDS which could be associated with the project. It included several recommendations regarding information, education and communication campaigns, condom distribution, and screening and treatment of STDs for those people attracted to the construction areas.

HIV/AIDS prevention needs to be the goal of all sectors of society, not just the domain of the public health sector, if we are truly to bring the epidemic under control and stop its frightening march through the subcontinent. In the rush for economic growth we must not create a breeding ground for human tragedy in the shape of a worsening HIV/AIDS epidemic in the future.

ACKNOWLEDGMENTS

The author would like to thank Klaus von Grebmer, Rosemary O'Neill, and participants at the symposium "HIV/AIDS in Africa: Reviewing the Past, Understanding the Present, and Charting the Future," held at the University of Illinois at Urbana-Champaign, July 14–17, 1999, for their comments on an earlier draft. The author alone is responsible for the final outcome.

NOTES

1. Healthier children and more educated girls reduce the fertility rate and number of children per household. The falling fertility rate results in a population shift from one which is dominated by children and young people to one dominated, for a period of time, by people in their working years. This means more people working and fewer people dependent. For a fuller discussion of the impacts of the demographic transition see David E. Bloom, David Canning, and Jaypee Sevilla, 2001Economic growth and the demographic transition. National Bureau of Economic Research. Working Paper Series (U.S.); No. 8685:1-[86], December.

2. The eight countries comprised: Burkina Faso (1993), Central African Republic (1994–5), Côte d'Ivoire (1994), Haiti (1994–5), Kenya (1993), Tanzania (1994), Uganda (1995), Zimbabwe (1994) and N.E. Brazil (1991).

3. Based on a forecast of 1.9 percent per capita private consumption in World Bank 1998, plus 3 percent for population growth.

4. The IFPRI impact model is a set of country or regional models linked through trade that determines supply, demand, and prices for agricultural commodities. For a full description, see Rosegrant et al. 1995.

5. This section draws on Brown 1996.

6. Burden of disease analysis relies on Disability Adjusted Life Years (DALYs), an indicator of the time lived with disability and the time lost due to premature mortality. Years lost from premature mortality are estimated with respect to a standard expectation of length of life. Years lived with a disability are translated into an equivalent time loss through multiplication by a set of weights that reflect reduction in functional capacity. Therefore, DALYs are an effort to combine in a single indicator mortality and morbidity. For further discussions on this topic see Anand, Sudhir, 1998 DALYs: efficiency versus equity. World Development (U.K.); 26:307–310, February.

7. The discount rate used is 5 percent.

8. This statement is based on healthy life years saved compiled for Ghana in International Journal of Epidemiology (1981) for other diseases.

9. This figure is based on a calculation of high adult HIV seroprevalence levels of 11 percent in 1995.

10. This assumes there is an optimal production mix of workers and other inputs such as capital. Each additional worker added to this mix will be less productive than the previous one.

11. For a discussion of Solow-type growth models see a macroeconomic text book such as Section 3.3 of

Dornbusch R., S. Fischer and R. Startz, Macreconomics, 7th edn, Irwin McGraw-Hill.

12. Zero implies there is no decline in labor productivity; 2 implies the loss of productive labor of both the infected individual and a caregiver.

13. Savings may be reduced not only by the direct cost of health care expenditures to treat AIDS-related morbidity but also by social sector spending to care for orphans, or by public health programs to prevent the spread of HIV.

14. Population growth is assumed to decline by 0.7 percent, conservative by U.S. Bureau of the Census estimates.

15. Population growth is assumed to decline by 1.2 percent, conservative by U.S. Bureau of the Census estimates.

16. Sticky wages are slow to adjust in the presence of surplus labor and thus unemployment results.

17. A true comparison would involve estimating economic growth in the same economy for the same period both with and without the AIDS pandemic. By definition one state does not exist – if there is an AIDS epidemic it is impossible to estimate economic growth for that period "without AIDS." An alternative often used in project or program evaluation is to use a "control case" which is chosen to be as similar as possible to the treatment case. However, realistically it is hard to "pair up" economies as AIDS and non-AIDS economies as each is unique.

Chapter 22

Rising Tide of AIDS Orphans in Southern Africa

Jayati Ghosh and Ezekiel Kalipeni

Introduction

Many of the people dying from AIDS are be-tween 15 and 49 years and often leave children behind. For example, in 1999 alone, 1 million children aged 0–14 found themselves with one parent or both dead. In terms of cumulative AIDS orphans, it was estimated that by 1999 there were 13.2 million AIDS orphans through-out the world. Of these orphans, 12.1 million were in sub-Saharan Africa alone (UNICEF 2000; see Figure 22.1). Orphans constitute one of the worst catastrophes faced by sub-Saharan African countries as millions of children lose one parent or both to AIDS. Orphans are vul-nerable to a host of problems such as malnu-trition, face social stigma, absence of parental guidance, limited access to education, and are more likely to be employed in the informal economy (Muller and Abbas 1990; Muller et al. 1999; Ntozi and Mukiza-Gapere 1995; Black 1991). In addition, they may lose their inheritance, be forced to migrate, may become homeless, and be involved in crime (Ntozi 1997; Ntozi and Mukiza-Gapere 1995; Lugalla and Kibassa forthcoming).

In this chapter the emphasis will be placed on the southern African countries of Angola, Botswana, Lesotho, Madagascar, Malawi, Mo-zambique, Namibia, South Africa, Swaziland, Zambia, and Zimbabwe. This region was selected based on the fact that many of its countries are experiencing the highest rates of HIV/AIDS infection in the world and have borne the brunt of the devastating effects of the AIDS crisis. It is also estimated that by 2010 between 60 and 85 percent of all orphans in this region are likely to be designated as AIDS orphans. The central aim of this chapter is to highlight the ravages of the HIV/AIDS epidemic with special reference to orphans in the southern part of Africa.

HIV/AIDS in Southern Africa and Its Impacts

Before the advent of AIDS, about 2 percent of all children in countries of southern Africa were orphans. However, by 1997, the propor-tion of children with one or both parents dead had skyrocketed to 7 percent in many African countries and in some cases reached an as-tounding 11 percent (UNAIDS). At country level, by the year 2000 about 10 percent of all children in Botswana under 15 years of age had been orphaned due to the death of the mother or both parents. Many of these orphans

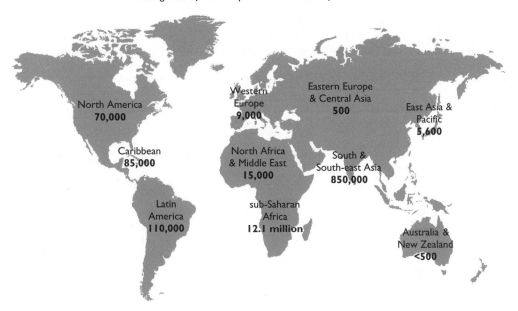

Figure 22.1 *Cumulative number of children estimated to have been orphaned by AIDS at age 14 or younger at the end of 1999*

Source: UNAIDS 2000.

Note: By the end of 1999 there were 13.2 million children worldwide who had lost their mother or both parents to AIDS before the age of 15 years, of whom 12.1 million were in Africa.

attribute the loss of parent(s) to AIDS. The proportion of AIDS orphans was about 52 percent in Zambia and 61 percent in Zimbabwe. In the countries of Lesotho and Malawi AIDS orphans, expressed as percentage of all maternal and or double orphans, stood at 36.1 and 31.2 percent, respectively. In other words, a third of all orphaned children were estimated to have lost parent(s) to AIDS. In 1999 about 8 percent of South African children were orphans, of whom 60 percent were estimated to have lost parent(s) to AIDS.

What these data indicate is a dramatic increase in the percent of AIDS orphans between 1990 and 2000. Based on USAID estimates, by 2000, in Botswana, 70 percent of orphans can attribute the loss of parent(s) to AIDS. Botswana is estimated to experience an increase in percent of orphaned children, reaching about 20.3 percent by 2010, 90 percent of whom will be AIDS orphans. In the countries of Lesotho, Malawi, and South Africa it is estimated that between 61 and 69 percent of all orphans will be designated as AIDS orphans. In Lesotho, 8.2 percent of children below 15 years of age will lose their

parent(s), with 79.3 percent estimated to be AIDS orphans. In Zambia, AIDS will be the leading cause behind 78 percent of all orphans (UNAIDS 2000b). Already, more than half a million children in Zambia have lost a mother or both parents to AIDS. The number is expected to double by 2014. With the proportion of orphaned children rising to more than 38 percent, Zambia leads as one of the most orphaned countries in the world (Baggaley and Needham 1997). In Zimbabwe, another hardest-hit country, 85 percent of orphaned children will lose their parent(s) to AIDS. These startling figures clearly reflect the severity and urgency of the problem in the southern African region.

According to the United States Census Bureau (1999), there will be more adults in their sixties and seventies in Botswana in 20 years' time than there will be adults in their forties and fifties. This implies that a small number of young adults – the group that has traditionally provided care for both children and the elderly – will have to support large numbers of young and old people. As UNAIDS (1999g) notes, many of these young adults will themselves be debilitated by AIDS and may even require care from their children or elderly parents rather than providing it.

The scenario in the case of Botswana will repeat itself in other southern African countries. For example, in Lesotho, a landlocked country of southern Africa which in 1997 had a population of 2.1 million, at the end of 1999 23.6 percent of its adult population was HIV positive. About 31 percent of pregnant women were HIV positive and by the end of 1999 there were about 35,000 AIDS orphans within this tiny country. Data showing the grim situation in which southern African countries find themselves are given in Table 22.1.

Already adult and child deaths are on the increase in these countries. Figures 22.2 and 22.3 give estimated deaths in children (<15 years) from HIV/AIDS during 1999 and the estimated cumulative number of orphans in southern Africa alive and dead in 1997. It has been noted that even without analyzing the data on death rates, countries with severe longstanding HIV epidemics such as those in southern Africa know from the massive increase in funerals that deaths are on the rise. Data in Table 22.1 confirm this sad truth of rising orphan deaths. The social and economic impacts of the epidemic cannot be overemphasized. The thousands of premature deaths of the economically active sector of the population aged 15–49 can only be expected to have a dramatic impact on virtually every aspect of social and economic life. While it is difficult to measure the precise impact of HIV at a national level in most hard-hit countries, a great deal of information does exist about how the epidemic is affecting everything from households to the public and private sectors of the economy (UNAIDS 1999g). Many surveys show that there has been a dramatic decrease in income for households having a family member with AIDS (Van de Walle 1990). This implies curtailed spending on school education and food consumption, while expenditure on health care may go up for the household as a whole.

Rising Tide of Orphans

Oppong (1998b), in applying vulnerability theory to Ghana's HIV/AIDS situation, points out that adverse life circumstances such as hunger and disease do not affect social groups uniformly. Oppong and other authors (cf. Baylies and Lyons in this volume) further argue that while all human beings are biologically susceptible to infection by different diseases such as HIV/AIDS, certain social and economic factors place some individuals and social groups in situations of increased vulnerability. In short, the vulnerability perspective deals, among other things, with issues of differential access to resources. This fact alone is crucial in the survival of AIDS orphans.

In embracing this perspective, we take the definition of orphans offered by agencies such as UNAIDS, WHO, and UNICEF. These agencies define AIDS orphans as those children who are under the age of 15 years and have lost a parent or both parents to AIDS. These children may be classified into maternal, paternal, or double orphans. It is to be noted that most countries collect and report data on maternal or double orphans. Since most countries do not gather information on the number of paternal orphans, there is limited data available about this group. Therefore UNICEF and UNAIDS estimates might actually understate the magnitude of the orphan problem as they do not include the orphaned children who may have lost their father only. Thus in this chapter we use data reported by these agencies which refers to maternal or double orphans.

In order to understand better the workings of vulnerability theory, let us look at the HIV/AIDS prevention efforts in Africa. As Packard and Epstein (1991) note, to encourage efforts to combat the spread of HIV/AIDS through sex education, just like efforts to control population growth in Africa through birth control, or tuberculosis through segregation, is to work against strong social, political, and economic forces, and not simply culturally determined patterns of behavior. The general ineffectiveness of AIDS prevention programs in Africa does not just stem from lack of funding, but from an unwillingness to look beyond simplistic approaches that focus on the peculiarities of individual sexual behavior rather than the social, economic, and political contingencies which make certain social groups such as orphans and poor women vulnerable. The reality of sexual behaviors is much more complicated. Poverty is one factor that limits the

Table 22.1 Estimates of HIV/AIDS statistics in southern Africa in 1999

Country	Population in 1999 ('000)		Estimated number of people living with AIDS			Pregnant women's rate (%)	Orphans cumulative	Estimated AIDS deaths(adults and children) in 1999	Deaths in children age 0–14 in 1999 (high estimate)
	Total	Adults age 15–49	Adults & children	Adults age 15–49	Adult rate(%)				
Angola	12,497	5,389	160,000	150,000	2.78	1.2	98,000	15,000	4,400
Botswana	1,592	775	290,000	280,000	35.80	39.1	66,000	24,000	5,100
Lesotho	2,108	998	240,000	240,000	23.57	31.3	35,000	16,000	4,900
Madagascar	15,502	7,199	11,000	10,000	0.15	0.0	2,600	870	240
Malawi	10,674	4,733	800,000	760,000	15.98	18.5	390,000	70,000	22,000
Mozambique	19,222	8,607	1,200,000	1,100,000	13.22	9.9	310,000	98,000	32,000
Namibia	1,689	790	160,000	150,000	19.54	22.7	67,000	18,000	3,500
South Africa	39,796	20,630	4,200,000	4,100,000	19.94	24.5	420,000	250,000	74,000
Swaziland	981	480	130,000	120,000	25.25	30.3	12,000	7,100	2,000
Zambia	8,974	4,137	870,000	830,000	19.95	25.9	650,000	99,000	24,000
Zimbabwe	11,509	5,771	1,500,000	1,400,000	25.06	24.0	900,000	160,000	38,000
Southern Africa total	124,544	59,509	9,561,000	9,140,000	15.36	–	2,950,000	757,970	210,140
Sub-Saharan Africa total	596,272	273,488	24,500,000	23,400,000	8.57	–	12,000,000	2,200,000	610,000
Global total	5,958,849	3,082,548	34,300,000	33,000,000	1.07	–	13,200,000	2,800,000	670,000

Source of data: Compiled from "Table of Country-Specific HIV/AIDS Estimates and Data" at the UNAIDS homepage (http://www.unaids.org/epidemic_update/ report/index.html#table). For country-specific data see UNAIDS/WHO 2000a, 2000b, 2000c, 2000d, 2000e, 2000f, 2000g.

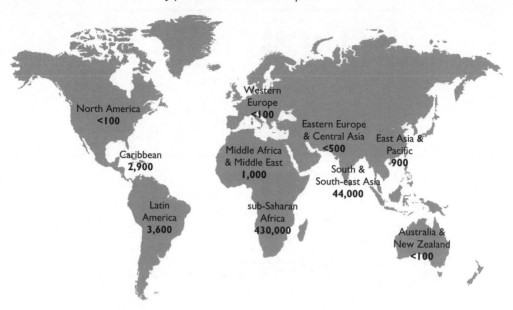

Figure 22.2 *Estimated deaths in children (<15 years) from HIV/AIDS during 1999*
Source: UNAIDS 2000.
Note: During 1999 there were 480,000 deaths of children less than 15 years of age from HIV/AIDS, of whom 430,000 were in Africa.

number and amount of resources available and gender is another (Kalipeni and Craddock 1998). As Craddock (2000) and Kalipeni and Craddock (1998) argue, for women in particular, jobs are scarce, resources such as government training projects or agricultural extension services are directed toward men, and local income-earning opportunities are generally unavailable. Scarce job opportunities for men mean that migrancy is high among many southern African countries as jobs are sought in neighboring countries or in regions far away from the home country. The result is that prostitution is one of the few income-earning occupations open to many women who must find a way to feed not just themselves but their children in the absence of their husband's or any other means of support. In short, vulnerability, whether it be that of an individual, an orphan, or a country, has a lot to do with the well-being of members of society. Individuals in certain social groups are more vulnerable than others. Poorer countries can ill afford the provision of employment and health care facilities. This theme will be used to guide the discussion in this chapter.

According to Hunter and Williamson (1998), the impact of the HIV/AIDS crisis is expected to peak by 2010 in the countries of southern Africa. These authors expect the already large numbers of orphaned children to continue to increase at dramatic rates thereafter. According to Hunter and Williamson (1998) and many other researchers, when children lose their mothers the loss is associated with psychosocial consequences (see, for example, Preble 1990; Ankrah 1996; Aspaas 1999; Dane and Levine 1994; Mok and Cooper 1997; Siegel and Gorey 1994). In such cases they lose the love and care of parents and may be forced to live with extended family members. Paternal orphans, on the other hand, face economic hardships as the income level of the family drops with the loss of the father. The problems are further magnified in case of double orphans.

A careful examination of Table 22.1 and Figure 22.3 shows the magnitude of the orphan problem in southern Africa. As noted earlier, according to UNAIDS, by the end of 1999 there were a cumulative total of 13.2 million orphans worldwide. Of these, the majority (over 90

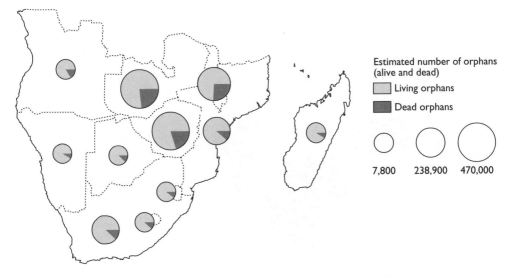

Figure 22.3 *Estimated cumulative number of orphans in southern Africa, alive and dead, 1997*
Source: UNAIDS 1998

percent) were in sub-Saharan Africa. Of the 12 million orphans in sub-Saharan Africa, 25 percent (about 3 million) were concentrated in the 11 countries of southern Africa. In 1999 alone, over 200,000 children below age 14, many of them orphans, had died. Indeed, as shown in Figure 22.3, a sizable portion of orphans throughout southern Africa have since died of AIDS, malnutrition, and other diseases (see also Gregson et al. 1999). Figures 22.4a and 22.4b show the geographic distribution of orphans in sub-Saharan Africa. These two maps, which show the total number of orphans as a percent of children under age 15 in each country, are a mirror of the distribution of HIV/AIDS cases. The intensity of the distribution of HIV/AIDS cases between 1990 and 2000 shifted from the north (i.e., Uganda, Democratic Republic of Congo) toward the south (i.e., Malawi, Zambia, Zimbabwe, Botswana, and South Africa). Hence the imperative of examining carefully the repercussions of this epidemic on orphans in southern Africa.

Impact of the AIDS Pandemic on Orphans in Southern Africa

The impact of AIDS on orphans, the economy, and society is very complex and manifold. It not only involves the immediate loss of loved ones but also there are long-term implications that can ravage economic and social progress that countries have achieved over the past few decades (Danziger 1994).

Impact on nutrition level

As Hunter and Willamson (1998) note, in many African countries a significant proportion of the population has limited access to proper nutrition. This is further compounded in the case of AIDS orphans. In many cases when parent(s) die, the income level of households drops, which puts strain on the amount of resources that can be spent on buying food (Barnett and Blaikie 1992). In some cases this may begin while the HIV-infected parent(s) may be living but a significant amount of money is used for their treatment. Additionally, food intake of children may be lowered by the fact that as the economically active age group succumbs to AIDS and shortage of agricultural labor ensues, there is decline in the production of food crops (Barnett and Blaikie 1992). Barnett and Blaikie (1992) also note that in some cases in Uganda, for example, when parents die, children may lose the land their parents cultivated to unscrupulous relatives, resulting in limited access to food. Scholars

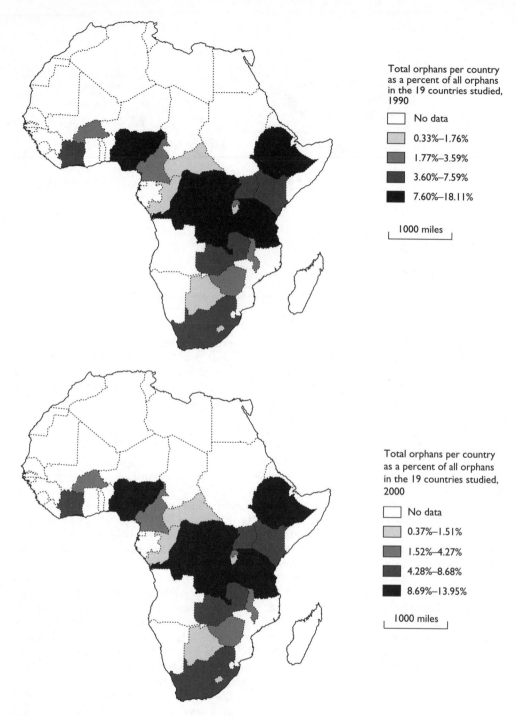

Figure 22.4 *Distribution of orphans in sub-Saharan Africa (orphans as percent of children under age 15 in each country).*
(a) 1990; (b) 2000.
Source: Authors; data from UNAIDS.

Table 22.2 *Economic growth indicators in selected southern African countries*

Country	Per capita GNP (US $)	Stunted children (%)	Ratio primary school enrolment (gross)	
			Male	Female
Botswana	3,310	22	111	112
Lesotho	680	44	92	102
Malawi	210	48	142	128
South Africa	3,210	23	117	115
Zambia	370	42	92	86
Zimbabwe	720	32	115	111

Source: UNAIDS/WHO 2000a, 2000b, 2000c, 2000d, 2000e, 2000f, 2000g.

such as Danziger (1994), Ntozi (1997), and Ankrah (1993) have also noted the lack of access to productive resources such as land for orphans whose parents have died, mainly due to the confiscation of their parents' land by older members of society. The overall result is lowering of nutrition level for AIDS orphans (Hunter and Willamson 1998). Some studies (see, for example, Ryder et al. 1994; Castle 1996) have shown that maternal AIDS orphans are more likely to have unequal access to food in the event that the father marries again. All of these add to the vulnerability of children to malnutrition which results in long-term impacts such as impediment of physical and mental development. It can also lead to lowering productivity of these children when they reach working age. Another issue that needs to be mentioned here is that some of these orphans may be infected by HIV and in such instances access to proper nutrition is of paramount importance.

One impact of lack of adequate nutrition is stunting. In southern Africa stunting is a major problem that affects many children. In Botswana and South Africa, which reported per capita income of over $3,000, less than 30 percent of children experienced moderate to severe levels of stunting (Table 22.2). In the former country the commitment on the part of the government to allocate resources toward child health and nutrition helped to lower malnutrition during the 1970s and 1980s (UNICEF and UNAIDS 1999). However, these achievements will be reversed as the AIDS pandemic continues to devastate the country. In Zim-

babwe, according to UNICEF reports (1999f), about 32 percent of children were stunted. The problem is more severe in the countries of Lesotho, Malawi, and Zambia where over 40 percent of children were stunted (Table 22.2). Although data are not available which would help to shed light on the percentage of AIDS-orphaned children who are affected by malnutrition, it can be argued that AIDS orphans are more likely to be vulnerable to malnutrition because of lack of food availability. In countries with already high levels of stunted children in existence, AIDS orphans can further add to the dilemma.

Lack of access to education

Improving the level of education is key to promoting economic growth and development. In the case of most African countries and in light of increasing external debt, structural adjustment programs, and growing poverty, governments are increasingly finding it difficult to allocate resources toward education. For example, Zambia no longer provides free primary education to children and therefore parents find it financially hard to send children to schools (UNICEF and UNAIDS 1999). The AIDS pandemic is already having a considerable negative impact on the education of AIDS orphans (Kamali et al. 1996; Okeyo 1995). Children are more likely to drop out of schools due to financial difficulties, illness, and the social stigma of parents dying from AIDS, or lack of willingness on the part of guardians to send these children to school

(Lugalla and Kibassa forthcoming). In general, school enrollment in sub-Saharan African countries is low and some disparity does exist between male and female rates (Kalipeni 1997). According to UNICEF (1999a), the primary school enrollment ratio between males and females for Botswana was 111 to 112 while for Lesotho the ratio was 92 males to 102 females. On the other hand, in all the other countries the ratio between male and female enrollment is skewed toward males. Primary enrollment data suggests that in Malawi there are 142 males to 128 females, about 117 males to 115 females in South Africa, 92 males to 86 females in Zambia, and 115 males to 111 females in Zimbabwe (Table 22.2).

Indeed, recent research from eastern and southern Africa confirms the sad truth that the gender disparity in education has been on the increase, in part due to AIDS-orphaned girls who often end up dropping out of school due to lack of school fees and, more importantly, to take care of sick parents or become parents to their siblings once the parents are dead (see, for example, Sherr et al. 1996; Ntozi and Mukiza-Gapere 1995; Ntozi 1997; Lugalla and Kibassa forthcoming). Many communities are now facing troubling scenarios: grandmothers struggling to care for orphans; households headed by children, many of them primary-school age, who are caring for younger siblings; and worse, children with nowhere at all to turn. AIDS-orphaned girls in cities as well as rural areas have increasingly joined street children and are heavily dependent on commercial sex for survival incomes. Many of them suffer many of the insults of an unhealthy environment characterized by inadequate shelter and clothing, poor sanitation, a decline in nutritional status, loss of health care, increased demands for their labor, reduced opportunities for education, loss of inheritance, homelessness, discrimination, physical abuse, and violent crimes such as robbery, theft, rape, incest, and assault (see Olenja and Kimani forthcoming; Le Roux 1996; Ayaya and Esamai, 2001). In some countries such as Malawi and Zambia, young girls have been dependent on sugar daddies to keep themselves in school (Kalipeni 2000). The need for school fees and other school supplies is very high for girls who have lost both parents while in secondary school, which often raises their vulnerability to the HIV/AIDS crisis. In some cases girls have literally been married off at very young ages, as older men are increasingly giving preference to younger girls as brides in the hopes that such brides are free of HIV (Hunter and Williamson 1998).

Another tragic consequence of the epidemic is the decline in the number of teachers as many have succumbed to this disease. The impact on education is therefore twofold: first, the supply of teachers has been eroded and thus class sizes have increased, ultimately diminishing the quality of education. Secondly, it is adversely affecting family budgets, reducing the money available for school fees which results in higher dropout rates. For example, in Zambia, deaths among teachers have increased rapidly over the past decade. UNAIDS reports that in the first ten months of 1998, Zambia lost 1,300 teachers – the equivalent of around two-thirds of all new teachers trained annually. Thus with limited education, AIDS orphans, particularly girls, continue to be trapped in a vicious cycle of vulnerability to HIV and poverty.

Orphans and extended family networks

The majority of African societies are characterized by the presence of strong ties with extended family members. As more children lose their parent(s) to AIDS they are being taken care of by their grandparents, uncles, and aunts. The extended family members provide valuable support to AIDS-orphaned children (Ryder et al. 1994). Indeed, throughout sub-Saharan Africa child fostering is a culturally sanctioned activity whereby biological parents allow their children to be reared in other households or by other adults (Aspaas 1999; Isiugo-Abanihe 1985; Bledsoe 1990b). As Aspaas (1999) and Isiugo-Abanihe (1985) note, child fosterage has several advantages to both the biological parents and the fostering household. Fosterage serves to reallocate resources within the extended family or among related kin so that the survival of individual households is ensured and ties with the extended kin are strengthened. Other motivations for child fostering may include education and economic considerations. Families living in urban areas and with ample resources will take in foster children from rural areas in order to send them to school in the urban environment, for example. The biological parents are provided with a means for managing the consequences of high fertility. The fostering family in a rural setting gains in terms of farm labor as well as household chores from the fostered children. Women with no children gain companionship and when the child grows to adulthood he/she may provide social and economic advancement. Thus, the practice of fostering children is seen as contributing to benefits for both the biological and fostering families (Bledsoe 1990b; Castle 1996; Foster et al. 1996).

However, the AIDS epidemic has brought fostering into crisis. Crisis fostering occurs when a death or some tragedy hits the natal family, depleting essential resources. Such a family is likely to send a child to another household for fostering. In this case the politically and economically motivated rationale as well as the mutual benefits under normal fosterage are de-emphasized or dismissed (Aspaas 1999). In the case of AIDS orphans in southern Africa, the situation is clearly an example of crisis fostering exacerbated by the escalating deaths of the economically active and parenting age group (ages 15–44). As the AIDS pandemic has worsened, the number of orphans has increased dramatically, putting the traditional child fostering system in a crisis mode. Traditionally, when parents die, children are sent to live with another member of the extended family, but the challenge of absorbing ever-increasing numbers of children into households that have limited resources has surpassed the material ability of most households, regardless of the willingness or desire to help (Aspaas 1999). It is clear from research in southern and eastern Africa that the traditional way of caring for orphans is now beyond the extended family's ability to cope (Ankrah 1993; Hunter 1990; Rutayuga 1992; Seeley et al. 1993).

A study in five African countries heavily affected by the AIDS epidemic has found a high incidence of AIDS-orphaned children suffering from intense poverty in rural areas as well as in urban areas. Those in urban areas were often roaming as gangs on the streets (Okeyo 1995). Although there is no clear-cut

evidence that many of these children are AIDS orphans, Okeyo notes that the fact that there is a growing number of street children, orphaned or not, provides a clear indication that the extended family system is overstretched and unable to provide support to these children. He further admonishes that worsening economic conditions, which have resulted in massive poverty in African countries, combined with weakened communities due to HIV/AIDS could easily lead to social upheaval. In short, many southern African countries are experiencing the rapid growth of orphans and street children so that family structures are no longer able to cope. Families and communities can barely fend for themselves given severe economic constraints, let alone take care of orphans (UNAIDS 1999g).

Trapped in the vicious cycle of poverty and vulnerability

Controlling poverty is crucial for human development. In spite of continued efforts on the parts of different African governments and international organizations, a large segment of the continent's population continues to live in poverty. Rising HIV prevalence rates and deaths from AIDS will increase the number of people living below the poverty line, especially AIDS orphans. It has been established that poverty plays a critical role in the contraction and development of AIDS (Farmer 1992b). In the developing and developed countries the poor are more likely to be infected by HIV and develop AIDS than those in societies with access to resources (Ryder et al. 1994). Some of the characteristics of poverty are low levels of education and poor nutrition which result in low labor productivity. It has already been indicated that AIDS orphans are likely to receive lower education and experience nutritional deficiency and therefore will continue to be trapped in poverty (Over et al. 1996). The percentage of population living below the poverty line, in southern Africa, ranges between 68 percent in Zambia and 25 percent in Zimbabwe (World Bank 2000b). In general, rural poverty tends to be higher than urban poverty and that has in the past dictated migration from rural to urban areas. These numbers are likely to be pushed up as the

AIDS pandemic puts more strain on limited resources. As a result, AIDS orphans will be trapped in the cycle of poverty in both rural and urban areas. Poverty is already intense in rural areas and as the orphans begin to migrate to cities, they will join the already burgeoning numbers of street children in urban economies that are themselves in crisis. In order to support themselves a vast majority will have to work at all sorts of odd jobs. Many are already dependent on the informal sector of the economy, such as commercial sex for girls, just to make a living for the day. In short, the orphans as they continue to grow up in poverty are being forced to undertake high risk behavior patterns such as crime, use of drugs, and prostitution which increases their susceptibility to HIV. According to UNICEF and UNAIDS (1999), nearly 75,000 children live in the streets of the capital city of Lusaka, Zambia; many of these children are orphans and often they are exploited for sex. Another dimension that is already apparent in many countries of southern Africa is the rise in orphan-headed households. Such households are particularly vulnerable to poverty and HIV, as clearly illustrated in the chapter by Emma Guest in this volume.

Rising to the Challenge

It is common knowledge that children who have lost a mother or both parents to AIDS face a more difficult future than that of other orphans due to the social stigma that a death from AIDS often entails in many African societies. Despite the enormity of the crisis and its devastating impacts, countries and communities across Africa are rising to the challenge (see, for example, the Health Technical Services Project of TvT Associates n.d.). Although the situation is grim, there is a glimmer of hope. Richer countries of southern Africa such as Botswana and South Africa are in the process of redoubling their efforts to contain the epidemic, although it will take years for this to bear fruit. Uganda and Senegal offer some hope. Uganda, for example, has turned a major epidemic around due to its extraordinary effort of national mobilization which has seen the AIDS prevalence rate drop from a

high of 14 percent to 8 percent by 2000. Senegal has managed to slow transmission.

In addressing the problem of orphans, governments of southern African countries and international organizations are taking concerted action. For example, in Malawi, the government decided early on to support community-based programs and has had a National Orphan Care Task Force since 1991. Across the country, community-based organizations are setting up childcare centers to improve the care of children and increase their learning opportunities (UNAIDS 1999g). The government of Malawi realized early on that because communities are in the best position to assess their own needs, they would play an important role in addressing the AIDS orphan crisis. One of the main government strategies in Malawi was therefore to promote and support community-based programs. As such, many NGOs and community-based organizations work closely with government ministries and district authorities to plan and carry out orphan programs. Many of these programs attempt to reintegrate orphans and street children with their parents, extended families, foster families, and communities. Some programs have devised innovative ways of sustainably reintegrating orphans into their communities through the provision or acquisition of necessary skills for the child to prepare him/her for the future. This ensures that orphans do not feel inferior in their communities and have the necessary skills to survive and live a productive and secure life. For an example of such a program that has proven to be successful in mitigating the plight of orphans and street children in Uganda see Wakiraza (forthcoming). Indeed the community-based approach, one of many models that have been implemented throughout Africa, has shown great promise in a number of countries (for example, Tanzania, Uganda, and Kenya) in caring for orphans (Mukoyogo and Williams 1991), hence its adoption by many southern African countries. For example, in Zambia, which has the largest proportion of AIDS orphans in the world, nongovernmental organizations such as CARE International Zambia and the Family Health Trust are working hard to fill gaps by providing food, clothing, and school fees to orphans and their families. The idea is to scale up home-based care and other forms of community-based orphan support so that orphans and other vulnerable children can be integrated into families and social networks (see http://carezambia.org/index.asp). Government ministries are working in concert with non-governmental, religious, and community organizations and donor agencies in scaling up community-led responses and household coping mechanisms.

Following the community-based approach, in Zimbabwe, where 7 percent of all children under 15 are orphaned by AIDS, a National Policy on the Care and Protection of Orphans has been developed, which advocates that orphans should be placed in institutions only as a last resort and should be cared for by the community whenever possible. In South Africa, many non-governmental organizations are mushrooming up and providing much-needed support to orphans. The South African Ministry of Health (MOH) has joined hands with local and international key partners such as USAID and its collaborators to lessen the plight of orphaned children. In the year 2000 the government of South Africa allocated R450 million (U.S. $64 million) over the next three years to community and home-based care for children orphaned by HIV/AIDS (UN Integrated Regional Information Network 2000). Throughout South Africa, there are about 165 community-based centers which care for and support such children and their families.

In all of these countries, laws to protect the rights of orphans are being devised. For example, Zimbabwe's government policy notes that all children, including orphans, should receive education and there should be laws and guidelines to enforce this right. Under this policy, the property rights of orphans should be safeguarded by legislation, and care and protection of orphans must comply with the Convention on the Rights and Welfare of the Child.

Conclusion

Although the statistics presented in this paper paint a grim picture, responses to the AIDS epidemic in general and more specifically responses to the crisis of orphans raise a glimmer of hope. The reduction of HIV prevalence rates in Uganda from a high of 14 percent in the early 1990s to around 8 percent today is testament to the fact that strong prevention campaigns do work (United Nations Department of Public Information and UNAIDS 2001). Recent data from Zambia's HIV sentinel surveillance system show that the percentage of HIV-positive pregnant girls aged 15–19 living in the capital, Lusaka, has on average dropped by almost half in the past six years. Comparisons between studies of sexual behaviors conducted in 1990, 1992, 1996, and 1998 suggest that these falling HIV rates are due in part to a decrease in the prevalence of some types of risky sexual behaviors in urban areas (UNAIDS 1999g). Furthermore, it is gratifying to see so many non-governmental organizations get involved in addressing the plight of orphans.

However, many of the initiatives to address the plight of orphans are still in their infancy and are in no way commensurate with the enormity of this problem (Brough 2000; Office of National AIDS Policy 1999). There is great need for human, financial, and organization resources in order for these efforts to make a dent in the suffering of orphans. The resources to deal with this problem aren't there. Poverty, which has been deepened by global economic trends, particularly structural adjustment programs and debt, means that AIDS programs get lip-service from the respective governments of southern Africa. Often these programs receive funding at levels insufficient for effective implementation and enforcement. Nevertheless, current government and non-governmental initiatives to deal with the problem of orphaned children in southern Africa are very encouraging. Indeed, a number of scholars have pointed out that the cost of doing nothing for the AIDS orphans will be phenomenal in the near future (Sowell 2000; Thiuri 1996).

Chapter 23

Excerpt from *Children of AIDS: Africa's Orphan Crisis*: A Mother to Her Brothers: A Child-headed Household's Story, Johannesburg, South Africa

Emma Guest

"Our relatives don't come. They don't want to see us. I don't know why. Some of them came before my parents died. Some of them. Right now, they don't come. No one visits us. I don't know why. They live close but we don't see them. When we last saw them, it was at the funeral. That was the last time. I feel angry because ... Why don't they come to visit us?"

Molatela is a gorgeous 17-year-old from Sebokeng, a township outside Johannesburg where some of the worst massacres of the apartheid era were perpetrated. She has a shy, appealing smile and she cares about her appearance. She keeps up with fashion and frequently changes her hair. She lives in a small, box-like house; one of thousands lined up along the township's dusty roads. Under the same roof are her four brothers. The oldest, Ngwako is 21, followed by Matome who is 14 and Nakampe who is nine. Pheega, the baby of the family, is three and HIV positive.

One week in July 1999, they lost both of their parents to AIDS. The family of children is now going it alone. Under the circumstances they are not doing badly.

No relatives offered to take them in. Extended family relations were strained before their parents died and even if relatives had offered, the children would have been reluctant because it would have meant leaving the family home and being split up. They want to stick together.

Molatela has become the family's new mother. When she speaks, she repeats phrases with an air of slight bewilderment.

"My father died first and we buried him on Saturday ..." She trails off and looks panicky, "I've forgotten the date ... The funeral was very big. And after we'd buried him, my mum died at 12 o'clock on the Sunday. She was so ill in hospital that they didn't tell her that my father had died. They didn't tell her. But I don't know whether she knew, because the day before my father died, I went to the hospital to see her and she told me that she'd dreamt about him. In the dream she saw that he'd died. I told her, 'No, my father hasn't died.' On the Tuesday, the family came to tell me that my father had died. It was winter.

"My mum was always sick. Maybe since '95. But my father was only sick since June this year and he died in July. Very quick. It was a shock. I didn't know he was sick too.

"At my mother's funeral, there were so many people. Maybe 200. There were four buses on the way to the graveyard and there were lots more at home who didn't go to the grave because there just weren't enough buses. Some of the neighbors helped me to cook for the people."

For four years, Molatela and her brothers cared for their mother at home, and later their father too. She learnt about AIDS through caring for her mother, not from teachers or leaflets and posters. She knows nothing of taking extra care when handling blood and other bodily fluids. No one has taught her.

"I found out my mother had AIDS, one time when she was cooking and she cut herself with a knife. When her blood came out, she said, 'No, don't help me.' But she didn't tell me she had AIDS. I couldn't understand why she wouldn't let me help her with her blood. Another time she said, 'I have AIDS.' She was trying to tell me, but I thought she was joking. Finally one day, I over-heard her telling her friends. They were talking together and I heard her say, 'I have HIV.' My brothers heard it too. After she'd told these friends, they went out crying, and I said to myself, 'OK.' My parents didn't actually tell us but I talked with my brothers about it. I said, 'I heard them talk about AIDS. They say they have AIDS.' And my brothers said they heard it too.

"I didn't know AIDS. I didn't know what it was, but when I saw them sick, I believed they had it because they got so thin. And their tongues were . . . sort of . . . furry and they had purple spots on their arms. They coughed a lot and were always sleeping. Sometimes, she was OK. Sometimes she was so sick she'd go to the hospital. Then she'd come back better and then she'd go to the hospital again. When she was better she was herself and we could laugh. And she would cook. She could really cook.

"I remember how I often used to go into town, shopping with my mum. And one time we went out to dinner at Nando's [a chillied chicken restaurant]. Just us, the girls. We were joking, laughing. It was a special day.

"My mother was a cleaner in somebody's house. But only for one month. After that, she was sick and my father told her to stop working. He was a mechanic. He fixed trucks. Sometimes he'd go to work in another city and stay there a month, maybe two. But he'd always come back to us.

"I have a good memory of December 31 last year. We were at home. We were listening to music and my father was dancing to jazz. We were laughing. Everyone was dancing and laughing."

The children's home is secure. The parents had paid off the bond before they died. They have running water, a flushing toilet, a stereo, television, and fridge. They have enough space. Most importantly, the house contains memories of their parents, some happy, some painful.

"Sometimes it seemed like when my mum was better, Pheega was sick. When he was better, she was sick. All the time, there was sickness.

"I looked after my parents until they died. My big brother helped with my father. He washed him and I washed my mother. No one else helped us . . . They didn't come. I don't know why.

"Before they died, my mum told her friends about having AIDS. Some of them were frightened and didn't come to our house again. I didn't tell anyone about what was going on at home because some people, when they knew that my mum was dying of AIDS, they looked at me like . . . I don't know what. So I didn't tell. I knew that's how they would act.

"But I did tell my best friend, Precious. When I told her, she understood because she'd helped me when my mother and father were always at home. She'd seen. She knew it was AIDS but she wasn't frightened.

"When they saw my mother was ill, some of the neighbors brought food. But some of them didn't come because they knew it was AIDS. They just didn't come any more. And some of them didn't come to the funeral. Even now, the neighbors don't speak to us. I tell myself if someone doesn't talk to me, there's nothing I can do to force her to talk to me. Some of them make me cry. Yes, they make me cry. Why won't they talk to us? Why won't they say, 'Good morning'?"

After a month of struggling in isolation, Molatela and her brothers were informally "adopted" by Gail Johnson, who runs Nkosi's Haven, a residential home for destitute, HIV-positive women and their children in Berea, a crowded, crumbling district in central Johannesburg.

Gail is flamboyant. She has bright, hennaed hair, big eye lashes and long pink nails. She lives at running pace, with one hand on the steering wheel and the other pressing a mobile phone to an ear. She sweeps into a room, constantly having "one of those days" and greets everyone with a theatrical, "Hello darling." She jokes, swears, and laughs heartily. She is also warm and fearless of emotional involvement with exceptionally needy babies and children. As well as two grown-up children of her own and an adopted, ten-year-old, HIV-positive son, Nkosi, Gail's home is also a registered place of safety for abused and abandoned children. The Child Protection Unit sometimes delivers them to her in the middle of the night. They are hers for anything up to six weeks. Sometimes longer.

Gail shows her emotions. On one occasion she is confronted with Mary, a 20-year-old woman, who arrives at her door with a baby she gave birth to the day before. She wants to abandon it and the hospital suggested she try Gail. A depressed-looking, older woman-friend accompanies her and holds the baby. Both women are unemployed and homeless. Mary's boyfriend has kicked her out because the baby is not his. She is adamant that she does not want this baby. She wants him looked after by a "proper mother." The older woman confirms Mary's determination to give the child up. She wants someone to take the baby before Mary abandons it in the street.

Both women look dejected as they eat food given to them. Mary's eyes search the faces of the people in the room, imploring them to understand and help her out. She does not seem to want to explore other options. It slowly emerges that she wants to return to her boyfriend. She cannot do that with the baby. She seems helpless and unhappy but she has made up her mind.

Gail fluctuates between caring and toughness. Again and again, she checks that Mary understands the implications of her decision and its permanence. Finally, Gail agrees to take the baby. She makes Mary promise to get herself to family planning every three months for a contraceptive injection until she is married and ready for children.

When it is time for Mary to leave, she says goodbye to her baby. Named "Gift" on his birth certificate, he is so new that his umbilical cord is still clipped with a peg. She cries. Gail cries, hugging the woman and asking if there is anything that can be done to keep them together. There is nothing to be done, and the women leave in sadness. Gail is bereft. She keeps repeating, "She gave away her baby."

It was a monumental decision to witness. The child lay, uncomprehending, in the midst of this maelstrom of emotion. Gail takes the little bundle home. Later, a detective from the Child Protection Unit visits with the necessary paperwork. He renames the baby "Tulani" (Quiet One). The next day, staff from Johannesburg Child Welfare Society turn up to take him away. Gail cannot understand why they have decided to place him in an institution to await adoption, rather than risk his bonding with her. She does not always agree with agency decisions.

Gail probably annoys some people because she is a bossy, outspoken white woman with scant regard for political correctness. But she gets things done. She has made a huge difference to the quality of life of one family of AIDS orphans in Sebokeng. She calls them "my babies." Once a week, she and the project's social worker, Mosibudi, drive out to see them with an abundance of food, clothes, and concern.

Without the kindness of strangers, the family of orphans was heading for disaster.

"Before Gail gave us food, we didn't have food," says Molatela. " 'Sometimes we didn't even have mealie meal [maize]. Then we'd have to borrow from the neighbors that day. Some would give me sugar. Some just said, 'No.' If they say they don't have sugar, there's nothing I can do. My father stopped working in June when he got sick. June, July, August, we had to ask neighbors for food. Sometimes we were hungry. Sometimes we'd go to sleep without eating because we didn't have money to buy food.

"At that time, I didn't know what to do. I talked to my big brother. I said, 'What can we do? We don't have food.' And he said to me, 'There's nothing we can do. Our relatives haven't come, and haven't given us money, so there's nothing we can do. We must just stay in the house.' He had no ideas. I didn't have ideas. So we just stayed together.

"We didn't want to go and live with relatives. My grandmother on my mother's side is dead and before my father died he told me about his mother. He said that she wanted to give him something that when you eat it you can die. They didn't get on because he didn't give her money. I told my big brother that she might poison us too. So we didn't want to live with her. When she visited us occasionally, like at the funeral, we were very scared."

Now Gail is there. She is a compassionate adult on the periphery of their lives. She gets Molatela to make lists of things they need. One visit there were brand-new school shoes and trousers for all of them. Molatela tried on her trousers. She is a voluptuous girl but the size she requested was vast. The gray school trousers hung off her. She looked embarrassed and mumbled that she would take them in. Matome tried on his shiny, unscuffed new shoes. He looked very pleased with them. The younger boys tucked into a tray of fruit.

Another week, Gail delivered towels, soap, and some cooked chickens donated by a hotel that usually supplies schools but had forgotten that it was the school holidays.

One of their first lists requested ice cream. They are optimistic children. It takes Gail over an hour to reach them in her hot little car. Another week, at the bottom of their list of necessities, in tiny apologetic writing, was a plea for sweets and *simbas* (crisps).

Initially, Gail took them food from the cupboards of Nkosi's Haven. A little later, she persuaded the children to do an interview with a local paper. Their story made the front page. "Orphaned by AIDS, five youngsters fight off the harsh realities of life," it announced. Readers sent donations. One of the children's relatives angrily asked Gail why she had sought publicity. Gail replied, "They were hungry." The woman was silent. The Welfare Department is not keen to hand out money when no adult lives with them. Gail has applied for a grant to be processed through Nkosi's Haven. In the meantime, her intervention is an ad hoc response to their desperate situation. It is not an operation that could be scaled up. Even from a distance, it is labor intensive and expensive looking after just this one family of orphans.

Seven years ago, Gail became Nkosi's foster mother. When his mother died of AIDS, Gail took him to the funeral in rural KwaZuluNatal. He is HIV positive but, having only been seriously ill once and having Gail to fight for his reinstatement in a school, which initially rejected him, he manages to lead a relatively normal life. He has, however, become the world's best-known child with HIV/AIDS since he made a speech at the International AIDS Conference in Durban in 2000 and urged people not to be afraid of people like him.

He is an extraordinarily charming and confident child. Every visitor to his home gets offered tea or coffee and polite conversation until his busy mother returns. He confides that Gail is tired and he wishes he could learn to cook so that he could help her more. He knows how lucky he is.

On one occasion, Gail takes Nkosi to visit the orphans. They need to see a healthy boy with HIV. On a previous visit, Nakampe had been weeping with anxiety that Pheega would die soon, like both his parents. Gail is proud to show off Nkosi's long, HIV-positive life. He survives, without the benefit of expensive antiretroviral drugs, on a regime of good nutrition and lots of love and care. She talks openly about AIDS, illness, and sex in front of Nkosi. She explains why she wants the orphans to see him. Nkosi is obliging. He is more worried that his face, which is painted like a dog after a school art class, will smudge.

Mosibudi joins the crowded car on this expedition. As well as counseling the residents at Nkosi's Haven, she also works at a hospital's AIDS clinic. She is unhappy because she has seen two of her patients die that day. They had been with her since 1994 and she has supported them through HIV to full-blown AIDS and now death. She is depressed and tetchy. "Don't ask me why 1 got involved with Gail, this Mother Theresa," she snaps.

But as the journey goes on, she relaxes and after an hour of banter with Gail she is a different woman. In the back seat, Nkosi grins at their rude jokes. Gail will not make the trip to Sebokeng on her own. She only feels safe going there accompanied by a black colleague.

Being able to speak South Sotho, the children's first language, Mosibudi takes charge. She instructs Gail not to unload any of the food from the car until she has assessed whether any of the children's grasping relatives are around. After their parents' funeral, the children saw nothing of granny or aunts until the latter heard that there were two women coming out from Johannesburg with food. The children had to put a lock on the fridge.

"There was only half a packet of chicken in the fridge, when we got involved a month after the parents had died," says Gail, angrily. "No housework had been done. All their clothes were dirty. The kids were neglected and depressed. This family was on the verge of collapse."

Gail first heard about Molatela and her brothers from a local community worker, Mushathama, whom she met by chance on an aeroplane. Now she visits them every week. She hopes to find them a freezer, so that she does not have to bring food so often. But she thinks they will need emotional support and advice for quite some time. Now that Gail is involved, Mushathama has virtually disappeared from the scene.

The children are not fools. Molatela has observed adult duplicity at close range. "My mother's sister came round to help with the ironing one day because she knew that Gail was coming. The rest of the time she didn't come."

When Nkosi is brought to visit, Molatela has prepared some food for him. Gail is embarrassed that her son is gobbling up the orphans' supplies. Mosibudi tells her that it is good that guests accept hospitality from them. It shows that at least some people are not worried about food being contaminated or catching HIV from their cutlery.

Molatela's relief at Gail's appearance in their lives is palpable. Suddenly there is an adult in the picture who cares enough to insist that they find a phone and get in touch when problems crop up. Gail was a stranger but she wanted to know them. She is also willing to help take care of Pheega, which lightens Molatela's burden.

Pheega gets chickenpox. Every inch of his little body is covered in angry, itchy spots. He wails with misery and makes Molatela stroke his back. He does not want to be removed from his siblings and taken home with Gail. Last time he was sick, he spent a fortnight at Gail's house being nursed back to health from a serious infection caused by a perforated eardrum. But he returned to his siblings much stronger. He also picked up some English while he was staying with her because she made him say "please" and "thank you."

Gail, an experienced foster mother, does not put up with misbehavior, regardless of whether the child has HIV or not. And this child, whose mother was sick throughout his life, has not known discipline. Molatela admits

that he gets his own way. No one said no to him, until he met Gail. He is a stubborn little thing. At first, he refused to eat and threw food and tantrums. He did not appreciate Gail telling him off. Gail thinks he is spoilt and needs to be socialized. She also loves him. He lets Gail hug him but his resistance to going with her again is clear.

His condition is worrying. Gail is horrified that no one told her when he fell ill. He has been feverish and spotty for three days. The problem is that, even though she wants to, she cannot take him at the moment because she cannot risk him infecting Nkosi in her home or any of the residents at Nkosi's Haven. Their compromised immune systems may not be up to dealing with Pheega's vicious-looking chickenpox.

A fortnight later Pheega lies on a mattress looking wretched. Molatela has been applying ointment to his skin. It gives his face a reddish tinge. He has visibly lost weight and he has wet himself. Molatela is worried.

Gail goes to a local pharmacy and buys numerous lotions and potions. She demands that the older siblings administer them to Pheega. She warns them that she will be cross if the bottle is not half-empty at her next visit. All the fruit and vegetables she provides are partly aimed at keeping Pheega's diet balanced. She once asked Molatela what he eats. The answer was, "Kellogg's. Three times a day."

Molatela may not know much about what her baby brother should eat to stay healthy, but she has definitely become his mummy.

> "I had to tell him that his mother and father aren't here, but he can call me his mother. He calls me Mummy. He didn't understand when they died until he saw them in the boxes. He saw them. Now he understands because he saw them in the coffins and being put in the ground. He told me, 'My mum died.' When he calls me Mummy, I say, 'Hello. What do you want?' It's strange because he calls our big brother Ngwako, Ngwako. He doesn't call him Father."

A month on from his battle with chickenpox, little Pheega looks a lot better. His cheeky grin has reappeared. He potters about waving at everyone. This particular crisis is over but the long-term prognosis remains bleak. Molatela amuses him, and herself, by donning a pair of comedy spectacles with a white plastic nose attached.

"Every day when we go to school, my cousin looks after Pheega. She's 24 but she's not working or going to school. She had a baby when she was a teenager so she left school. She's nice. She's not worried about looking after a child who's sick. But when he had chickenpox, I cared for him. I had to stay off school because he wanted me. He didn't want my cousin. He wanted me."

The older children decide that, during term time, Pheega should sometimes stay at Gail's home or Nkosi's Haven. They can visit him at weekends or he can accompany Gail and Mosibudi on their weekly visits to Sebokeng. He will not like this arrangement. However, if childcare arrangements with their cousin fail or he gets very ill, it will keep Molatela in school and keep Pheega as healthy and well-fed as possible.

From a distance, Ngwako might be mistaken for being quite tough. Close up, like Molatela, he has a beguiling "please like me" smile. At 21, he is the man of the family. Matome and Nakampe are still confused little boys. They are angry and argumentative one minute and tearful the next. They are all burdened beyond their years, but Molatela and Ngwako carry the largest load. They are still enrolled in school, but they often miss classes. Ngwako is only in his ninth year of education. In South Africa, classes include pupils of widely varied ages, because many missed years during the struggle against apartheid or have had to repeat years. It is not uncommon for people in their twenties to be studying beside teenagers. Ngwako struggles academically. It is unlikely that he will be out of school and looking for work for some time. Molatela has only one more year till she graduates, but family trauma makes it hard for her to concentrate on her studies.

"Before my parents died, when we were going to school there was no one to look after them. I was worried. At the end, my big brother didn't go to school. He told them that our parents were very sick, so he couldn't be in school. He stayed at home one week. Just one week. But the next week, when he went to school, they said they wanted to keep him out. I don't know why. They gave no reason. He's found another school to take him now.

"The thing I like most about my big brother is that he hasn't gone off with his friends. He is always at home with the family. Sometimes at the weekend he goes with his friends and they say, 'Don't look after your sister and your younger brothers.' But he tells them, 'No.'

"I worry about my younger brothers at the moment, because they don't want to go to school. I don't know why. When I talk to them, they say, 'We don't do anything at school. It's boring. So we won't go.' I talk to Ngwako about it and he says they must go to school the next day. In the morning they put on their uniform, but when I go to school, they don't go. When I come home at lunch, I ask them, 'Did you go to school?' They say, 'No.' They're very naughty. When I talk to them, they don't listen to me. They listen to big brother and he tries to be strict with them. I don't know why they don't listen to me.

"Sometimes, when I talk to them, they hit me and I must run away. They hurt me, sometimes. If I ask them, 'Can you wash your clothes today or do something else to help me?' they hit me because they don't want to do chores. Then I scream at them loudly and it makes them want to beat me more, so I have to run away. They listen to Ngwako. He and I are always talking with each other. We watch television together and we eat together. But it's me who must prepare food for them.

"Before my mum and my dad died, they didn't teach me about cooking or washing clothes or cleaning. Right now, I think of how things have changed. I knew I must cook and do the cleaning and other things like this, so I taught myself. No one told me how. It was very hard to learn to cook because I didn't know anything about it. Sometimes my brothers help me. Other times they don't want to. When I ask them, they say, 'I'm going to my friend's,' or 'I'm too busy.'

"Although I'm cooking, washing, cleaning till late, I never feel like leaving my family. When I'm not at school, I stay at home. I don't have time to go out. And I don't want my friends to visit me. Only my best friend, Precious, comes here. I don't want the others to visit me because after my mother and father died, some of them made themselves at home in our house, cooking and eating, without respect. Before my parents died, they'd come and just sit. They wouldn't make themselves so at home. It annoys me they behave differently.

"I don't know any other families like us. I talked to Precious about AIDS and she doesn't know anyone else like us either. But recently, my uncle (the one whose daughter looks after Pheega) told my grandmother (the one with the poison) that he has a I don't know what... on his private parts. He told my grandmother it was like he was having AIDS. That sign. He said he saw that sign on my father. But he does not know for sure that he has AIDS. He just saw this sign of AIDS or STDs [sexually transmitted diseases] on his private parts. Are they different things? Anyway, he's worrying about it. But he doesn't go and get the test. I think he is scared.

"Precious has been my friend for years. She comes to help me. When I'm worried about something, I talk to her about it and she comes to me. But, with some problems I first go to Ngwako. After I tell him, we decide whether to talk to Gail or Mushathama, our community worker. Like when we got the big electricity bill. It was R670 [about £67]. On Wednesday they switched off the lights at 12 o'clock and they wanted the money. I didn't go back to school. I talked to my big brother and then I went to Mushathama. It was a long way on the bus. Then I went with her to the office and she paid it. And we got light again on Thursday."

As well as love Molatela probably, sometimes, feels anger and resentment for her dead parents and needy siblings, but she does not admit it. She admits only the melancholy and resignation she feels. She frequently struggles to find the words to describe her experiences, but she does not cry.

Despite the trauma of losing her parents and the risk of losing her baby brother, Molatela seems remarkably resilient. Even as she holds the present together, she manages to look forward.

"When I finish school next year, I'm thinking of becoming a sound engineer in the music industry. I don't have any idea how but I think my subjects are right. I like science and technical drawing. My big brother doesn't know what he wants to do."

Since their basic needs have been taken care of, the improvement in this family's circumstances is dramatic. The first time Gail visited, the house was filthy and the children despairing. Within a month, some laughter has returned and the house has been cleaned up. Hand-washed clothes hang on the line in the yard. They have come a long way in a short time.

Molatela beams when Gail arrives at their door. Gail tells her she looks lovely and jokes that, perhaps, next time she will bring condoms with the fruit and vegetables because there will be boyfriends queuing up at the door. Actually, Gail fears for Molatela when word gets out that there is an attractive, lonely, and vulnerable orphan living there. She has talked to her about condoms and has told her brothers that they need to protect her but they have their own troubles. Gail and Mosibudi dash in and out with supplies and hugs but do not always have time to stop and listen to the children. Gail always asks how they are doing and whether they've had any trouble from neighbors or relatives. "No, no, we're fine," they reply almost in unison. They are still shy with Gail. She hugs them and kisses them and they respond gladly, but do not initiate physical affection.

Molatela has had her childhood interrupted. She is an extraordinary teenager. Having nursed her parents through terminal illness, she has become a substitute mother for her siblings. She is doing the best she can to wash, cook, and clean for a family of five, keep herself and her rebellious younger brothers in school, keep an HIV-positive three-year-old well, while dealing with her own grief at the loss of her parents. With food parcels and weekly visits from caring outsiders, the family is coping, more or less.

They have not so much been abused by the adult world, as neglected by it. The stigma surrounding their parents' death and Pheega's HIV status has kept people away. They remain vulnerable.

"If I knew other people like us and they needed advice, I'd tell them that they must look after themselves. They must be independent and make sure they go to school every day and always eat. Maybe if there's a big brother or sister, they must look after their younger brothers and sisters. And I would say to the big brother or sister, you mustn't take the advice of your friends because friends don't care for the family group... I'm thinking of Ngwako's friends... And maybe, if they are lucky like us, they can find someone who can help them... like Gail."

Chapter 24

Concluding Remarks: Beyond Epidemiology

Joseph R. Oppong and Jayati Ghosh

Twenty years into the epidemic, after numerous books, research articles, and academic conferences, the world has not been able to stop HIV/AIDS. Clearly a major part of the problem is political. National budget priorities, allocations for health versus other sectors, funding for antiretrovirals, affordable and effective treatment of sexually transmitted diseases, efforts to destigmatize AIDS – these are all clear political questions, contested beyond the realm of HIV/AIDS. As former U.S. President Clinton argued in his speech at the Barcelona AIDS Conference, what is lacking is not the money, or the knowledge, or the science, or the strategic skill to end this epidemic; rather, the people with the power to turn this epidemic around seem to have other priorities (Clinton 2002). To avoid repeating the cycle of more AIDS deaths, more research, more money, more AIDS deaths, a change in the scope and focus of research is required. This is the message throughout this volume. In this closing chapter, we identify some directions for future research aimed at breaking this cycle.

First, the contributors to this volume recognize that HIV/AIDS is complexly embedded in the social, economic, cultural, and political fabrics of society, requiring multiple points of analytical entry with various optics addressing the regionally varied contexts underlying transmission, experience, local attitudes and understanding of the disease. Previous research has prioritized and focused on sexuality – sexual practices and mobility. More recent research on HIV vulnerability has begun to uncover the salient roles played by gender politics, poverty, colonialism, global economics, migration, and war. The contributors to this book have added to this more recent trend in AIDS research while also understanding that these optics are inextricably related to each other and demand the fullest analytical integration possible in the search for clearer understanding and effective intervention.

Multidisciplinary approaches are thus unavoidable if we are to make progress. The massive assault of HIV/AIDS requires the active collaboration of all – experts, communities, those living with AIDS, and governments. The assumption that experts or governments can plan and implement decisions for "the poor victims" of AIDS needs to be problematized. As Kesby points out in this volume, input from patients and relatives, caregivers, and the population at risk is critical for any effective intervention strategy to be successful. After all, those who live with the disease daily should be heard. Treatment regimens should be planned with input from those who would benefit. The creation and implementation of education programs targeting populations at risk should include as active participants those presently sick with the disease.

Previous research and intervention programs have overexploited the behavioral paradigm, but the solution resulting from this research approach – behavior change – has not worked; where there are claims of success, these are seriously contested. Behavior change, including increased use of condoms and sex education, has been credited for Uganda's apparent recent decline in HIV infection. However, other researchers, including Baylies in this volume, argue that the decline in the number of people living with HIV/AIDS may be due more to increased deaths from AIDS-related illness rather than a decline in new cases. Furthermore, much previous research centered on sex workers, STD patients, blood donors, drug users, army personnel, and truck drivers. Yet as the research in this volume shows, occupational groups may not be as critical as economic and social groups.

Moreover, as has been shown several times in this volume (Zulu, Ezzeh, and Amooh-Dodoo; Oppong and Mensah; Lyons; Mbugua and Rugalema), poverty and disease burden are inextricably linked. Behavior change requires more than mere information dissemination. For many people, ignorance of HIV transmission through unprotected sex is not the problem. Pressing immediate need, whether in the form of food, medicines, clothing, or school supplies for children, supersedes the more abstracted and variable risk of HIV. As one commercial sex worker (CSW) in Ghana indicated, "I pray to God daily to protect me, and hope that my current client does not have the disease." Unless the poverty that produced this risky behavior is removed, short-term survival will continue to come before longer-term risk of HIV in the prioritizations of everyday practice.

In short, the message driven home by this volume is that both theoretical as well as methodological restructuring of research is under

way but has a long way to go in order to effect meaningful disruptions of current transmission patterns and experience of disease. Top-down research objectifying individuals and their sexual behavior must embrace bottom-up research that incorporates individuals as knowledgeable subjects with insights into the disease and their location within the coordinates of risk. Grassroots research that produces action is required.

Many fundamental research tasks remain. The spread of HIV/AIDS is associated with high levels of migration, but the direct relationship between migration and HIV remains unclear. Poverty, lack of employment opportunities, and economic restructuring are recognized as important trajectories. Traditionally, labor has used migration as a mechanism to adjust to economic crisis due to a drop in labor demand. Workers move from agriculture to other economic sectors such as manufacturing, construction, and service or to centers of high labor demand such as urban areas or the mining towns of southern Africa. By facilitating intra-country movements, including rural–urban migration, the expansion of infrastructure enhances opportunities for the spread of HIV. Despite this complex relationship, previous research has focused on HIV prevalence rates among highly migratory population groups. Research needs to illuminate what factors push individuals to migrate in the first place, and the forms and configurations of that migration, in order to unravel more fully the links between migration and HIV infection. Such research should include involuntary migration, refugee-producing conflicts, and natural disasters.

Further research is also needed to establish the true spatial pattern of HIV/AIDS, particularly in rural areas. Because HIV testing sites are often located in distant urban centers, access for rural residents is limited. Thus reporting of HIV prevalence or AIDS-related deaths privileges urban areas. As Oppong and Mensah argue in this volume, the low rural prevalence of the disease in parts of Africa may be a simple artifact of the data collection process and ascertaining the true extent of rural HIV is extremely difficult. Related to this, the paucity of comprehensive testing data makes the reported spatial pattern of

HIV/AIDS simply spurious. Further research should focus on studying HIV/AIDS at local and district levels, although traditionally, funding limitations have precluded such studies.

Other important questions need to be addressed. The relationship between global economic policies, national growth strategies, local poverty, and HIV/AIDS needs further amplification and action. Economic growth strategies pursued by sub-Saharan Africa over the past decades have not produced the desired results. Many of the problems such as lack of employment, poor performance in the agricultural sector, lack of industrialization, and high levels of poverty are embedded in local economic policies and global economic trends begun during colonial administrations and continuing in postcolonial periods. Corruption, crime, and political instability, by impeding economic growth, have increased vulnerability to HIV/AIDS. As delineated by Brown, it is also evident that AIDS is having deleterious impacts on the economies of hardhit African countries and the ability of individuals within them to generate adequate income. Apparently poverty produces AIDS and AIDS produces poverty.

Disproportionate funding for biomedical approaches has marginalized other interpretations and approaches, leaving many questions inadequately examined. Controversies over vaccines and access to antiretrovirals persist, with the resulting scenario that while millions are dying of AIDS, others are reaping huge profits from the same disease. How religion impacts vulnerability to HIV/AIDS is under-researched. In fact, the whole cultural interpretation and understanding of AIDS and related phenomena is a ripe area for investigation. Does a spatially varied fatalism expressed in the inevitability of death impact risky behavior? How does the concept of death in the local culture impact risky behavior? How is the most visible evidence of HIV/AIDS presence, AIDS orphans, impacting society, behavior, and communities? Which strategies work best for orphans? Does this vary regionally, culturally?

Finally, the AIDS epidemic has been so devastating because too many individuals see people with AIDS as different – sex workers, drug addicts, homosexuals, poor, from another country, continent, or race. Such denial, stigma, and shame associated with the disease reflected in these labels make it difficult for people to acknowledge their disease, but also conceal the vulnerability of those outside these groups. Consequently, many people, unaware that they have the disease, spread it inadvertently, while those who know they have the disease suffer secretly to avoid the shame and stigma. The stigma surrounding the disease deserves scrutiny, for the role it plays in increasing HIV infection, number of AIDS deaths, and the social and physical misery accruing to those living with AIDS. AIDS is a human problem. Let us deal with it, wherever it is found.

Between the 2000 Durban AIDS Conference and the 2002 Barcelona conference, an estimated 6 million people died from AIDS (Mandela 2002). During the Barcelona Conference, in the most authoritative work on the subject (Stover et al. 2002), a group of international experts convened by UNAIDS and WHO concluded that an expanded global response to the AIDS epidemic based on 12 essential interventions could prevent some 29 million new HIV infections among adults by 2010.[1] Implementation of the full package by 2005 could cut new infections by 64 percent, lowering the number of adults infected each year from over four million currently to approximately 1.5 million. However, a three-year delay could reduce these potential gains by 50 percent. Over the first four years, the total cost of bringing prevention programs to scale is estimated to be U.S. $8.4 billion. From 2005 onwards, the program will cost an estimated U.S. $4.8 billion annually. The full costs of scaling-up and sustaining the effort to 2010 are estimated to be U.S. $27 billion, or a total of some U.S. $1,000 per infection averted. Unfortunately, few African countries have a GNP per capita of $1,000 or more. In fact, in mainland sub-Saharan Africa in 2000, only five countries – Botswana, Gabon, Namibia, South Africa, and Swaziland – could afford this bill, assuming they spent the entire GNP per capita on AIDS prevention (World Bank 2002). For the vast majority of African countries, then, this package of prevention is unaffordable. The din of high unemployment, poverty, malaria, tuberculosis, political instability, war, drought, starvation, is too loud, too harsh. Yet the establishment of a Global Fund for AIDS has thus far raised only a fraction of needed resources from U.S., European, and Japanese governments. So, the cycle may continue of more AIDS deaths, more research, more money, more AIDS deaths, until political will is mobilized toward compassionate collaborations among governments, organizations, corporations, physicians, researchers, communities, and individuals. For those currently living with AIDS in Africa, that time cannot come soon enough.

NOTE

1. The 12 prevention interventions include mass media campaigns; public sector condom promotion and distribution; condom social marketing; voluntary counseling and testing programs; prevention of mother-to-child transmission; school-based programs; programs for out-of-school youth; workplace programs; treatment of sexually transmitted infections; peer counseling for sex workers; outreach to men who have sex with men; and harm reduction programs for injecting drug users.

Bibliography

Abdool-Karrim, S., Ziqubu-Page, I., and Arendse, R., 1994 Bridging the Gap: Potential for a Health Care Partnership between African Traditional Healers and Biomedical Personnel in South Africa. Pinelands, South Africa: Publications of the Medical Association of South Africa.

ABEL, 1991 Educating Girls: Strategies to Increase Access, Persistence, and Achievement. Advancing Basic Education and Literacy (ABEL) Project. Project No. 936–5832.

Abrahamsen, R., 1997 Gender Dimensions of AIDS in Zambia. Journal of Gender Studies 6(2):177–189.

Acuda, S. W., 1982 Drug and Alcohol Problems in Kenya Today: A Review of Research. East African Medical Journal 59(10):642–644.

Adamchak, D., Mbizo, M., and Tawanda, M., 1990 Male Knowledge of and Attitudes and Practices towards AIDS in Zimbabwe. AIDS 4(3):245–250.

Addai, I., 1999 Ethnicity and Sexual Behavior. Social Biology 46(1–2):17–32.

Addo-Yobo, E. O., and Lovel, H., 1991 How Well Are Hospitals Preventing Iatrogenic HIV? A Study of the Appropriateness of Blood Transfusions in the Ashanti Region, Ghana. Tropical Doctor 21(4):162–164.

Addo-Yobo, E. O., and Lovel, H., 1992 Hospital User's Knowledge about Blood Transfusion and Awareness and Attitudes towards AIDS/HIV Infection in a Region in Ghana. Journal of Tropical Pediatrics 38(2):94–95.

African Network on Ethics, Law and HIV, 1994 Dakar Declaration, drafted and endorsed by participants at the Intercountry Consultation of the African Network on Ethics, Law and HIV, organized in Dakar, Senegal, from June 27 to July 1, 1994 by the UNDP HIV and Development Programme.

African Religious Leaders, 2002 Recommendations on National Policy and Advocacy Strategies on Children and HIV/AIDS, June 11. Electronic document. http://www.hopeforafricanchildren.org.

Agadzi, V. K., 1989 HIV-AIDS: The African Perspective of a Killer Disease. Accra: Ghana Universities Press.

Aggleton, P., 1996 Global Priorities for HIV/AIDS Intervention Research. International Journal of STD & AIDS 7(Suppl. 2):13–16.

Agyei-Mensah, S., 2001 Twelve Years of HIV/AIDS in Ghana: Puzzles of Interpretation. Canadian Journal of African Studies 35(3):441–472.

Ahmed, S. I., 1992 Truck Drivers as Vulnerable Group in North East India. Second International Congress on AIDS in Asia and the Pacific. New Delhi, November [Abstract D624].

AIDS Analysis Africa 1995.

Ainsworth, M., and Over, M., 1994 AIDS and African Development. The World Bank Research Observer 9(2):203–240.

Ajayi, A., Marangu, L., Miller, J., and Paxman, J., 1991 Adolescent Sexuality and Fertility in Kenya: A Survey of Knowledge, Perceptions, and Practices. Studies in Family Planning 22(4).

Akeroyd, A. V., 1996 Some Gendered and Occupational Aspects of HIV and AIDS in Eastern and Southern Africa: Changes, Continuities and Issues for Further Consideration at the End of the First Decade. Edinburgh: Centre of African Studies, University of Edinburgh [Occasional Paper No. 60].

Akeroyd, A. V., 1997 Sociocultural Aspects of AIDS in Africa: Occupational and Gender Issues. *In* AIDS in Africa and the Caribbean. G. Bond, J. Kreniske, I. Susser, and J. Vincent, eds. pp. 11–32. Boulder, CO: Westview Press.

Akinsete, I., 2000 Nigeria Country Report. Paper presented at the Foundation for Democracy Regional Conference on Strategies to Combat the Spread of HIV/AIDS in West Africa, Abuja, Nigeria, June 4–9.

Akoto, S. A., 2000 The Spread of HIV/AIDS in Tema. Undergraduate dissertation, Department of Geography and Resource Development, University of Ghana, Legon.

Akuffo, F., 1987 Teenage Pregnancies and School Drop-Outs: The Relevance of Family Life Education and Vocational Training to Girls' Employment Opportunities. *In* Sex Roles, Population, and Development in West Africa. C. Oppong, ed. pp. 154–164. Portsmouth: Heinemann.

Allen, S., Lindan, C., Serufilira, A., Van De Perre, P., Rundle, A. C., Nsengumuremyi, F., Caraël, M., Schwalbe, J., and Hulley, S., 1991 Human Immunodeficiency Virus Infection in Urban Rwanda. JAMA: The Journal of the American Medical Association 266(12) (September 25):1657–1663.

Alpers, E. A., 1972 The Yao in Malawi. *In* The Early History of Malawi. B. Pachai, ed. London: Longman.

Alubo, S. O., 1994 Death for Sale: A Study of Drug Poisoning and Deaths in Nigeria. Social Science and Medicine 38(1):97–103.

Amanze, J., 1982 The Bimbi Shrine in the Upper Shire and its Relationships with the Yao Chiefs, 1830–1925. Journal of Science 9:37–50.

American Medical Association, 1990 Physician Characteristics and Distribution in the US. Chicago: American Medical Association.

Amnesty International, 1995 Women in Kenya: Repression and Resistance. London: Amnesty International.

Ampofo, A. A., 1993a Report from a Survey of Sexual Behavior and Knowledge Regarding AIDS among Out-of-School Youth in the Central Region of Ghana. Prepared for UNICEF.

——1993b Controlling and Punishing Women: Violence against Ghanaian Women. Review of African Political Economy 56:102–111.

Ampofo, A. A., 1995 Women and AIDS in Ghana: "I Control My Body (or Do I)?", Ghanaian Sex Workers and Susceptibility to STDs, especially AIDS. *In* Women's Position and Demographic Change in Sub-Saharan Africa. P. Makwina-Adebusoye and A. Jensen, eds. Liège: Ordina Editions.

AMREF, n.d. Study of Lorry Drivers along Mombasa–Nairobi Highway. Nairobi: AMREF.

Anacleti, O., 1996 The Regional Response to the Rwandan Emergency. Journal of Refugee Studies 9(3):303–311.

Anarfi, J., 1992 Sexual Networking in Selected Communities in Ghana and the Sexual Behaviour of Ghanaian Female Migrants in Abidjan, Côte D'Ivoire. *In* Sexual Behaviour and Networking: Anthropological and SocioCultural Studies on the Transmission of HIV. Tim Dyson, ed. pp. 233–247. Liège: Editions Derouaux-Ordina (for IUSSP).

Anarfi, J. K., 1990 International Migration of Ghanaian Women to Abidjan, Côte d'Ivoire: A Demographic and Socio-economic Study. Ph.D. dissertation, Regional Institute for Population Studies, University of Ghana.

Anarfi, J. K., Appiah, E. N., and Awusabo-Asare, K., 1997 Livelihood and the Risk of HIV/AIDS Infection in Ghana: The Case of Female Itinerant Traders. Health Transition Review 7(Suppl.):225–242.

Angell, M., 1997 The Ethics of Clinical Research in the Third World. The New England Journal of Medicine 337(12):847–849.

Ankomah, A., 1998 Condom Use in Sexual Exchange Relationships among Young Single Adults in Ghana. AIDS Education and Prevention 10(4):303–316.

Ankomah, A., and Ford, N., 1994 Sexual Exchange: Understanding Pre-Marital Heterosexual Relationships in Urban Ghana. *In* AIDS: Foundations for the Future. P. Aggleton, P. Davies, and G. Hart, eds. pp. 123–135. London: Taylor & Francis.

Ankrah, E., 1991 AIDS and the Social Side of Health. Social Science and Medicine 32(9):967–980.

Ankrah, E., 1996 AIDS Socio-economic Decline and Health: A Double Crisis for the African Woman. *In* AIDS as a Gender Issue: Psychosocial Perspectives. L. Sherr, C. Hankins and L. Bennett, eds. pp. 99–118. London: Taylor & Francis.

Ankrah, E. M., 1989 AIDS: Methodological Problems in Studying its Prevention and Spread. Social Science & Medicine 29(3):265– 276.

Ankrah, M., 1993 The Impact of HIV/AIDS on the Family and Other Significant Relationships: The African Clan Ravished. AIDS Care 5:5–21.

Anonymous, 1988 The Bamako Initiative. Lancet ii:1177–1178.

Anonymous, 1990 Structural Adjustment and Health in Africa. Lancet 335:885–886.

Anonymous, 1992 Current and Future Dimensions of the H/V/AIDS Pandemic: A Capsule Summary. Geneva: WHO.

Anonymous, 1993a Africa: Make or Break. Boston: Oxfam America.

—— 1993b 1.5 Million New HIV Infections in Africa Pushes Global Total to over 15 Million. Geneva: WHO Press Release, December 10.

Anonymous, 1994 Did HIV Contribute to the Breakdown of Society in Rwanda? A Question Worth Asking. AIDS Analysis Africa 4(5) (September/October).

Anonymous, 1997 HIV Trends and Migration in East Africa. Migration and Health Newsletter. Geneva: ILO, January.

Aryeetey-Attoh, S., 1997 Geography and Development in Sub-Saharan Africa. *In* Geography of Sub-Saharan Africa. S. Aryeetey-Attoh, ed. pp. 223–261. Upper Saddle River, NJ: Prentice Hall.

Asiimwe-Okiror, G., Opiyo, A. A., Musinguzi, J., Madraa, E., Tembo, G., and Caraël, M., 1997 Change in Sexual Behaviour and Decline in HIV Infection among Young Pregnant Women in Urban Uganda. AIDS 11(14):1757–1763.

Aspaas, H. R., 1999 AIDS and Orphans in Uganda: Geographical and Gender Interpretations of Household Resources. Social Science Journal 36(2):201–226.

Asthana, S., 1994 Economic Crisis, Adjustment and the Impact on Health. *In* Health and Development. D. R. Philips and Y. Verhasselt, eds. pp. 50–64. London: Routledge.

AVSI, 1998 Where Is My Home? Children in War. Kampala: AVSI (Collection of children's drawings depicting war and disorder in the north).

Awusabo-Asare, K., 2000 The Challenges of HIV/AIDS in Ghana. Paper Presented at the 51st Annual New Year School, University College of Education of Winnoba, 3rd January.

Awusabo-Asare, K., and Anarfi, J. K., 1997 Postpartum Sexual Abstinence in the Era of AIDS in Ghana: Prospects for Change. Health Transition Review 7(Suppl.):257–70.

Ayaya, S. O., and Esamai, F. O., 2001 Health Problems of Street Children in Eldoret, Kenya. The East African Medical Journal 78(12):624–630.

Azikiwe, U., 1992 Women Education and Empowerment. Nsukka: Fulladu Publishing Company.

Baggaley, R. C., and Needham, D., 1997 Africa's Emerging AIDS-Orphans Crisis. Canadian Medical Association Journal 156(6):873– 875.

Baggaley, R. C., Sulwe, J., Chilala, M., and Mashambe, C., 1999 HIV Stress in Primary School Teachers in Zambia. Bulletin of the World Health Organization 77(3):284–287.

Baggaley, R. C., Sulwe, J., Kelly, M, Macmillan, M. N., and Godfrey-Faussett, P., 1996 HIV Counsellors' Knowledge, Attitudes and Vulnerabilities to HIV in Lusaka, Zambia, 1994. AIDS Care 8(2):155–166.

Baker, C. A., 1975 The Government Medical Service in Malawi, 1891–1974. Journal of History of Medicine 20(3):296–311.

Baleta, A., 1999 South African Government Faces Furious Zidovudine Debate. (News) The Lancet, March 13, 353(9156):908.

Balmer, D. H., 1994 The Phenomenon of Adolescence: An Ethnographic Inquiry. Nairobi: Naresa Monograph No. 4.

Balthazar, G. M., 1994 The Prevalence Rate of HIV/AIDS Increases with the Proximity to the Kenya/Uganda Border. Unpublished report. Kenya National AIDS & STDs Control Programme, Ministry of Health.

Balthazar, G. M., and Okeyo, T. M., 1996 The HIV Sentinel Surveillance System in Kenya: Methodology, Results and Uses. Paper presented at the International Conference on AIDS, July 7–12, 11(1):150 (Abstract No. Mo.C.1550).

Banda, H. K., and Young, T. K., 1946 Our African Way of Life. London: Lutterworth.

Bandawe, C. R. n.d. Preliminary Recommendation to the Malawi Government Ministries of Health and Education and Culture, following a Study of AIDS-Related Behaviors among Secondary School Students in Malawi. Blantyre: Department of Community Health, University of Malawi College of Medicine.

Barnett, T., and Blaikie, P., 1992 AIDS in Africa – Its Present and Future Impact. New York: Guilford Press.

Barnett, T., and Piers, B., 1992 AIDS in Africa: Its Present and Future Impact. London: Belhaven Press.

Barnett, T., and Whiteside, A., 1998 The Jaipur Paradigm, HIV/AIDS, Society and Economy: Case Studies and a Conceptual Framework. Unpublished MS.

Barongo, L. R. et al., 1992 The Epidemiology of HIV-1 Infection in Urban Areas, Roadside Settlements and Rural Villages in Mwanza Region, Tanzania. AIDS 6:1521–1528.

Barton, T. C., 1991 Sexuality and Health in Sub-Saharan Africa: An Annotated Bibliography. Nairobi: African Medical and Research Foundation (AMREF).

Barton, T. C., and Wamai, G., 1994 Equity and Vulnerability: A Situation Analysis of Women, Adolescents and Children in Uganda, 1994. Kampala: UNICEF.

Bassett, M., and Mhloyi, M., 1991 Women and AIDS in Zimbabwe: The Making of an Epidemic. International Journal of Health Services 21(1):143–156.

Bassett, M., and Sherman, J., 1994 Female Sexual Behavior and the Risk of HIV Infection: An Ethnographic Study in Harare, Zimbabwe. Washington, DC: International Center for Research on Women.

Bassett, M. T., Emmanuel, J. C., Katzenstein, D. A. et al., 1990 HIV Infection in Urban Men in Zimbabwe. VI International Conference on AIDS, San Francisco, June [Abstract Thc 581]:45.

Batliwala, S., 1994 The Meaning of Women's Empowerment; New Concepts of Action. *In* Population Politics Reconsidered: Health Empowerment and Rights. G. Sen, A. Germain, and L. Chen, eds. pp. 127–138. Boston: Harvard University Press.

Bauni, E. K., and Jarabi, B. O., 2000 Family Planning and Sexual Behavior in the Era of HIV/AIDS: The Case of Nakuru District, Kenya. Studies in Family Planning 31(1):69–78.

Bawah, A. A., Akweongo, P., Simmons, R., and Phillips, J. F., 1999 Women's Fears and Men's Anxieties: The Impact of Family Planning on Gender Relations in Northern Ghana. Studies in Family Planning 30(1):54–66.

Bayer, R., 1998 The Debate over Maternal–Fetal HIV Transmission Prevention Trials in Africa, Asia and the Caribbean: Racist Exploitation or Exploitation of Racism? American Journal of Public Health 88 (4):567–570.

Baylies, C., 1999 International Partnership in the Fight against AIDS, Addressing Need and Redressing Injustice? Review of African Political Economy 26(81):387–394.

Baylies, C., Forthcoming Reconciling Individual Costs with Collective Benefits: Women Organising against AIDS in Mansa. *In* AIDS, Sexuality and Gender in Africa: Collective Strategies for Protection against AIDS in Tanzania and Zambia. C. Baylies and J. Bujra, with the Gender and AIDS Group, eds. London: Routledge.

Baylies, C., and Bujra, J., 1995 Discourses of Power and Empowerment in the Fight against HIV/AIDS in Africa. *In* AIDS: Safety, Sexuality and Risk. P. Aggleton, P. Davies, and G. Hart, eds. pp. 194–222. London: Taylor & Francis.

Baylies, C., and Bujra, J., 1997 Social Science Research on AIDS in Africa: Questions of Content, Methodology and Ethics. Review of African Political Economy 24(73):380–388.

Baylies, C., and Bujra, J., 2000 AIDS, Sexuality and Gender in Africa: Collective Strategies and Struggles in Tanzania and Zambia. London: Taylor & Francis.

Baylies, C., and Bujra, J., with the Gender and AIDS Study Group, 2001 AIDS, Sexuality, and Gender in Africa: The Struggle Continues. London: UCL Press.

Baylies, C., and Bujra, J., with the Gender and AIDS Group, Forthcoming AIDS, Sexuality and Gender in Africa: Collective Strategies for Protection against AIDS in Tanzania and Zambia. London: Routledge.

Beck, U., 1992 Risk Society: Towards a New Modernity. London: Sage.

Becker, C., Dozon, J-P., Obbo, C., and Toure, M., 1999 Introduction. *In* Experiencing and Understanding AIDS in Africa. C. Becker, J-P. Dozon, C. Obbo, and M. Toure, eds. pp. 11–19. Dakar: Codesria, Karthala, IRD.

Bedele, D. K., 1993 Population and Agricultural Landuse in the Manya Krobo District. Ph.D. dissertation, Department of Geography, University of Ghana.

Bello, W., Cunningham, S., Rau, B., 1994 Dark Victory: The United States, Structural Adjustment and Global Poverty. Oakland: Institute for Food and Development Policy.

Bemba, S., 1984 Cinquante Ans de Musique du Congo-Zaïre. Paris: Présence Africaine.

Benatar, S., and Singer, P., 2000 A New Look at International Research Ethics. British Medical Journal 321:824–826.

Benjamin, J. A., 1996 AIDS Prevention for Refugees: The Case of Rwandans in Tanzania. AIDSCAPTIONS (National Library of Medicine) 3(2):4–9.

BenMayor, R., 1991 Testimony, Action Research and Empowerment, Puerto Rican Women and Popular Education. *In* Women's Words: The Feminist Practice of Oral History. S. Gluck and D. Patal, eds. pp. 159–174. London: Routledge.

Bennett, O., Bexley, J., and Warnock, K., 1995 Arms to Fight, Arms to Protect. London: Panos Publications.

Berer, M., and Ray, S., 1993 Women and HIV/AIDS: An International Resource Book. Information, Action and Resources on Women and HIV/AIDS, Reproductive Health and Sexual Relationships. UK: Harper and Collins Publishers.

Bernault, F., 1996 Démocraties Ambiguës en Afrique Centrale. Congo-Brazzaville, Gabon: 1940–1965. Paris: Karthala.

Bertrand, J., and Bakutuvwidi, M., 1991 Sexual Behaviour in 10 Sites in Zaire. Journal Of Sex Research 28:347–364.

Bevan-Pritchard, H. G., 1930 Malawi National Archive (MNA) M2/5/16.

Black, M., 1991 Report on a Meeting about AIDS and Orphans in Africa. New York: International Child Development Center, UNICEF.

Black, R. E., Collins, S., and Boroughs, D. L., 1992 The Hidden Costs of AIDS. US News and World Report July 27, 49–59.

Blair, C., Ojakaa, D., Ochola, S. A., and Gogi, D., 1997 Barriers to Behaviour Change: Results of Focus Group Discussions Conducted in a High HIV/AIDS Incidence Area of Kenya. *In* Confronting the AIDS Epidemic. Davidson C. Umeh, ed. pp. 45–55. Trenton, New Jersey: Red Sea Press.

Blanc, A., and Way, A., 1998 Sexual Behavior and Contraceptive Knowledge and Use among Adolescents in Developing Countries. Studies in Family Planning 29(2):106–116.

Bledsoe, C., 1990a Transformation in Sub-Saharan African Marriage and Fertility. Annals of the American Academy of Political and Social Science 510:115–125.

—— 1990b The Policies of Children: Fosterage and the Social Management of Fertility among the Mende of Sierra Leone. *In* Births and Power: Social Change and the Politics of Reproduction. W. P. Handwerker, ed. pp. 51–84. Boulder, CO: Westview Press.

BLM (Banja La Mtsogolo) Annual Report, 1997. MNA.

Block, R., 2001 AIDS Activists Win Skirmish in South Africa. Wall Street Journal March 7, A17.

Bloom, B. R., 1998 The Highest Attainable Standard: Ethical Issues in AIDS Vaccines. Science 279:186–188.

Bloom, D., and Mahal, A. S., 1997 Does the AIDS Epidemic Threaten Economic Growth? Journal of Econometrics 77:105–124.

Bockie, S., 1993. Death and the Invisible Powers: The World of Kongo Belief. Bloomington: Indiana University Press.

Bodenheimer, T., 2000 Uneasy Alliance – Clinical Investigators and the Pharmaceutical Industry. New England Journal of Medicine 342.

Bonacci, M. A., 1992 Senseless Casualties: The AIDS Crisis in Asia. Washington, DC: International Voluntary Services and Asia Resource Center.

Bond, G. C., Kreniske, J., Susser, I., and Vincent, J. eds., 1997 AIDS in Africa and the Caribbean. Boulder, CO: Westview Press.

Bond, G. C., and Vincent, J., 1997a AIDS in Uganda: The First Decade. *In* AIDS in Africa and the Caribbean. G. C. Bond, J. Kreniske, I. Susser, and J. Vincent, eds. pp. 85–98. Boulder, CO: Westview Press.

—— 1997b Community Based Organizations in Uganda: A Youth Initiative. *In* AIDS in Africa and the Caribbean. G. C. Bond, J. Kreniske, I. Susser, and J. Vincent, eds. pp. 99–113. Boulder, CO: Westview Press.

Bond, V., 1997 "Between a Rock and a Hard Place": Applied Anthropology and AIDS Research on a Commercial Farm in Zambia. Health Transition Review 7 (Suppl.): 69–83.

Bond, V., and Dover, P., 1997 Men, Women and the Trouble with Condoms: Problems Associated with Condom Use by Migrant Workers in Rural Zambia. Health Transition Review 7(Suppl.):377–391.

Bone, D.S., 1982 Islam in Malawi. Journal of Religion in Africa, 13(2):126–138.

Bongmba, E., 1998 Toward a Hermeneutic of Wimbum Tfu. African Studies Review 41(3):165–191.

Boohene, E., Tsodzai, J., Hardee-Cleaveland, K., Weir, S., and Janowitz, B., 1991 Fertility and Contraceptive Use among Young Adults in Harare, Zimbabwe. Studies in Family Planning 22(4):264–271.

Bose, K., 1994 Spotlight on International Organizations: The World Bank. Health Policy and Planning 9:95–99.

Brabin, L., Kemp, J., Obunge, O. K., et al., 1994 Reproductive Tract Infections and Abortion among Adolescent Girls in Rural Nigeria. Lancet 346:530–536.

Brandful, J. A., Ampofo, W. K., Apeagyei, F. A., Asare-Bediako, K., and Osei-Kwasi, M., 1997 Predominance of HIV-1 among Patients with AIDS-Related Complex in Ghana. East African Medical Journal 74(1):17–20.

Brennan, T., 1999 Proposed Revisions to the Declaration of Helsinki – Will They Weaken the Ethical Principles Underlying Human Research? The New England Journal of Medicine 341(7):527–530.

British Broadcasting Corporation, 2001 39 Pharmaceutical Companies Drop Case against South Africa. Electronic document. http://News.bbc.co.uk/hi/english/world/africa/newsid 1285000/1285097.stm.

Brittain, V., 2002 Calvary of the Women of Eastern Democratic Republic of Congo. Review of African Political Economy 93–94 (September–December).

Brokensha, D., Patton, J., and Conant, F., 1987 Social Factors in the Transmission of AIDS in Africa. Report prepared for the Directorate for Health, Bureau of Science and Technology, Agency for International Development. Binghampton, NY: Institute for Development Anthropology.

Brockerhoff, M., Biddlecom, A., and Saha, T., 1996. Migration, Sexual Behaviour and HIV Diffusion in Kenya. Paper presented at the Annual Meeting of the Population Association of America, New Orleans, May 9–11.

Brockerhoff, M., and Brennan, E., 1998 The Poverty of Cities in Developing Countries. Population and Development Review 24(1):75–114.

Brough, D., 2000 Plight of Africa's AIDS Orphans Worsening. Daily Mail and Guardian February 17. Electronic document. http://www.mg.coza/news/2000feb2/17-aids2.html.

Brown, D., 1994 World Bank to Emphasize AIDS as Economic Threat. Washington Post November 28, A7.

Brown, L. R., 1996 The Potential Impact of AIDS on Population and Economic Growth Rates. Food, Agriculture, and the Environment Discussion Paper 15. Washington DC: International Food Policy Research Institute.

Brown, M., 1995 Ironies of Distance: An Ongoing Critique of the Geographies of AIDS. Environment and Planning D: Society and Space 13:159–183.

Bujra, J., and Baylies, C., 1999 Solidarity and Stress: Gender and Local Mobilization in Tanzania and Zambia. *In* Families and Communities Responding to AIDS. P. Aggleton, G. Hart, and P. Davies, eds. pp. 35–52. London: UCL Press.

Bullock, C., 1950 The Mashona and the Matabele. Cape Town: Juta & Co..

Burans, J. P., McCarthy, M., El Tayeb, S. M. et al., 1990 Serosurvey of Prevalence of Human Immunodeficiency Virus amongst High Risk Groups in Port Sudan, Sudan. East African Medical Journal 67:650–655.

Bureau of Statistics, 1990 Tanzania Population Census 1988 Regional Profile (Kagera). Dar es Salaam: Government Printer.

Burke, T., 1996 Lifebuoy Men, Lux Women: Commodification, Consumption, and Cleanliness in Modern Zimbabwe. London: Leicester University Press.

Butchart, A., 1998 The Anatomy of Power: European Constructs of the African Body. London: Zed Books.

Butcher, K., and Kievelitz, U., 1997 Planning with PRA: HIV and STD in a Nepalese Mountain Community. Health Policy and Planning 12(3):253–261.

Buvé A., 2000 HIV/AIDS in Africa: Why so Severe, Why so Heterogeneous? Programs and abstracts of the 7th Conference on Retroviruses and Opportunistic Infections, January 30–February 2, San Francisco, CA. Abstract S28.

Bwayo, J. J., Mutere, A. N., and Omari, M. A., 1991 Long Distance Truck Drivers: 2: Knowledge and Attitudes Concerning Sexually Transmitted Diseases and Sexual Behaviour. East African Medical Journal 68(9):714–719.

Bwayo, J. J., Oman, A. M., Mutere, A. N. et al., 1991 Long Distance Truck Drivers: 1. Prevalence of Sexually Transmitted Diseases (STD's). East African Medical Journal 68:425–429.

Caldwell, J. C., 1995 Understanding the AIDS Epidemic and Reacting Sensibly to it. Social Science and Medicine 41(3):299–302.

Caldwell, J. C., and Caldwell, P., 1993 The Nature and Limits of the Sub-Saharan AIDS Epidemic: Evidence from Geographic and Other Patterns. Population and Development Review 19(4):817–848.

Caldwell, J. C., and Caldwell, P., 1996 The African AIDS Epidemic. Scientific American 274(3): 62–63, 66–68.

Caldwell, J. C., Caldwell, P., and Quiggin, P., 1989 The Social Context of AIDS in Sub-Saharan Africa. Population and Development Review 15(2):185–234.

Callaway, H., 1992 Ethnography and Experience: Gender Implications in Fieldwork and Texts. *In* Anthropology and Autobiography: ASA Monograph 29. J. Okely and H. Callaway, eds. pp. 29–49. London: Routledge.

Cameron, C., and Shepard, J., 1992 The Cost of AIDS Care and Prevention. *In* AIDS in the World. J. M. Mann, D. J. M. Tarantola, and T. W. Netter, eds. Cambridge: Harvard University Press.

Campbell, C., 1992 Learning to Kill? Masculinity, the Family and Violence in Natal. Journal of Southern African Studies 18(3):614–628.

Campbell, C., 1995a The Social Identity of Township Youth: An Extension of Social Identity Theory (Part 1). South African Journal of Psychology 25(3):150–159.

—— 1995b The Social Identity of Township Youth: Social Identity Theory and Gender (Part 2). South African Journal of Psychology 25(3):160–167.

Campbell, C., 1997 Migrancy, Masculine Identities and AIDS: The Psychosocial Context of HIV Transmission on the South African Gold Mines. Social Science and Medicine, 45(2):273–281.

Campbell, C., 2003 Letting Them Die: Why HIV/AIDS Prevention Programmes Often Fail. Bloomington: Indiana University Press, Oxford: James Currey.

Campbell, C., and Williams, B., 1996 Academic Research and HIV/AIDS in South Africa. South African Medical Journal 86(L):55–60.

Campbell, C., and Williams, B., 1999 Beyond the Biomedical and Behavioural: Towards an Integrated Approach to HIV Prevention in the Southern African Mining Industry. Social Science and Medicine 48:1625–1639.

Campbell, C. A., 1995 Male Gender Roles and Sexuality: Implications for Women's AIDS Risk and Prevention. Social Science and Medicine 41(2):197–210.

Caraël, M., 1996 Women, AIDS and Sexually Transmitted Diseases in Sub-Saharan Africa: The Impact of Marriage Change. *In* Population and Women. United Nations, ed. pp. 125–140. New York: United Nations.

Caraël, M., 1997 Urban–Rural Differentials in HIV/STDs and Sexual Behaviour. *In* Sexual Cultures and Migration in the Era of AIDS: Anthropological and Demographic Perspectives. Gilbert Herdt, ed. pp. 107–126. Oxford: Oxford University Press.

Caraël, M., and Allen, S., 1995 Women's Vulnerability to HIV/STD in Sub-Saharan Africa: An Increasing Evidence. *In* Women's Position and Demographic Change in Sub-Saharan Africa. P. Makinwa and A.-M. Jensen, eds. pp. 201–222. Liège, Belgium: International Union for the Scientific Study of Population (IUSSP).

Caraël, M., Buve, A., and Awusabo-Asare, K., 1997 The Making of HIV Epidemics: What Are the Driving Forces? AIDS 11 (Suppl. B):S23–S31.

Carswell, J. W., Lloyd, C., and Howells J., 1989 Prevalence of HIV-1 in East African Lorry Drivers. AIDS 3:759–761.

Castle, S., 1996 The Current and Intergenerational Impact of Child Fostering on Children's Nutritional Status in Rural Mali. Human Organization 55:193–205.

Catholic Church, 1991 AIDS: A Christian Response. Balaka: Montfort Press.

Celentano, D. D., Akarasewi, P., Sussman, L. et al., 1994 HIV-1 Infection among Lower Class Commercial Sex Workers in Chiang Mai, Thailand. AIDS 8:533–537.

Center for International Health Information in the United States, 1998 Country Health Statistics Report. Alexandria, VA: Center for International Health Information in the United States.

Central Bureau of Statistics (Kenya), 2000 Economic Survey 2000. Nairobi: Government Printers.

Centre for Social Research (CSR), 1999 Two Decades of Social Research: A Directory. Zomba: Centre for Social Research.

Chabot, J., Harnmeijer, J-W., and Streetfland, P. H., eds., 1995 African Primary Health Care in Times of Economic Turbulence. Amsterdam: Royal Tropical Institute.

Chaima, C., 1994 Knowledge, Attitudes, Beliefs and Behaviour Regarding the Sexual Activities of Girls in TA Kalolo, Lilongwe District, Malawi. Copy at CSR, Zomba.

Chamber of Mines, 1993 Statistical Tables 1993. Johannesburg: Chamber of Mines.

Chambers, R., 1994a Participatory Rural Appraisal (PRA): Analysis of Experience. World Development 22(9):1253–1268.

—— 1994b Participatory Rural Appraisal (PRA): Challenges, Potentials and Paradigm. World Development 22(10):1437–1454.

Chambers, R., 1997 Whose Reality Counts: Putting the Last First. London: Intermediate Technology Publications.

CHANGE, 1999 Non-Consensual Sex in Marriage: Information Package Number One – April 1999. London: CHANGE.

Channock, M., 1985 Law, Custom and Social Order: The Colonial Experience in Malawi and Zambia. Cambridge: Cambridge University Press.

Chanock, M. L., 1972 Development and Change in the History of Malawi. *In* The Early History of Malawi. B. Pachai, ed. London: Longman.

Chavunduka, G., 1973 Paths to Medical Care in Highfield, Rhodesia. The Society of Malawi Journal 26(2):25–45.

Cheesbrough, J. S., 1986 Acquired Immunodeficiency Syndrome in Malawi. Malawi Medical Journal 3:5–13.

Chenault, K., Carey, J., and Magnusson, P., 1999 Will the AIDS Plague Change U.S. Trade Policy? Business Week September 13 (3646):58.

Chikwem, J. O., Mohammed, I., Okara, G. C., Ukwandu, N. C., and Ola, T. O., 1997 Prevalence of Transmissible Blood Infections among Blood Donors at the University of Maiduguri Teaching Hospital, Maiduguri, Nigeria. East African Medical Journal 74(4):213–216.

Chilivumbo, A., 1975 The Cultural Consequences of Population Change in Malawi. *In* The Consequences of Population Change. Report on a seminar held in Bucharest, Romania, August 14–17, 1974. Washington, DC: The Center for the Study of Man, Smithsonian Institution.

Chilongozi, D. A., Costello, C., Daly, C., Liomba, N. G., and Dallabetta, G., 1996 Sexually Transmitted Diseases: A Survey of Case Management in Malawi. International Journal of STD and AIDS 7:269–275.

Chimombo, S., 1989 Dreams, Conversion and Nthara's Man of Africa. Journal of Religion in Africa XIX(1):49–70.

Chiphangwi, J. D, Keller, M., Wirima, J., Ndovi, E., Taylor, E., Saah, A., and Polk, B. F., 1988 Prevalence of HIV Infection in Pregnant Women in Malawi. Seminar paper. [Abstracts] in Fourth International AIDS Conference, Stockholm. Stockholm: Ministry of Health and Social Affairs.

Chirimuuta, R., and Chirimuuta, R., 1989 AIDS, Africa, and Racism. London: Free Association Books.

Chirwa, W., and Kanyongolo, E., 2000 The State of Democracy in Malawi. Seminar paper, Chancellor College, July.

Chirwa, W. J., 1988 Aliens and AIDS in Southern Africa: The Malawi–South Africa Debate. African Affairs 97:53–79.

Chisiza, D., 1961 Africa: What Lies Ahead? New Delhi: Indian Council for Africa.

Chisvo, M., and Munro, L., 1994 A Review of Social Dimensions of Adjustment in Zimbabwe, 1990–1994. Unpublished paper.

Chiwaya, W. B., n.d. Bar Girls Study in Mangochi District. Zomba: Centre for Social Research (CSR).

Christakis, N., and Fox, R., 1992 Informed Consent in Africa. The New England Journal of Medicine 327 (15):1101–1102.

Choopanya, K., Vanichseni, S., Plangsringarm, K. et al., 1991 Risk Factors and HIV Seropositivity among Injecting Drug Users in Bangkok. AIDS 5:1509–1513.

Chowdhury, A. N., 1991 AIDS Prevention: What Are We Talking about? Journal of Indian Medical Association 89:304–305.

Ciekawy, D., and Geschiere, P., 1998 Containing Witchcraft: Conflicting Scenarios in PostColonial Africa. African Studies Review 41(3):1–14.

Civic, D., and Wilson, D., 1996 Dry Sex in Zimbabwe and Implications for Condom Use. Social Science and Medicine 42(1):91–98.

Clark, P., 2000 Passionate Engagements: A Reading of Sony Labou Tansi's Private Ancestral Shrine. Research in African Literatures 31(3):39–68.

Cleland, J., and Ferry, B., 1995 Sexual Behavior and AIDS in the Developing World. London: World Health Organization/Taylor & Francis.

Cleland J., and Way, P., 1994 Social and Demographic Dimensions of AIDS: An Introduction. Health Transition Review 4 (Suppl.):1–10.

Clifford, J., 1986 Introduction: Partial Truths. *In* Writing Culture: The Poetics and Politics of Ethnography. J. Clifford and G. Marcus, eds. pp. 1–26. Berkeley: University of California Press.

Cleland, J. G., Ali, M. M., and Capo-Chichi, V., 1999 Post-Partum Sexual Abstinence in West Africa: Implications for AIDS-Control and Family Planning Programs. AIDS 13(1):125–31.

Clinton, W. J., 2002 Action against AIDS: For the Global Good. Closing remarks, Barcelona XIV International AIDS Conference. Electronic document. http://www.kff.org/aids2002/transcript/transcript_webcast_12_a1.htm.

Cohen, D., 1998a The HIV Epidemic and Sustainable Human Development. HIV and Development Program Issues Paper #29. New York: UNDP.

—— 1998b Socio-Economic Causes and Consequences of the HIV/AIDS Epidemic in Southern Africa. HIV and Development Program Issues Paper #31. New York: UNDP.

Cohen, D., and Reid, E., 1996 The Vulnerability of Women: Is This a Useful Construct for Policy and Programming? [UNDP HIV and Development Programme Issues Paper #28]. United Nations Development Program. Electronic document. http://www.undp.org/hiv/issue28E.html.

Cohen, M. E., 1992 Prevention. *In* AIDS in the World. J. M. Mann, D. J. M. Tarantola, and T. W. Netter, eds. Cambridge: Harvard University Press.

Cohen, M. S., 2000 Prevention of Sexual HIV Transmission. Medscape Conference Summaries from the XIII International AIDS Conference, Durban, South Africa, July 9–15, 2000.

Colson, E., 1958 Marriage and the Family among the Plateau Tonga of Northern Rhodesia. Manchester: Manchester University Press.

Colson, E., 1960 Social Organization of the Gwembe Tonga. Manchester: Manchester University Press.

Colson, E., and Gluckman, M., 1961 Seven Tribes of British Central Africa. Manchester: Manchester University Press.

Comaroff, J., 1982 Medicine: Symbol and Ideology. *In* The Problem of Medical Knowledge. P. Wright and A. Treacher, eds. Edinburgh: Edinburgh University Press.

Comaroff, J., 1993 The Diseased Heart of Africa: Medicine, Colonialism, and the Black Body. *In* Knowledge, Power, and Practice: The Anthropology of Medicine and Everyday Life. S. Lindenbaum and M. Lock, eds. pp. 305–329. Berkeley: University of California.

Comaroff, J., and Comaroff, J., eds., 1993 Modernity and its Malcontents. Chicago: University of Chicago Press.

Connor, E., Sperling, R., Gelber, R., Kiselev, P., Scott, G., O'Sullivan, M. J., Vandyke, R., Bey, M., Shearer, W., Jacobson, R., Jimenez, E., O'Neill, E., Bazin, B., Delfraissy, J-F., Culnane, M., Coombs, R., Elkins, M., Moye, J., Stratton, P., and Balsley, J., 1994 Reduction of Maternal–Infant Transmission of Human Immunodeficiency Virus Type 1 with Zidovudine Treatment. The New England Journal of Medicine 331 (18):1173–1180.

Cornia, G. A., Jolly, R., and Stewart, F., eds., 1987 Adjustment with a Human Face. Oxford: Clarendon Press.

Cornwall, A., and Jewkes, R., 1995 What Is Participatory Research? Social Science and Medicine 41(12):1667–1676.

Costello, A., Watson, F., and Woodward, D., 1994 Human Face or Human Faúade? Adjustment and the Health of Mothers and Children. London: Centre for International Development.

Costello, A., and Zumla, A., 2000 Moving to Research Partnerships in Developing Countries. British Medical Journal 321:827–829.

Craddock, S., 2000 Gender, Identity, and Risk: Rethinking the Geography of AIDS. Transactions of the Institute of British Geographers 25:153–168.

Creenblatt, R. M., Lukehart, S. A., Plummer, F. A. et al., 1988 Genital Ulceration as a Risk Factor for Human Immunodeficiency Virus Infection. AIDS 2:47–50.

Crisp. J., 1996 AIDS Programmes in the Mining Industry: An Overview. *In* HIV/AIDS Management in South Africa: Priorities for the Mining Industry. B. Williams and C. Campbell, eds. Johannesburg: Epidemiology Research Unit.

Cuddington, J. T., 1993a Modeling the Macro-Economic Effects of AIDS, with an Application to Tanzania. World Bank Economic Review 7(2):178–189.

—— 1993b Further Results on the Macro-Economic Effects of AIDS: The Dualistic, Labor Surplus Economy. World Bank Economic Review 7(3):403–417.

Cuddington, J. T., and Hancock, J. D., 1994 Assessing the Impact of AIDS on the Growth Path of the Malawian Economy. Journal of Development Economics 43:363–368.

Cunnison, I., 1959 Luapula Peoples of Northern Rhodesia: Custom and History in Tribal Politics. Manchester: Manchester University Press.

Dabis, F., Msellati, P., Meda, N. et al. 1999 6-Month Efficacy, Tolerance, and Acceptability of a Short Regimen of Oral Zivoduvine to Reduce Vertical Transmission of HIV in Breastfed Children in Côte d'Ivoire and Burkina Faso. Lancet 353(9155):786–792.

Daily Graphic of Ghana, 2000 The Police Service AIDS Control Program. Daily Graphic of Ghana, March 4.

Daily Graphic of Ghana, 2000 Korle Bu Treats AIDS Patients with Herbal Drugs. Daily Graphic of Ghana, December 7.

Dak, O., 1968 A Geographical Analysis of the Distribution of Migrants in Uganda. Kampala, Makerere University College, Department of Geography Occasional Paper No. 11.

Daley, S., 1998 AIDS Is Everywhere, but Africa Looks Away. New York Times, December 4: A,1.

Dallabeta, G. A., Odaka, N., Hoover, D., Chiphangwi, J. D., Liomba, G., Miotti, P., and Saah, A., 1991 High Socio-Economic Status Is a Risk Factor for HIV-1 Infection, but not for STDs in Malawi. Unpublished MS.

Dane, B. O., and Levine, C., 1994 AIDS and the New Orphans: Coping with Death. Westport, CT: Auburn House.

Danziger, R., 1994 The Social Impact of HIV/AIDS in Developing Countries. Social Science and Medicine 39(7):905–917.

David, Petit [Pseudonym], 1995 Sony Labou Tansi: La Mort et Demie? La Rue Meurt. Brazzaville: June.

Dawson, M. C., 1992 Socio-Economic Change and Disease: Smallpox in Colonial Kenya. *In* The Social Basis of Health and Healing in Africa. S. Feireman and J. M. Janzen, eds. Berkeley: University of California Press.

De Bethune, X., Alfani, S., and Lahaye, I. P., 1989 The Influence of an Abrupt Price Increase on Health Service Utilization: Evidence from Zaire. Health Policy and Planning 4:76–81.

De Boeck, F., 2001 Garimpeiro Worlds: Digging, Dying and "Hunting" for Diamonds in Angola. Review of African Political Economy 90, 549–562.

De Boeck, F., n.d., On Being Shege in Kinshasa: Children, the Occult and the Street in Kinshasa. Seminar paper in the Program on Contested Childhood, International Institute, University of Michigan, Ann Arbor, October 24, 2001.

De Cock, K. M., Lucas, S. B., Lucas, S., Agness, J., Kadio, A., and Gayle, H. D., 1993 Clinical Research, Prophylaxis, Therapy, and Care for HIV Disease in Africa. American Journal of Public Health 83:1385–1389.

De Cock, K. M., Porter, A., Odehouni, K. et al., 1989 Rapid Emergence of AIDS in Abidjan, Ivory Coast. Lancet ii:408–411.

De Vos, P., 2000 The Constitution Made Us Queer: The Sexual Orientation Clause in the South African Constitution and the Emergence of Gay and Lesbian Identity. *In* Sexuality in the Legal Arena. C. Stychin and D. Herman, eds. pp. 194–207. London: The Athlone Press.

De Zalduondo, B.O., Msamanga, G. I., and Chen, L.C., 1989 AIDS in Africa: Diversity in a Global Pandemic. Daedalus 118(3):165–204.

Declaration of Helsinki IV, 1989, 41st World Medical Assembly, Hong Kong, September.

Decosas, J. F., 1996 HIV and Development. AIDS 10 (Suppl. 3):S69–S74.

Decosas, J. F., and Adrien, A., 1999 The Future of HIV/AIDS Programming in the Pan African Program. Technical discussion paper prepared for the Canadian International Development Agency.

Decosas, J. F., Kane, J. K., Anarfi, K. D., Sodji, K. D. R., and Wagner, H. U., 1995 Migration and HIV-AIDS. The Lancet 346(8978):826–828.

DelAmo, J. et al., 1998 Disease Progression and Survival in HIV1 Infected Africans in London. AIDS 12(10):1203–1209.

Dell, S., 1984 Stabilization: The Political Economy of Overkill. *In* The Political Economy of Development and Underdevelopment. 3rd edition. C. K. Wilber, ed. New York: Random House.

Demery, L., and Walton, M., 1998 Are Poverty Reduction and Other 21st Century Social Goals Attainable? Washington, DC: The World Bank.

Desjeux, D., 1987 Strategies Paysannes en Afrique Noire: Le Congo. Essai sur la Gestion de l'Incertitude. Paris: L'Harmattan.

Development, 2001 Special Issue: Violence Against Women and the Culture of Masculinity. Development 44(3):1–143.

Devésa, J.-M., 1996 Sony Labou Tansi. Ecrivain de la Honte et des Rives Magiques du Kongo. Paris: L'Harmattan.

Devisch, R., 1996 "Pillaging Jesus": Healing Churches and the Villagisation of Kinshasa. Africa 66(4):555–583.

Dhadphale, M., Mengech, H. N. R., Synme, D., and Acuda, S. W., 1982 Drug Abuse among Secondary School Pupils in Kenya: A Preliminary Survey. East African Medical Journal 59:152–156.

Diallo, M. O., Ettiene-Traore, V., Maran, M., Kouadio, J., Brattegard, K., Makke, A., Van Dyck, E., Laga, M., and De Cock, K. M., 1997 Sexually Transmitted Diseases and Human Immunodeficiency Virus Infections in Women Attending an Antenatal Clinic in Abidjan, Côte d'Ivoire. International Journal of STD and AIDS 8(10):636–638.

Dixon-Mueller, R., 1993 The Sexuality Connection in Reproductive Health. Studies in Family Planning 24(5):269–282.

Dodoo, F. N.-A., and Ampofo, A. A., 2001 AIDS-Related Knowledge and Behavior among Married Kenyan Men: A Behavioral Paradox? Journal of Health and Human Services Administration (forthcoming).

Dommen, C., 2002 Raising Human Rights Concerns in the World Trade Organization: Actors, Processes and Possible Strategies. Human Rights Quarterly 24(1):1–49.

Donnelly, J., 2002 World's AIDS Crisis Worsening, Report Says. Boston Globe Online, June 16. Electronic document. http://www.boston.com/dailyglobe2/167/nation/World.

Douglas, M., and Wildavsky, A., 1982 Risk and Culture. Berkeley: University of California Press.

Dowell, W., 1999 Ethics and AIDS Drugs. Time, July 12, 154(2):49.

Dozon, J.-P., and Fassin, D., 1989 Raisons Epidemiologique et Raisons d'état: Les Enjeux Socio-Politiques du SIDA en Afrique. Sciences Sociales et Santé VII(1):21–36.

Drake, A. M., 1976 Illness, Ritual, and Social Relations among the Chewa of Central Africa. Ph.D. dissertation, Duke University.

Dube, N., and Wilson, D., 1995 Peer Education Programmes among HIV-Vulnerable Communities in Southern Africa. *In* HIV/AIDS Management in South Africa: Priorities for the Mining Industry. B. Williams and C. Campbell, eds. Johannesburg: Epidemiology Research Unit.

Dubos, R., 1965 Man Adapting. New York: Charles Scribner.

Dunbar Moodie, T., 1988 Migrancy and Male Sexuality on the South African Gold Mines. Journal of Southern African Studies 14(2):228–256.

Dunbar Moodie, T., 1994 Going for Gold: Men, Mines and Migration. Johannesburg: Witwatersrand University Press.

Duncan, M. E., Gerard, T., Andrée, P. et al., 1990 First Coitus before Menarche and Risk of Sexually Transmitted Disease. The Lancet 335:338–340.

Duncan, S., and Savage, M., 1989 Space, Scale and Locality. Antipode 21:179–206.

Dunton, C., and Palmberg, M., 1996 Human Rights and Homosexuality in Southern Africa. Current African Issues 19. 2nd edition. Uppsala: Nordiska Afrikainstitute.

Eboko, F., 1999 Logiques et Contradictions Internationales dans le Champ du Sida au Cameroun. *In* Le Sida des Autres. Claude Fay, ed. pp. 123–140. Editions De l'Aube, IRD. Economist, 1997 334(8036):19.

Economist, 1999 AIDS in the Third World: A Global Disaster. Economist (UK) 350(January 2–8):42–44.

Edwards, M., 1989 The Irrelevance of Development Studies. Third World Quarterly 11:116–136.

Ehrenreich, R., 1997 The Scars of Death: Children Abducted by the Lord's Resistance Army in Uganda. New York & Middot: Human Rights Watch.

Ekambaram, S., 2000 South Africa: "Health Before Profits" Campaign. Women's International Network News 26(1):23.

Ekwempu, C. C., Maine, D., Olorukoba, M. B., Essien, E. S., and Kisseka, M. N., 1990 Structural Adjustment and Health in Africa [Letter]. Lancet 336:56–57.

Ellsworth, E., 1989 Why Doesn't This Feel Empowering? Working through the Repressive Myths of Critical Pedagogy. Harvard Educational Review 59(3):297–324

Elmendorf, A. E., and Roseberry, W., 1993 Structural Adjustment: What Effect on Health? On Vulnerability to HIV? IX International Conference on AIDS, Berlin, June [Abstract WS-D20-4].

Emah. E., 1998 Nigeria's NGOs Foster a Caring Community. Impact on HIV 1(1):1–7.

Epprecht, M., 1998 "Good God Almighty, What's This!": Homosexual "Crime" in Early Colonial Zimbabwe. *In* Boy-Wives and Female Husbands: Studies in African Homosexualities. S. O. Murray and W. Roscoe, eds. pp. 197–221. New York: St Martin's Press.

Epstein, H., 1999 Something Happened. New York Review of Books, December 2: 24–28.

Epstein, H., 2002 The Hidden Cause of AIDS. New York Review of Books, May 9, 49(8):43–49.

Ernst, W, and Harris, B., 1999 Race, Science, and Medicine, 1700–1960. New York: Routledge Press.

Ewens, G., 1994 Congo Colossus: The Life and Legacy of Franco and OK Jazz. Norfolk, England: Buku Press.

Falobi, O., 1999. Pre-ICASA 4 Services Under Strain – Nigeria. International Conference on AIDS and STDs in Africa.

Faleyimu, B. L., Ogunniyi, S. O., Urbane, L. A., and Faleyimu, A. I., 1999 Sexual Networking and AIDS Education in the Workplace and the Community: The Case of Oil Locations in Nigeria. National HIV Prevention Conference (United States), Aug 29–Sep 1 (Abstract No. 158).

Falola, T., 1996 Africa in Perspective. *In* Africa Now. S. Ellis, ed. London: Heinemann.

Family Health International, AIDS Control and Prevention Project (AIDSCAP), 1997a Final Report, vol. 2. August 21, 1991 – December 31, 1997. Arlington, VA: USAID, Contract No. HRN-5972-C-4001-00.

——1997b Final Report for the AIDSCAP Program in Rwanda, October 1993 to April 1997. Arlington, VA: USAID.

Famine Early Warning System (FEWS Project), 1996 Flight of Refugees from Zaire: Roots of the Problem, Special Report 7. Arlington, VA: USAID.

Fanon, F., 1970 Black Skin, White Masks. St Albans: Paladin.

Farmer, P., 1992a New Disorder, Old Dilemmas: AIDS and Anthropology in Haiti. *In* The Time of AIDS, Social Analysis, Theory and Method. G. Herdt and S. Lindenbaum, eds. pp. 287–318. London: Sage Publications.

—— 1992b AIDS and Accusation: Haiti and the Geography of Blame. Berkeley: University of California Press.

Farmer, P., 1994 AIDS-Talk and the Constitution of Cultural Models. Social Science and Medicine 38(6):801–809.

Farmer, P., 1999a Infections and Inequalities: The Modern Plagues. Berkeley: University of California Press.

—— 1999b AIDS and Social Scientists, Critical Reflections. *In* Experiencing and Understanding AIDS in Africa. C. Becker, J-P. Dozon, C. Obbo, and M. Toure, eds. pp. 33–39. Dakar: Codesria, Karthala Editions, IRD.

Farmer, P., Lindenbaum, S., and Good, M., 1993 Women, Poverty, and AIDS: An Introduction. Cultural Medical Psychiatry 17:387–397.

Farmer, P.E., Connors, M., Simmons, J., eds., 1996 Women, Poverty, and AIDS: Sex, Drugs, and Structural Violence. Monroe, ME: Common Courage Press.

Fassin, D., 1994 Le Domaine Privé de la Santé Publique: Pouvoir, Politique et Sida au Congo. Annales Histoire et Sciences Sociales 4:745–775.

Faux, J., 2002 A Deal Built on Sand. The American Prospect 13(1):A22–24.

Feierman, S., and Janzen J. M., eds., 1992 The Social Basis of Health and Healing in Africa. Berkeley: University of California Press.

Feinberg, R., 1992 Defunding Latin America: Reverse Transfers by the Multilateral Lending Agencies. *In* The Political Economy of Development and Underdevelopment. 5th edition. C. K. Wilber and K. P. Jameson, eds. New York: McGraw Hill.

Fendell, N., 1963 Public Health and Urbanization in Africa. Public Health Report 78:574–579.

Fernandes, W., and Tandon, R., eds., 1981 Participatory Research and Evaluation, Experiments in Research as a Process of Liberation. Delhi: Indian Social Institute.

Finkel, D., 2000 Few Drugs for the Needy. Washington Post, November 11: A1.

Foreman, M., 1998a AIDS and Men – Old Problem, New Angle. [Panos H/V/AIDS Briefing No. 6] London: The Panos Institute. Electronic document. http://www. onewodd.org/panos/index, htm.

Foreman, M., ed., 1998b AIDS and Men: Taking Risks or Taking Responsibility. London: Panos/Zed Books.

Forster, P. G., 1994 Culture, Nationalism, and the Invention of Tradition in Malawi. The Journal of Modern African Studies 32(3):477–498.

Forsythe, S., and Rau, B., 1998 Evolution of Socio-economic Impact Assessments of HIV/AIDS. AIDS 12(Suppl.):S47–S55.

Forsythe, S., Sokal, D., Lux, L., and King, T., 1993 An Assessment of the Economic Impact of AIDS in Kenya. Washington, DC: Family Health International/AIDSCAP.

Forsythe, S., Rau, B. et al., 1996 AIDS in Kenya: Socio-economic Impact and Policy Implications. Arlington, VA: Family Health International [AIDSCAP] and USAID.

Foster, C., Makufa, C., Drew, R., Kambeu, S., and Saurombe, K., 1996 Supporting Children in a Community-Based Orphan Visiting Programme. AIDS Care 8:39–403.

Foucault, M., 1977 Discipline and Punish. New York: Pantheon.

Foundation for Democracy in Africa (The), 2000 Proceedings of the Regional Conference on HIV/AIDS in West Africa. Abuja, Nigeria, 5–8 June. Electronic document. http://www. democracy-africa.org/hivconf.htm.

Francois, E. M., 1992 The Iatrogenic Factor in the AIDS Pandemic in Africa: The Case of Ghana. International Conference on AIDS, July 19–24, 8(3):165 (Abstract No. Puc 8077).

Frankenberg, R., 1995 Learning from AIDS: The Future of Anthropology. *In* The Future of Anthropology: Its Relevance to the Contemporary World. A. Ahmed and C. Shore, eds. pp. 110–133. London: Athlone Press.

Freedman, B., 1987 Equipoise and the Ethics of Clinical Research. The New England Journal of Medicine 317(3):141–145.

French, H. F., 1994 The World Bank: Now Fifty, but How Fit? World Watch 7:10–18.

Frieden, J., 1991 Debt, Development and Democracy. Princeton: Princeton University Press.

Gaga, E. H., 1982 Bunda Hill. Society of Malawi Journal 35(2):61–63.

Gage, A., and Bledsoe, C., 1994 The Effects of Education and Social Stratification on Marriage and the Transition to Parenthood in Freetown, Sierra Leone. *In* Nuptiality in Sub-Saharan Africa: Contemporary Anthropological and Demographic Perspectives. C. Bledsoe and G. Pison, eds. pp. 148–166. London: Oxford University Press.

Gage, A., and Meekers, D., 1994 Sexual Activity before Marriage in Sub-Saharan Africa. Social Biology 41(1–2):44–60.

Gaelesiwe, L., 1999 Men Talking Dirty in Botswana: A Way to Fight AIDS. [Panos News and Features-PANOS-BOTSWANAJ1]. London: The Panos Institute. Electronic document. http://oneworld.org/panos/news/6may99.htm.

Gaisie, K., 1993 Zambia Demographic and Health Survey 1992. Lusaka: Central Statistical Office.

Garret, L., 1994 The Coming Plague: Newly Emerging Diseases in a World Out of Balance. New York: Farar, Strauss and Giroux.

Gashau, W., Hall, T. L., and Hearst, N., 1992 Awareness Regarding AIDS and HIV Seroprevalence in Nigerian Long Distance Truck Drivers. VIII International Conference on AIDS, Amsterdam, July [Abstract P0D522 1].

Gay, J., 1985 "Mummies and Babies" and Friends and Lovers in Lesotho. Journal of Homosexuality 11(3–4):97–116.

Geelhoed, G. W., 1991 Migration of African AIDS from Town to Country. African Urban Quarterly 6(1&2):45–51.

Geise, L. L., and Elias, C., 1995 Transforming AIDS Prevention to Meet Women's Needs: A Focus on Developing Countries. Social Science and Medicine 40(7):931–943.

Geisler, G., 1995 Troubled Sisterhood – Women and Politics in Southern Africa: Case Studies from Zambia, Zimbabwe and Botswana. African Affairs 94(377):545–578.

Geisler, G., 1997 Women Are Women or How to Please Your Husband: Initiation Ceremonies and the Politics of "Tradition" in Southern Africa. African Anthropology IV(1):92–128.

Gelfand, M., 1965 The Normal Man: A New Concept of Shona Philosophy. NADA IX(2):78–93.

Geschiere, P., 1997 The Modernity of Witchcraft: Politics and the Occult in Postcolonial Africa. Charlottesville: University Press of Virginia.

Geschiere, P., 1998 Globalization and the Power of Indeterminate Meaning: Witchcraft and Spirit Cult in Africa and East Asia. Afrika Zamani 5 and 6:143–176.

Gevisser, M., 1998 The "Unsaying" of Indigenous Homosexualities in Zimbabwe: Mapping a Blindspot in an African Masculinity. Journal of Southern African Studies 24(4):631–651.

Gevisser, M., and Cameron, E., eds., 1994 Defiant Desire: Gay and Lesbian Lives in South Africa. London: Routledge.

Ghana National AIDS Control Program, 1995 AIDS in Ghana: Background Projections, Impacts, Interventions. Accra: Ghana Ministry of Health.

Ghana National AIDS Control Program, 1999 HIV/AIDS in Ghana: Background, Projections, Impacts, Interventions. Accra: Ghana Ministry of Health.

Ghana National AIDS Control Program, 2000 HIV Sentinel Surveillance 1999. Accra: Ghana Ministry of Health.

Ghana Statistical Service, 1989 Ghana Demographic and Health Survey 1988. Accra: Ghana Statistical Service.

Ghys, P. D., Diallo, M. O., Ettine-Traore, V., Yeboue, K. M., Gnaore, E., Lorougnon, F. et al., 1995 Genital Ulcers Associated with Human Immunodeficiency Virus – Related Immunosuppression in Female Sex Workers in Abidjan, Ivory Coast. Journal of Infectious Diseases 175(2):1371–1374.

Gibbs, J. L., ed., 1988 Peoples of Africa: Cultures of Africa South of the Sahara. Prospect Heights, IL: Waveland Press.

Gilbert, M., 1994 The Politics of Location: Doing Feminist Research at "Home." Professional Geographer 46(1):90–96.

Gill, H. S., and Aliyu, A. T., 1992 Social Impact of AIDS in Northern Nigeria. International Conference on AIDS, July 19–24, 8(2):D493 (Abstract No. Pod 5627).

Gillis, M., Perkings, D. H., Roemer, M., and Snodgrass, D. R., 1992 Economics of Development. 3rd edition. New York: Norton.

Gillmore, M., Butler, S., Lohr, M., and Gilchrist, L., 1992 Substance Use and Other Factors Associated with Risky Sexual Behavior among Pregnant Adolescents. Family Planning Perspectives 24(6):255–268.

Gilman, S., 1985 The Hottentot and the Prostitute: Toward an Iconography of Female Sexuality. *In* Difference and Pathology: Stereotypes of Sexuality, Race, and Madness. pp. 76–108. Ithaca, NY: Cornell University Press.

Girvan, N., 1984 Swallowing the IMF Medicine in the Seventies. *In* The Political Economy of Development and Underdevelopment. 3rd edition. C. K. Wilber, ed. New York: Random House.

Global AIDS News, 1993 Effective Prevention Could Halve New HIV Infections. Geneva: GPA/WHO (No. 3).

Glynn, J., Caraël, M., Bertran, A. et al., 2001 Why Do Young Women Have a Much Higher Prevalence of HIV Than Young Men? A Study in Kisumu, Kenya and Ndola, Zambia. AIDS 15(Suppl. 4):S51–S60.

Goddard, K., 2001 Being Positive about AIDS in Zimbabwe. Voices from Africa. UN Non-Governmental Liaison Services. Electronic document. http://www.unsystem.org/ngls/documents/publications.en/voices. africa/number10/a12goddard.htm

Godwin, P., 1995 The HIV/AIDS Epidemic and its Impact on Human Development. Paper presented at the Third International Conference on AIDS in Asia and the Pacific, Chang Mai, Thailand, September 17–21.

Goliber, T., 1997 Population and Reproductive Health in Sub-Saharan Africa. Population Bulletin 52(4). Washington, DC: Population Reference Bureau.

Gomez, M. P., Bain, R. M., Dean, S., McNeil, P., and Read, S. E., 1997 Zidovudine Reduces Vertical Transmission of HIV in the Bahamas. Presented at Conference on Global Strategies for the Prevention of HIV Transmission from Mothers to Infants, Washington, DC, September 3–6.

Good, C., 1995 Incentives Can Lower the Incidence of HIV-AIDS in Africa. Social Science and Medicine 40(4):419–424.

Gordon, A. A., 1996 Population Growth and Urbanization. *In* Understanding Contemporary Africa. A. A. Gordon and D. L. Gordon, eds. pp. 167–194. Boulder, CO: Lynne Rienner.

Gordon, G., and Kanstrup, C., 1992 Sexuality – the Missing Link in Women's Health. IDS Bulletin 23(1):29–37.

Gordon, P., and Crehan, K., n.d. Dying of Sadness: Gender, Sexual Violence and the HIV Epidemic. Gender and the HIV Epidemic. New York: UNDP HIV and Development Program. Electronic document. http://www.undp.org/hiv/publications/gender/violencee.htm, accessed March 22, 2000.

Gormley, N., and Bondi, L., 1999 Ethical Issues in Practical Contexts. *In* Geography and Ethics: Journeys Through a Moral Terrain. J. Proctor and D. Smith, eds. pp. 251–262. London: Routledge.

Goss, J., and Leinback, T., 1996 Focus Groups as Alternative Research Practice: Experience with Transmigrants in Indonesia. Area 28:115–123.

Gough, D., 1998 Beaten Wives Challenge Custom. The Guardian (London), December 31: 14.

Gould, P., 1993 The Slow Plague: A Geography of the AIDS Pandemic. Cambridge, MA: Blackwell Press.

Gould, P., and Wallace, R., 1994 Spatial Structures and Scientific Paradoxes in the AIDS Pandemic. Geografiska Annaler 76B(2):105–116.

Government of Kenya, 1999 AIDS in Kenya: Background, Projections, Impact, Interventions, and Policy. Nairobi: National AIDS/STDs Control Programme, Ministry of Health.

Gray, R. H., Kiwanuka, N., Quinn, T. C. et al., 2000 Male Circumcision and HIV Acquisition and Transmission: Cohort Studies in Rakai, Uganda (Rakai Project Team). AIDS 14(15): 2371–2381.

Green, E., 1988 AIDS in Africa: An Agenda for Behavioral Scientists. *In* AIDS in Africa. R. Rockwell and N. Miller, eds. New York: Lewiston.

Gregson, S., Anderson, R., Ndlovu, J., Zhuwau, T., and Chandiwana, K., 1997 Recent Upturn in Mortality in Rural Zimbabwe: Evidence for an Early Demographic Impact of HIV-1 Infection? AIDS 11(10):1269–1280.

Gregson, S., Terciera, N., Kakowa, M. et al., 2001 Study of Bias in Antenatal Clinic HIV-1 Surveillance Data in a High Contraceptive Prevalence Population in Sub-Saharan Africa. AIDS 16:643–652.

Gregson, S., Zaba, B., and Garnett, G. P., 1999 Low Fertility in Women with HIV and the Impact of the Epidemic on Orphanhood and Early Childhood Mortality in Sub-Saharan Africa. AIDS 13(Suppl. A):S249–S257.

Grootaers, J.-L., ed., 1998 Mort et Maladie au Zaïre. Tervuren/Paris: CEDAF-ASDOC/L'Harmattan.

Gruénais, M.-é., 1993 Dire ou ne pas Dire. Enjeux de l'Annonce de la Séropositivité au Congo. Atelier sur Les Sciences Sociales face au Sida en Afrique, Abidjan, Ivory Coast.

Gumodoka, B., Favot, I., Berege, Z. A., and Dolmans, W. M. V., 1997 Occupational Exposure to the Risk of HIV Infection among Health Care Workers in Mwanza Region, United Republic of Tanzania. Bulletin of the World Health Organization 75(2):133–140.

Gupta, G., and Weiss, F., 1993 Women's Lives and Sex: Implications for AIDS Prevention. Cultural Medical Psychiatry 17:399–412.

Guthrie, M., 1967–71 Comparative Bantu. 3 vols. Hampshire: Gregg Press.

Guyer, J., and Belinga, E., 1995 Wealth in People and Wealth in Knowledge: Accumulation and Composition in Equatorial Africa. Journal of African History 36:91–120.

Hagenbucher-Sacripanti, F., 1994 Représentations du SIDA et Médecines Traditionelles dans la Région de Pointe-Noire (Congo). Paris: ORSTOM éditions.

Hagey, R., 1997 The Use and Abuse of Participatory Action Research. Chronic Diseases in Canada 18:1–4.

Haraway, D., 1988 Situated Knowledges: The Science Question in Feminism as a Site of Discourse on the Privilege of Partial Perspective. Feminist Studies 14(3):575–599.

Haraway, D., 1996 Modest Witness at Second Millennium. New York: Routledge.

Harpham, T., 1986 Health and the Urban Poor. Health Policy and Planning 1:5–18.

Harries, T., 1990 Symbols and Sexuality: Culture and Identity on the Early Witwatersrand Gold Mines. Gender and History 2(3):318–336.

Harris, L., 1988 The JMF and Mechanisms of Integration. *In* Survival and Change in the Third World. B. Crow, M. Thorpe, H. Bernstein, et al., eds. New York: Oxford University Press.

Harris, N., 1986 The End of the Third World. Harmondsworth: Penguin.

Hassig, S. E., Perrins, J., Baende, E., Kahotwa, M., Bishagara, K., Kinkela, N., and Kapita, B., 1990 An Analysis of the Economic Impact of HIV Infection among Patients at Mama Yeo Hospital, Kinshasa, Democratic Republic of the Congo. AIDS 4:883–887.

Hawkes, S., 1992 Travel and HIV/AIDS. AIDS Care 4(4):446–449.

Hayes, M., 1992 On the Epistemology of Risk: Language, Logic and Social Science. Social Science and Medicine 35(4):401–407.

Health Technical Services Project of TvT Associates, n.d. Children on the Brink: Strategies to Support Children Isolated by HIV/AIDS. Arlington, VA: Health Technical Services Project of TvT and the Pragma Corporation for the HIV/AIDS Division of USAID.

Heise, L. L., and Elios, C, 1995 Transforming AIDS Prevention to Meet Women's Needs: A Focus on Developing Countries. Social Science and Medicine 40(7):931–944.

Heise, L. L., Raikes, A., Watts, C., and Zwi, A. B., 1994 Violence against Women: A Neglected Public Health Issue in Less Developed Countries. Social Science and Medicine 39(9): 1165–1179.

Helander, B., and Richards, P., eds., Forthcoming No Peace, No War: Anthropological Studies of Low-Intensity Violent Conflicts.

Helitzer-Allen, D., 1994 An Investigation of Community-Based Communication Networks for Adolescents Girls for HIV/STD Prevention Messages in Rural Malawi. Washington, DC: International Center for Research on Women.

Helitzer-Allen, D., 1996 Beliefs and Practices During Pregnancy in a Bantu Community in Malawi. In Cultural and Demographic Aspects of Health Care in Contemporary Sub-Saharan Africa. E. Kalipeni and P. Thiuri, eds. Langley Park, MD: International Association of African Scholars Publishers.

Herdt, G., 1992 Introduction. In The Time of AIDS, Social Analysis, Theory and Method. G. Herdt and S. Lindenbaum, eds. pp. 3–26. London: Sage Publications.

Herman, T., and Mattingly, D., 1999 Community, Justice and the Ethics of Research: Negotiating Reciprocal Research Relations. In Geography and Ethics: Journeys Through a Moral Terrain. J. Proctor and D. Smith, eds. pp. 209–222. London: Routledge.

Hersak, D., 2001 There Are Many Kongo Worlds: Particularities of Magico-Religious Beliefs among the Vili and Yombe of Congo-Brazzaville. Africa 71(4):614–640.

Hewitt, K., 1998 Excluded Perspectives in the Construction of Disaster. London: Routledge.

Hintzen, P. C., 1995 Structural Adjustment and the New International Middle Class. Transition 24:53–73.

Ho, D., 1997 It's AIDS, Not Tuskegee. Time 150(13):83.

Hoad, N., 1998 Tradition, Modernity and Human Rights: An Interrogation of Contemporary Gay and Lesbian Rights' Claims in Southern African Nationalist Discourses. Development Update 2(2):32–43.

Hobsbawm, E., and Ranger, T., eds., 1991 The Invention of Tradition. Cambridge: Canto (Cambridge University Press).

Hodgson, A. G. O., 1913 Notes on the Achewa and Angoni of the Dowa District. Journal of the Royal African Institute 63:123–165.

Hogg, M., and Abrams, D., 1988 Social Identifications. London: Routledge.

Hogg R. S., Strathdee, S. A., Craib, K. J. P., O'Shaughnessy, M. V., Montaner, J. S. G., and Schechter, M. T., 1994 Lower Socio-economic Status and Shorter Survival following HJV Infection. Lancet 344:1120–1124.

Hooper, E., 1999 The River: A Journey to the Source of HIV and AIDS. New York: Little, Brown.

Hope Sr, K. R., 1995 The Socio-Economic Context of AIDS in Africa. Journal of Asian and African Studies 30:80–89.

Hours, B., 1986 African Medicine as an Alibi and Reality. In African Medicine in the Modern World. Edinburgh: Edinburgh University, CAS Seminar No. 27.

Hrdy, D. B., 1987 Cultural Practices Contributing to the Transmission of Human Immunodeficiency Virus in Africa. Review of Infectious Diseases 9:1112–1118.

Huband, M., 1991 The Price of Sex. Africa Rep 36: 69.

Hubbard, D., 1991 A Critical Discussion of the Law on Rape in Namibia. In Putting Women on the Agenda. S. Bazili, ed. pp. 134–179. Braamfontein: Iravan Press.

Hubley, J., 1988 Understand Behaviour: The Key to Successful Health Education. Tropical Doctor 18:134–138.

Hughes, C. C., 1963 Public Health in Non-Literate Societies. In Man's Image in Medicine and Anthropology. I. Galdston, ed. New York: International Universities Press.

Human Rights Watch Interview, 1997a World Vision's Gulu Traumatized Children of War Project. Gulu, May 30.

—— 1997b Concerned Parents of Aboke. Lira, May 27.

Hunt, C., 1989 Migrant Labour and Sexually Transmitted Disease: AIDS in Africa. Journal of Health and Social Behaviour 30(4):353–373.

Hunt, C. W., 1996 Social vs. Biological: Theories on the Transmission of AIDS in Africa. Social Science and Medicine 42(9):1283–1296.

Hunter, S., and Williamson, J., 1998 Children on the Brink: Strategies to Support Children Isolated by HIV/AIDS. Electronic document. http://www.info.usaid. gov/pop_health/aids/brink.pdf.

Hunter, S. S., 1990 Orphans as a Window on the AIDS Epidemic in Sub-Saharan Africa: Initial Results and Implications of a Study in Uganda. Social Science and Medicine 31:681–690.

Hyden, G., 1969 Political Development in Rural Tanzania: A West Lake Study. Nairobi: East African Publishing House.

IDS (Institute of Development Studies), 1996 Introductory PRA Methodology Pack. Sussex: Sussex University, Institute of Development Studies.

IDS (Institute of Development Studies), 1997a The SHIP: Sexual Health Information Pack; Using Participatory Learning Approaches in Sexual Health Work. Sussex: Sussex University, Institute of Development Studies.

—— 1997b PRA and Gender Topic Pack. Sussex: Sussex University, Institute of Development Studies.

IIED (International Institute for Environment and Development), 1995 PLA Notes 23. Special Issue on Participatory Approaches to HIV/AIDS Programs. London: International Institute for Environment and Development.

Ijsselmuiden, C., and Faden, R., 1992 Research and Informed Consent in Africa – Another Look. The New England Journal of Medicine 326 (12):830–833.

Ireland, D., 1999 AIDS Drugs for Africa. Nation 269(10), October 4: 5–6.

IRIN-CEA, 1999. Update 709 for Central and Eastern Africa. July 7.

Irwin, K., Bertrand, J., Mibandumba, N., Mbuyi, K., Muremeri, C., Mukoka, M., Munkolenkole, K., Nzilambi, N., Bosenge, N., Ryder, R., Peterson, H., Lee, N., Wingo, P., O'Reilly, K., and Rufo, K., 1991 Knowledge, Attitudes and Beliefs about HIV Infection and AIDS among Health Factory Workers and their Wives, Kinsasha, Zaire. Social Science and Medicine 32(8):917–930.

Isiugo-Abanihe, C. U., 1985 Child Fosterage in West Africa. Population and Development Review 11:53–73.

Jackson, L. A., 1993 Friday the 13th University of Zimbabwe Mini-Skirt Saga. Southern Africa Political and Economic Monthly Dec'92/Jan'93: 25–26.

Jacobs, S. M., and Howard, T., 1987 Women in Zimbabwe: Stated Policy and State Action. *In* Women, State, and Ideology: Studies from Africa and Asia. H. Afshar, ed. London: Macmillan.

Janzen, J. M., 1982 Lemba, 1650–1930: A Drum of Affliction in Africa and the New World. New York: Garland.

Janzen, J. M., and MacGaffey, W., 1974 An Anthology of Kongo Religion: Primary Texts from Lower Zaire. Lawrence, KS: University of Kansas Press.

Jeater, D., 1993 Marriage, Perversion and Power: The Construction of Moral Discourse in Southern Rhodesia 1894–1930. Oxford: Clarendon Press.

Jochelson, K., Mothibeli, M., and Leger, J. P., 1991 Human Immunodeficiency Virus and Migrant Labour in South Africa. International Journal of Health Services 21(1):157–173.

Johnson, B., and Covello, V., eds., 1987 The Social and Cultural Construction of Risk. Dordrecht: Reidel.

Johnston, H., 1897 The Natives of British Central Africa. New York: Negro University Press.

Joint United Nations Programme on HIV/AIDS and the World Health Organization, 1999 AIDS Epidemic Updates. Geneva, Switzerland: Joint United Nations Programme on HIV/AIDS and the World Health Organization.

Joint United Nations Programme on HIV/AIDS, 2000 Ethical Considerations in HIV Preventive Vaccine Research. UNAIDS Guidance Document, Geneva.

Jonfar, E. et al., 1991 Participatory Modeling in North Omo, Ethiopia: Investigating the Perceptions of Different Groups through Models. RRA Notes 14:24–25.

Jost, T., 2000 The Globalization of Health Law: The Case of Permissibility of Placebo-Based Research. American Journal of Law and Medicine 26:176–186.

Kabeer, N., 1994 Reversed Realities: Gender Hierarchies in Development Thought. London and New York: Verso.

Kaijage, F., 1993 AIDS Control and the Burden of History in Northwestern Tanzania. Population and Environment 14(3):279–300.

Kakhongwe, P., 1997 Directory of AIDS Service Organizations in Malawi. Copy at CSR.

Kaleeba, N., Kalibala, S., Kaseje, M., Ssebbanja, P., Anderson, S., Van Praag, E., Tembo, G., and Katabira, E., 1997 Participatory Evaluation of Counseling, Medical and Social Services of the AIDS Support Organization (TASO) in Uganda. AIDS Care 9(1):13–26.

Kalipeni, E., 1995 The AIDS Pandemic in Malawi: A Somber Reflection. 21st Century Afro Review 1(2):73–110.

Kalipeni, E., 1997. Gender and Regional Differences in Schooling between Boys and Girls in Malawi. East African Geographical Review 19(1):14–32.

Kalipeni, E., 2000 Health and Disease in Southern Africa: A Comparative and Vulnerability Perspective. Social Science and Medicine 50(7–8):965–983.

Kalipeni, E., and Craddock, S., 1998. Mapping the Face of AIDS in Southern and Eastern Africa: Patterns and Prevention Strategies. Paper presented at the Applied Geography Conference, Louisville, Kentucky, November 24–29.

Kalipeni, E., and Oppong, J. R., 1998 The Refugee Crisis in Africa and Implications for Health and Disease: A Political Ecology Approach. Social Science and Medicine 46(12):1637–1653.

Kalumba, K., 1990 Impact of Structural Adjustment Programmes on Household Level Food Security and Child Nutrition: The Zambian Experience. University of Zambia, Unpublished MS.

Kaluwa, O. L., Feluzi, H. G., Songwe, A. C., and Zingani, A. M., 1995 1995 Sentinel Surveillance Report. Zomba: Centre for Social Research.

Kamali, A., Seeley, J. A., Nunn, A. J. et al., 1996 The Orphans Problem: Experience of a Sub-Saharan Africa Rural Population in the AIDS Epidemic. AIDS Care 8:509–515.

Kambou, G., Devarajan, S., and Over, M., 1992 The Economic Impact of AIDS in an African Country: Simulations with a Computable General Equilibrium Model of Cameroon. Journal of African Economies 1(1):109–130.

Kamenga, M., Ryder, R. W., Jingu, M. et al., 1991 Evidence of Marked Sexual Behavior Change Associated with Low HIV-1 Seroconversion in 149 Married Couples with Discordant HIV Serostatus. AIDS 5(1):61–67.

Kammeren, C. A., and Symonds, P. V., 1992 Hill Tribes Endangered at Thailand's Periphery. Cultural Survival Quarterly 16:23–25.

Kamwendo, G., and Kamowa, O., 1999 HIV/AIDS and a Return to Traditional Cultural Practices in Malawi. *In* AIDS and Development in Africa: A Social Science Perspective. R. H. Kempe, ed. New York: The Haworth Press.

Kandawire, J. A. K., 1979 Thangata: Forced Labour or Reciprocal Assistance? Zomba: Chancellor College (Copy in Chancellor College (CC) Library, Zomba).

Kanji, N., 1989 Charging for Drugs in Africa: UNICEF's "Bamako Initiative." Health Policy and Planning 4:110–120.

Kanji, N., Kanji, N., and Manji, F., 1991 From Development to Sustained Crisis: Structural Adjustment, Equity and Health. Social Science and Medicine 33:985–993.

Kaplan, R. D., 1994 The Coming Anarchy. The Atlantic Monthly 273(2):44–76.

Karim, A. Q., and Karim, S. S., 1999 South Africa: Host to a New and Emerging HIV Epidemic. Sexually Transmitted Infections 75:139–147.

Karim, A. Q., Preston-Whvte, E., and Zuma, N., 1993 Prevention of HIV Infection for Women by Women in Natal, South Africa. Durban, South Africa: Research Institute for Diseases in a Tropical Environment.

Karim, S., 1998 Placebo Controls in HIV Perinatal Transmission Trials: A South African's Viewpoint. American Journal of Public Health 88(4):564–566.

Karlen, A., 1995 Plague's Progress: A Social History of Man and Disease. London: Victor Gollancz.

Kaspin, D., 1993 Chewa Visions and Revisions of Power: Transformation of the Nyau Dance in Central Malawi. *In* Modernity and its Malcontents. J. Comaroff and J. Comaroff, eds. Chicago: University of Chicago Press.

Katjiuanjo, P., Titus, S., Zauana, M., and Boerma, J. T., 1993 Namibia Demographic and Health Survey 1992. Windhoek: Ministry of Health and Social Services.

Katz, C., 1994 Playing the Field; Questions of Fieldwork in Geography. Professional Geographer 46(1):54–102.

Kay, K., 1997 Commercial Farmers Union. Harare: AIDS Control Project.

Kendall, L., 1998 When a Woman Loves a Woman in Lesotho: Love, Sex, and the (Western) Construction of Homophobia. *In* Boy-Wives and Female Husbands: Studies of African Homosexualities. S. O. Murray and W. Roscoe, eds. pp. 223–242. New York: St Martin's Press.

Kenyatta, J., 1946 Facing Mount Kenya. London: Secker and Warbug.

Kesby, M., 1999 Locating and Dislocating Gender in Rural Zimbabwe: The Making of Space and the Texturing of Bodies. Gender Place and Culture 6(1):27–47.

Kesby, M., 2000a Participatory Diagramming as a Means to Improve Communication about Sex in Rural Zimbabwe: A Pilot Study. Social Science and Medicine 50(12):1723–1741.

——2000b Participatory Diagramming: Deploying Qualitative Methods through an Action Research Epistemology. Area 32(4):423–435.

Khasiani, S. A., 1985 Adolescents' Fertility in Kenya with Special Reference to High School Teenage Pregnancy and Childbearing. Unpublished thesis, Population Studies Research Institute, University of Nairobi, Nairobi, Kenya.

Kiama, W., 1998 Where Are Kenya's Homosexuals? [Panos News and Features, PANOS-KENYA/I]. London: The Panos Institute. Electronic document. http://www.onewodd.org/panos/news/15aug98.htm].

Kigongo, D. et al., 1992 HIV Prevalence Patterns among Migrants and Those Reporting Travel: A Two Year Follow Up in Rakai District, Uganda (Rakai Project, Columbia University and Makerere University). Paper presented at a Conference in Yaounde, Cameroon, 1992.

Killewo, J., Dahlgren, L., and Sandstrom, A., 1994 Socio-Geographical Patterns of HIV-1 Transmission in Kagera Region, Tanzania. Social Science and Medicine 38:129–134.

Killewo, J. Z. J. et al., 1990 Prevalence of HIV-1 Infection in the Kagera Region of Tanzania: A Population Based Study. AIDS 4(11):1081–1085.

Kim, J., Millen, J., Irwin, A., and Gershman, J., 2000 Dying for Growth: Global Inequality and the Health of the Poor. Monroe, ME: Common Courage Press.

King, E. M., 1990 Educating Girls and Women: Investing in Development. Washington, DC: The World Bank.

King, K., 1987 Primary Schooling and Developmental Knowledge in Africa. Seminar paper presented at the African Futures: 25th Anniversary Conference, Centre of African Studies, University of Edinburgh.

King, M., and King, E., 1992 The Story of Medicine and Disease in Malawi. Blantyre: Montfort Press.

King, M., and King, E., 2000 The Great Rift: Africa, Surgery, AIDS, Aid. Cambridge: ARCO Books.

King, P., 1997 A Partnership to Resolve the Conundrum. British Medical Journal 314 (22): 890–891.

Kinnaird, V., and Hyma, B., 1993 In Search of Working Models of Gender Sensitive Participatory Research. Environments 22(1):9–20.

Kippax, S., and Crawford, J., 1993. Flaws in the Theory of Reasoned Action. *In* The Theory of Reasoned Action: Its Application to AIDS-Preventive Behaviour. D. Terry, C. Galbois and M. McCamish, eds. Oxford: Pergamon.

Kiragu, K., 1991 The Correlates of Sexual and Contraceptive Behavior among In-School Adolescent in Kenya. Ph.D. Dissertation, The Johns Hopkins University, Baltimore, MD.

Kirunga, C. T., and Ntôzi, J. P. M., 1997 Socio-economic Determinants of HIV Serostatus: A Study of Rakai District, Uganda. HTR Supplement to Vol. 7:175–188.

Kisekka, M. N., 1990 AIDS in Uganda as a Gender Issue. Women and Therapy 10(3):35–53.

Kishindo, P. A. K., 1990 Knowledge, Attitudes and Beliefs on AIDS. Monograph. CC Library, Zomba.

Kishindo, P. A. K., 1994 Land Tenure: The Case of the Salima District, Central Malawi. Malawi Journal of Social Science 16:57–67.

Kisumu Department of Community Health, 1997 Draft Report of Kisumu Study Site: Multi-Center Study, Phase One, December 1996– March 1997. Unpublished report.

Kitchen, R., 1999 Morals and Ethics in Geographical Studies of Disability. *In* Geography and Ethics: Journeys through Amoral Terrain. J. Proctor and D. Smith, eds. pp. 223–236. London: Routledge.

Kitzinger, J., 1994 Focus Groups: Methods or Madness. *In* Challenge and Innovation: Methodological Advances in Social Research on HIV/AIDS. M. Boulton, ed. pp. 159–175. London: Taylor & Francis.

Klitsch, M., 1992 Rural Ugandan Women's HIV Infection Rates Seem Related to Trade Routes. International Family Planning Perspectives 18(2):79.

Konde-Lule, J. K., 1991 The Effects of Urbanization on the Spread of AIDS in Africa. African Urban Quarterly 6(1&2):13–18.

Konde-Lule, J. K., 1995 The Declining HIV Seroprevalence in Uganda: What Evidence? Health Transition Review 5(Suppl.): 27– 33.

Konde-Lule, J. K., Tumwesigye, M. N., and Lubanga, R. G., 1997 Trends in Attitudes and Behaviour Relevant to AIDS in a Ugandan Community. East African Medical Journal 74(7):406–410.

Konde-Lule, J. K., Wawer, M. J., Sewankambo, N. K. et al., 1997 Adolescents, Sexual Behavior and HIV-1 in Rural Rakai District, Uganda. AIDS 11(6):791–799.

Kornblit, A. L., 1994 Domestic Violence: An Emerging Health Issue. Social Science and Medicine 39(9):1181–1188.

Kreiss, J., Koech, D, Plummer, F., Holmes, K, Lightfoote, M., Piot, P., Ronald, A., Ndinya-Achola, J. O., D'Costa, L., Roberts, P., Ngugi, E., and Quinn, T., 1986 AIDS Virus Infection in Nairobi Prostitutes: Spread of the Epidemic to East Africa. The New England Journal of Medicine 314(7):414–418.

Krzywicki, J., 1997 Un Témoignage Important: Sony Labou Tansi Vu par J.-M. Devésa. Studies of the Department of African Languages & Cultures 21:51–61.

Kustner, H., 1994 The Relationship between the Growth Rate of the Pool of HIV Infections and the Incidence of Full-Blown AIDS, South Africa, 1990–1993. Epidemiological Comments 21:239–243.

Lackritz, E. M., Djomand, G., Vetter, K. M., Zadi, F., Diaby, L., and De Cock, K. M., 1993 Beyond Blood Screening: Reducing Unnecessary Transfusions and Improving Laboratory Services in Côte d'Ivoire. International Conference on AIDS, June 6–11, 9(1):92 (Abstract No WS-C11-2).

Laga, M., Alary, M., Nzilambi, N. et al., 1994 Condom Promotion, Sexually Transmitted Diseases Treatment, and HIV Decline among Female Zairian Sex Workers. Lancet 344:246–248.

Lamptey, P., and Tarantola, D. (Co-chairs), 1998 MAP Monitoring the AIDS Pandemic: The Status and Trends of the HIV/AIDS Epidemics in the World. Veyrier Du Lac, France: Marcel Merieux Foundation, June 23–25.

Lankoande, S., Meda, N., Sangare, L. et al., 1998 Prevalence and Risk of HIV Infection among Female Sex Workers in Burkina Faso. International Journal of STD and AIDS 9(3):146–150.

Larson, A., 1990 The Social Epidemiology of Africa's AIDS Epidemic. Africa Affairs 89(354):5–25.

Last, J. M., 1988. A Dictionary of Epidemiology. London: Oxford University Press.

Latif, A., Katzenstein, D., Bassett, M., Houston, S., Emmanuel, J., and Marowa, E., 1989 Genital Ulcers and Transmission of HIV among Couples in Zimbabwe. AIDS 3(8):519–523.

Lather, P., 1991 Getting Smart: Feminist Research and Pedagogy with/in the Postmodern. London: Routledge.

Laurie, W., 1958 A Pilot Scheme of Venereal Disease Control in East Africa. British Journal of Venereal Disease 34:16–21.

Laver, S., Van Den Borne, B., Kok, G., and Woelk, G., 1997 A Pre-Intervention Survey to Determine Understanding of HIV and AIDS in Farm Worker Communities in Zimbabwe. AIDS Education and Prevention 9(1):94–110.

Layraud, V., 1988 Sony Labou Tansi ou "L'Aventure Ambiguë" du Théâtre. Mémoire de D.E.A. sous la Direction de M. Alain Ricard. Institut Des Sciences de l'Information et de la Communication, Université Bordeaux-III.

Le Roux, J., 1996. Street Children in South Africa: Findings from Interviews on the Background of Street Children in Pretoria, South Africa. Adolescence 31(122):423–431.

Leacock, E., and Lee, R., eds., 1982 Politics and History in Band Societies. Cambridge: Cambridge University Press.

Learmonth, A., 1988 Disease Ecology: An Introduction. London: Basil Blackwell.

Lee, R., 1979 The !Kung San: Men, Women and Work in a Foraging Society. Cambridge: Cambridge University Press.

Lee, R., 1993 The Dobe Ju "Hoansi. New York, NY: Harcourt Brace.

Lele, U., 1990 Structural Adjustment, Agricultural Development and the Poor: Some Lessons from the Malawian Experience. World Development 18(9):1207–1219.

Lema, V. M., and Hassan, M. A., 1994 Knowledge on Sexually Transmitted Diseases: HIV Infection and AIDS among Sexually Active Adolescents in Nairobi, Kenya and its Relationships to their Behavior and Contraception. Medical Journal 71:122–128.

Lensink, R., 1996 Structural Adjustment in Sub-Saharan Africa. Harlow, Essex: Longman Group UK Ltd.

Leon, The Hon. R., Davies A., Salamon, M., and Davies, J., 1995 Commission of Inquiry into Safety and Health in the Mining Industry. Pretoria: Department of Mineral and Energy Affairs.

Leonard, A., and Muia, E., 1998 Community-Based AIDS Prevention and Care in Africa, Building on Local Initiatives: Results of Four Action-Research Interventions in East and Southern Africa. New York: Population Council.

Lesetedi, L. T., Mompati, G. D., Khulumani, P., Lesetedi, G. N., and Rutenberg, N., 1989 Botswana Family Health Survey II, 1988. Gaborone: Central Statistical Office, Ministry of Finance and Development Planning.

Leurs, R., 1996 Current Challenges Facing Participatory Rural Appraisal. Public Administration and Development 16:57–72.

Lewin, K., 1958 Group Decisions and Social Change. *In* Readings in Social Psychology. E. McCaby, ed. New York: Holt, Reinhart & Wilson.

L'Herminez, R. H., Hofs, M. A. G., and Chiwaya, W. B., 1992 AIDS in Mangochi District: Clinical Presentations. Malawi Medical Journal 8(3):113–117.

Lindan, C., Allen, S., Caraël, M. et al., 1991 Knowledge, Attitudes and Perceived Risk of AIDS among Urban Rwandan Women: Relationship to HIV Infection and Behavior Change. AIDS 5:993–1002.

Linden, I., and Linden, J., 1974 Catholics, Peasants and Chewa Resistance in Nyasaland 1889–1939. London: Richard and Clay.

Lindenbaum, S., 1992 Knowledge and Action in the Shadow of AIDS. *In* the Time of AIDS: Social Analysis, Theory and Method. G. Herdt and S. Lindenbaum eds. pp. 319–332. London: Sage Publications.

Loewenson, R., 1993 Structural Adjustment and Health Policy in Africa. International Journal of Health Services 23:717–730.

Loff, B., and Black, J., 2000 The Declaration of Helsinki and Research in Vulnerable Populations. Medical Journal of Australia 172:292–295.

Logie, D., 1993 Zimbabwe: Health or Debt. Lancet 341:950.

Logie, D. L., and Woodroffe, J., 1993 Structural Adjustment: The Wrong Prescription for Africa? British Medical Journal 307:41–44.

London, L., 1998 AIDS Control and the Workplace: The Role of Occupational Health Services in South Africa. International Journal of Health Services 28(3):575–591.

Lone, P., 1987 AIDS and Labour Policy. South African Labour Bulletin 12:80–88.

Long, L. D., 1997 Refugee Women, Violence and HIV. *In* Sexual Cultures and Migration in the Era of AIDS: Anthropological and Ethnographic Perspectives. G. Herdt, ed. pp. 87–103. Oxford: Clarendon Press.

Long, N., 1992 Conclusion. *In* Battle Fields of Knowledge: The Interlocking of Theory and Practice in Social Research and Development. N. Long and A. Long, eds. pp. 268–277. London: Routledge.

Long, N., and van rer Ploeg, J., 1989 Demythologizing Planned Intervention: An Actor Perspective. Journal of the European Society of Rural Sociology 29:226–249.

Lugalla, J. L. P., and Kibassa, C. G., Forthcoming Poverty, AIDS, and Street Children in East Africa. Lewiston, NY: Edwin Mellen Press.

Lurie, P., Hintzen, P., and Lowe, P., 1995 Socio-economic Obstacles to HIV Prevention and Treatment in Developing Countries – The Roles of the International Monetary Fund and the World Bank. AIDS (6):539–546.

Lurie, P., and Wolfe, S., 1998 Inappropriate Use of Placebos in Human Experiments: Testimony before the Committee on Government Reform and Oversight, U.S. House of Representatives, April 22. Electronic document. http://www.citizen.org/hrg/publications/1438.htm.

Lurie, P., and Wolfe, S., 1999a Letter to Dr. Jose Esparza, Joint UN Programme on HIV/AIDS, Comments on the Guidance Document on Ethical Considerations in International Trials of HIV Preventive Vaccines, January 15. Electronic document. http://www.citizen.org/hrg/publications/1471.htm.

—— 1999b Letter to Dr. Delon Human, World Medical Association, March 29. Electronic document. http://www.citizen.org/hrg/publications/1477.htm.

Lurie, P., Wolfe, S., Jordan, W., Annas, G., Grodin, M., and Silver, G., 1997 Letter to Secretary Donna Shalala, Department of Health and Human Services, April 22. Electronic document. http://www.citizen.org/hrg/publications/1415.htm.

Lwanda, J. L., 1993 Kamuzu Banda of Malawi. Glasgow: Dudu Nsomba Publications.

Lwanda, J. L., 1995 A Sabbatical Year Report to the Postgraduate Dean, Glasgow University.

Lwanda, J. L., 1996 Promises, Power Politics and Poverty. Glasgow: Dudu Nsomba Publications.

Lwanda, J. L., 1999 The Traditional in the Popular: Lyrical Ambiguities in Malawi's Socio-Medical Discourse, 1961–1999. Seminar paper presented at the Commonwealth Studies Department, Stirling University, December.

Lwanda, J. L., 2000 Breaking the silence. Letter. British Journal of General Practice 50:1009.

Lwanda, J. L., 2002 Politics, Culture and Medicine in Malawi: Historical Continuities and Ruptures with Special Reference to HIV/AIDS. Ph.D. dissertation, Edinburgh University.

Lwihula, G. K., 1990 Social Cultural Factors Associated with the Transmission of HIV Virus in Tanzania. Unpublished MS, Muhimbili Medical Center, Faculty of Medicine, Department of Behavioural Sciences, P.O. Box 65015, Dar es Salaam.

Lyons, M., 1996 Foreign Bodies: The History of Labour Migration as a Threat to Public Health in Uganda. *In* African Boundaries: Barriers, Conduits and Opportunities. P. Nugent and A. I. Asiwaju, eds. pp. 131–144. London: Pinter.

MacGaffey, J., 1986 Women and Class Formation in a Dependent Economy: Kisangani Entrepreneurs. *In* Women and Class in Africa. C. Robertson and I. Berger, eds. New York: Africana Publishing Company.

MacGaffey, J., and Bazenguissa-Ganga, R., 2000 Congo-Paris: Transnational Traders on the Margins of the Law. Oxford: James Currey for IAI.

MacGaffey, J. with Vwakyanakazi, M., Rukarangira, Wa N., Schoepf, B. G. et al., 1991 The Real Economy of Zaire: The Contribution of Smuggling and Other Unofficial Activities to National Wealth. London: James Currey and Philadelphia: University of Pennsylvania Press.

MacGaffey, W., 1986 Religion and Society in Central Africa: The Bakongo of Lower Zaire. Chicago: The University of Chicago Press.

MacGaffey, W., 1994 Kimbanguism and the Question of Syncretism in Zaire. *In* Religion in Africa. T. Blakeley et al., eds. pp. 241–256. London: James Currey/Heinemann.

Macheke, C., 1996 AIDS Awareness Programmes on the Mines: A Postal Survey. *In* HIV/AIDS Management in South Africa: Priorities for the Mining Industry. B. Williams and C. Campbell, eds. Johannesburg: Epidemiology Research Unit.

Macheke, C., and Campbell, C., 1995 Mineworkers' Perceptions of HIV/AIDS: "Knowledge," Uncertainties and Contextual Background. *In* Epidemiology Research Unit Report Series, No 34. Johannesburg: Epidemiology Research Unit.

Machida, T., 1992 Sisters of Mercy. *In* Amazon to Zami. M. Reinfelder, ed. pp. 118–129. New York: Cassell.

Madan, T., 1987 Community Involvement in Health Policy: Socio-Structural and Dynamic Aspects of Health Beliefs. Social Science and Medicine 25(6):615–620.

Madge, C., 1997 Ethics of Research in the Third World. *In* Postgraduate Fieldwork in Developing Areas: A Rough Guide. 2nd edition. E. Robson and K. Willis, eds. pp. 113–124. Keele: University of Keele Press,.

Maguire, P., 1987 Doing Participatory Research: A Feminist Approach. Amherst, MA: Center for International Education, University of Massachusetts.

Maina, G., 1995 Youth Peer Survey in Kenya. Planned Parenthood Challenges 1:24–25.

Makiadi, L., 1987 Attention Na SIDA. African Sun Music.

Makiadi, L., 1994 Les Rumeurs. Sonodisc CDS 6981 SD 30.

Malamba, S. S., Wagner, H. U., Maude, G., Okongo, M., Nunn, A. J., Kengeya-Kayondo, J. F., and Mulder, D. W., 1994 Risk Factors for HIV-1 Infection in a Rural Ugandan Community: A Case-Control Study. AIDS 8(2):253–257.

Malawi AIDS Control Programme Manual, 1989. Lilongwe: Ministry of Health.

Malawi Ministry of Health, 1991 Bibliography of Health Information in Malawi. Lilongwe: MOH.

Malawi National Family Planning Strategy (NFPS), 1994. Lilongwe, Malawi.

Malawi National Statistical Office, 1994 Demographic and Health Survey 1992. Zomba: Malawi National Statistical Office.

Malawi Vision 2020, 1997. Lilongwe: UNDP/Malawi Government.

Maliyamkono, T., and Bagachwa, M. S. D., 1990 The Second Economy in Tanzania. London: James Currey.

Maluwa-Banda, D. W., 2000 HIV/AIDS-Related Knowledge and Self-Reported Sexual Behaviour of Secondary School Students in Southern Malawi: Implications for AIDS Education and Counselling. Seminar paper, Chancellor College, July 2000.

Maman, S., Campbell, J., Sweat, M. D., and Gielden, A. C., 2000 The Intersections of HIV and Violence: Directions for Future Research and Interventions. Social Science & Medicine 50: 459–478.

Mandela, N., 2002 Care, Support and Destigmatization. Closing Remarks. Barcelona XIV International AIDS Conference. Electronic document. http://www.kff.org/aids2002/transcript/transcript_webcast_12_a2.html

Mandevu, R., 1995 Botswana: Where Young Girls Are, Easy Prey. AIDS Analysis Africa 5(4): 12–13.

Manji, F., Moses, S., Bradley, J. E., and Nagelkerke, N. J. D., 1992 Impact of User Fees on Attendance for Sexually Transmitted Diseases. VIII International Conference on AIDS. Amsterdam, July [Abstract Pod 5581].

Mann, J. M., 1996 Human Rights and AIDS: The Future of the Pandemic. *In* AIDS Education: Interventions in Multicultural Societies. I. Schenker, G. Sabar-Friedman and F. Sy, eds. pp. 1–7. New York: Plenum Press.

Mann, J. M., Francis, H., Davachi, F. et al., 1986 Risk Factors for Human Immunodeficiency Virus Seropositivity among Children 1–24 Months Old in Kinshasa, Zaire. Lancet ii:654–657.

Mann, J. M., Gruskin, S., and Grodin, M., eds., 1999 Health and Human Rights: A Reader. New York and London: Routledge.

Mann, J. M., Nzilambi, N., Piot, P. et al., 1988 HIV Infection and Associated Risk Factors in Female Prostitutes in Zaire. AIDS 2(4):249–254.

Mapanje, J., 1981 Of Chameleons and Gods. London: Heinemann.

Mapanje, J., and White, L., eds., 1983 Oral Poetry from Africa. London: Heinemann.

Marks, S., 1987 Not Either an Experimental Doll: The Separate Worlds of Three South African Women. Bloomington: University of Indiana Press.

Martin-Granel, N., 2000 Le Quatrième Coté du Triangle, or Squaring the Sex: A Genetic Approach to the "Black Continent" in Sony Labou Tansi's Fiction. Research in African Literatures 31(3):69–99.

Marwick, M. G., 1965 Sorcery in its Social Setting. Manchester: Manchester University Press.

Matchaba, P., 1999 Af-Aids@Hivnet.Ch, [207] RE: Zambia: "Debt for Development Agreement" to Combat HIV-AIDS [200].

Matrix Development Consultants, 1993 Nairobi's Informal Settlements: An Inventory. A report prepared for USAID/REDSO/ESA. Nairobi: USAID.

Matu, J., Kidandy, J., Okech, M, and Omollo, M., 1996 Women Fighting AIDS in Kenya (WOFAK), Nairobi, Kenya. Paper presented at the International Conference on AIDS, Nairobi, Kenya, July 7–12, 11(2):490 (Abstract No. Pub.D.1337).

Maxwell, K. B., 1983 Bemba: Myth and Ritual: The Impact of Literacy on an Oral Culture. New York: Peter Lang.

Mayaud, P., Msuya, W., Todd, J., Kaatano, G., West, B., Begkoyian, G., Grosskurth, H., and Mabey, D., 1997 STD Rapid Assessment in Rwandan Refugee Camps in Tanzania. Genitourinary Medicine 73(1):33–38.

Mayoux, L., 1995 Beyond Naivety: Women, Gender Inequality and Participatory Development. Development and Change 26:235–258.

Mazrui, A., 1986 The Africans. New York: Little-Brown Publishers.

Mazrui, A., 1990 Cultural Forces in World Politics. Oxford: James Currey.

Mbidde, E., 1998 Bioethics and Local Circumstances. Science 279(5348):155.

Mbizvo, M., and Adamchak, D., 1991 Family Planning Knowledge, Attitudes, and Practices of Men in Zimbabwe. Studies in Family Planning 22(1):31–38.

Mbizvo, M., and Adamchak, D., 1992 Male Fertility Regulation: A Study on Acceptance among Men in Zimbabwe. Central African Journal of Medicine 38(2):52–57.

McAfee, K., 1991 Storm Signals: Structural Adjustment and Development Alternatives in the Caribbean. London: Zed Books.

McAulife, E., 1994 AIDS: The Barriers to Behaviour Change. Zomba: Center for Social Research.

McCracken, J., 1977 Politics and Christianity in Malawi. Cambridge: Cambridge University Press.

McCracken, J., 1998 Blantyre Transformed: Class, Conflict and Nationalism in Urban Malawi. Journal of African History 39:247–269.

McFadden, P., 1992 Sex, Sexuality and the Problems of AIDS in Africa. *In* Gender in Southern Africa: Conceptual and theoretical Issues. R. Meena, ed. pp. 157–195. Harare: Sapes Books.

McGeary, J., 2001 Death Stalks a Continent. Time Magazine, February 12:36–53.

McGreal, C., 1992 The Last Emperor. Esquire, October:129–133.

McLean, G.R., 1997 A Case for Goodwill. British Medical Journal 314 (22):890–891.

McNamara, R., n.d. Female Genital Health and the Risk of HIV Transmission. New York: UNDP, HIV and Development Programme [Issues paper No.3]. Electronic document. http://www.undp.org/hiv/publications/issues/english/issue03e.htm, accessed March 27, 2000.

McPake, B., 1993 User Charges for Health Services in Developing Countries: A Review of the Economic Literature. Social Science and Medicine 36(11):25–30.

Mechanic, D., 1990 Promoting Health. Society January/February:16–22.

Meda, N., Ndoye, I., M'Boup, S. et al., 1999 Low and Stable Rate HIV Rates in Senegal: Natural Course of the Epidemic or Evidence for Success of Prevention? AIDS 13:1397–1405.

Meda, N., Sangare, L., and Lankoande, S., 1998 The HIV Epidemic in Burkina Faso: Current Status and Knowledge Level of the Population about AIDS, 1994–1995. Rev. of Epidemiol Sante Publique 46(1):14–23.

Meda, N., Zoundi-Guigui, M. T., Van De Perre, P. et al., 1999 HIV Infection among Pregnant Women in Bobo-Dialousso, Burkina-Faso: Comparison of Voluntary and Blinded Seroprevalence Estimates. International Journal of STD and AIDS 10(11):738–740.

Medecins Sans Frontières (MSF) 2000 MSF in the DRC: Medical Data. MSF Belgium, 25 January.

Meekers, D., and Calvès, A.-E., 1997 "Main" Girlfriends, Girlfriends, Marriage, and Money: The Social Context of HIV Risk Behaviour in Sub-Saharan Africa. Health Transition Review 7(Suppl.):361–375.

Meester, L. F., Abbink, C. P. B., Van Der Ploeg, C., Van Vliet and Habbema, J. D. F., 1997 Decision Making on STD Control in Nyanza Province: Possibilities for Support by the Model STDSIM. Paper presented at a workshop organized by Erasmus University of Rotterdam, Kisumu, Kenya, September 25–26.

Mehrotra, M., Burde, D., Banerjee, D., and Pardiwala, T., 1999 AIDS: An Expression of Gender-based Violence. New York: UNDP. Electronic documents. http://undp.org/rblac/gender/aidsgender.htm.

Meursing, K., 1997 A World of Silence: Living with HIV in Matabeleland, Zimbabwe. Amsterdam: Royal Tropical Institute.

Meursing, K., and Sibindi, F., 1995 Condoms, Family Planning and Living with HIV in Zimbabwe. Reproductive Health Matters 5:56–67

Meursing, K., Vos, T., Coutinho, O., Moyo, M., Mpofu, S., Oneke, O., Mundy, V., Dube, S., Mahlangu, T., and Sibindi, F., 1995 Child Sexual Abuse in Matabeleland, Zimbabwe. Social Science and Medicine 41(12):1693–1704.

Mgalla, Z., Schapink, D., and Boerma, J. T., 1998 Protecting Schoolgirls against Sexual Exploitation: A Guardian Programme in Mwanza, Tanzania. Reproductive Health Matters 6(12):19–30.

Mhloyi, M. M., 1990 Perceptions on Communication and Sexuality in Marriage in Zimbabwe. Women and Therapy: A Feminist Quarterly 10(3):61–73.

Mhloyi, M. M., 1994 Racing against Time. In HIV and AIDS: The Global Inter-Connection. E. Reid, ed. pp. 13–25. West Hartford, CA: Kumarian Press.

Mhloyi, M. M., 1995 Racing against Time. In HIV & AIDS: The Global Interconnection. Elizabeth Reid, ed. pp. 13–25. West Hartford, CT: Kumarian Press for UNDP.

Miles, L., 1993 Women, AIDS, and Power in Heterosexual Sex: A Discourse Analysis. Women's Studies International Forum 16(5):497–511.

Ministry of Health, 1997 Programme National de Lutte contre le Sida. Kigali, Rwanda: Department of Epidemiology, Ministry of Health.

Ministry of Health (Kenya), 2001 AIDS in Kenya: Background, Projections, Impact, Interventions, and Policy. 6th edition. Nairobi: National AIDS and STD Control.

Minkin, S. F., 1991 Iatronic AIDS: Unsafe Medical Practices and the HIV Epidemic. Social Science and Medicine 33(7):786–790.

Miotti, P., Dallabeta, G. A., Chiphangwi, J. D., Liomba, G., and Saah, A. J., 1992 A Retrospective Study of Childhood Mortality and Spontaneous Abortion in HIV-1 Infected Women in Urban Malawi. International Journal of Epidemiology 21(4):792–799.

Misihairambwi, P., 1997 The Women's AIDS Support Network Youth Programme in Zimbabwe. Paper given at a workshop on Community Responses to HIV in Southern Africa, Sheffield College, October 4.

Mitchell, J. C., 1952 A Note on the African Conception of Causality. The Nyasaland Journal 5(2):51–58.

Mitchell, J. C., 1956 The Yao Village. Manchester: Manchester University Press.

Mkamanga, E., 2000 Suffering in Silence. Glasgow: Dudu Nsomba Publications.

Mkandawire, A., 1997 Living My Destiny. Glasgow: Dudu Nsomba Publications.

Mok, J., and Cooper, S., 1997 The Needs of Children Whose Mothers Have HIV Infection. Archives of Disease in Childhood 77(6):483–487.

Mokgoro, J. Y., 1998 Ubuntu and the Law in South Africa. Buffalo Human Rights Law Review 4:15–23.

Molapo, M., 1995 Job Stress, Health and Perceptions of Migrant Mineworkers. *In* Crossing Boundaries: Mine Migrancy in a Democratic South Africa. J. Crush and W. James, eds. pp. 88–100. Cape Town: Creda.

Montavon, C., Bibollet-Ruche, F., Robertson, D. et al., 1999 The Identification of a Complex A/G/I/J Recombinant HIV Type 1 Virus in Various West African Countries. AIDS Research and Human Retroviruses 15(18):1707–1712.

Moodie, R., and Aboagye-Kwaneng, T., 1993 Confronting the HIV Epidemic in Asia and the Pacific: Developing Successful Strategies to Minimize the Spread of HIV Infection. AIDS 7:1543–1551.

Moodley, D., Bobat, R. A., Coutsoudis, A., and Coovadia, H. M., 1994 Caesarian Section and Vertical Transmission of HIV-1. Lancet 344:338.

Moore, H., 1994 Households and Gender in a South African Bantustan: A Comment. African Studies 53(1):137–142.

Moore, P. S., Allen, S., Sowell, A. L. et al., 1993 Role of Nutritional Status and Weight Loss in HIV Seroconversion among Rwandan Women. Journal of Acquired Immune Deficiency Syndrome 6:611–616.

Morgan, D., 1997 Focus Groups as Qualitative Research. 2nd edition. London: Sage Publications.

Morrell, R., 1998 Of Boys and Men: Masculinity and Gender in Southern African Studies. Journal of Southern African Studies 24(4):605–630.

Morris, B., 1985 Chewa Conceptions of Disease: Symptoms and Etiologies. The Society of Malawi Journal 38(1):14–43.

Moses, S., Bailey, R. C., and Ronald, A. R., 2000. Male Circumcision: Assessment of Health Benefits and Risks. Sexually Transmitted Infections 74(5):368–373.

Moses, S., Bradley, J. E., Nagelkerke, N. J. et al., 1990 Geographical Patterns of Male Circumcision Practices in Africa: Association with HIV Seroprevalence. International Journal of Epidemiology 19(3):693–7.

Moses, S., Manji, F., Bradley J. E., Nagelkerke, N. J., Malisa, M. A., and Plummer, F. A., 1992 Impact of User Fees on Attendance at a Referral Centre for Sexually Transmitted Diseases in Kenya. Lancet 340:463–466.

Moses, S., Muia, E., Bradley, J. E. et al., 1994 Sexual Behavior in Kenya: Implications for Sexually Transmitted Disease Transmission and Control. Social Science and Medicine 39(12):1649–1656.

Moses, S., Plummer, F. A., Ngugi, E. N., Nagelkerke, N. J. D., Anzala, A. O., and Ndiya-Achola, J. O., 1991 Controlling HIV in Africa: Effectiveness and Cost of an Intervention in a High-Frequency STD Transmitter Core Group. AIDS 5(4):407–411.

Mosse, D., 1994 Authority, Gender and Knowledge: Theoretical Reflections on the Practice of Participatory Rural Appraisal. Development and Change 25:497–526.

Moyo, I., Ray, S., Chisvo, D., Gumbo, N., Low, A., Katsumbe, T., and Mbengeranwa, O., 1993 Behavioral Patterns Which May Predispose to HIV Infection or Further Transmission and Possible Intervention Strategy in the City of Harare: Part II. Central African Journal of Medicine 39(11):217–221.

Moyo Magazine, 1986. Lilongwe: Ministry of Health.

Mphande, L., 1996 Dr Hastings Kamuzu Banda and the Malawi Writers Group: The (Un)Making of a Cultural Tradition. Research in African Literatures 27:80–101.

Msapato, K. M., Kumwenda, K. M, Chirwa, B. Z., Chalira, A. M., and Mzembe, C. P., 1990 Study of Knowledge and Aspects of Attitudes of School Teenagers in Mzimba District about HIV Infection/AIDS. Lilongwe: Health Research Unit, Ministry of Health, Malawi.

Msiska, A. W. C., 1995 The Spread of Islam in Malawi and its Impact on Yao Rites of Passage, 1870–1960. Society of Malawi Journal 48(1):49–86.

Msonthi, J., 1982 Herbal Medicines Used by Traditional Birth Attendants in Malawi. Tropical Geography 34:81–85.

Msukwa, L. A. H., 1981 Meeting the Basic Health Needs of Rural Malawi: An Alternative Strategy. Norwich: Geo Books.

Muizarubi, B., Cole, L., Outwater, A., and Lamson, N., 1991 Targeting Truckers in Tanzania. AIDS & Society (April/May):4.

Mukoyogo, M. C., and Williams, G., 1991 AIDS Orphans: A Community Perspective from Tanzania. London: ACTIONAID, AMREF, and WORLD in Need.

Mukuna, K. W., 1992 The Genesis of Urban Music in Zaire. African Music: Journal of International Library of African Music 7(2):72–84.

Mukuna, K. W., 1999 The Evolution of Urban Music in Democratic Republic of Congo during the 2nd and 3rd Decades (1975–1995) of the Second Republic – Zaire. African Music: Journal of International Library of African Music 7(4):73–87.

Mulder, D., Nunn, A., Kamali, A., and Kengeya-Kayondo, J., 1995 Decreasing HIV-1 Seroprevalence in Young Adults in a Rural Ugandan Cohort. British Medical Journal 311:833–836.

Mulindi, S. A. Z., Onsongo, J., Gatai, M., and Kenya, P., 1998 Situation Analysis. Supported by UNAIDS and DFID.

Muller, O., and Abbas, N., 1990 The Impact of AIDS Mortality on Children's Education in Kampala (Uganda). AIDS Care 2:77–80.

Muller, O. et al., 1992 HIV Prevalence, Attitudes and Behaviour in Clients of a Confidential HIV Testing and Counseling Centre in Uganda. AIDS 6:869–874.

Muller, O., Sen, G., and Nsubuga, A., 1999 HIV/AIDS, Orphans, and Access to School Education in a Community of Kampala, Uganda. AIDS 13(1):146–147.

Munguti, K., Grosskurth, H., Newell, J., Senkoro, K., Mosha, F., Todd, J., Mayaud, P., Gavyole, A., Quigley, M., and Hayes, R., 1997 Patterns of Sexual Behavior in a Rural Population in North-Western Tanzania. Social Science and Medicine 44(10):1553–1561.

Murdoch W. W., 1980 The Poverty of Nations. Baltimore: Johns Hopkins University Press.

Musgrave, S. et al., 1991 Patterns of HIV-1 Prevalence among Migrants and Those Reporting Travel in Rakai District, Uganda. Paper presented at the 6th International Conference on AIDS in Africa, Dakar, December.

Musopole, A. C., 1996 Needed: A theology Cooked in an African Pot. *In* Theology Cooked in an African Pot. K. Fiedler, P. Gundani, and H. Mijoga, eds. Zomba: ATISCA/CLAIM.

Mwale, G., and Burnard, P., 1992 Women and AIDS in Rural Africa: Rural Women's Views of AIDS in Zambia. Aldershot: Avebury.

Mwale, J. K., 1977 Aspects of Non-Formal Education, Traditional Customs and Beliefs of the Chewa People of Central Malawi. Unpublished MS, copy in CC Library, Zomba.

Mwangulube, K., Simgogo, P., and Nowa, S., 1997 Baseline Survey for Malawi Prisons AIDS Interventions Report. Unpublished MS, copy at the Malawi National AIDS Control Programme Headquarters in Lilongwe.

Nabaitu, J., Bechengana, C., and Seeley, J., 1994 Marital Instability in a Rural Population in South-West Uganda: Implications for the Spread of HIV-1 Infection. Africa 62(2):243–251.

Nabarro, D., and McConnell, C., 1989 The Impact of AIDS on Socio-economic Development. AIDS 3 (Suppl. 1):S265–S272.

Nabila, J., 1988 Urbanization in Ghana. Accra: Population Impact Project, University of Ghana.

Nachimas, D., and Nachimas, C., 1981 Research Methods in the Social Sciences. New York: St. Martin's Press.

Namate, D. E., and Kornfield, R., 1997 Condom Use among Urban Workers and their Wives. Unpublished MS, copy at Malawi National AIDS Control Programme Headquarters in Lilongwe.

Nast, Heidi, 1994 Women in the Field: Critical Feminist Methodologies and Theoretical Perspectives. Professional Geographers 46(1):54–102.

NASTLP [Zambia National AIDS/STD/TB & Leprosy Programme] and UNICEF, 1996 HIV/AIDS Bibliography: An Annotated Review of Research on HIV/AIDS in Zambia. Lusaka.

Nation (The) 1999 Uganda's Lesson with AIDS. The Nation (Nairobi) June 3.

Nation Correspondent, 1999 Kenya Domestic Violence Campaign is Creating Awareness. The Nation (Nairobi), April 21. Electronic document. http://www.africanews.org/women/stories/19990421_feat1.html.

National Aids Control Programme (NACP), 1999 Malawi National AIDS Control Programme Sentinel Survey Report. Lilongwe: MOH.

National AIDS and STDs Control Programme and National Council for Population Development, 1998 AIDS in Kenya: Background Projections, Impact, Interventions. Nairobi: Ministry of Health and Ministry of Planning and National Development.

National AIDS Coordination Programme, 1998a National HIV/AIDS Policy Document (2nd Draft Document). Harare, Zimbabwe: Ministry of Health and Child Welfare.

—— 1998b HIV/AIDS in Zimbabwe: Background, Projections, Impact, Interventions. Harare, Zimbabwe: Ministry of Health and Child Welfare.

National Council for Population and Development et al., 1993 Kenya Demographic and Health Survey, 1993. Nairobi and Columbia, MD: National Council for Population and Development, Ministry of Home Affairs and National Heritage, Central Bureau of Statistics, Office of the Vice President, Ministry of Planning and National Development, Demographic and Health Surveys, Macro International.

National Council for Population and Development et al., 1998 Kenya Demographic and Health Survey, 1998 Preliminary Report. Nairobi and Columbia, MD: National Council for Population and Development, Central Bureau of Statistics and Macro International, Inc.

National Research Council (NRC), 1996 Preventing and Mitigating AIDS in Sub-Saharan Africa: Research and Data Priorities for the Social and Behavioral Sciences. Washington, DC: National Academy Press.

National Statistical Office, 1994 Demographic and Health Survey of Malawi 1992. Zomba, Malawi: National Statistical Office.

Ndiaye, M., n.d. A Healthy Diet for Better Nutrition for People Living with HIV/AIDS. Nairobi: Network for African People Living with HIV/AIDS (NAP+).

Ndibwani, A., Henry, E., and Saka, J. D. K., 1998 Proceedings of the Workshop on Research Priorities in Medicinal Plants and Traditional Medicine in Malawi. Seminar held at Chancellor College, Zomba, March 25–26.

Ndinya-Achola, J. O., Ghee, A. E., Kihara, A. N., Krone, M. R., Plummer, F. A., Fisher, L. D., and Holmes, K. K., 1997 High HIV Prevalence, Low Condom Use and Gender Differences in Sexual Behavior among Patients with STD-Related Complaints at a Nairobi Primary Health Care Clinic. International Journal of STD and AIDS 8:506–514.

Neequaye, A. R., Neequaye, J. E., Biggar, R. J., Mingle, J. A., Drummond, J., and Waters, D., 1997 HIV-1 and HIV-2 in Ghana, West Africa: Community Surveys Compared to Surveys of Pregnant Women. West African Journal Medicine 16(2):102–108.

Nelson, N., and Wright, S., eds., 1995 Power and Participatory Development: Theory and Practice. London: Intermediate Technology Publications.

Nelson, R. E., Celentano, D. D., Suprasert, S. et al., 1993 Risk Factors for HIV Infection among Young Adult Men in Northern Thailand. Journal of American Medical Association 270: 955–960.

New Vision, December 13, 1996.

New Vision, 1997a Uganda–Zaire Border Closed. New Vision, January 20.

——1997b Zaire Border Trade Booms (Buranga Border). New Vision, January 1.

——1997c June 20.

New Vision, 1998 Ugandan Minister for Regional Cooperation, Ms Rebecca Kadaga, Said in an Address to the East African Law Society. New Vision, April 13.

New Vision, 1999 Sex Booming in Rural Uganda. New Vision, May 31.

N'Galy, B., Ryder, R. W., Bila, K. et al., 1988 Human Immunodeficiency Virus Infection among Employees in an African Hospital. New England Journal of Medicine 319:1123–1127.

Ngimbi, I. V., 1997 Jeunesse, Funérailles et Contestation Socio-Politique en Afrique. Paris, L'Harmattan.

Ngugi, E., Wilson, D., Sebstad, J., Plummer, F., and Moses, S., 1996 Focused Peer-Mediated Educational Programs among Female Sex Workers to Reduce Sexually Transmitted Diseases and HIV Transmission in Kenya and Zimbabwe. Journal of Infectious Diseases 174 (Suppl. 2):S240–S247.

Nguyen, V.-K., 2002 Antiretrovirals, Biomedical Globalism and Therapeutic Economy. Oikos and Anthropos: A Workshop on Rationality, Technology, and Infrastructure, Prague, April 26–27. Electronic document. http://ls.berkeley.edu/dept/anth/econ1.pdf, June 10, 2002.

Nicoll, A., and Brown, P., 1994 HIV: Beyond Reasonable Doubt. New Scientist 141 (January 15):24–28.

Nigeria AIDS Bulletin No 15, May 20, 2000.

Njau, W., 1993 Factors Associated with Pre-Marital Teenage Pregnancy and Childbearing in Kiambu and Narok Districts. Dissertation, University of Nairobi, Nairobi, Kenya.

Njovana, E., and Watts, C., 1996 Gender Violence in Zimbabwe: A Need for Collaborative Action. Reproductive Health Matters 7:46–53.

Nkinya-Achola, J., 1997 High HIV Prevalence, Low Condom Use and Gender Differences in Sexual Behavior among Patients with STD-Related Complaints at a Nairobi Primary Health Care Clinic. International Journal of STD and AIDS 7:506–514.

Nlandu-Tsasa, C., 1997 La Rumeur au Zaire de Mobutu. Paris: L'Harmattan.

Ntozi, J. P., 1997 Effect of AIDS on Children: The Problem of Orphans in Uganda. Health Transition Review 7(Suppl.):23–40.

Ntozi, J. P., and Ahimbisibwe, F. E., 1999 Some Factors in the Decline of AIDS in Uganda. *In* The Continuing HIV/AIDS Epidemic in Africa. John C. Caldwell, James P. M. Ntozi, and I. O. Orubuloye, eds. pp. 93–107. Canberra: Health Transition Centre, Australian National University.

Ntozi, J. P., and Mukiza-Gapere, J., 1995 Care for AIDS Orphans in Uganda: Findings from Focus Group Discussions. Health Transition Review 5(Suppl.):245–252.

Nunn, A. J., Kengenya-Kayondo, J. F., Malamba, S. S. et al., 1994 Risk Factors for HIV-1 Infection in Adults in a Rural Ugandan Community: A Population Study. AIDS 8(1):81–86.

Nyang', J., and Obudo, F. O., 1996 Knowledge, Attitude and Practice (KAP) Survey on HIV/AIDS at Workplace in Kisumu District. Kisumu. Unpublished mimeo.

Nzila, N., Laga, M., Thiam, A. B. et al., 1991 HIV and Other Sexually Transmitted Diseases among Female Prostitutes in Kinshasa. AIDS 5:715–722.

Nzilambi, N., De Cock, K. M., Forthal, D. N. et al., 1988 The Prevalence of Infection with Human Immunodeficiency Virus over a 10-Year Period in Rural Zaire. New England Journal of Medicine 318:276–279.

Nzioka, C., 1994 AIDS Policies in Kenya: A Critical Perspective on Prevention. *In* AIDS: Foundations for the Future. P. Aggleton, P. Davies and G. Hart, eds. pp. 159–175. London: Taylor & Francis.

Nzongola-Ntladja, G., 2002 The Congo from Leopold to Kabila: A People's History. London: Zed Books.

Nzyuko, S., Lurie, P., McFarland, W., Leyden, W., Nyamwaya, D., and Mandel, J. S., 1997 Adolescent Sexual Behavior along the Trans-Africa Highway in Kenya. AIDS 11(Suppl. 1): S21–S26.

Oakes, P., Haslam. A., and Turner. J., 1994 Stereotyping and Social Reality. Oxford: Blackwell.

Obbo, C., 1991 HIV Solution: Men Are the Solution. Unpublished MS.

—— 1993a HIV Transmission: Men Are the Solution. Population and Environment 14(3):211–243.

—— 1993b: HIV Transmission Through Social and Geographical Networks in Uganda. Social Science and Medicine 36(7):949–955.

—— 1999 Social Science Research: Understanding and Action. In Experiencing and Understanding AIDS in Africa. C. Becker, J.-P. Dozon, C. Obbo, and M. Toure, eds. pp. 67–78. Paris: Karthala, IRD.

Obudho, R. A., 1997 Nairobi: National Capital and Regional Hub. In The Urban Challenge in Africa: Growth and Management of its Large Cities. Carole Rakodi, ed. pp. 292–334. Tokyo, Japan: United Nations University Press.

Odida, I. O., 1999 Non-Consensual Sex in Marriage and Other Forms of Sexual Abuse: The Uganda Case. London: CHANGE.

Odujinrin O. M., and Adegoke O. A., 1995. AIDS: Awareness and Blood Handling Practices of Health Care Workers in Lagos, Nigeria. European Journal of Epidemiology 11(4):425–430.

Office of National AIDS Policy, 1999 Report on the Presidential Mission on Children Orphaned by AIDS in Sub-Saharan Africa: Findings and Plan of Action. pp. 1–35. Washington, DC: Office of National AIDS Policy.

Ofori-Amoah, B., 1995 Development Research and Africa's Development Crisis. Review of Human Factor Studies 1(1):26–44.

Ogara, A. I., Nnamani, J. I., and Ameh, E. L., 1998 Knowledge, Attitude and Practice Related to HIV/AIDS and STDs in Rural Schools in Nigeria. International Conference on AIDS 12:428 (Abstract No. 23433).

Ogungbemi, S., 1992 A Philosophical View on Witchcraft in Africa. Journal of Humanities 6:1–16.

Okeyo, T. M., 1995 AIDS Orphans – a New Epidemic with Disaster Implications. Discovery and Innovation 7(1):1–2.

Okie, S., 1992 Truck Drivers Find Brothels along their Route Stocked with Condoms, Sex Education Counselors. Washington Post, 7 April: 7.

Okumu, M. I., Chege, I. N., Youri, P., and Oranga, H. O., 1994 Female Adolescent Health and Sexuality in Kenyan Secondary Schools: A Survey Report. African Medical and Research Foundation, February.

Olenja, J. M., and Kimani, V. N., Forthcoming Poverty, Street Life and Prostitution: The Dynamics of Child Prostitution in Kisumu, Kenya. In Poverty, AIDS, and Street Children in East Africa. J. L. P. Lugalla and C. G. Kibassa, eds. Lewiston, NY: Edwin Mellen Press.

Oliver, M., 1997 Emancipatory Research: Realistic Goal or Impossible Dream? In Doing Disability Research. C. Barnes and G. Mercer, eds. pp. 15–31. Leeds: The Disability Press.

Oliver, M., 1999 Final Accounts and the Parasite People. In Disability Discourse. M. Corker and S. French, eds. pp. 183–223. Buckingham: Open University Press.

Omorodion, F. I., 1999 Sexual Networking among Market Women in Benin City, Bendel State Nigeria. In The Continuing HIV/AIDS Epidemic in Africa. J. C. Caldwell and J. P. M. Ntozi, eds. pp. 9–18. Canberra: Health Transition Centre, Australian National University.

Oppong, C., 1995 A High Price to Pay for Education, Subsistence or a Place in the Job. Health Transition Review 5(Suppl.):35–56.

Oppong, J. R., 2003 Medical Geography of Sub-Saharan Africa. In Geography of Sub-Saharan Africa. Samuel Aryeetey-Attoh, ed. pp. 324–362. Upper Saddle River, NJ.: Prentice Hall.

Oppong, J. R., 1998a The Medical Consequences of Social Change: A Political Ecology of Health Care in Contemporary Ghana. Paper presented at the Department of Geography Friday Colloquium, University of Illinois at Urbana-Champaign, January 30, 1998.

——1998b A Vulnerability Interpretation of the Geography of HIV/AIDS in Ghana 1986–1995. Professional Geographer 50(4):437–448.

Oppong J. R., and Williamson, D. A., 1996 Health Care between the Cracks: Itinerant Drug Vendors and HIV/AIDS in West Africa. African Rural and Urban Studies 3(2): 13–34.

Orubuloye, I. O., 1992 Sexual Behavior, STDs and HIV/AIDS Transmission: The Role of Long Distance Drivers and Itinerant Female Hawkers in Nigeria. International Conference on AIDS, July19–24, 8(2):D425 (Abstract No. Pod 5230).

Orubuloye, I. O., Caldwell, J. C., and Caldwell, P., 1992 Diffusion and Focus in Sexual Networking: Identifying Partners and Partners' Partners. Studies in Family Planning 23(6 Pt 1):343–351.

Orubuloye, I. O., Caldwell, J. C., and Caldwell, P., 1994 Diffusion and Focus in Sexual Networking: Identifying Partners and Partners' Partners. *In* Sexual Networking and AIDS in Sub-Saharan Africa: Behavioral Research and the Social Context. I. Orubuloye, J. C. Caldwell, G. Santow, P. Caldwell, and J. Anarfi, eds. pp. 33–44. Canberra: Health Transition Centre, Australian National University.

Orubuloye, I. O, Caldwell, J. C., Santow, G., Caldwell, P., and Anarfi, J., eds., 1994 Sexual Networking and AIDS in Sub-Saharan Africa: Behavioural Research and the Social Context. Canberra: Health Transition Centre, Australian National University.

Ouma, V., 1996 A Spatio-Temporal Analysis of HIV/AIDS Diffusion in Kenya: 1986–1993. MA dissertation, Department of Geography, University of Illinois at Urbana-Champaign.

Over, M., 1992 The Macroeconomic Impact of AIDS in Sub-Saharan Africa. Washington, DC: Africa Technical Department, Population, Health, and Nutrition Division Technical Working Paper 3, World Bank.

Over, M., 1998 Towards Estimating the Impact of AIDS on Social Welfare: A Methodological Note with an Application to Malawi. DECRG Mimeo, World Bank.

Over, M., Bertozzi, S., Chin, J., N'Galy, B., and Nyamuryekunge, K., 1988 The Direct and Indirect Cost of HIV Infection in Developing Countries: The Cases of Democratic Republic of the Congo and Tanzania. *In* The Global Impact of AIDS. A. F. Fleming et al., eds. New York: Alan R. Liss.

Over, M., Mujinja, P., Ainsworth, M. et al., 1996 Coping with AIDS: Summary of Research Results on the Economic Impact of Adult Mortality from AIDS and Other Causes on Households in Kagera, Tanzania. Bukoba, Tanzania: World Bank/University of Dar es Salaam Research Project.

Owuamanam, D., 1983 Peer and Parental Influence on Sexual Activities of School-Going Adolescent in Nigeria. Adolescence 18(69):169–179.

Oyo, R., 1999 Health-Nigeria: HIV Spreads at the Rate of One Person per Minute. Inter Press Service, December 6, http://www.aegis.com/news/ips/1999/IP991205.html.

Pachai, B., ed., 1972 The Early History of Malawi. London: Longman.

Pachai, B., ed., 1973 The History of the Nation. London: Longman.

Pachai, B., ed., 1975 Land and Politics in Malawi. Ontario: Limestone Press.

Packard, R. M., 1987 Tuberculosis and Industrial Health Policy on the Witwatersrand, 1902–1932. Journal of Southern African Studies 13(2):187–209.

Packard, R. M., 1989 White Plague, Black Labour: Tuberculosis and the Political Economy of Health and Disease in South Africa. Pietermaritzburg: University of Natal Press.

Packard, R. M., and Coetzee, D., 1995 White Plague: Black Labour Revisited: TB and the Mining Industry. *In* Crossing Boundaries: Mine Migrancy in a Democratic South Africa. J. Crush and W. James, eds. pp. 101–115. Cape Town: Creda.

Packard, R. M., and Epstein, P., 1991 Epidemiologists, Social Scientists, and the Structure of Medical Research on AIDS in Africa. Social Science and Medicine 33(7):771–794.

Painter, T., 1999 Livelihood Mobility and AIDS Prevention in West Africa: Challenges and Opportunities for Social Scientists. *In* Experiencing and Understanding AIDS in Africa. C. Becker, J-P. Dozon, C. Obbo, and M. Toure, eds. pp. 645–665. Dakar: Codesria, Karthala, IRD.

Pan African News Agency, September 21, 1998.

Panos Dossier, 1990 Triple Jeopardy: Women & AIDS. London: The Panos Institute.

Parker, M., 1991 South Africa: Undermined by AIDS. South June/July:17–18.

Parker, R., 1996 Empowerment, Community Mobilization and Social Change in the Face of HIV/AIDS. AIDS 10 (Suppl. 3):S27–S31

Parker, R., Barbosa, R., and Aggleton, P., eds., 2000 Framing the Sexual Subject. pp. 110–115. Berkeley: University of California Press.

Parrinder, E. G., 1956 African Ideas of Witchcraft. Folklore 67:142–150.

Patai, D., 1991 US Academics and Third World Women: Is Ethical Research Possible? *In* Women's Words: The Feminist Practice of Oral History. S. Gluck and D. Patai, eds. pp. 137–153. London: Routledge.

Patel, S., 1996 From Seed to a Tree: Building Community Organization in India's Cities. *In* Gender in Popular Education: Methods for Empowerment. S. Walters and L. Manicom, eds. pp. 89–98. London: Zed Books.

Pattman, R., 1995 Discourses of Sex, AIDS, and Sex/AIDS Education in Zimbabwe. Unpublished Ph.D. dissertation, Institute of Education, University of London.

Patton, C., (1997) From Nation to Family: Containing African AIDS. *In* The Gender/Sexuality Reader: Culture, History, and Political Economy. R. N. Lancaster and M. di Leonardo, eds. pp. 279–290. New York: Routledge.

Peeters, M., Gaye, A., Mboup, S. et al., 1996 Presence of HIV-1 Group O Infection in West Africa. AIDS 10(3):343–344.

Peeters, M., Gueye, A., Mboup, S. et al., 1997 Geographical Distribution of HIV-1 Group O Viruses in Africa. AIDS 11(4):493–498.

Peltzer, K., 1986 Some Contributions of Traditional Healing Practices. Ph.D. dissertation, Hannover University, copy in Chancellor College Library, Zomba, Malawi.

Perlman, D., 1992 One More Problem for Third World. San Francisco Chronicle, July 20.

Phillips, O., 1997 Zimbabwean Law and the Production of a White Man's Disease. Social and Legal Studies 6(4):471–492.

Phillips, O., 1999 Sexual Offences in Zimbabwe: Fetishisms of Procreation, Perversion, and Individual Autonomy. Unpublished Ph.D. thesis, University of Cambridge.

Phillips, O., 2000 Constituting the Global Gay: Issues of Individual Subjectivity and Sexuality in Southern Africa. *In* Sexuality in the Legal Arena. C. Stychin and D. Herman, eds. pp. 17–33. London: The Athlone Press.

Phiri, D., 1998 Ulangizi. Balaka: Sounds of Malawi, IY 1098043.

Phiri, I. A., 1997 Women, Presbyterianism and Patriarchy: Religious Experience of Chewa Women in Central Malawi. Blantyre: Kachere/CLAIM.

Phiri, K., 1983 Some Changes in the Matrilineal Family System among the Chewa of Malawi since the Nineteenth Century. Journal of African History 23:257–274.

Phiri, K., 1998 Dr Banda's Cultural Legacy and its Implications for a Democratic Malawi. *In* Democratisation in Malawi: A Stocktaking. K. Phiri and K. Ross, eds. Blanytre: Kachere/CLAIM.

Phiri, K., and Ross, K., eds., 1998 Democratisation in Malawi: A Stocktaking. Blanytre: Kachere/CLAIM.

Pickering, H., and Nunn, A. J., 1997 A Three-Year Follow-Up Survey of Demographic Changes in a Ugandan Town on the Trans-African Highway with High HIV-1 Seroprevalence. Health Transition Review, 7(Suppl.):41–47.

Pickering, H., Okongo, M., Bwanika, K., Nnalusiba, B., and Whitworth, J., 1996 Sexual Mixing Patterns in Uganda: Small-Time Urban/Rural Traders. AIDS 10(5):533.

Pickering, H., Quigley, M., Hayes, R. J. et al., 1993 Determinants of Condom Use in 24,000 Prostitute/Client Contacts in the Gambia. AIDS 7:1093–1098.

Pillai, V., and Benefo, K., 1995 Teenagers in Zambia: Sexual Activity among School Going Females. International Journal of Contemporary Sociology 32(1):125–132.

Piot, P., 1997 Business in a World of HIV/AIDS. Electronic document. http://www.unaids.org/ unaids/speeches/davspc.html

Piot, P., 1999 HIV/AIDS and Violence against Women. Presentation to the United Nations Commission on the Status of Women, Forty-Third Session: Panel on Women and Health, March 3, 1999. Electronic document. http://www. unaids.org/unaids/speeches/ny3march99. html.

Piot, P., and Caraël, M., 1988 Epidemiological and Sociological Aspects of HIV-Infection in Developing Countries. British Medical Bulletin 44(1):66–88.

Pitts, M., and Jackson, H., 1993 No Joking Matter: Formal and Informal Sources of Information about AIDS in Zimbabwe. AIDS Education and Prevention 5(3):212–219.

Pool, R., Washija, R., and Maswe, M., 1995 Promiscuity, Acquiescence and Exchange: Sexual Relationships in the Fishing Villages of Magu District, Tanzania. Abstract Wec260 of paper presented at the IXth International Conference on AIDS & STDs in Africa, Kampala, December 10–14.

Potts, D., 1995 Shall We Go Home? Increasing Urban Poverty in African Cities and Migration Processes. The Geographical Journal 16:245–64.

Preble, E., 1990 Impact of HIV/AIDS on African Children. Social Science and Medicine 31(6): 671–680.

Prieur, A., 1990 Norwegian Gay Men: Reasons for the Continued Practice of Unsafe Sex. AIDS Education and Prevention 2(2):109–115.

Proceedings of a Symposium, 1999 The Declaration of Helsinki: A Symposium to Review Current Proposals for Change. Victorian Institute of Forensic Medicine, Monash University, Melbourne.

Quinn, T. C., Mann, J., Curran, J. et al., 1986 AIDS in Africa: An Epidemiologic Paradigm. Science 234:955–963.

Radcliffe-Brown, A. R., 1950 African Systems of Kinship and Marriage. New York: Oxford University Press.

Raikes, A., 1989 Women's Health in East Africa. Social Science and Medicine 28(5):447–459.

Rangeley, W. H. J., 1948 Notes on Chewa Tribal Law. Nyasaland Journal 1(3):5–58.

Ray, S., Gumbo, N., and Mbizvo, M., 1996 Local Voices: What Some Harare Men Say about Preparation for Sex. Reproductive Health Matters 7:34–45.

Rayner, S., 1992 Cultural Theory and Risk Analysis. *In* Social Theories of Risk. S. Krimsky and D. Golding, eds. Westport: Praeger.

Reeves, H., 1998 Stepping Stones to the Transformation of Gender Relations? Development and Gender in Brief, Issue 7 Health and Well-Being. Brighton: BRIDGE (Institute of Development Studies, University of Sussex).

Reid, E., 1992 Gender, Knowledge and Responsibility. *In* AIDS in the World. J. M. Mann, D. Tarantola, and T. W. Netter, eds. Cambridge, MA: Harvard University Press.

Reid, E., 1994 Approaching the HIV Epidemic: The Community's Response. AIDS Care 6(5): 551–557.

Reid, E., 1996a: HIV and Development in Multicultural Contexts. Issue Paper 20. New York: HIV and Development Programme, UNDP.

—— 1996b HIV and Development; Learning from Others. *In* AIDS as a Gender Issue: Psycho-social Perspectives. L. Sherr, C. Hankins and L. Bennett, eds. London: Taylor and Francis.

Reid, E., 1997 Placing Women at the Center of the Analysis. *In* AIDS in Africa and the Carribean. G. Bond, J. Kreniske, I. Susser, and J. Vincent, eds. pp. 159–165. Boulder, CO: Westview Press.

Report of a workshop held at the Royal Society of Medicine, London, 1999 Revising the Declaration of Helsinki: A Fresh Start. Bulletin of Medical Ethics 151:13–17.

Republic of Kenya, 1991 National Development Plan 1994–96. Nairobi: Government Printer.

Republic of Kenya, Ministry of Health, 1997 Sessional Paper No. 4 of 1997 on AIDS in Kenya. Nairobi: Republic of Kenya, Ministry of Health.

Republic of Zambia, 1997 Mid-Term Review of the Second Medium Term Plan (MTP II) for the Prevention and Control of HIV/AIDS in Zambia. Lusaka.

Richards, A. I., 1956 Chisungu: A Girl's Initiation Ceremony among the Bemba of Northern Rhodesia. London: Faber and Faber Limited.

Rivers, K., and Aggleton, P. 1999 Men and the HIV Epidemic. Gender and the HIV Epidemic. New York: UNDP HIV and Development Program. Electronic document. http://www.undp.org/hiv/publications/gender/mene.htm>, accessed March 22, 2000.

Robb, C., 1999 Can the Poor Influence Policy? Participatory Poverty Assessments in the Developing World. Washington DC: The World Bank.

Roles, N. C., 1966 Tribal Surgery in East Africa during the XIXth Century. East African Medical Journal 43(12):570–594.

Romaniuk, A., 1967 La Fécondité des Populations Congolaises. Paris: Mouton.

Rosegrant, M. W., Agcaoili-Sombilla, M., and Perez, N. D., 1995 Global Food Projections to 2020: Implications for Investment. Food, Agriculture, and the Environment Discussion Paper 5. Washington, DC: International Food Policy Research Institute.

Rosenbaum, E., and Kandel, D. B., 1990 Early Onset of Adolescent Sexual Behavior and Drug Involvement. Journal of Marriage and the Family 52:783.

Rosenberg, C., 1992 Framing Disease: Illness, Society, and History. In Framing Disease: Studies in Cultural History. C. Rosenberg and J. Golden, eds. New Brunswick: Rutgers University Press.

Rosenstock, I. M., Stetcher, V. J., and Becker, M. H., 1988 Social Learning Theory and the Health Belief Model. Health Education Quarterly 15:178–183.

Ross, A. C., 1996 Blantyre Mission and the Making of Modern Malawi. Blantyre: Kachere/CLAIM.

Ross, J., Stover, J., and Willard, A., 1999 Profiles for Family Planning and Reproductive Health Programs for 116 Countries. Washington, DC: The Futures Group International.

Rotberg, R., 1966 The Rise of Nationalism in Central Africa: The Making of Malawi and Zambia. Harvard: Harvard University Press.

Rothman, D., 2000 The Shame of Medical Research. The New York Review of Books XLVII (19):60–64.

Rowley, J. T., Anderson, R. M., and Ng, T. W., 1990 Reducing the Spread of HIV Infection in Sub-Saharan Africa: Some Demographic and Economic Implications. AIDS 4:47–56.

Rude, D., 1999 Reasonable Men and Provocative Women: An Analysis of Gendered Domestic Homicide in Zambia. Journal of Southern African Studies 25(1):7–27.

Rugalema, G., 1997 Asserting Life in the Presence of Death: How Young Tanzanians View their Life Chances in Environments of High HIV Prevalence. Project document, Agrarian Technology Group (TAO), Wageningen Agricultural University.

Rugalema, G., 1999a Adult Mortality as Entitlement Failure: AIDS and the Crisis of Rural Livelihoods in a Buhaya Village, Bukoba District, Tanzania. Doctoral dissertation submitted to the Institute of Social Studies, The Hague (also published in August 1999 by Shaker Publishers, Maastricht).

—— 1999b HIV/AIDS and the Commercial Agriculture Sector of Kenya: Impact, Vulnerability, Susceptibility and Coping Strategies. Rome: Consultancy Report, FAO.

Rugalema, G. H., Johnsen, F. H., and Rugambisa, J., 1994 The Homegarden Agroforestry System of Bukoba District, North-Western Tanzania: 2. Constraints to Farm Productivity. Agroforestry Systems 26:205–214.

Rukarangira, Wa N., Ngirabakunzi, K. D., Bihini, Y., and Kitembo, M., 1990 Evaluation of the AIDS Information Program Using Mass Media Campaign in Lubumbashi, Zaire. Abstract FD 844, VI International AIDS Conference, San Francisco, June 20–24.

Rukarangira, Wa N., and Schoepf, B. G., 1991 Unrecorded Trade in Shaba and Across Zaire's Southern Borders. In The Real Economy of Zaire. J. MacGaffey, ed. pp. 72–96. London: James Currey and Philadelphia: University of Pennsylvania Press.

Runganga, A., Pitts, M., and McMaster, J., 1992 The Use of Herbal and Other Agents to Enhance Sexual Experience. Social Science and Medicine 35(8):1037–1042.

Rundstrom, R., and Deur, D., 1999 Reciprocal Appropriation: Towards an Ethics of Cross-Cultural Research. *In* Geography and Ethics: Journeys Through a Moral Terrain. J. Proctor and D. Smith, eds. pp. 237–250. London: Routledge.

Rushing, W. A., 1995 The AIDS Epidemic: Social Dimensions of an Infectious Disease. Boulder, CO: Westview Press (see Chapter 3 of this book).

Rushton, J. P., and Bogaert, A. F., 1989 Population Differences in Susceptibility to AIDS: An Evolutionary Analysis. Social Science and Medicine 28:1211.

Russell, S. S., Jacobsen, K., and Stanley, W. D., 1990 International Migration and Development in Sub-Saharan Africa, Vol. I: Overview, Vol. II: Country Analyses. World Bank Discussion Papers, Africa Technical Department Series, 101. Washington, DC: World Bank.

Rutayuga, J. B., 1992 Assistance to AIDS Orphans within the Family/Kinship System: A Program for East Africa. AIDS Education and Prevention (Fall, Suppl.):57–68.

Ryder, R. W., Hassig, S. E., Kamega, M. et al., 1989 Perinatal Transmission of HIV-1 to Infants of Seropositive Women in Zaire. New England Journal of Medicine 320 (22 June): 1637–1642.

Ryder, R. W., Kamenga, M., Nkusu, M., Batter, V., and Heyward, W. L., 1994 AIDS Orphans in Kinshasa, Zaire: Incidence and Socio-economic Consequences. AIDS 8(5):673–679.

Ryder, R. W., Ndilu, M., Hassig, S. E. et al., 1990 Heterosexual Transmission of HIV-1 among Employees and their Spouses at Two Large Businesses in Zaire. AIDS 4:725–732.

Sabatier, R., 1996 Migrants and AIDS: Themes of Vulnerability and Resistance. *In* Crossing Borders: Migrations, Ethnicity and AIDS. M. Haour-Knipe and R. Rector, eds. pp. 86–111. London: Taylor and Francis.

Sachs, A., 1994 The Last Commodity: Child Prostitution in the Developing World. World Watch 7:24–30.

Sachs, J., 2001 Macroeconomics and Health: Investing in Health for Economic Development. Commissioned report. Geneva: World Health Organization (WHO).

Sadik, N., 1992 World Population Continues to Rise. *In* Third World 92/93. 14th edition. Guildford: Duskin Publishing.

Sanders, D., and Sambo, A., 1991 AIDS in Africa: The Implications of Economic Recession and Structural Adjustment. Health Policy and Planning 6:157–165.

Sassan-Morokro, M., Greenberg, A. E., Coulibaly, I. M., Coulibaly, D., Sidibe, K., Ackah, A., Tossou, O., Gnaore, E., Wiktor, S. Z., De Cock, K. M., 1996 High Rates of Sexual Contact with Female Sex Workers, Sexually Transmitted Diseases, Condom Neglect among HIV-Infected and Uninfected Men with Tuberculosis in Abidjan, Côte d'Ivoire. Journal of Acquired Immune Deficiency Syndrome and Human Retrovirology 11(2):183–187.

Schoepf, B. G., 1978 Women in the Informal Economy of Lubumbashi: The Case of the Ndumba. Paper presented at the IV International Congress of African Studies, Kinshasa, December.

Schoepf, B. G., 1983 Health for Rural Women. Community Action (Zimbabwe) 1(1): 26–27.

Schoepf, B. G., 1986 CONNAISSIDA: AIDS Control Research and Interventions in Zaire. Proposal submitted to the Rockefeller Foundation, November 12.

Schoepf, B. G., 1988 Women, AIDS and Economic Crisis in Central Africa. Canadian Journal of African Studies 22(3):625–644.

Schoepf, B. G., 1991a Ethical, Methodological and Political Issues of AIDS Research in Central Africa. Social Science and Medicine 33(7):749–763.

——1991b Representations du Sida et Pratiques Populaires a Kinshasa. Anthropologie et Societes 15(2–3):149–166.

Schoepf, B. G., 1992a Women at Risk: Case Studies from Zaire. *In* The Time of AIDS: Social Analysis, Theory and Method. G. Herdt and S. Lindenbaum, eds. pp. 259–286. Newbury Park, CA: Sage Publications Inc.

——1992b: AIDS, Sex and Condoms: African Healers and the Reinvention of Tradition in Zaire. Medical Anthropology 14:225–242.

——1992c: Sex, Gender and Society in Zaire. *In* Sexual Behaviour and Networking: Anthropological and Sociocultural Studies on the Transmission of HIV. T. Dyson, ed. pp. 353–375. Liège: Editions Derouaux-Ordina.

Schoepf, B. G., 1993 AIDS Action-Research on AIDS with Women in Kinshasa. Social Science and Medicine 37(11):1401–1413.

Schoepf, B. G., 1995 Culture, Sex Research and AIDS Prevention in Africa. *In* Culture and Sexual Risk: Anthropological Perspectives on AIDS. H. T. Brummelhuis and G. Herdt, eds. pp. 29–51. Luxembourg: Gordon and Breach Publishers.

Schoepf, B. G., 1998 Inscribing the Body Politic: Women and Aids in Africa. *In* Pragmatic Women and Body Politics. M. Lock and P. Kaufert, eds. pp. 98–126. Cambridge: Cambridge University Press.

Schoepf, B. G., 2000 Theoretical therapies, Remote Remedies: SAPs and the Political Ecology of Poverty and Health in Africa. *In* Dying for Growth: Global Inequality and the Health of the Poor. J. Kim, J. Millen, A. Irwin, and J. Gershman, eds. pp. 91–126. Monroe, ME: Common Courage Press.

Schoepf, B. G., 2001 International AIDS Research in Anthropology: A Critical Perspective on the Crisis. Annual Review of Anthropology 30:335–361.

Schoepf, B. G., 2002 "Mobutu's Disease": A Social History of AIDS in DRC. Review of African Economy: 93–94.

Schoepf, B. G., 2004 Gender, Sex and Power: A Social History of AIDS in Mobutu's Zaire. MA: Blackwell.

Schoepf, B. G., and Mariotti, A. M., 1975 Politics of theory: Participant Observation in the United States. *In* Women Cross-Culturally: Challenge and Change. R. Rohrich-Leavitt, ed. pp. 389–419. The Hague: Mouton.

Schoepf, B. G., Rukarangira, Wa N., Payanzo, N., Walu, E., and Schoepf, C., 1988a AIDS, Women and Society in Central Africa. *In* AIDS, 1988 AAAS Symposium Papers. R. Kulstad, ed. pp. 175–181. Washington, DC: American Association for the Advancement of Science.

Schoepf, B. G., Rukarangira, Wa N., Schoepf, C. et al., 1988b AIDS and Society in Central Africa: A View from Zaire. *In* AIDS in Africa: Social and Policy Impact. N. Miller and R. Rockwell, eds. pp. 211–235. Lewiston, NY: Mellen Press.

Schoepf, B. G., Schoepf, C., and Millen, J. V., 2000 Theoretical Therapies, Remote Remedies: SAPs and the Political Ecology of Health in Africa. *In* Dying for Growth: Global Inequality and the Health of the Poor. J. Y. Kim, J. V. Millen, A. Irwin, and J. Gershman, eds. pp. 91–125, 440–457 & References. Monroe, ME: Common Courage Press.

Schoepf, B. G., and Walu, E., 1991 Women's Trade and Contribution to Household Budgets in Kinshasa. *In* The Real Economy of Zaire. J. MacGaffey, ed. pp. 124–151. London: James Currey and Philadelphia: University of Pennsylvania Press.

Schoepf, B. G., Walu, E. V., Rukarangira, Wa N. et al., 1991 Gender, Power and Risk of AIDS in Central Africa. *In* Women and Health in Africa. M. Turshen, ed. pp. 187–203. Trenton, NJ: Africa World Press.

Schoepf, B. G., Walu, E., Russell, D., and Schoepf, C., 1991 Women and Structural Adjustment in Zaire. *In* Structural Adjustment and African Women Farmers. C. Gladwin, ed. pp. 151– 168. Gainesville: University of Florida Press.

Schoffeleers, J. M., 1979 Guardians of the Land: Essays on Central African Territorial Cults. Gweru: Mambo.

Schoffeleers, J. M., 1997 Religion and the Dramatisation of Life. Blantyre: Kachere/CLAIM.

Schoffeleers, J. M., 1999 The AIDS Pandemic, the Prophet Billy Chisupe, and the Democratisation Process in Malawi. Journal of Religion in Africa 29(4):406–441.

Schoffeleers, J. M., and Roscoe, A. A.,1985 Land of Fire: Oral Literature from Malawi. Blantyre: Popular Publications.

Schoofs, M., and Waldholz, M., 2000 Drug Firms, Senegal Set HIV Drug Pact. Wall Street Journal, October 24: A3.

Schoofs, M., and Waldholz, M., 2001 New Regimen: AIDS-Drug Price War Breaks Out in Africa, Goaded By Generics. Wall Street Journal, March 7: A1.

Scott, S., and Mercer, M., 1994 Understanding Cultural Obstacles to HIV/AIDS Prevention in Africa. AIDS Education and Prevention 8:81–89.

Seale, J., 1986 Infectious AIDS. Nature 320:391.

Sebunya, C., 1995 The Educated Still Think Ignorance Is Bliss. AIDS Analysis Africa 5(3):16.

Seeley, J., Kajura, E., Bachengana, C., Okongo, M., Wagner, U., and Mulder, D., 1993 The Extended Family and Support for People with AIDS in a Rural Population in South West Uganda: A Safety Net with Holes? AIDS Care 5:117–122.

Seeley, J., Kengeya-Kayondo, J., and Mulder, D., 1992 Community-Based HIV/AIDS Research – Whither Community Participation? Unsolved Problems in a Research Programme in Rural Uganda. Social Science and Medicine 34(10):1089–1095.

Seidel, G., 1993 The Competing Discourses of HIV/AIDS in Sub-Saharan Africa: Discourses of Rights and Empowerment versus Discourses of Control and Exclusion. Social Science and Medicine 36(3):175–194.

Seidman, G., 1984 Women in Zimbabwe: Post-Independence Struggles. Feminist Studies 10(3):(Fall).

Serwadda, D., Gray, R., Kiwanuka, N., Sewakambo, N. K., Kelly, R., and Wawer, M., 2000 Potential Efficacy of Male Circumcision for HIV Prevention in Rakai, Uganda. Program and Abstracts of the XIII International AIDS Conference, July 9–14, Durban, South Africa. Abstract Moorc194.

Serwadda D., Wawer, M. J., Musgrave, S. D., Sewankambo, N. K., Kaplan, J. E., and Gray, R. H., 1992 HIV Risk Factors in Three Geographical Strata of Rural Rakai District, Uganda. AIDS 6(9):983–989.

Serwadda, D., Mhalu, F., Karita, E., and Moses, S., 1994 HIV and AIDS in East Africa. *In* AIDS in Africa. M. Essex, S. Mboup, P. Kanki, and M. Kalengayi, eds. New York: Raven Press.

Setel, P., 1996 AIDS as a Paradox of Manhood and Development in Kilimanjaro, Tanzania. Social Science and Medicine 43(8):1169–1178.

Setel, P., 1999 Local Histories of Sexually Transmitted Diseases and AIDS in Western and Northern Tanzania. *In* Histories of Sexually Transmitted Diseases and HIV/AIDS in Sub-Saharan Africa. P. W. Setel, M. Lewis, and M. Lyons, eds. pp. 119–142. Westport, CT: Greenwood Press.

Setel, P. W., Lewis, M., and Lyons, M., eds., 1999 Histories of Sexually Transmitted Diseases and HIV/AIDS in Sub-Saharan Africa. Westport, CT: Greenwood Press.

Shannon, G. W., and Pyle, G. F., 1989 The Origin and Diffusion of AIDS: A View from Medical Geography. Annals of the Association of American Geographers 79(1):1–24.

Shannon, G. W., Pyle, G., and Bashushur, R. L., 1991 The Geography of AIDS. New York: Guilford Press.

Sharma, Rohit 2000 AIDS Vaccine Research Focuses on Subtypes in Developed World. British Medical Journal 321(7264):787.

Shaw, C., 1995 Colonial Inscriptions: Race, Sex and Class in Kenya. Minneapolis: University of Minnesota Press.

Shaw, R., 2000 "Tok Af, Lef Af": A Political Economy of Temne Techniques of Secrecy and Self. *In* African Philosophy as Cultural Inquiry. I. Karp and D. A. Masolo, eds. pp. 25–49. Bloomington, Indiana University Press.

Shepard, D. S., 1997 Levels and Determinants of Expenditures on HIV/AIDS in Five Developing Countries. Background papers to Confronting Aids. Electronic document. http://www.worldbank.org/.

Shepperson, G., and Price, T., 1958 Independent African. Edinburgh: Edinburgh University Press.

Sherr, L., Hankins, C., and Bennett, L., 1996 AIDS as a Gender Issue: Psychosocial Perspectives. London: Taylor & Francis.

Shire, C., 1994 Men Don't Go to the Moon: Language, Space and Masculinities in Zimbabwe. *In* Dislocating Masculinities: Comparative Ethnographies. A. Cornwall and N. Lindisfarne, eds. pp. 147–158. London: Routledge.

Short, P., 1974 Banda. London: Routledge & Kegan Paul.

Shostak, M., 1981 Nisa: The Life and Words of !Kung Woman. Cambridge, MA: Harvard University Press.

Siegel, K., and Gorey, E., 1994 Childhood Bereavement due to Parental Death from Acquired-Immunodeficiency-Syndrome. Journal of Development and Behavioral Pediatrics 15(3)(Suppl.):S66–S70.

Singh, S., 2000 Only the Rich Can Live. World Press Review 47(2):30.

Singh, Y. N., Joshi, R., and Rustagi, C., 1992 Truck Drivers: Their Possible Role in Disseminating HIV in Rural India. Second International Congress on AIDS in Asia and the Pacific, New Delhi, November [Abstract D626].

Sitas, A., 1985 From Grassroots Control to Democracy: A Case Study of the Impact of Trade Unionism on Migrant Workers' Cultural Formations. Social Dynamics 11(1):32–43.

Siziya, S., and Hakim, J. G., 1996 Differential Human Immunodeficiency Virus Risk Factors among Female General Nurses, Nurse Midwives and Office Workers/Teachers in Zambia. Central African Journal of Medicine 42(4):114–117.

Siziya, S., Hakim, J. G., Rusakaniko, S., Matchaba-Hove, R. B., and Chideme-Maradzika, J., 1996 Non-Condom Use among Female Nurses in Zambia. Central African Journal of Medicine 42(7):188–191.

Slack, P., 1992 Epidemics and Ideas: Essays on Historical Perception of Pestilence. Cambridge: Cambridge University Press.

Sliep, Y., 1995 Malawi After Banda: Building New Bridges. AIDS Analysis Africa 5(1):4–5.

Slutsker, L., Cabeza, J., Wirima, J., and Steketee, R., 1994 HIV-1 Infection among Women of Reproductive Age in a Rural District in Malawi. AIDS 8:1337–1340.

Smallman-Raynor, M., Cliff, A., and Haggett, P., 1992 International Atlas of AIDS. London: Blackwell.

Smallman-Raynor, M. R., and Cliff, A. D., 1991 Civil War and the Spread of AIDS in Central Africa. Epidemiology and Infection 103:69–80.

Smith, D., and Blanc, M., 1997 Grassroots Democracy and Participation: A New Analytical and Practical Approach. Environment and Planning D, Society and Space 15:281–303.

Smith, D. C., 1990 Thailand: AIDS Crisis Looms. Lancet 335:781–782.

Smith, M., and Katner, H., 1995. Quasi-Experimental Evaluation of Three AIDS Prevention Activities for Maintaining Knowledge, Improving Attitudes, and Changing Risk Behaviors of High School Seniors. AIDS Education and Prevention 7(5):391–402.

Soros, G., 2002 On Globalization. New York: Public Affairs.

Southall, A., ed., 1961 Social Change in Modern Africa. London: Oxford University Press.

Sowell, R. L., 2000 AIDS Orphans: The Cost of Doing Nothing. AIDS Care 11(6):15–16.

Specter, M., 1998 Doctors Powerless as AIDS Rakes Africa. New York Times, August 6: A,1.

Stacey, J., 1991 Can There Be a Feminist Ethnography? *In* Women's Words: The Feminist Practice of Oral History. S. Gluck and D. Patai, eds. pp. 111–119. London: Routledge.

Staeheli, L., and Lawson, V., 1994 A Discussion of "Women in the Field": The Politics of Feminist Fieldwork. Professional Geographer 46(1):54–102.

Standing, G., 1989 Global Feminization through Flexible Labor. World Development 17(7): 1077–1096.

Stanecki, K. A., and Way, P. O., 1996 The Dynamic HIV/AIDS Pandemic. *In* AIDS in the World II: Global Dimensions, Social Roots, and Responses. J. M. Mann and D. J. M. Tarantola, eds. pp. 41–56. New York: Oxford University Press.

Stannus, H. S., 1910 Some Notes on Some Tribes of British Central Africa. Journal of the Royal Anthropological Institute of Great Britain and Ireland Journal 40:285–334.

Stark, E., 1977 The Epidemic as a Social Event. International Journal of Health Services 7:681–705.

Stauffer, P., 1999 Making Lab Tests More Accurate: Ghanaian Effort Offers Model Process. Impact on HIV 1(2), Family Health International. Electronic document. http://www.fhi.org/en/aids/impact/iohiv/ioh12/ioh125.html.

STD/AIDS Control Programme, Ministry of Health, 1996 A Report on Declining Trends in HIV Infection Rates in Sentinel Surveillance Sites in Uganda. Entebbe, Uganda: Ministry of Health.

Steen, R., Vulsteke, B., De Cotto, T. et al., 2000 Evidence of Declining STD Prevalence in a South African Mining Community following a Core Group Intervention. Sexually Transmitted Diseases 27:1–8.

Stein, Z., 1990 HIV Prevention: The Need for Methods Women Can Use. American Journal of Public Health 80:460–462.

Stevenson, D., 1964 The Health Services of Malawi. MD thesis 2504, Glasgow University.

Stewart, F., 1989 Recession, Structural Adjustment and Infant Health: The Need for a Human Face. Transactions of Royal Society of Tropical Medicine and Hygiene 834:30–31.

Stewart, G., 2000 Rumba on the River: A History of the Popular Music of the Two Congos. London: Verso.

Stiglitz, J., 2002 A Fair Deal for the World. New York Review of Books XLIX (9):24–28.

Stiglitz, J. E., 1993 Economics. New York: Norton.

Stock, R., 1995 Africa South of the Sahara – a Geographical Interpretation. New York: Guilford Press.

Stockdale, J., 1995 The Self and Media Messages: Match or Mismatch? In Representations of Health, Illness and Handicap. I. Markova and R. Farr, eds. London: Harwood.

Stockhausen, K., 2000 The Declaration of Helsinki: Revising Ethical Research Guidelines for the 21st Century. Medical Journal of Australia 172:252–253.

Stover, J., Walker, N., Garnett, G. P., Salomon, J. A., Stanecki, K. A., Ghys, P. D., Grassly, N. C., Anderson, R. M., and Schwartländer, B., 2002 Can We Reverse the HIV/AIDS Pandemic with an Expanded Response? The Lancet 360:73–77.

Streefland, P., Harnmeijer, J-W., and Chabot, J., 1995 Implications of Economic Crisis and Structural Adjustment Policies for PHC in the Periphery. In African Primary Health Care in Times of Economic Turbulence. J. Chabot, J-W. Harnmeijer and P.H. Streefland, eds. pp. 11–18. Amsterdam: Royal Tropical Institute.

Studdert, D., and Brennan, T., 1998 Clinical Trials in Developing Countries: Scientific and Ethical Issues. Medical Journal of Australia 169:545–548.

Stychin, C. F., 1998 A Nation by Rights: National Cultures, Sexual Identity Politics and the Discourse of Rights. Philadelphia: Temple University Press.

Sunday Vision, 1997 Bigger Sex Back to Lyantonde. Sunday Vision, September 28.

Sundkler, B., 1980 Bara Bukoba: The Church and the Society in Tanzania. London: C. Hurst.

Swantz, M. L., 1985 Women in Development: A Creative Role Denied? London: C. Hurst.

Sweat, M., and Denison, J., 1995 Reducing HIV Incidence in Developing Countries with Structural and Environmental Interventions. AIDS 9(Suppl. A):S251–S257.

Taha, T. E., Dallabeta, G., Chiphangwi, J. D., Mtimavalye, L. A. R, Liomba, N. G., Kumwenda, N., Hoover, D., and Miotti, P., 1998 Trends of HIV-1 and Sexually Transmitted Diseases among Pregnant and Postpartum Women in Urban Malawi. Unpublished MS, copy at College of Medicine Library, Blantyre.

Tajfel, H., 1981 Human Groups and Social Categories: Studies in Social Psychology. Cambridge: Cambridge University Press.

Taljaard, R., Taljaard, D., Auvert, B., and Neilssen, G., 2000 Cutting It Fine: Male Circumcision Practices and the Transmission of STDs in Carletonville. Program and Abstracts of the XIII International AIDS Conference, Durban, South Africa, July 9–14, 2000. Abstract Moorc195.

Talle, A., 1995 Bar Workers at the Border. *In* Young People at Risk: Fighting AIDS in Northern Tanzania. K. Knut-Inge, P. M. Biswalo, and A. Talle, eds. pp. 18–30. Scandinavia: Scandinavian University Press.

Tansi, S. L., 1995 Le Commencement des Douleurs. Paris: éditions Du Seuil.

Tansi, S. L., n.d. Congrès Mondial Des Peuples Kongo.

Tanzania Gender Networking Programme (TGNP) and SARDC-WIDSAA, 1997 Beyond Inequalities: Women in Tanzania. Dar-Es-Salaam and Harare: TGNP and SARDC.

TAP (Tanzania AIDS Project), 1994 National Assessment of Families and Children Affected by AIDS. Dar es Salaam: USAID.

Tastemain, C., and Coles, P., 1993 Can a Culture Stop AIDS in its Tracks? New Scientist 139 (September 11):13–14.

Tawil, O., Verster, A., and O'Reilly, K., 1995 Enabling Approaches for HIV/AIDS Prevention: Can We Modify the Environment and Minimize the Risk? AIDS 9:1299–1306.

Taylor, C. C., 1995 Rwanda Baseline Assessment. Prepared for AIDSCAP.

Tembo, K. C., 1993 Village Health Committees as Instruments for Primary Health Care Promotion. Society of Malawi Journal 46(1):38–42.

Tembo, K. C., and Phiri, T. B., 1993 Sexually Based Cultural Practices Implicated in the Transmission of HIV/AIDS. Society of Malawi Journal 46(1):43–48.

Temple, R., 1982 Government Viewpoint of Clinical Trials. Drug Information Journal 16: 10–17.

Temple, R., 1996 Problems in Interpreting Active Control Equivalence Trials. Accountability in Research 4:267–275.

Tevera, D. S., 1997 Structural Adjustment and Health Care in Zimbabwe. *In* Issues and Perspectives on Health Care in Contemporary Sub-Saharan Africa. E. Kalipeni and P. Thiuri, eds. pp. 227–242. Lewiston, NY: The Edwin Mellen Press.

Thiuri, P. J., 1996 AIDS Orphans Care: A Policy Challenge for Sub-Saharan Africa. African Rural and Urban Studies 3(2):163–192.

Thomas, T. S. W., 1930 Despatch from Governor to Colonial Office. Zomba: MNA M680/30.

Thompson, T. J., 1995 Christianity in Northern Malawi: Donald Fraser's Missionary Methods and Ngoni Culture. Leiden: E. J. Brill.

Tibaijuka, A. K., 1984 An Analysis of Smallholder Banana/Coffee Farms in Kagera, Tanzania. Causes for the Decline in Productivity and Strategies for Revitalization. Ph.D. dissertation, Swedish University of Agricultural Sciences, Uppsala.

Tibaijuka, A. K., 1997 AIDS and Economic Welfare in Peasant Agriculture: Case Studies from Kagabiro Village, Kagera Region. World Development 25(6):963–975.

Timaeus, I., and Lush, L., 1995 Intra-Urban Differentials in Child Health. Health Transition Review 5(2):163–190.

Time Bomb Ticks South of the Sahara, 1-7-1999. Electronic document. Af-Aids-Admin @Hivnet.Ch.

Tlou, S. D., 1990 Health Status of Botswanan Women. Women's Studies International Forum 12(2):167–174.

Todaro, M., 1989a Urbanization and Rural–Urban Migration: Theory and Policy. *In* Economic Development in the Third World. M. Todaro, ed. pp. 263–289, chapter 9. New York: Longman.

——1989b Economic Development in the Third World. New York: Longman.

Treichler, P., 1992a Beyond Cosmo: AIDS, Identity, and Inscriptions of Gender. Camera Obscura 28:21–78.

——1992b AIDS, HIV and the Cultural Construction of Reality. *In* The Time of AIDS, Social Analysis, Theory and Method. G. Herdt and S. Lindenbaum, eds. pp. 65–98. London: Sage Publications.

Treichler, P., 1999 How to Theory in an Epidemic: Cultural Chronicles of AIDS. Durham: Duke University Press.

Tritton, A. S., 1962 Islam. London: Hutchison and Company.

Tsoka, M. G., 1999 Analysis of the HIV/AIDS Epidemic and the High Population Growth in Malawi. Paper for the Policy Analysis Project for Dr. A Conroy, Project Coordinator, Office of the Vice President, Lilongwe 3. Copy at the Centre for Social Research, Zomba.

Turshen, M., 1984 The Political Ecology of Disease in Tanzania. New Brunswick: Rutgers University Press.

Turshen, M., 1989 The Politics of Public Health. London: Zed Books.

Turshen, M., ed., 1991 Women and Health in Africa. Trenton, NJ: Africa World Press.

Turshen, M., 1999a West African Workshop on Women in the Aftermath of Civil War. Review of African Political Economy 26(79):123–131.

—— 1999b Privatizing Health Services in Africa. New Brunswick: Rutgers University Press.

Ugalde, A., 1985 Ideological Dimensions of Community Participation in Latin American Health Programs. Social Science and Medicine 21(1):41–53.

Ulin, P., 1992 African Women and AIDS: Negotiating Behavioral Change. Social Science and Medicine 34(1):63–73.

UN Integrated Regional Information Network, 2000 South Africa Allocates US $64 Million for AIDS Orphans. October 20, 2000.

UN Population Institute, 2001 World Population Data Sheet. Electronic document. http://www.iisd.ca.

UNAIDS, 1997a Multi-Center Study, Phase One: Qualitative Information (A Draft Report of Kisumu Study Site). Kisumu, Kenya: Department of Community Health.

—— 1997b Refugees and AIDS: UNAIDS Point of View. Geneva: UNAIDS.

UNAIDS, 1998a AIDS in Africa, Johannesburg, November 30, 1998. Electronic document. http://www.unaids.org/ highband/fact/saepap98.htm.

—— 1998b AIDS and the Military. [UNAIDS Point of View, in UNAIDS Best Practice Collection]. Electronic document. http://www. unaids.org/highband/.

—— 1998c UNAIDS/WHO Working Group on Global HIV/AIDS and STD Surveillance. Geneva: UNAIDS.

—— 1998d Country Epidemiological Fact Sheet on HIV/AIDS and Sexually Transmitted Diseases. New York: UNAIDS.

—— 1998e AIDS and the Military. Geneva: UNAIDS Best Practice Collection. Electronic document. http://www.unaids.org/publications/documents/sectors/military/militarypve.pdf.

UNAIDS, 1999a Syntheses of Comparative Analysis: General Population. Preliminary Report. Geneva: UNAIDS.

—— 1999b Sexual Behavior Change for HIV: Where Have the Theories Taken Us? Geneva: UNAIDS.

—— 1999c AIDS Epidemic Update: December 1999. Electronic document. http://www.unaids.org.

—— 1999d Meeting Statement on the Africa Partnership against HIV/AIDS, April 23/24, 1999. Electronic document. http://www.unaids.org/unaids/doc/london%2sdoutcome.htm.

—— 1999e Acting Early to Prevent AIDS: The Case of Senegal. Geneva: UNAIDS. Electronic document. http://www.unaids.org/bestpractice/collection/country/senegal/senegal.html.

—— 1999f Gender and HIV/AIDS: Taking Stock of Research and Programs. Geneva: UNAIDS. Electronic document. http://www.unaids.org/publications/documents/human/gender/una99e16.pdf.

—— 1999g Report on the Global HIV/AIDS Epidemic: AIDS in a New Millennium: A Grim Picture with Glimmers of Hope. Electronic document. http://www.unaids.org/epidemic_update/report/epi_report_ chap_millenium.htm.

UNAIDS, 2000 AIDS Epidemic Update. Electronic document. www.unaids.org.

—— 2000a Report on the Global HIV/AIDS Epidemic – June 2000. Geneva: UNAIDS.

—— 2000b Report on the Global HIV/AIDS Epidemic. Geneva: UNAIDS. Electronic document. http://www.unaids.org/epidemic_update.

——2000c Cameroon Epidemiological Fact Sheet on HIV/AIDS and Sexually Transmitted Infections. Geneva: UNAIDS. Electronic document. http://www.unaids.org/hivaidsinfo/statistics/june00/fact_sheets/pdfs/cameroon.pdf.

——2000d Benin Epidemiological Fact Sheet on HIV/AIDS and Sexually Transmitted Infections. Geneva: UNAIDS. Electronic document. http://www.unaids.org/hivaidsinfo/statistics/june00/fact_sheets/pdfs/benin.pdf.

——2000e Liberia Epidemiological Fact Sheet on HIV/AIDS and Sexually Transmitted Infections. Geneva: UNAIDS. Electronic document. http://www.unaids.org/hivaidsinfo/statistics/june00/fact_sheets/pdfs/liberia.pdf.

——2000f Sierra Leone Epidemiological Fact Sheet on HIV/AIDS and Sexually Transmitted Infections. Geneva: UNAIDS. Electronic document. http://www.unaids.org/hivaidsinfo/statistics/june00/fact_sheets/pdfs/sierraleone.pdf.

——2000g Nigeria Epidemiological Fact Sheet on HIV/AIDS and Sexually Transmitted Infections. Geneva: UNAIDS. Electronic document. http://www.unaids.org/hivaidsinfo/statistics/june00/fact_sheets/pdfs/nigeria.pdf.

——2000h Civil Society Essential to Fighting AIDS. Press Release 2000. Electronic document. http://www.unaids.org/whatsnew/press/eng/cotonou091000.html.

——2000i Nigeria Pivotal in African AIDS Response. Press Release 2000. Electronic document. http://www.unaids.org/whatsnew/press/eng/abuja300300.html.

——2000j International Partnership against AIDS in Africa. Weekly Bulletin #35. Electronic document. http://www.unaids.org/africapartnership/bulletin/apb271100.html.

——2000k AIDS Devastates Health Sector in Africa. Electronic document. http://www.unaids.org/whatsnew/press/eng/ouagadougou070500.html.

——2000l: Men and AIDS – A Gendered Approach: 2000 World AIDS Campaign. New York: UNAIDS. Electronic document. http://www.unaids.org/wac/2000/campaign.html>], accessed March 20, 2000.

UNAIDS, 2001a Epidemic Update. Electronic document. http://www.unaids.org.

——2001b Home page. Electronic document. http://www.unaids.org/accessed 12/02/01.

UNAIDS, 2003 Epidemic Update. Washington, DC.

UNAIDS and Economic Commission for Africa (ECA), 2000. AIDS in Africa: Country by Country. Africa Development Forum 2000. Geneva, Switzerland: UNAIDS. Electronic document. http://www.unaids.org/wac/2000/wad00/files/AIDS_in_Africa.htm.

UNAIDS/WHO, 2000a HIV/AIDS: The Global Epidemic. Electronic document. http://hivinsite.ucsf.edu/social/ un2098.401c.html.

——2000b Epidemiological Fact Sheet on HIV/AIDS and Sexually Transmitted Diseases, Botswana. Electronic document. http://www.unaids.org/hivaidsinfo/statistics/fact_sheets/pdfs/Botswana_en.pdf.

——2000c Epidemiological Fact Sheet on HIV/AIDS and Sexually Transmitted Diseases, Lesotho. Electronic document. http://www.unaids.org/hivaidsinfo/statistics/fact_sheets/pdfs/Lesotho_en.pdf.

——2000d Epidemiological Fact Sheet on HIV/AIDS and Sexually Transmitted Diseases, Malawi. Electronic document. http://www.unaids.org/hivaidsinfo/statistics/fact_sheets/pdfs/Malawi_en.pdf.

——2000e Epidemiological Fact Sheet on HIV/AIDS and Sexually Transmitted Diseases. South Africa. Electronic document. http://www.unaids.org/hivaidsinfo/statistics/fact_sheets/pdfs/Southafrica_en.pdf.

——2000f Epidemiological Fact Sheet on HIV/AIDS and Sexually Transmitted Diseases, Zambia. Electronic document. http://www.unaids.org/hivaidsinfo/statistics/fact_sheets/pdfs/Zambia_en.pdf.

——2000g Epidemiological Fact Sheet on HIV/AIDS and Sexually Transmitted Diseases, Zimbabwe. Electronic document. http://www.unaids.org/hivaidsinfo/statistics/fact_sheets/pdfs/Zimbabwe_en.pdf.

UNAIDS/WHO Working Group on Global HIV/AIDS and STD Surveillance, 1999 Infection Reaches Unprecedented Levels in Sub-Saharan Africa. New York: UNAIDS and WHO.

Ungeheuer, F. D., 1993 The Master Detective Still on the Case (Work of L. Montagnier). Time 140 (August 3):34.

UNICEF, 1994 State of the World's Children Report, 1994. New York: Oxford University Press.

UNICEF, 1996 State of the World's Children Report, 1996. New York: Oxford University Press.

UNICEF, 1999a UNICEF Country Statistics: Botswana. Electronic document. http://www.unicef.org/statis/Country_1page23.html.

——1999b UNICEF Country Statistics: Lesotho. Electronic document. http://www.unicef.org/statis/Country_1page98.html.

——1999c UNICEF Country Statistics: Malawi. Electronic document. http://www.unicef.org/statis/Country_1page105.html.

——1999d UNICEF Country Statistics: South Africa. Electronic document. http://www.unicef.org/statis/ Country_1page160.html.

——1999e UNICEF Country Statistics: Zambia. Electronic document. http://www.unicef.org/statis/Country_1page192.html.

——1999f UNICEF Country Statistics: Zimbabwe. Electronic document. http://www.unicef.org/statis/Country_1page193.html.

UNICEF, 2000 The State of the World's Children 2000. Electronic document. http://www.unicef.org/sowcOO/.

UNICEF and UNAIDS, 1999 Children Orphaned by AIDS: Front-Line Responses from Eastern and Southern Africa. Electronic document. http://w.unaidss.org/whatsnew/press/eng/pressarc99/newyork12199.html#top.

United Nations, 1998 World Urbanization Prospects: The 1996 Revision. New York: United Nations, Department of Economic and Social Affairs, Population Division.

United Nations Department of Public Information and UNAIDS, 2001 Fact Sheets: United Nations Special Session on HIV/AIDS, 25–27 June New York: Global Crisis and Global Action. New York: UNAIDS.

United Nations Development Program, 1990 Human Development Report. New York: Oxford University Press.

United Nations Development Program, 1991 Human Development Report. Oxford: Oxford University Press.

United Nations Development Program, 1999 Human Development Report. New York: Oxford University Press.

U.S. Bureau of the Census, 1994. AIDS Database. Washington, DC: U.S. Bureau of the Census.

U.S. Bureau of the Census, 1999 HIV/AIDS in the Developing World Washington, DC: Government Printing House.

Vail, L., ed., 1999 The Creation of Tribalism in Southern Africa. London: University of California Press.

Van de Walle, E., 1990 Impact of AIDS in Sub-Saharan Africa. Milbank Quarterly 68(1).

van der Straten, A., King, R., Grinstead, O., Serufihira, A., and Allen, S., 1995 Couple Communication, Sexual Coercion, and HIV Risk Reduction in Kigali, Rwanda. AIDS 9(8):935–944.

Varmus, H., and Satcher, D., 1997 Ethical Complexities of Conducting Research in Developing Countries. The New England Journal of Medicine 337(14):1003–1005.

Vaughan, M., 1991 Curing their Ills: Colonial Power and African Illness. Palo Alto: Stanford University Press and Cambridge: Polity Press.

Villarreal, M., 1992 The Poverty of Practice: Power, Gender and Intervention from an Actor Orientated Perspective. *In* Battle Fields of Knowledge: The Interlocking of theory and Practice in Social Research and Development. N. Long and A. Long, eds. pp. 245–267. London: Routledge.

Vogel, C., and Wondergem, P., 1995. Baseline Survey (KABB): AIDS/STD Prevention Program for Rwandan Refugees, Benaco Camp, Tanzania, April 4.

Vogelman, L., and Eagle, G., 1991 Overcoming Endemic Violence against Women in South Africa. Social Justice 18(1–2):209–229.

Vos, T., 1994 Attitudes to Sex and Sexual Behavior in Rural Matabeleland Zimbabwe. AIDS Care 6(2):193–203.

Waddington, C. I., and Enyimayew, K. A., 1989 A Price to Pay: The Impact of User Charges in Ashanti-Akim District, Ghana. International Journal of Health Planning and Management 4:17–47.

Waite, G., 1992 Public Health in Pre-Colonial East Central Africa. *In* The Social Basis of Health and Healing in Africa. S. Feierman, and J. M. Janzen, eds. Berkeley: University of California Press.

Wakiraza, C., Forthcoming Reintegration of Street Children: A Critical Look at Sustainable Success. *In* Poverty, AIDS, and Street Children in East Africa. J. L. P. Lugalla and C. G. Kibassa, eds. Lewiston, NY: Edwin Mellen Press.

Waldby, C., 1996 AIDS and the Body Politic: Biomedicine and Sexual Difference. London and New York: Routledge.

Walker, P. T., Hebblethwaite, M. J., and Bridge, J., 1983 Project for Banana Pest Control and Implementation in Tanzania: A Report to the Government of Tanzania. Dar-Es-Salaam.

Wallman, S., 1997 Appropriate Anthropology and the Risky Inspiration of 'Capability'. Brown: Representations of What, by Whom, and to What End? *In* After Writing Culture: Epistemology and Praxis in Contemporary Anthropology. A. James, J. Hockey and A. Dawson, eds. pp. 244–263. London: Routledge.

Wallman, S., 1998 Ordinary Women and Shapes of Knowledge: Perspectives on the Context of STD and AIDS. Public Understanding of Science 7:169–185.

Wangel, A. M., 1995 AIDS in Malawi – a Case Study: A Conspiracy of Silence? MSc thesis, London School of Hygiene and Tropical Medicine.

Watney, S., 1989 Missionary Positions: AIDS, "Africa," and Race. Critical Quarterly 31(3): 45–63.

Watts, C., Keogh, E., Ndlovu, M., and Kwaramba, R., 1998 Withholding of Sex and Forced Sex: Dimensions of Violence against African Women. Reproductive Health Matters 6(12):57–65.

Weeks, D. C., 1992 The AIDS Pandemic in Africa. Current History 91:208–213.

Weeks, J., 1989 Sex, Politics, and Society; the Regulation of Sexuality since 1800. Harlow: Longman.

Weinstein, K. I., Ngallaba, S., Cross, A. R., and Mburu, F. M., 1995 Tanzania Knowledge, Altitudes and Practices Survey 1994. Dar es Salaam: Bureau of Statistics, Planning Commission and Maryland: DHS, Macro International Inc.

Weiss, B., 1993 Buying Her Grave: Money, Movement and AIDS in North-West Tanzania. Africa 63(1):19–35.

Weiss, G. N., 1993 The Distribution and Density of Langerhans Cells in the Human Prepuce: Site of a Diminished Immune Response? Israel Journal of Medical Science 29:42–43.

Weiss, G. N., and Weiss, E. B., 1994 A Perspective on Controversies over Neonatal Circumcision. Clinical Pediatrics 33(12):726–30.

Weiss, H. A., Quigley, M. A., and Hayes, R. J., 2000 Male Circumcision and Risk of HIV Infection in Sub-Saharan Africa: A Systematic Review and Meta-Analysis. AIDS 14(15): 2361–2370.

Welbourn, A., 1991 RRA and the Analysis of Difference. RRA Notes 14:14–23.

Welbourn, A., 1992 Rapid Rural Appraisal, Gender and Health – Alternative Ways of Listening to Needs. IDS Bulletin 23(1):8–18.

Werner, A., 1906 The Natives of British Central Africa. London: Archibald Constable.

Wernette, M., 1994 UNAIDS Planning Management Specialist, Geneva, Focal Point.

White, B. W., 2002 Rumba and Other Cosmopolitanisms in the Belgian Congo (1949–1999). *In* Musique, Joie et Crise dans le Cosmotropole Africain. B. W. White, ed. Numéro Spécial de Cahiers d'études Africaines, Spring/Summer.

White, L., 1989 Magomero: Portrait of an African Village. Cambridge: Cambridge University Press.

White, L., 1990 The Comforts of Home: Prostitution in Colonial Nairobi. Chicago: The University of Chicago Press.

WHO, 1998 Weekly Epidemiological Report 73:373–380. Geneva: World Health Organization.

Whyte, S. R., 1997 Questioning Misfortune: The Pragmatics of Uncertainty in Uganda. Cambridge: Cambridge University Press.

Wilke, M., and Kleiber, D., 1991 AIDS and (Sex-) Tourism. VII International Conference on AIDS, Florence, June [Abstract MD 4037].

Wilkinson, D., and Gilks, C. F., 1998 Increasing Frequency of Tuberculosis among Staff in a South African Hospital: Impact of the HIV Epidemic on the Supply Side of Health Care. Transactions of the Royal Society of Tropical Medicine and Hygiene 92:500– 502.

Williams, B., and Campbell, C., 1996 Mines, Migrancy and HIV in South Africa – Managing the Epidemic. South African Medical Journal 86:1249–1251.

Williams, G., and Ray, S., 1993 Work against AIDS. London: Action AID; Nairobi: AMREF.

Williamson, J., 1956 Salt and Potashes in the Life of the Chewa. Nyasaland Journal 9: 82–87.

Wilmhurst, P., 1997 Scientific Imperialism. British Medical Journal 314 (7084):840–841.

Wilson, D., Greenspan, R., and Wilson, C., 1989 Knowledge about AIDS and Self-Reported Behavior among Zimbabwean Secondary School Pupils. Social Science and Medicine 28(9):957–961.

Wilson, D., Sibanda, B., Mboyi, L., Msimanga, S., and Dube, G., 1990 A Pilot Study for an HIV Prevention Program among Commercial Sex Workers in Bulawayo, Zimbabwe. Social Science and Medicine 31(5):609–618.

Witte, K., Cameron, K. A., and Nzyuko, S., 1996 HIV/AIDS along the Trans-Africa Highway in Kenya: Examining Risk Perceptions, Recommended Responses, and Campaign Materials (Final report of focus groups conducted with commercial sex workers, truck drivers and their assistants, and young men aged 18–23, at Malaba, Mashinari, and Simba Truckstops in Kenya). Unpublished report.

Woelk, G., 1992 Cultural and Structural Influences in the Creation of and Participation in Community Health Programs. Social Science and Medicine 35(4):419–424.

Wolfe, S., and Lurie, P., 1997 Letter to Secretary Donna Shalala, Department of Health and Human Services, October 23. Electronic document. http://www.citizen.org/hrg/PUBLICATIONS/1430.htm.

Wondergem, P., and Brady, B., 1994a AIDS/STD Program for Rwandan Refugees: Health System and Community Assessment: Benaco Camp, Ngara District, Tanzania. AIDSCAP Task Order 5004-007, August 8 – September 2. Arlington, VA: John Snow Inc.

—— 1994b AIDS/STD Program for Rwandan Refugees: Health System and Community Assessment – Benaco Camp, Ngara District, Tanzania. AIDSCAP August 8 – September 2.

Wood, K., Maforah, F., and Jewkes, R., 1998 "He Forced Me to Love Him": Putting Violence on Adolescent Sexual Health Agendas. Social Science and Medicine 47(2):233–242.

World Bank, 1990 World Development Report. Washington, DC: Oxford University Press.

World Bank, 1992a Malawi: Population Sector Study. Washington, DC: World Bank.

—— 1992b Tanzania: AIDS Assessment and Planning Study. Washington, DC: World Bank.

World Bank, 1993a World Development Report: Investing in Health. New York: Oxford University Press.

—— 1993b World Development Report 1993: Investing in Health. Oxford: Oxford University Press.

World Bank, 1995 Country Briefs. Washington DC: World Bank.

World Bank, 1997a Confronting AIDS: Public Priorities in a Global Epidemic. Washington, DC: Oxford University Press for World Bank.

—— 1997b World Development Report. New York: Oxford University Press.

World Bank, 1999 HIV and AIDS in Africa: The World Bank's Response. Washington, DC: World Bank.

World Bank, 2000a World Development Indicators 2000 (Life Expectancy and Mortality, Table 2.18). Electronic document. http://www.worldbank.org/data/databytopic/databytopic.html.

——2000b Entering the 21st Century. World Development Report 1999/2000. Washington, DC: Oxford University Press.

World Bank, 2002 African Development Indicators 2002. Washington, DC: World Bank.

World Health Organization, 1992 Current and Future Dimensions of the HIV/AIDS Pandemic: A Capsule Summary. Geneva: WHO.

World Health Organization, 2001 Health in the Democratic Republic of Congo. Situation Report. Geneva: WHO.

World Health Organization, 2002 WHO Takes Major Steps to Make HIV Treatment Accessible. Electronic document. www.GlobalFundATM.org/journalists/press%20 releases/who

X1th International Conference on AIDS and STDs in Africa [ICASA], 1999 Abstract Book, Looking Into the Future, September 12–16, 1999, Lusaka, Zambia.

Xinhua News Agency, June 28, 1999.

Yoshida, K., 1993 Masks and Secrecy among the Chewa. African Arts 26(2):34–45.

Youri, P., ed., 1993 Female Adolescent Health and Sexuality Study in Kenyan Secondary Schools: A Survey Report. Nairobi: African Medical Research Foundation.

Zambian Daily Times, June 24, 1998.

Zimmerman, R., Pesta, J., and Block, R., 2001 Cipla AIDS-Drug Offer Changes Outlook. The Wall Street Journal, February 8: B13.

Zwi, A. B., and Bachmayer, D., 1990 HIV and AIDS in South Africa: What Is an Appropriate Public Health Response? Health Policy and Planning 5:316–326.

Zwi, A. B., and Cabral, J., 1991 Identifying "High Risk Situations" for Preventing AIDS. British Medical Journal 303:1527–1529.

Index

Index compiled by Frank Pert